GREEN CHEMISTRY FOR SUSTAINABLE BIOFUEL PRODUCTION

GREEN CHEMISTRY FOR SUSTAINABLE BIOFUEL PRODUCTION

Edited by
Veera Gnaneswar Gude, PhD

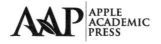

Apple Academic Press Inc.
3333 Mistwell Crescent
Oakville, ON L6L 0A2 Canada

Apple Academic Press Inc.
9 Spinnaker Way
Waretown, NJ 08758 USA

© 2018 by Apple Academic Press, Inc.

First issued in paperback 2021

Exclusive worldwide distribution by CRC Press, a member of Taylor & Francis Group

No claim to original U.S. Government works

ISBN-13: 978-1-77463-134-8 (pbk)
ISBN-13: 978-1-77188-639-0 (hbk)

Library and Archives Canada Cataloguing in Publication

Green chemistry for sustainable biofuel production / edited by Veera Gnaneswar Gude, PhD.

Includes bibliographical references and index.
Issued in print and electronic formats.
ISBN 978-1-77188-639-0 (hardcover).--ISBN 978-1-315-09935-4 (PDF)

1. Biomass energy. 2. Green chemistry. I. Gude, Veera Gnaneswar, 1978-, editor

| TP339.G74 2018 | 660.028'6 | C2018-900011-2 | C2018-900012-0 |

Library of Congress Cataloging-in-Publication Data

Names: Gude, Veera Gnaneswar, 1978- editor.
Title: Green chemistry for sustainable biofuel production / editor, Veera Gnaneswar Gude, PhD.
Description: Toronto ; New Jersey : Apple Academic Press, 2018. | Includes bibliographical references and index.
Identifiers: LCCN 2017061143 (print) | LCCN 2018000089 (ebook) | ISBN 9781315099354 (ebook) | ISBN 9781771886390 (hardcover : alk. paper)
Subjects: LCSH: Biomass energy. | Green chemistry.
Classification: LCC TP339 (ebook) | LCC TP339 .G74 2018 (print) | DDC 660.028/6--dc23
LC record available at https://lccn.loc.gov/2017061143

Apple Academic Press also publishes its books in a variety of electronic formats. Some content that appears in print may not be available in electronic format. For information about Apple Academic Press products, visit our website at **www.appleacademicpress.com** and the CRC Press website at **www.crcpress.com**

DEDICATION

To my late father Gude Bhaskar Rao,
my mother Gude Fathima,
my sister Gude Veera Nirmala Kalyani,
my brothers Gude Veera Kiran and Gude Veera Chitti Karunakar,
and to Preeti Muire

CONTENTS

ABOUT THE EDITOR

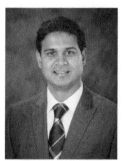

Veera Gnaneswar Gude, PhD

*Associate Professor of Civil and Environmental
Engineering, Mississippi State University,
Mississippi, USA*

Veera Gnaneswar Gude, PhD, is a faculty member of
Civil and Environmental Engineering Department at
Mississippi State University. He has published over
125 scientific research articles focusing on biofuels,
desalination, and water/wastewater treatment topics. He is the author of the
book *Microwave-Mediated Biofuel Production* published by CRC Press in
2017. He holds two patents on novel processes in biofuels and desalination
technical areas respectively. He is an editor or editorial board member of
several reputed scientific journals in the areas of biofuels, environmental
engineering and science, desalination and water research. He also serves on
numerous scientific advisory boards and committees across the world.

LIST OF CONTRIBUTORS

María González Alriols
Biorefinery Processes Research Group (BioRP), Chemical and Environmental Engineering Department, University of the Basque Country UPV/EHU, Plaza Europa, 1, 20018, Donostia-San Sebastián, Spain

P. N. Amaniampong
IC2MP UMR CNRS 7285, Université de Poitiers, ENSIP, B1, 1 rue Marcel Doré TSA

Marta Amirsadegh
Department of Chemical and Materials Engineering, California State Polytechnic University Ponoma, Ponoma, CA, 91768, USA

María Angeles Andres
Biorefinery Processes Research Group (BioRP), Chemical and Environmental Engineering Department, University of the Basque Country UPV/EHU, Plaza Europa, 1, 20018, Donostia-San Sebastián, Spain

N. Araji
IC2MP UMR CNRS 7285, Université de Poitiers, ENSIP, B1, 1 rue Marcel Doré TSA

Michele Aresta
Department of Chemical and Biomolecular Engineering, NUS, 117858 Singapore, SG / Department of Chemical Engineering, University of Bath, BA27AY Bath, UK

R. Behling
IC2MP UMR CNRS 7285, Université de Poitiers, ENSIP, B1, 1 rue Marcel Doré TSA

Dorin Boldor
Department of Biological and Agricultural Engineering, Louisiana State University Agricultural Center, Baton Rouge, LA 70803, United States

G. Chatel
University of Savoie Mont Blanc, LCME, F-73000 Chambéry, France

Sarah C. Davis
Voinovich School of Leadership and Public Affairs, Ohio University, Athens, OH (45701), USA

Florian Delrue
CEA Cadarache, Groupe Biomasse 3G, Cité des Energies, Saint-Paul-lez-Durance, F-13108 France

Angela Dibenedetto
Department of Chemistry, University of Bari, 70126 Bari, IT / CIRCC, via Celso Ulpiani 27, 70126 Bari, IT

Xabier Erdocia
Biorefinery Processes Research Group (BioRP), Chemical and Environmental Engineering Department, University of the Basque Country UPV/EHU, Plaza Europa, 1, 20018, Donostia-San Sebastián, Spain

Dhan Lord Fortela
Department of Chemical Engineering, University of Louisiana at Lafayette, Lafayette, LA, 70504, USA

Todd French
Dave C. Swalm School of Chemical Engineering, Mississippi State University, Mississippi State, MS, 39759, USA

Parag R. Gogate
Chemical Engineering Department, Institute of Chemical Technology, Matunga, Mumbai – 400019, India

Martin Gross
Department of Food Science and Human Nutrition – AGLS, Iowa State University, Ames, IA 50011, USA

Esther Grossman
Voinovich School of Leadership and Public Affairs, Ohio University, Athens, OH (45701), USA

Veera Gnaneswar Gude
Assistant Professor of Civil and Environmental Engineering, Mississippi State University, Mississippi, USA

Rafael Hernandez
Department of Chemical Engineering, University of Louisiana at Lafayette, Lafayette, LA, 70504, USA

Cannayen Igathinathane
Department of Agricultural and Biosystems Engineering, North Dakota State University, 1221 Albrecht Boulevard, Fargo, ND 58102, USA

Alexander Jones
Voinovich School of Leadership and Public Affairs, Ohio University, Athens, OH (45701), USA

Jalel Labidi
Biorefinery Processes Research Group (BioRP), Chemical and Environmental Engineering Department, University of the Basque Country UPV/EHU, Plaza Europa, 1, 20018, Donostia-San Sebastián, Spain

Adam F. Lee
European Bioenergy Research Institute, Aston University, Birmingham B4 7ET, UK

Kim E. Miller
Voinovich School of Leadership and Public Affairs, Ohio University, Athens, OH (45701), USA

Ashish V. Mohod
Chemical Engineering Department, AISSMS College of Engineering, Kennedy Road, Pune – 411 001, India

Andro Mondala
Department of Chemical and Paper Engineering, Western Michigan University, Kalamazoo, MI 49008, USA

Pranjali D. Muley
Department of Biological and Agricultural Engineering, Louisiana State University Agricultural Center, Baton Rouge, LA 70803, United States

Kok Siew Ng
Centre for Environmental Strategy, University of Surrey, Guildford, UK

Emmanuel Revellame
Department of Industrial Technology, University of Louisiana at Lafayette, Lafayette, LA, 70504, USA

M. Toufiq Reza
Department of Mechanical Engineering, Ohio University, Athens, OH 45701, USA

Abbey Rodjom
Voinovich School of Leadership and Public Affairs, Ohio University, Athens, OH (45701), USA

Jhuma Sadhukhan
Centre for Environmental Strategy, University of Surrey, Guildford, UK

Matt Sanderson
Northern Great Plains Research Laboratory, USDA-ARS, 1701 10th Avenue SW, Mandan, ND 58554, USA

Ashik Sathish
Department of Food Science and Human Nutrition – AGLS, Iowa State University, Ames, IA 50011, USA

Mobolaji Shemfe
Centre for Environmental Strategy, University of Surrey, Guildford, UK

Atal Shivhare
European Bioenergy Research Institute, Aston University, Birmingham B4 7ET, UK

Kaitlin C. Straker
Voinovich School of Leadership and Public Affairs, Ohio University, Athens, OH (45701), USA

S. Valange
IC2MP UMR CNRS 7285, Université de Poitiers, ENSIP, B1, 1 rue Marcel Doré TSA

K. De Oliveira Vigier
IC2MP UMR CNRS 7285, Université de Poitiers, ENSIP, B1, 1 rue Marcel Doré TSA, 41105, 86073 Poitiers Cedex 9, France

Zhiyou Wen
Department of Food Science and Human Nutrition – AGLS, Iowa State University, Ames, IA 50011, USA

Karen Wilson
European Bioenergy Research Institute, Aston University, Birmingham B4 7ET, UK

LIST OF ABBREVIATIONS

ACC	annual capital charge
AD	anaerobic digestion
APR	aqueous phase reforming
ASE®	accelerated solvent extraction
ASP	aquatic species program
ASTM	American Society for Testing and Materials
BD	Bligh and Dyer
BES	bioelectrochemical systems
BGFC	biomass gasification fuel cell
BIGCC	biomass-integrated gasification combined cycles
BOD	biochemical oxygen demand
BTL	biomass to liquids
CAL-B	Candida Antarctica lipase B
CBP	consolidated biomass processing
CC	capital cost
CEPCI	chemical engineering plant cost index
CNT	carbon nanotubes
CO	carbon monoxide
COD	chemical oxygen demand
CODH	carbon monoxide dehydrogenases
COP	cost of production
CRP	conservation reserve program
CSTR	continuous stirred tanked reactor
DAF	dissolved air flotation
DAGs	diacylglycerides
DCF	discounted cash flow
DDGS	distillers' dry grain with solubles
DME	dimethyl ether
DS	degree of substitution
DSILs	double-salt ionic liquids
DW	dry weight
EFB	empty fruit bunches
EHL	enzymatically hydrolyzed lignin

EP	economic potential
EPA	eicosapentaenoic acid
EROEI	energy returned on energy invested
EROI	Energy Return on Investment
EU	European Union
FAME	fatty acid methyl esters
FAS	fatty acid synthase
FAs	fatty acids
FDH	formate dehydrogenases
FFAs	free fatty acids
FFB	fresh fruit bunches
FTS	Fischer Tropsch synthesis
GC-FID	gas chromatography with flame ionization detection
GH	glycosidic hydrolases
GHG	greenhouse gas
HB	humid biomass
HDO	hydrodeoxygenation
HMF	hydroxymethylfurfural
HRT	hydraulic retention time
HTL	hydrothermal liquefaction
IEA	international energy agency
IL	ionic liquid
LCA	life cycle assessment
LCA	life-cycle analysis
LHHW	Langmuir-Hinshelwood-Hougen-Watson
LUC	land use change
MAGs	monoacylglycerides
MCC	microcrystalline cellulose
MECs	microbial electrolysis cells
MESs	microbial electrosynthesis systems
MFCs	microbial fuel cells
MSW	municipal solid waste
MTBE	methyl *tert*-butyl ether
MTO	methyltrioxorhenium
MV	microwave
NEB	net energy balance
NER	net energy ratio

NG	natural gas
NO	nitrogen oxides
NPV	net present value
ODP	oxidation ditch process
OFMSW	organic fraction of municipal wastes
OLR	organic loading rate
PBR	photo-bioreactors
PCET	proton-coupled electron transfers
PET	polyethylene terephthalate
PHA	polyhydroxyalkanoate
PLs	phospholipids
POM	partial oxidation of methane
POME	palm oil mill effluent
PS	primary sludge
RFS	renewable fuels standard
ROI	return on investment
SBRs	sequencing batch reactors
SC-CO$_2$	supercritical carbon dioxide
SCFAs	short chain fatty acids
SCO	single cell oils
SE	steam-explosion
SFE	supercritical fluid extraction
SHF	separate hydrolysis and fermentation
SOFC	solid oxide fuel cells
SRT	solids retention time
SRWC	short rotation woody crops
SSCF	simultaneous saccharification and cofermentation
SSF	simultaneous saccharification and fermentation
TAGs	triacylglycerides
TEA	techno-economic analysis
TRL	technology readiness level
UASB	upflow anaerobic sludge blanket reactor
US	ultrasounds
USA	United States of America
VOCs	volatile organic compounds
VOP	value on processing
WAS	waste activated sludge

Wes	wax esters
WF	water footprint
XH	xylitol dehydrogenase
XR	xylose reductase

PREFACE

Petroleum-based fuels are currently serving the modern world and it has been the case over the past century. However, due to rapid population growth and industrialization, these petroleum sources—once considered as inexhaustible—are diminishing at much faster rate than the natural processes can replenish them. This combined with several interrelated impending global crises, namely, climate change, chemicals, energy, and environmental pollution, raises the need for alternative energy supplies such as biofuels from renewable resources. This book focuses on chemistry related to biofuels research and their sustainable development. Biofuels can be broadly categorized as any fuels that are of biomass origin such as bioethanol, biodiesel, biogas, biooils, and syngas. Understanding the fundamental chemistry of these renewable biofuels and developing appropriate technologies for implementation will provide sustainable solutions for the future.

Efficient synthesis of renewable fuels remains a challenging and important field of research. Embracing the principles of green chemistry and engineering may result in a sustainable route for their production. Green chemistry provides unique opportunities for innovation via product substitution, new feedstock generation, catalysis in aqueous media, utilization of microwaves or ultrasound, waste minimization and scope for alternative or natural solvents. The potential use of waste products as a new resource and development of integrated processes producing multiple high value bioproducts from biomass is highly desirable to improve the economics of the renewable fuels.

Renewable fuel research and process development requires interdisciplinary approaches involving chemists and physicists from both scientific and engineering backgrounds. This book includes chapters contributed by both research scientists and research engineers with significant experience in biofuel chemistry and process development. This book is organized into four sections covering detail topics related to: (i) biofuel feedstock challenges and potential; renewable fuels from carbon sources; (ii) process intensification and green chemistry through the use of microwave irradiation, hydrodynamic cavitation, hydrothermal processes and ionic liquids; (iii) evaluation of nonconventional and emerging sustainable feedstock such as microalgae, oleaginous microorganisms from wastewater sludge, and biorefinery configurations with bioelectrochemical systems as a central technology; and finally (iv) energy-efficiency analysis, techno-economic aspects and life-cycle impacts and inventories of various biofuel production processes.

ACKNOWLEDGMENTS

I would like to thank the publisher for the opportunity to disseminate the knowledge contained in this book. Contributing authors of this book are thanked for their excellent scientific contributions, patience, and cooperation throughout the publication process.

I would like to express my appreciation to the colleagues in the Civil and Environmental Engineering Department, the Bagley College of Engineering, and the Office of Research and Economic Development at Mississippi State University for their support. Collaborations with colleagues in Swalm School of Chemical Engineering (Dr. Todd French, Dr. Rafael Hernandez, now at University of Louisiana; and Dr. Andro Mondala, now at Western Michigan University; and Mr. William Holmes, now at University of Louisiana) and Department of Chemistry (Dr. David Wipf) and United States Department of Agriculture—Agricultural Research Service (Dr. John Brooks) are gratefully acknowledged. My sincere thanks and gratitude are extended to my doctoral and postdoctoral advisors Dr. Nagamany Nirmalakhandan, Dr. Ricardo Jacquez, Dr. Shuguang Deng, and Dr. Adrian Hanson of New Mexico State University for their continuous support in my professional career. Prof. Shuguang Deng is particularly acknowledged for introducing me to biofuels research during my postdoctoral research studies at New Mexico State University. Dr. Prafulla Patil was instrumental in developing my knowledge in this area. My graduate research students at Mississippi State University are appreciated for their diligent efforts and energy in work environment and research contributions, especially Dr. Edith Martinez-Guerra for her work on microwave and ultrasound enhanced biodiesel production from microalgae and other waste sources. Dr. Bahareh Kokabian and Ms. Sara Fast are also acknowledged for their contributions in microbial desalination and advanced oxidation processes research, respectively. Finally, I would like to thank Ms. Preeti Muire for her support, care and love.

—*Veera Gnaneswar Gude, PhD*

PART I

BIOFUELS FROM RENEWABLE AND ALTERNATIVE FEEDSTOCK AND GREEN PROCESSES

CHAPTER 1

GREEN CHEMISTRY AND ENGINEERING FOR SUSTAINABLE BIOFUEL PRODUCTION

VEERA GNANESWAR GUDE

Associate Professor of Civil and Environmental Engineering, Mississippi State University, Starkville, Mississippi, USA

CONTENTS

ABSTRACT

This chapter provides the background for the green chemistry and green engineering principles that could be instrumental in sustainable biofuel process development. These principles are summarized into four major thrusts and three process steps. The major thrusts include: use of alternative or renewable feedstocks; use of less hazardous chemicals and environmentally friendly solvents; develop reaction conditions to increase the selectivity for the product; and minimizing the energy consumption for chemical transformations. These major thrusts can be implemented through the "green design" process steps, which involve identification of challenges and investigation of opportunities for innovation in green chemistry methods followed by implementation of sustainable processes; and evaluation of process performance, and redesign or refinement of process elements. This chapter also provides background for and highlights of the important contributions from the other authors in these thrust areas.

1.1   INTRODUCTION

At present most of the world's fuel and energy needs are derived from fossil fuel sources. These resources are expected to diminish within the next 50 years at the current rate of consumption [1]. Fossil fuel utilization is based on exothermic chemical reactions that generate heat and CO_2. An estimated 30 billion tons of CO_2 are released annually worldwide through the combustion of fossil fuels. This causes an increase of CO_2 content in the atmosphere and the oceans. While the presence of CO_2 is vital to biomass production, higher concentrations can be problematic. For instance, the atmospheric CO_2 concentration has increased from about 280 ppm to more than 400 ppm in 2009 from the time of industrial revolution posing many climate change and global warming issues [2]. To address this carbon conundrum, chemically feasible and cost-effective solutions should be developed for efficient use of the limited fossil resources including sustainable processes that convert biomass and CO_2 into fuels and value-added chemicals on a large scale.

The need for the share of renewable biofuels in the current energy budget can never be overstressed considering the global energy demands and associated environmental pollution and resource depletion issues [3]. Biofuel production can only be sustainable if they are derived from local and inexhaustible sources using innovative and energy- and resource-efficient process technologies [4]. They should also provide superior benefits when compared to their counter parts in terms of climate change and environmental pollution. Green chemistry and engineering principles can be of immense help to develop sustainable processes for biofuel production.

1.2   GREEN CHEMISTRY AND ENGINEERING PRINCIPLES

Green chemistry and engineering practices seek to maximize efficiency and minimize health and environmental hazards throughout the life cycle of a product [5, 6]. The major goal for developing the green chemistry and engineering principles is focused on promoting cleaner and faster syntheses that is based on environmentally conscious design and responsible resource utilization.

As shown in Table 1.1, the majority of the principles of green chemistry and engineering represent the same objective and thus the same action plan for safer and "greener" chemistry [7]. Common goals among the two sets of principles can be summarized into the following four major thrusts.

- Use of alternative or renewable feedstocks and important chemicals;
- Efficient conversion of raw materials using environmentally friendly catalysts and solvents;
- Develop and design to promote reaction conditions that increase the selectivity for the product;
- Maximize energy efficiency and integrate processes for chemical transformations.

Green chemistry principles and metrics can influence the entire life cycle of biofuels significantly. Green metrics such as E-factor (environmental factor which refers to a weight ratio of waste to product), atom economy (refers to transformation of most of the atoms in reactants to

TABLE 1.1   Principles of Green Chemistry [1] and Green Engineering [2]

Green Chemistry	Green Engineering
1. Waste prevention	1. Inherent rather than circumstantial
2. Atom economy	2. Prevention instead of treatment
3. Less hazardous chemical syntheses	3. Design for separation
4. Designing safer chemicals	4. Maximize efficiency
5. Safer solvents and auxiliaries	5. Output-pulled versus input-pushed
6. Design for Energy efficiency	6. Conserve complexity
7. Use of renewable feedstocks	7. Durability rather than immortality
8. Reduce derivatives	8. Meet need, minimize excess
9. Catalysis	9. Minimize material diversity
10. Design for degradation	10. Integrate material and energy flows
11. Real-time analysis for pollution prevention	11. Design for commercial "Afterlife"
12. Inherently safer chemistry for accident prevention	12. Renewable rather than depleting

products) and mass reaction efficiency (main product amount divided by balance sheet total input) can be used as simple tools determine the greenness of biofuel production.

To reduce, reuse and recycle the chemicals and materials, it is imperative to develop nonfossil fuel based raw materials, to minimize waste production and to increase energy efficiency of chemical reactions or processes and separation operations. Considering catalyst development, it is desirable to replace rare, expensive, and/or toxic chemicals/materials with earth-abundant, inexpensive, and benign chemicals/materials. Recycling of chemicals/materials that cannot be replaced; development of nonpetroleum based sources of important raw materials; elimination of waste products and enhancements in efficiencies of chemical reactions and processes; discovery of new separation science that will facilitate recycling and production of valuable chemicals/materials; and development and characterization of low cost and sustainable materials with improved properties, are all critical for implementing green chemistry and engineering principles. Other processes that involve reduced use of toxic components, such as solvents, carbon emissions, and pollutants; processes under ambient conditions, as opposed to extreme temperatures, pressures or other harsh conditions and finally increased conservation of natural resources, such as water, raw material, and energy.

1.3 SUSTAINABLE BIOFUEL PROCESS DEVELOPMENT ("GREEN DESIGN")

Further, the process of sustainable biofuel production can be simplified into three steps resulting in an iterative process:

1. Identify challenges and investigate opportunities;
2. Invent green chemistry methods and implement sustainable processes; and
3. Review or Evaluate process performance and redesign/refine the process if necessary.

These steps will be discussed in detail in Section 1.4. Figure 1.1 shows the relationship between the book content and the steps involved in sustainable biofuel process development.

Chapters 2, 3, 4, 9, 10   **Chapters 5, 6, 7, 8**

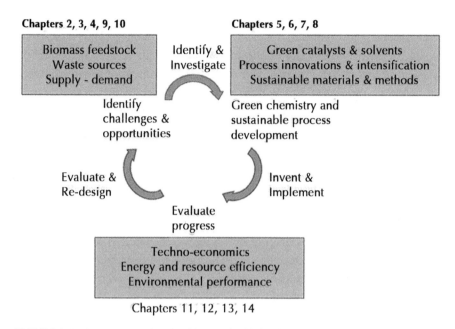

FIGURE 1.1 Process steps involved in sustainable biofuel production.

1.4 BOOK STRUCTURE

This book is divided into 14 chapters and Chapter 1 provides the context and background for sustainable biofuel production in general. It also covers the overarching theme of this book and highlights the organization and structure of this edited book and the content of the contributed chapters in detail.

1.4.1 PART 1: BIOFUELS FROM RENEWABLE AND ALTERNATIVE FEEDSTOCK AND GREEN PROCESSES

A large variety of biofuel feedstocks are discussed in this section. They are separated into four major categories: (1) high-efficiency feedstocks (e.g., palm oil, sugar cane); (2) moderate efficiency feedstocks (e.g., corn, soybean, rapeseed, sugar beet); (3) feedstocks under development (e.g., sweet sorghum, Jatropha); and (4) dedicated energy feedstocks (e.g., switchgrass, miscanthus, short rotation crops, algae, waste) [8]. While choosing the appropriate feedstock various factors related to sustainability should be considered. It is also important to understand the limitations of the feedstock related to their characteristics and their effects on the process development and overall process economics (Chapter 2). Alternative feedstock such as recycling spent carbon can be an important endeavor considering this effect (Chapter 3). Further, development of green catalysts and catalytic processes for biofuel production can enhance the overall efficiencies and process economics and sustainable production (Chapter 4).

Chapter 2 describes the biofuel feedstock challenges and limitations and potential for future developments in production and utilization of various biofuel feedstock types (dedicated energy crops), potential for production and challenges in consumption and management of crop stands, land availability, conversion process, competing use, and economics of utilization; opportunities in processing for biofuels and bioproducts using green-processing technologies (direct conversion, drop-in strategies, valorization of waste products) high-value products, advanced feedstock supply and distributed preprocessing systems, energy security, and perennial crops role in sustainability.

Chapter 3 focuses on establishing a circular economy through carbon recycled biofuels. This chapter includes biorefinery concepts based on natural and man-made carbon recycling with conversion processes, biotechnology options and performance indicators. Direct carbon conversion from concentrated sources or natural sources such as biomass was discussed. A variety of pretreatment and conversion technologies for biofuel production from cellulose biomass, lipid containing biomass, and aquatic biomass were presented for bioethanol production and lipids suitable for further transformation.

Chapter 4 elaborates on the novel catalytic processes for biofuels and chemical production. It also presents a detailed account on a range of heterogeneously catalyzed processes, including esterification, transesterification, Fischer-Tropsch synthesis and hydrodeoxygenation, and associated inorganic nanocatalysts, for transformation of lignin, carbohydrate and oil feedstocks. Design of robust catalytic materials, with mass transport properties tailored for the rapid diffusion of bulky molecules, high selectivity and minimal deactivation, is a particular focus of discussions.

1.4.2 PART 2: GREEN CHEMISTRY AND PROCESS INTENSIFICATION

Part 2 discusses about recent advances in green process development involving utilization of microwave and ultrasound irradiations and development of hydrodynamic cavitational reactors for process intensification, which results in increased energy-efficiency and product recovery. Process intensification and product recovery enhancement can also be achieved using water as green organic solvent at elevated pressures and temperatures. Further, selective recovery and reuse of solvents can be accomplished through a sustainable design of ionic liquids. This section presents four chapters on process intensification techniques involving microwave irradiation (Chapter 5), hydrodynamic cavitation (Chapter 6), hydrothermal processing (Chapter 7), and ionic liquids (Chapter 8), respectively.

Chapter 5 presents the use of advanced microwave technology for organic synthesis, highlighting a number of advantages over conventional methods. This chapter discusses the application of advanced microwave technology for biodiesel production through transesterification reaction with an overview of microwave theory of dielectric heating mechanism for biodiesel synthesis. The benefits of microwave processing are discussed in terms of reduced reaction and processing times, lower oil/solvent ratio, enhanced product selectivity, reduced catalyst consumption, and increased overall process efficiency. Process optimization, reaction kinetics under microwave heating and in-situ transesterification concepts are also presented.

Chapter 6 discusses the use of hydrodynamic cavitational phenomenon as a process intensification approach to eliminate the limitations of mass transfer in biodiesel production. It covers the basic mechanism and fundamentals of hydrodynamic cavitation, different reactor configurations, overview of different applications and important design and operational guidelines for the maximizing the extent of intensification. The use of sustainable feedstock such as nonedible oils and waste cooking oils was discussed. Possible combinations and the potential for scale up of hydrodynamic cavitation reactors for biodiesel synthesis were discussed with recent applications and guidelines for design and operational parameters for maximizing the intensification.

Chapter 7 presents the hydrothermal processes as green, renewable, and sustainable pathways for biofuel and bioenergy production. The dual role of water moisture as solvent and as catalyst during hydrothermal processes was discussed. Thermodynamic properties of liquid water and processes under inert atmosphere are discussed for different biofuels production. Hydrothermal carbonization, hydrothermal liquefaction, supercritical water gasification processes are presented in detail; in addition, wet air oxidation and supercritical water oxidation are also discussed. Reaction mechanism, chemistry, and kinetics and economic and environmental impacts of hydro-thermal processes were presented on a comparative basis.

Chapter 8 describes the investigations in strategies and innovations based on ionic liquids in terms of dissolution and pretreatment methods and their uses as reaction solvents, catalysts and extraction solvents in biorefinery. Use of ionic liquids for the valorization of cellulose, lignin and vegetable oil with emphasis on their impact on the reactivity and reaction pathways to further improve chemical yields is discussed. Additionally, several parameters involved in these processes such as the choice of the anion or/and cation of ionic liquids are thoroughly discussed. Recyclability, renewability and sustainability aspects related to biorefinery processes are also included.

1.4.3   PART 3: RENEWABLE FEEDSTOCK UTILIZATION AND BIOREFINERY CONCEPTS

Energy- and process-efficient feedstocks are not necessarily sustainable feedstock. Some feedstock such as sugarcane for bioethanol production have shown to be unsustainable due to the potential undesirable impacts in the land usage and greenhouse gas emission effect. Alternative feedstock such as activated sludge and renewable feedstock like microalgae are considered in detail. However, these are not exceptional in terms of the above mentioned. If biofuel production can be integrated with other beneficial processes via integrated biorefinery schemes, overall sustainability objectives can be met. Therefore, in this section two chapters (Chapters 9 and 10) discuss the use of alternative (wastewater activated sludge, i.e., oleaginous microorganisms) and renewable feedstock (microalgae), followed by a third chapter (Chapter 11), which discusses the various possibilities of integrated biorefinery concepts.

Chapter 9 presents microalgae as a promising feedstock for a variety of biofuels production including high value added chemicals and health products. This chapter focuses on algal biofuel production, which involves five essential steps: cultivation, harvesting, extraction of lipids and their conversion into biodiesel, separation, and purification. Concepts such as open raceway ponds, photobioreactors, biofilm-based systems, and conversion processes were discussed in detail. A special focus on the use of thermo-chemical-based methods such as hydrothermal liquefaction is presented with current hurdles to commercialization and proposition of possible solutions.

In Chapter 10, biofuel production from activated sludge and wastewater treatment are discussed. Wastewater treatment operations present numerous opportunities for integration of sustainable bioenergy production technologies. This chapter outlines and discusses research efforts in utilization of activated sludge, municipal and industrial wastewaters, and treatment facilities for the production of biofuels such as biodiesel and renewable diesel and nonfood-based lipid feedstock. Extraction, transesterification and catalytic cracking processes for renewable diesel production are discussed. Municipal and industrial wastewater sources as carbon and nutrient rich media for oleaginous yeasts to produce substantial quantities of microbial oils is presented. Similar discussion on lipid-rich activated sludge microbial biomass biodiesel or renewable diesel production is also included.

Chapter 11 explores the possibilities of integrating bioelectrochemical systems through biorefinery configurations for simultaneous bioelectricity and valuable chemical production. Electrochemical devices to harvest electrical energy from the microbial decomposition of organic substrates involving synergetic benefits of wastewater treatment and resource recovery were discussed. This chapter also provides a perspective on the production of fuels, electricity, and chemicals using bioelectrochemical systems. Working principles of bioelectrochemical systems, the integration of biorefineries with bioelectrochemical systems for the enhanced production of biofuels and valuable chemicals, state-of-the-art thermodynamic feasibility models and methods for evaluating the economic viability of the integrated systems are presented.

1.4.4 PART 4: ENERGY EFFICIENCY, TECHNO-ECONOMICS AND LIFE CYCLE ASSESSMENT OF BIOFUEL PRODUCTION

Finally it is crucial to evaluate the overall performance of biofuel production processes and major environmental issues associated with their production. The issues include energy consumption, greenhouse gas emissions, land use, water consumption, eutrophication, and air quality as shown in Figure 1.2. It is vital that these impacts are evaluated and quantified in order to provide a rational basis for assessing the long-term viability and acceptability of individual biofuel supply chain options. Tools such as material and energy balances (Chapter 12), techno-economics (Chapter 13), and life cycle inventory analysis (Chapter 14) can help assess the long-term feasibility

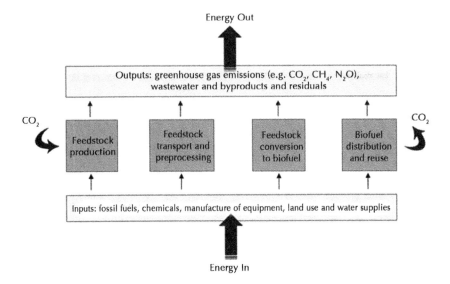

FIGURE 1.2 Generic scheme for environmental impacts and life cycle assessment of biofuel production.

and sustainability of the biofuel production systems which can be used for developing frameworks for sustainable biofuel production.

Chapter 12 elaborates on the energy efficiencies and economic feasibilities of various biofuel production processes based on the global inputs and outputs. Energy inputs for cultivation, harvesting, transport and conversion steps and energy outputs from the biofuel products and byproducts are taken into account to determine the overall energy efficiencies. This chapter also includes evaluation of greenhouse gas emissions and other environmental impacts associated with biofuel production.

Chapter 13 presents a techno-economic analysis (TEA) of microalgae for biofuel production. TEA can help identify best possible pathways and critical optimum process parameters for economic biofuel production. The major issues that render microalgal biofuel production uncompetitive are discussed in detail. This chapter suggests research efforts on screening and selecting highly efficient microalgae strains, utilization of waste streams for meeting the water and nutrient requirements and valorization of entire biomass for biofuel and valuable byproduct recovery and covalorization based on sensitivity analysis of microalgae biofuel productivity.

Chapter 14 provides critical perspectives on complexities associated with land use change for bioenergy production and associated poorly described land development and environmental impacts. Multi-use landscape scenarios incorporating agriculture, bioenergy, and fossil fuels are recommended for optimized production of all resources and for reducing environmental impacts of energy and agricultural sectors. A comparison of life cycle analysis studies for different bioenergy production schemes is provided in this chapter. A standardized analysis is suggested for efficient biofuel production while reducing waste generation and climate change mitigation.

1.5   CONCLUDING REMARKS

The principles of green chemistry and engineering serve as the fundamental building blocks for sustainable biofuel process development. It is also crucial to understand the fundamental chemistry involved in various process reactions required for biofuel production. Consideration and implementation of green chemistry principles and green metrics will result in maximum resource recovery with minimum environmental degradation. The chapters included in this book discuss various options for alternative and renewable feedstock utilization, process intensification, and challenges involved in biofuel production followed by evaluation of energy efficiency, techno-economics, and life cycle impacts and inventory analysis for various biofuel production processes.

KEYWORDS

- **environmental impact**
- **green chemistry**
- **green engineering**
- **life cycle assessment**
- **renewable feedstock**
- **sustainable biofuels**

REFERENCES

1. Amouroux, J., Siffert, P., Massué, J. P., Cavadias, S., Trujillo, B., Hashimoto, K., & Wang, X. (2014). Carbon dioxide: A new material for energy storage. *Progress in Natural Science: Materials International, 24*(4), 295-304.

2. Anastas, P. T., & Warner, J. C. (2000). Principles of green chemistry. *Green Chemistry: Theory and Practice,* Oxford University Press: New York, USA.

3. Anastas, P. T., & Zimmerman, J. B. (2003). Peer reviewed: design through the 12 principles of green engineering. *Environmental Science and Technology, 37*(5), 94A–101A.

4. Gude, V. G. (2015). Synergism of microwaves and ultrasound for advanced biorefineries. *Resource-Efficient Technologies, 1*(2), 116–125.

5. Gude, V. G., Patil, P., Martinez-Guerra, E., Deng, S., & Nirmalakhandan, N. (2013). Microwave energy potential for biodiesel production. *Sustainable Chemical Processes, 1*(1), 1.

6. Lee, A. F., Bennett, J. A., Manayil, J. C., & Wilson, K. (2014). Heterogeneous catalysis for sustainable biodiesel production via esterification and transesterification. *Chemical Society Reviews, 43*(22), 7887-7916.

7. Mason, T. J. (2007). Sonochemistry and the environment–Providing a "green" link between chemistry, physics and engineering. *Ultrasonics Sonochemistry, 14*(4), 476–483.

8. Mulvihill, M. J., Beach, E. S., Zimmerman, J. B., & Anastas, P. T. (2011). Green chemistry and green engineering: a framework for sustainable technology development. *Annual Review of Environment and Resources, 36*, 271–193.

CHAPTER 2

BIOFUEL FEEDSTOCK: CHALLENGES AND OPPORTUNITIES

CANNAYEN IGATHINATHANE[1] and MATT SANDERSON[2]

[1]Department of Agricultural and Biosystems Engineering, North Dakota State University, 1221 Albrecht Boulevard, Fargo, ND 58102, USA

[2]Northern Great Plains Research Laboratory, USDA-ARS, 1701 10th Avenue SW, Mandan, ND 58554, USA

CONTENTS

ABSTRACT

Use of locally grown renewable biofuel feedstocks for production of various fuel, energy, and bioproducts through green chemistry pathways aligns well with the global interest and presents great opportunities, in terms of possible environmental benefits, energy security, and new jobs stimulus, along with its associated challenges. Even though studies indicate uncertainties, a sustainable biomass availability and the processing technologies have been demonstrated to displace a significant amount of petroleum. Biofuel feedstock utilization in future might address the energy security and sustainability issues, such as providing the uninterrupted availability of energy sources at an affordable price through efficient production and conversion, scientific-technological innovations, stakeholder investments, and favorable governmental actions. This chapter provides a brief overview of challenges and opportunities for biofuel feedstock production and utilization in different sections that include biofuel feedstocks types, potential, production status, and consumption; challenges in production and utilization including establishment and management of crop stands, land availability, conversion process, competing use, and economics of utilization; opportunities in processing for biofuels and bioproducts using green-processing technologies, high-value products, environmental benefits analysis, modern concepts of biorefinery, advanced feedstock supply and distributed preprocessing systems, energy security, and perennial crops role in sustainability; and finally the conclusions and future directions.

2.1 INTRODUCTION

Utilization of bio-based feedstocks for biofuels, energy, and value-added products is recognized as environment-friendly and sustainable. The use of bio-based feedstocks presents great opportunities for stakeholders, but also presents challenges, technical and otherwise. A cleaner way of using the biofuel feedstocks is to use benign technologies, such as utilization of green chemistry. Green chemistry is defined as a technology that efficiently uses raw materials, eliminates waste and avoids the use of toxic and/or hazardous solvents and reagents in the manufacture and application of chemical products [26, 97]. One of the guiding principles of green chemistry, out of widely accepted 12 principles, is the use of renewable material feedstocks and energy sources [3]. Thus, the use of biofuel feedstocks that are locally grown falls in line with the green chemistry requirements.

In the renewable energy options portfolio, biofuel feedstock derived from biomass is unique in its ability to generate solid, liquid, and gaseous fuels, which can be stored and transported [45]. The environmental con-cerns caused by the use of fossil fuels, especially the contribution to climate change, make biomass an important source of energy that can displace fossil fuels. Biofuel feedstocks (renewable material of biological origin), which can be produced in a sustainable way and in short production cycle compared to fossil sources, as input material aligns well with the goals of green chemistry hence presents good opportunities. The proven advantages of the application of biofuel feedstocks have spurred global interest and nations have realized the role of greener technologies and the applicability of biofuel feedstocks among other renewable sources for a sustainable supply of nations bioenergy demands. Our goal in this chapter is to briefly review some of the challenges and opportunities associated with the use of biomass feedstocks in green chemistry applications. We provide a broad overview of some global issues, followed by types of biomass and their availability and a closer examination of the use of perennial bioenergy crops for feedstock production, status of feedstock production and consumption, and challenges in sustainable feedstock production. Finally, the opportunities of processing feedstocks for sustainable biofuels and bioproducts processing, which covers green processing, high-value bioproducts, environmental benefits, sustainability, and energy security are discussed.

2.1.1   GLOBAL INTEREST IN BIOFUEL FEEDSTOCK UTILIZATION

A principal driver of bioenergy development is the concern over global climate change. Mitigating the global annual emissions of greenhouse gasses (GHGs) by 2020 holding the increment in the global average temperature to well below 2°C, above preindustrial levels by reducing emissions through various pathways was emphasized in the recent United Nations, Paris Framework Convention on Climate Change [36]. It was also observed that biomass could play a significant role in meeting the global energy demands and achieving the GHG mitigation goals.

Biomass derived from agricultural and forestry activities represents a huge potential inventory that can be processed through available pathways to produce biofuels as well as bioenergy and bioproducts with lower GHG emissions, especially CO_2, compared with emissions from fossil fuels [8, 68]. The global interest in various applications of biofuel feedstocks is because of a combination of many driving and influencing factors such as [85]:

- transformation of the worldwide energy market towards increasing utilization of homegrown energy sources;
- recognition of the current role and future potential of bioenergy;
- increasing concern about oil prices and supply vulnerability;
- bio-economy related development and employment opportunities;
- growing interest driven by energy security concerns;
- implications of global climate change; and
- favorable renewable energy policies including government incentives, directives, and targets.

Policies dedicated to promoting the production and use of bioenergy from forests have been developed and implemented in European Union (EU) [14, 105], where biomass and renewable waste constitute just under two-thirds (64.2%) of the 2013 renewable energy production in the EU-28 countries [32]. For the renewable energy adoption, the EU 2020 policy targets for renewable energy sources and GHG emissions reduction constituted the main drivers [99]. In local energy production from solid fuels, the EU's 28 countries showed a steady decrease (15.3 EJ in 1990 to 6.0 EJ in 2015), while the renewable energy sources have more than doubled (3.0 EJ in 1990 to 8.6 EJ in 2015) during 1990 to 2015 [32]. The increase in consumption of bioenergy by EU is expected to continue because biomass is the only renewable energy solution for all energy sectors such as transportation, power, and heating and cooling (AEBIOM's 2015 statistical report). It was estimated based on pellet markets demand in energy and transportation sectors that the EU demand for woody biomass will increase from 105 to 305 Tg [99]. This trend in UN countries substantiates their commitment to moving towards bioenergy and highlights the opportunities of bioenergy utilization.

Other developing countries also invest in green technologies and renewable feedstocks for their energy needs because (i) the high cost of importing fossil fuels, (ii) the need to develop energy self-reliance, (iii) the need to reduce environmental pollution, and (iv) the availability of new technologies that enable the use of locally grown feedstocks for bioenergy production. The predominant use of biofuel feedstocks in the under-developed countries is cooking and water heating [27]. Thus, introducing simpler and mature technologies in these countries represents opportunities to develop well-distributed local biomass processing facilities (e.g., for densification, wood chips, wood mulch, biogas).

Several nations set and revise mandates on the usage of renewable energy from biofuel feedstocks as they plan to move towards a bio-economy (Figure 2.1). For example, the US Energy Independence and Security Act (EISA) developed a revised Renewable Fuels Standard (RFS) that mandates usage of renewable fuels equivalent to 136×10^6 m^3 (36 billion gallons) per year by 2022 [99a]. Also, the California's Low Carbon Fuel Standard (2007) sets a reduction of at least 10% in the carbon intensity of California's transportation fuels by 2020 [35]. This report indicates that this target seems plausible through low carbon fuel options, though these advanced technologies require further innovation in fuel and/or vehicle technologies.

Furthermore, the RFS mandates allocations of specific biofuels, such as cellulosic, advanced, biomass-based biodiesel, and conventional biofuels. Achieving these targets requires involvement from the stakeholders (e.g., feedstock producers, biorefinery processors, biofuel suppliers, traders, retailers). Current and planned global mandates of different countries range from 2% to 25% for ethanol and 1% to 20% for biodiesel (Figure 2.1). Thus, these targets represent great opportunities in terms of export, research and development, and local job creation including farming, preprocessing, logistics, biochemical engineering, and microbiology. For example, it was estimated that the 2007 EISA would result in the creation of nearly 2 million new jobs in the U.S. within 12–18 years [113].

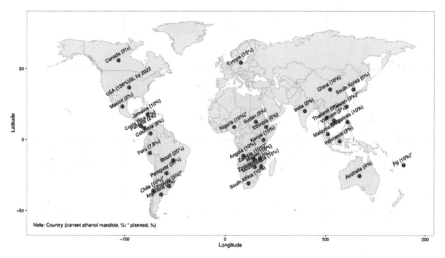

FIGURE 2.1 Global Renewable Fuel Alliance global biofuel mandate map showing the current or planned targets (Adapted from Global Renewable Fuel Alliance – http://globalrfa.org/biofuels-map/).

2.1.2   TYPES OF BIOFUEL FEEDSTOCKS

2.1.2.1   Potential Feedstock Categories

Potential biomass feedstock resources include primary forest and agriculture resources and secondary resources including wastes (Figure 2.2). Of these several of the feedstocks are already in use (e.g., corn grain for ethanol, oilseed crops for biodiesel, fuelwood for energy), the algal biomass also represent great potential for industrial applications. Currently, most biomass for energy consumption comes from wood, including firewood, forestry wastes (e.g., logging residues), and wood processing wastes (e.g., sawdust, construction waste). In terms of feedstocks used for liquid fuels, corn grain and soybean are the primary feedstocks for ethanol and biodiesel, respectively [116]. Near-term opportunities for expanding feedstock supplies include the sustainable collection of agricultural residues, such as corn stover or wheat

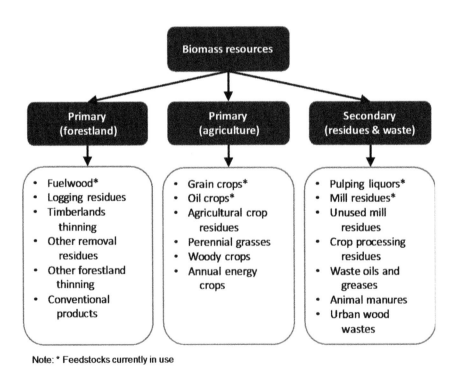

Note: * Feedstocks currently in use

FIGURE 2.2   Possible biomass resources types available for various utilization applications (Adapted from Ref. [115]).

straw along with efficiently using wastes from various agricultural (e.g., sugarcane bagasse), forestry (e.g., logging residues, forest thinnings), and industrial wastes.

On the availability of biomass feedstocks after meeting the demands for food, feed, fiber, and timber, the U.S. 2016 Billion-Ton Report [116] outlines the various categories of biomass feedstocks currently in use and their future potential through different scenarios (Table 2.1). The major potential feedstock categories include (i) forestry resources from private and federal lands, (ii) agricultural residues of major crops, (iii) energy crops, where widespread industrial application is not present now, (iv) waste resources from agricultural, forestry, municipal solid waste (MSW), other removal residues and supplies, and (v) algal biomass (Table 2.1.)

A decline in the forestry resources and an increase in agricultural residues were projected from 2017 to 2040. Dedicated energy crops are expected to play a major role in the future starting from 2030 with increasing contribution trend based on future market demand (Table 2.1). Waste resources derived from various categories of sources that represent low-cost opportunities without requiring additional inputs in terms of land or fertilizer [116]. These sources include agricultural secondary wastes, MSW (garbage consisting of yard trimmings and paper products), forest and wood wastes, and other supplies and several candidate feedstocks feature in these categories (Table 2.1). Though the immediate use of these wastes is industrial heat, based on the nature of these feedstocks these can also be processed into biofuels and bioproducts.

Environmental tradeoffs, however, may be involved with the use of forestry wastes or crop residues. For example, the use of thinnings or other residues from forestry may entail long-term risks to the environment, such as physical damage to soils and biodiversity loss [43]. Other types of residues, such as from corn or wheat production, have received extensive attention as feedstocks [76]. The exploitation of this feedstock supply, however, is constrained by potential negative effects on soil organic matter, greater risks of wind and water erosion, and soil compaction among other factors [94, 125, 130].

Algae (single cell or filamentous) biomass represents another attractive feedstock, which can be grown on freshwater, saline, or suitable waste stream, because of its high biomass yield per unit area and time and its non-competition with the food supply. The lipids, proteins, and carbohydrates contents can be processed into a variety of biogas and biofuel end products (e.g., hydrogen, methane, ethanol, renewable diesel, jet fuel), and the

TABLE 2.1 U.S. Potential Feedstocks Available (Forest, Agricultural, and Waste Biomass) at ≤$60 Dry Mg^{-1} Under Base-Case (1% Annual Yield Increase) and High-Yield* (3% Annual Yield Increase) Scenarios (Adapted from [116]).

Feedstock	Base-case scenario (dry Tg)			High-yield scenario (dry Tg)*		
	2017	2030	2040	2017	2030	2040
Forestry resources (e.g., sawtimber, pulpwood, other roundwood, whole-tree biomass, logging residues—all timberland—private 83% and federal 17%)	93	88	88	86	79	69
Agricultural residues (e.g., corn stover, wheat straw, oat straw, barley straw, sorghum stubble)	94	135	160	95	158	181
Energy crops (e.g., herbaceous—switchgrass, miscanthus, energy cane, biomass sorghum; woody—willow, eucalyptus, poplar, pine)	–	217	373	–	345	668
Waste resources (e.g., agricultural secondary waste—sugarcane residue, soybean hulls, cotton gin trash, etc.; MSW - garbage fraction; forest and wood wastes—other removal residues, residue thinning, mill residue, urban wood waste, etc.; other supplies—biosolids, used cooking oils, food processing waste, etc.)	124	127	129	124	127	129
Total scenario potential	**311**	**567**	**750**	**305**	**709**	**1047**
Total scenario (currently used: 331 dry Tg + potential)	**642**	**898**	**1081**	**636**	**1040**	**1378**

Algae (colocated facility; freshwater and saline media combined; price range $540–$3185 dry Mg^{-1})

	Present 2014 (dry Tg)	Future (dry Tg)
Ethanol plant producing waste CO$_2$	20	22
Coal electric generating unit (EGU)	66	20
Natural gas EGU	33	-
Total	**119**	**42**

residual biomass into high-value coproducts (e.g., livestock and aquaculture feed, biofertilizers). Algal biofuels are moving toward commercial applications in states including Hawaii, California, New Mexico, Arizona, Florida, Texas, and Iowa [116]. Even though the algal biomass cost is much higher than terrestrial biomass, identifying resource colocation opportunities for algal biofuel facilities has the potential to reduce costs, use waste resources, and focus attention on appropriate technologies and locations for commercialization (Table 2.1).

2.1.2.2 Dedicated Energy Crops

Long-term, the development of sustainable perennial energy crops is highly desirable as a source of second-generation feedstocks. Short-rotation woody crops offer potential as perennial biomass feedstocks. *Populus*, *Salix*, and *Eucalyptus* species (among others) have been researched for their adaptability, persistence, and productivity as biomass species [24, 48]. Productivity levels of these crops range from 5 to 20 Mg biomass ha^{-1} yr^{-1}.

Worldwide, dedicated lignocellulosic feedstocks produced from perennial herbaceous crop (e.g., perennial grasses) production have been intensively and extensively researched as second-generation feedstocks. This section focuses on perennial grasses (both native and introduced species) as dedicated energy crops, because they are highly productive, adapted to stressful environments, and have been reported to efficiently use water and nutrients.

Switchgrass (*Panicum virgatum* L.) is a warm-season (C_4 photosynthetic pathway) perennial grass native to North America that has been intensively researched as a dedicated bioenergy crop [89]. Switchgrass has been grown as a forage crop and conservation plant for decades and farmers are familiar with its management [118]. It has broad adaptability across many environments and can be grown under a low-input system but can be highly productive with additional inputs [49]. Its productivity has been well documented in the U.S. [129], England [17], and in the rest of Europe [2, 28, 72]. Improved varieties developed specifically for biomass production such as 'BoMaster' [13] and 'Liberty' [119] have been released.

Miscanthus (specifically Giant *Miscanthus*; *Miscanthus x giganteus* Greef and Deuter) has also received a great deal of attention as a perennial energy crop. A C_4 grass native to Asia, *Miscanthus* has very high yield potential and has a low requirement for nitrogen fertilizer [18, 46]. Yields more than 40 Mg dry biomass ha^{-1} have been reported [5]. It is a sterile trip-loid and must be propagated vegetatively [95]. *Miscanthus* may not be as widely adapted across a range of environments as switchgrass. For example, Giant *Miscanthus* does not survive soil temperatures (at 5 cm depth) below $-3°C$ [19] and thus would likely not survive winters in northern locations such as the upper Midwest and northern Great Plains of the USA.

Prairie cordgrass (*Spartina pectinata* Link.) is a C$_4$ (warm-season), tall, rhizomatous, perennial grass that has not received the attention as switch-grass and miscanthus had as a potential bioenergy crop. Prairie cordgrass found predominantly in marshes, wet meadows, potholes, and drainage ways throughout the continental United States and most of the Canada [9]. It has a broad climatic adaptation and grows on a wide array of soil types [56]. Prairie cordgrass is recognized for its tolerance to salinity and valued for wetland revegetation, streambank stabilization, wildlife habitat, and forage. The above-ground biomass yields varied from 1.37 Mg ha^{-1} (mar-ginal lands) to 12.7 Mg ha^{-1} (Red River germplasm mature stands) with even higher belowground biomass [9]. Prairie cordgrass ethanol yields of 205–276 g kg^{-1} biomass and 1748–4368 L ha^{-1} as a dedicated energy are comparable with those of switchgrass, corn stover, and bagasse [63].

Big bluestem (*Andropogon gerardii* Vitman) is a perennial warm-season grass native to the U.S.; the dominant grass species of the Midwestern tall-grass prairie; used for prairie restoration, highway revegetation, and mine reclamation; and found abundant in lowland prairies, overflow sites, and sandy areas and also in open woods, prairies, meadows, along riverbanks, and roadsides [122]. Under drought conditions, big bluestem can be more productive than switchgrass [112]. Many of the tillers of big bluestem can remain vegetative which reduces investment in seed production [93], and the thicker stems than switchgrass avoids lodging and yields in late winter and spring harvests [111].

Indiangrass (*Sorghastrum nutans* (L.) Nash.) is a native, perennial, warm-season, tall grass (0.9 to 1.5 m) that once dominated the prairies of the central and eastern U.S., and can be used as erosion control, livestock forage, and wildlife habitat [77]. Because of slow germination, the yields of Indiangrass is lower than that of switchgrass or big bluestem; but once estab-lished its yields of 8–10 Mg ha^{-1} yr^{-1} were comparable to as switchgrass in dry years [112]. In addition, the less leaf content and low nutrient values of leaves of Indiangrass compared to switchgrass, big bluestem, and cordgrass [67], makes it more suitable for bioenergy uses [111].

Another C_4 grass of great potential as a biofuel feedstock is Napier grass (*Pennisetum purpureum* Schumach.) and is also known as elephant grass. Napier grass is a robust perennial grass that is naturalized widely in the world's tropical and subtropical regions and can be harvested year-round. The crop is capable of achieving high yields of 94 dry Mg ha^{-1} [78]. Napier grass presents a unique opportunity for fractionation into solid (cellulosic fibers) for biofuel production and liquid streams (nutrient-rich juice) for coproduct generation [108]. Therefore, along with other energy crops Napier grass represents a significant potential as a feedstock for large-scale renewable biofuel production. These perennial warm season grasses intrinsically have high light, water, and nitrogen use efficiency as compared with that of cool season species, along with benefits of reduced tillage, soil carbon sequestration, and protect against erosion [102]. Some of the lands taken out of agriculture and marginal lands appear suitable for the production of such perennial grasses or other types of energy crops.

Reed canarygrass (*Phalaris arundinacea* L.) is a C_3 (cool-season) grass that grows well on wet soils and has been used mainly as a forage crop [16]. It is adapted to temperate environments and can be highly productive as a perennial biomass crop [47, 107, 128]. Reed canarygrass, however, can be highly invasive in native wetlands causing adverse environmental consequences [37]. Invasiveness, however, does not appear to be related to plant breeding for improved cultivars [55]. Reed canarygrass can be difficult to establish from seed because of poor seedling vigor and the harvested biomass may contain high concentrations of ash (>10% of dry matter) [128]. Ash and mineral concentrations can be reduced by delaying harvest over winter until the following spring [65].

In tropical and subtropical regions of the world, species such as species of Napier grass (or) elephant grass '*Cenchrus purpureus* (Schumach.) Morrone,' energy cane '*Saccharum* spp.,' bermudagrass '*Cynodon dactylon* L.' [4], and sorghums '*Sorghum bicolor* L. Moench' [75, 40], and giant reed '*Arundo donax* L.' [73] have demonstrated to have extremely high biomass yield. However, giant reed is considered an invasive species in the USA.

Although monocultures of perennial grasses are highly productive and straightforward to manage, extensive landscape expanses of monocultural crops are not considered desirable for the delivery of multiple ecosystem services, such as wildlife or pollinator habitat [7]. The use of polycultures or mixtures of several species of grasses or other plant functional groups (e.g., legumes and other forbs) is thought to be a less input intensive approach to bioenergy cropping [21, 110]. Increasing the diversity of agricultural systems (including grasslands) may provide additional benefits or ecosystem services, such as enhanced nutrient cycling, more efficient use of resources, and reduced pest pressures [86, 90]. Several field experiments, however, have not demonstrated productivity benefits for mixtures planted and grown for biomass feedstock production. For example, monocultures of four warm-season perennial grasses yielded more biomass than polycultures of grasses, legumes, and forbs in Oklahoma [42]. Monocultures of several grasses yielded more than a polyculture of several grasses and forbs in Minnesota (Figure 2.3) [57]. In a farm-scale study of crop and landscape position effects on grass monoculture and mixture yields, productivity of grass monocultures was greater than mixtures of prairie plant species [131]. In a survey of 20 fields dedicated either to a switchgrass monoculture or a diverse mixtures of prairie plant species and a field plot experiment comparing mixtures of 1 to 30 prairie plant species, there was no significant relationship between species richness of the plantings and biomass yields [25]. Research at nine locations in Minnesota and North Dakota, however, indicated that some mixtures of prairie plants can be as productive as switchgrass monocultures [58]. There has been little research, however, that has addressed multiple ecosystem services beyond biomass productivity.

Ultimately, the selection of a dedicated perennial bioenergy crop will depend on the landscape, growing environment, soils, climate, and

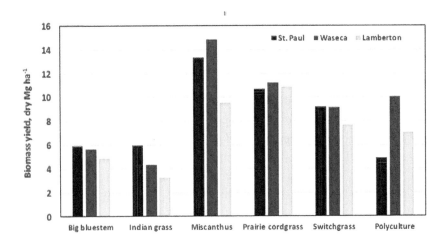

FIGURE 2.3 Biomass yields of warm-season perennial grasses in monocultures compared with a polyculture of 12 grass and forb species grown at three locations in Minnesota, USA (Adapted from Ref. [57]).

management along with market forces and agricultural policies [20]. A national or broadly distributed renewable energy industry will require multiple feedstocks distributed across the landscape locally and regionally across the country. The biorefining industry will need flexibility in the processes to accommodate multiple feedstocks within a locality or region. For example, a cellulosic biorefinery able to process switchgrass bales, corn stover, and perhaps mixed species biomass could potentially expand the fuelshed and facilitate a diverse agricultural landscape while maintaining multiple ecosystem benefits [83] (Figure 2.4) and avoid massive expanses of monocultural crops.

2.1.3 STATUS OF BIOFUEL FEEDSTOCK PRODUCTION AND CONSUMPTION

As the interest in the bio-economy grows at various rates among countries, a steady increase in feedstock production and consumption has been observed and future demand projections have been made. The current global

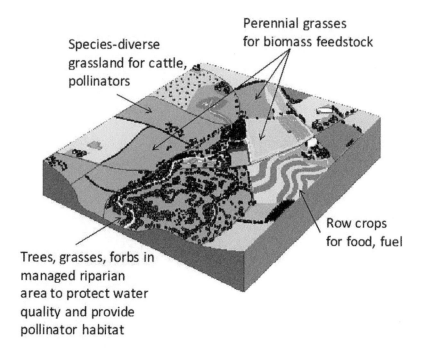

FIGURE 2.4 Hypothetical diverse farm landscape showing multiple crops distributed across the farm to take best advantage of soils and other natural resources.

bioethanol production data is an indication of the quantity of feedstocks used in generating the biofuel (Figure 2.5). The data show that the U.S. is the world leader in ethanol production (nearly 60% of global output), Brazil the second (25%), followed by the E.U. (6%), China (3%) and Canada (2%); which also show the availability of feedstocks and its usage for biofuels in these countries. However, this U.S. ethanol production is predominantly from the corn grain (1st generation biofuel), which will be supplemented by advanced biofuels such as lignocellulosic ethanol (2nd generation biofuel) and biofuels from microalgae (3rd generation biofuel).

Several studies have shown large uncertainties in the estimated current and future available supplies of biomass [80]. The U.S. DOE (2016) billion-ton biomass update demonstrated the feasibility of more than 898 Tg dry biomass (at \$66 dry Tg^{-1} base case scenario for 2030) available for use capable of displacing up to 30% of the petroleum consumption of the nation.

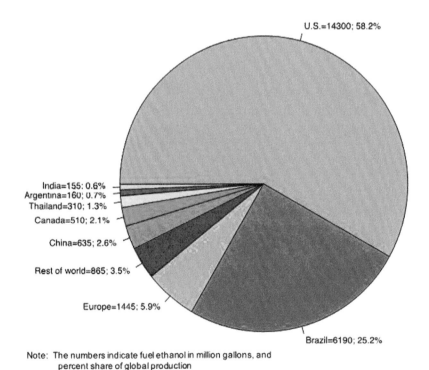

Note: The numbers indicate fuel ethanol in million gallons, and percent share of global production

FIGURE 2.5 Global 2014 ethanol production indicating the use of feedstocks in biofuel production (Adapted from RFA analysis of public and private estimates; Data from Ref. [52]).

Total energy produced from biomass sources (wood and wood-derived fuels, biomass waste, fuel ethanol, and biodiesel) and consumed in 2015 was 4.97 EJ and 4.95 EJ, which accounted for 5.4% and 4.8% of U.S. total primary energy (fossil fuels, nuclear electric power, and renewable energy sources) production and consumption, respectively [26]. This indicates the proportion of the energy from biomass at present and the scope for future growth.

It was estimated that about 42% of the U.S. biomass feedstock currently used (331 dry Tg) came from forest sources. The other prominent feedstocks include corn (*Zea mays* L.) grain for ethanol production, and specific forest (e.g., mill residues, fuel wood) and cropland (e.g., agricultural crop residues, cotton gin trash) biomass resources, while dedicated energy crops are virtually nonexistent at present in industrial scale but they can expand rapidly in response to market demand [116]. The U.S. total base-case scenario with 1% annual yield increase of feedstock available at ≤ $66 dry Mg^{-1} [116] are 311 and 750 dry Tg at 2017 and 2040, respectively; whereas the distribution of forestry resources is 30% and 12%, agricultural residues are 30% and 21%, energy crops is 0% and 50%, and waste resources are 40% and 17% at 2017 and 2040, respectively (Table 2.1). Obviously for the high-yield scenario, with 3% annual yield growth, increases the total feedstock potential to 1047 dry Tg (40% increase) at 2040. When included the currently used quantity of feedstocks, these projections increase by 331 dry Tg.

Brazil generated over 72 EJ (20 billion MWh) of power through biomass in 2012 [81]. Brazil's most abundant biomass feedstock is sugarcane '*Saccharum officinarum* L.' in agriculture, with pine '*Pinus spp.*' and eucalyptus '*Eucalyptus* spp.' dominating the forest resources. Brazil's sugarcane production estimates in the 2005–2006 harvest season reached 372 Gg, and its production has risen on average by 9.7% per year during 2001–2006 [121]. In Europe, their total supply of sustainable biomass in 2030 was predicted to be enough to fulfill their 10% bio-based economy demand [84].

2.2 CHALLENGES IN SUSTAINABLE PRODUCTION OF BIOFUEL FEEDSTOCK AND UTILIZATION

2.2.1 BIOFUEL FEEDSTOCK PRODUCTION CHALLENGES

Production challenges for dedicated bioenergy crops include rapid establishment of the crop, optimizing management inputs to result in economical feedstock yields with a positive energy balance, and efficient harvest, storage, and processing of the feedstock [89]. Ideally, bioenergy crop production should not compromise environmental quality but rather enhance ecosystem services, such as soil carbon storage, habitat for wildlife and pollinators, and nutrient cycling. Achieving both feedstock production and environmental quality goals may require tradeoffs in production practices and ecosystem service expectations.

2.2.1.1   Establishment of the Crop

Switchgrass has been studied as a bioenergy crop for more than two decades with considerable effort on improving seed germination and resulting plant establishment. Critical problems include overcoming seed dormancy to result in reliable germination and improving the ability of seedlings to withstand stresses (e.g., drought, weed competition) during establishment so that productive stands can be achieved in the seeding year. Approaches and solutions to seed germination difficulties include seed treatments to break dormancy, planting methods to naturally reduce dormancy, and plant selection and breeding to overcome dormancy genetically. Crop management solutions to establishment problems include planning appropriate crop rotations before seeding to reduce weed populations, using effective planting techniques to place seeds in a favorable seed bed, and management of weed competition after planting and establishment [89].

Miscanthus, another highly productive perennial grass proposed for feedstock production, presents a unique establishment challenge. The strain of *Miscanthus* studied for bioenergy production is a sterile triploid that must be planted vegetatively (i.e., by root or stem pieces) [95]. This presents challenges in producing viable vegetative pieces along with requirements for appropriate machinery and techniques for vegetative planting.

2.2.1.2   Management of Established Stands

The principal management concerns after establishment include fertilization and weed control. The critical fertilizer nutrient to manage for perennial grasses is nitrogen. Nitrogen fertilizer can greatly increase grass growth and biomass production. Fertilizer, however, is costly both economically and energetically. Therefore, effective fertilizer management is an optimization process.

Weed invasion and competition adversely affects bioenergy crops by not only by reducing production but also by reducing resultant feedstock quality for conversion. Effective weed management begins at seeding and establishment (see Section 2.2.1.1) to prevent initial invasions. In subsequent production years weed invasions must be managed either via herbicides or time harvest.

2.2.1.3   Land Availability

Producing biofuels on agricultural land can be viewed as competing with human food production [39]. To avoid food *vs* fuel competition for land, marginal agricultural lands have been suggested as an alternative land base [15]. In Europe, underused seminatural grasslands have been proposed as a noncompetitive land base [109, 120]. In the U.S., lands in the Conservation Reserve Program (CRP; a voluntary conservation program that pays farmers to retain environmentally sensitive land from agricultural production and planting species that will improve soil and environmental quality), which are often planted to mixtures of grasses and forbs, have been proposed to be repurposed for biofuel production and potentially avoid the C debt from land conversion [38, 66]. Research on conservation lands in Minnesota [59], South Dakota [74], and the northeastern U.S. [1] indicated significant biomass yield potentials. Because of relatively high commodity prices for grain crops in recent years, land in conservation programs such as CRP and other perennial grasslands have been converted to row crops [127] with potential adverse environmental consequences. In North Dakota, for example, land area in CRP has decreased dramatically in recent years (Figure 2.6).

Other degraded lands with potential for perennial bioenergy crop production include reclaimed surface mined lands. In the U.S., surface mined ("strip" mined) lands must be reclaimed to prevent erosion and other adverse environmental effects according to U.S. law (the Surface Mining and Reclamation Act). Reclamation efforts often use perennial grasses to restore vegetative cover [100]. Biomass production of switchgrass grown on biosolids-amended reclaimed mine land in West Virginia [34] and Virginia [12] ranged from 5 to 16 Mg dry biomass ha^{-1} and 3 to 7 Mg ha^{-1}, respectively.

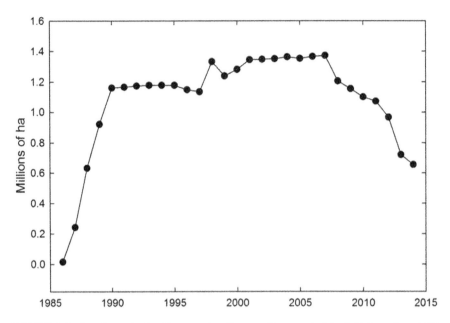

FIGURE 2.6   Land area in the Conservation Reserve Program in North Dakota from 1986 to 2014 ([36a]; http://www.fsa.usda.gov/programs-and-services/conservation-programs/reports-and-statistics/conservation-reserve-program-statistics/index).

2.2.2 *BIOFUEL FEEDSTOCK UTILIZATION CHALLENGES*

Biofuel feedstocks being biological in nature exhibit a high variation in their material properties, unlike other engineering materials. Biomass feedstocks related challenges include various issues associated with production, logistics, conversion, and economics (Table 2.2).

Even though existing harvesting and collection equipment can be used for traditional biomass crops, new designs of equipment are required to include other biomass and dedicated energy crops for efficient handling and processing (e.g., *Miscanthus*). In logistics, the terminology used such as "field to factory" sounds like a simple point-to-point transport of well-packaged biomass. But a closer look reveals the biomass in the form of bales is a dispersed source and calls for an additional in-field logistics operation of aggregating the bales [53]. For efficient in-field bale logistics, it was also found that formation of an increased number of bale stacks and increased multiple bales/trip hauled from the stacks (e.g., 6 bales/trip) make for efficient logistics [54].

TABLE 2.2 Biofuel Feedstock Utilization Challenges Component Sectors

Production
• Land availability – competing with other crops
• Land fertility – mostly marginal lands for energy crops
• Harvest and collection – sometimes specialized equipment required
• Competing use – food and feed
• Food *vs* fuel debate – products can be used for food
Logistics
• Wet material – needs energy intensive drying
• Dispersed resource – field to factory had additional field operations
• Infield logistics – aggregation of feedstocks in field
• Low bulk density – densification required
• Seasonality – not available in all seasons
• Not uniform product – mass and energy density variation
• Large transport distances – low energy density of feedstock
Conversion
• Recalcitrance of feedstock to enzymes
• Limited availability of specialized enzymes and catalyst
• Hydrolysis and fermentation issues
• Low solids loading
• High cost of chemicals used
• Non-uniform feedstock chemical properties
• Enzyme recovery and reuse issues
• Risk related with high pressure and high temperatures
• Low product production rates
• Large water requirement
• Several processes in developmental stage
• Scale-up issues
Economics
• At present not economical – compared to cheaper fossil fuels
• Adoption of biofuel "blend-wall"
• Affordable price of feedstocks at large quantities
• High logistics cost
• Current nonexistence of wide-spread market
• Uncertainty on feedstock supply and market availability
• Lack of necessary market penetration of biofuels and products

Further, much less attention has been paid in solving feedstock supply chain challenges, such as low bulk density of cellulosic biomass, compositional variability and seasonality of the feedstock, food *vs* fuel issues by processing cellulosic biomass (nonfood source), and local environmental concerns [31]. One way to address these challenges was the proposed concept of preprocessing distributed depots that condition and densify biomass into stable intermediate products that are compatible with existing supply and processing systems. An advanced feedstock supply system that will also produce merchandisable intermediates will be discussed later (Figure 2.10).

The conversion process, in addition, throws in several challenges (Table 2.2). Second generation biofuels (e.g., cellulosic ethanol) production is even more challenging than producing first generation biofuels (e.g., corn ethanol) due the complexity of the biomass involved in the process [6]. Other challenges associated with processing is converting biomass to liquid transportation fuel, namely pretreatment, hydrolysis, microbial fermentation, and fuel separation still exist and are being addressed in research and development.

There are also economics related challenges of biomass utilization (Table 2.2). All these challenges should be overcome to progress towards the bioeconomy, and several projects around the world have demonstrated successful deployment of specific technologies. Future research and assessments in the technical and economical fields should explore ways to address these challenges.

2.2.3   COMPETING USES FOR FEEDSTOCKS

Perennial grasses, such as switchgrass and reed canarygrass, traditionally have been used as hay and grazing crops for livestock. Thus, depending on markets, these traditional uses may compete with bioenergy feedstock use. Additionally, perennial grasses have been used in conservation to reduce soil erosion and filter nutrients in runoff water. Dedicated bioenergy crops potentially offer alternative revenue streams for farmers. Perennial grasses may also serve as dual crops producing both forage for livestock and a harvestable biomass crop depending on management [44].

2.2.4   ECONOMICS OF BIOFUEL FEEDSTOCK UTILIZATION

As there is an overall awareness of the benefits of renewable biofuel feedstocks in various applications, the interest and economic developmental activities are on the rise. Governmental programs also incentivize the development of the bio-economy. For example, the USDA "BioPreferred" program facilitates the development and expansion of markets for bio-based products and creating rural jobs. This program has a mandatory federal purchasing initiative (with an online catalog to assess bio-based content information, and to find and compare products) and a voluntary "USDA Certified Bio-based Product" label strategy. This initiative has grown rapidly and has 97 product categories representing about 14,200 products [41]. The economic impact of this program is evident from the 4.2 million jobs contributed and $393 billion value added (Figure 2.7). These bio-based products reported excludes the energy, livestock, food, feed, and pharmaceutical industries and had only a limited number of forest and textile fiber products. The use of bio-based products reduced the consumption of petroleum equivalents through replacement of chemical feedstocks and serving as substitutes for petroleum-based materials, which resulted in 1081 ML of petroleum displacement.

In the U.S. biofuel sector, across the economy, the ethanol industry supported more than 383,000 jobs (about 87,000 direct, 86,000 indirect, and the remainder induced) in 2012 [114]. Analysts agree that the biofuel sector could be a powerful jobs stimulus and new categories of jobs would be created (Table 2.3) through advanced biofuels and biopower when the industry expands beyond ethanol [117].

The feedstocks represented in these U.S. bio-based products and biofuels scenarios [117] were not exhaustive, and the inclusion of other potential feedstocks will likely expand the possibilities and impacts. Analyses have shown that necessary feedstocks in U.S. are available to support the bio-economy activities. A potential total supply when the currently used forestry, agricultural, and waste resources (e.g., corn grain, forestry products) included range from 642 to 1081 dry Tg at 2017 and 2040 at $\leq$ \$66 dry Mg^{-1}

U.S. Biobased products industries economic impact in 2014

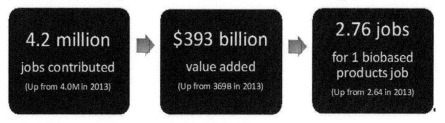

FIGURE 2.7 Economic impact of USDA "BioPreferred" program in 2014 in terms or jobs contributed and value added (Adapted from Ref. [41]).

TABLE 2.3   Job Categories and Avenues in Biofuels Sector (Adapted from Ref. [117])

Feedstocks	
• Farmers	• Seasonal workers
• Tree farm workers	• Mechanical engineers
• Harvesting equipment mechanics	• Equipment production workers
• Chemical engineers	• Chemical application specialists
• Chemical production workers	• Biochemists
• Agricultural engineers	• Genetic engineers and scientists
• Storage facility	
Conversion	
• Microbiologists	• Clean room technicians
• Industrial engineers	• Chemical and mechanical engineers
• Plant operators	
End use	
• Station workers	• Construction workers
• Codes and standards developers	• Regulation compliance workers
• Consultants	• Chemists
Transport of feedstocks and biofuels	
• Truck drivers	• Trucking filling station workers
• Pipeline operator	• Barge operators
• Railcar operators	• Train station operators

even in the base-case scenario. Thus the feedstock availability goes beyond 907 dry Tg (1 billion dry tons) in future (≥2030) with high-yield (3% annual yield increase) scenario as well as microalgae in the mix (Table 2.1).

2.3   OPPORTUNITIES IN FEEDSTOCK PROCESSING FOR SUSTAINABLE BIOFUELS AND BIOPRODUCTS

2.3.1   GREEN PROCESSING TECHNOLOGY OPPORTUNITIES

Various state-of-the-art green chemistry strategies for the valorization of waste biomass to platform chemicals are available [98] and these include:

- Drop-in strategy of complete deoxygenation to petroleum hydrocarbons and further processing using existing technologies,
- Direct conversion redox economic approach (e.g., carbohydrates to oxygenates by fermentation or chemo-catalytic processes),

- Three possible routes for producing a bio-based equivalent of the large volume polymer, polyethylene terephthalate (PET),
- Valorization of waste protein form an important source of amino acids as platform chemicals, which in turn can be converted to nitrogen containing commodity chemicals, and
- Valorization of glycerol, a coproduct of biodiesel manufacture from triglycerides, into commodity chemicals.

The collection and transport of relatively low-density waste biomass requires different strategies with respect to the logistics and economies of scale of biomass conversion. Mobile refineries that are brought to the source of biomass rather than bringing the biomass to the refinery can be one option [98]. The traditional metrics of sustainability of green chemistry include atom economy (conversion efficiency of the process in terms of all atoms involved) and environmental (E) factor (E factor = kg of waste / kg product). A higher E factor means more waste generated leading to greater negative environmental impact. But to suit the biomass utilization new metrics, such as materials efficiency, energy efficiency, land use, and process costs are proposed [98].

2.3.2   HIGH-VALUE BIOPRODUCTS OPPORTUNITIES

Biofuel feedstock refining processes, apart from producing biofuels, can generate high-value chemicals and products including plastics, polymers, and fibers, among many other outputs similar to petroleum refining to various chemicals and products. Plant-derived renewable feedstocks have the potential to replace petroleum-derived products by yielding basic chemical building blocks that can be refined into products of similar or better properties [29]. For example, U.S. researchers selected a list of 12 building block chemicals (Table 2.4) from the biomass feedstocks of practical importance from a condensed list of 30 potential candidates which were distilled from more than 300 candidate chemicals [124]. These building block chemicals can be subsequently processed into high-value bio-based chemicals, derivatives or products catering to various industries and applications (Table 2.4). Other potential chemicals form as a second-tier group of building block chemicals that can also be used for value-added chemicals production [124] (Table 2.4).

Established routes are available to produce several types of high-valued chemicals and specialized biofuels from a variety of feedstocks including cellulosic biomass having chemical structure with cellulose, hemicellulose,

TABLE 2.4 High-Valued Chemicals and Biofuels Derived from Biofuel Feedstocks (Data from: Refs. [29, 124])

First-tier building block chemicals (#12)	Second-tier group chemicals	Other biofuels	Applications
• 1,4-diacids (succinic, fumaric and malic)	• Gluconic acid	• Hydrogen	• Industrial
• 2,5-furan dicarboxylic acid	• Latic acid	• Methanol	• Transportation
• 3-hydroxy propionic acid	• Malonic acid	• Alkanes	• Textiles
• Aspartic acid	• Propionic acid	• Light alkanes	• Food
• Glucaric acid	• Triacids	• n-alkanes	• Environment
• Glutamic acid	• Citric acid	• Alcohols	• Communication
• Itaconic acid	• Aconitic acid	• Aromatics	• Housing
• Levulinic acid	• Xylonic acid	• Hydrocarbons	• Recreation
• 3-hydroxybutyrolactone	• Acetoin,	• Alkyl benzenes	• Health
• Glycerol	• Furfural	• Paraffins	• Hygiene
• Sorbitol	• Levoglucosan	• Coke	
• Xylitol/arabinitol	• Lysine	• Methyltetrahydrofuran	
	• Serine	• Levulinic esters	
	• Threonine	• Butanol	

and lignin (woody and agricultural feedstocks including wastes, residues, bagasse, corn grain, etc.) and triglycerides (vegetable oils, algae) following chemical, biological, and combined conversions [50]. Several types of specialized biofuels other than ethanol can be developed as well (Table 2.4). These fuels serve as gasoline and biodiesel either as direct use or as blends or as specialized fuel. Some of these specialized fuels are of high-value and suited to special applications.

The U.S. Department of Energy target of 50% production of chemical building blocks coming from plant-derived biomass by 2050 [29] emphasizes the opportunity and significance of green chemistry products from biomass feedstocks, such as various small-market specialty high-value chemicals based on feedstocks' unique biochemical structure. Similar opportunities exist to exploit various unique biomass feedstocks from around the world for the production of numerous unique high-value chemicals.

2.3.3   ENVIRONMENTAL BENEFITS

Bioenergy sustainability encompasses issues related to feedstock availability, process technology and efficiency, environmental, social, and economic impacts throughout the entire bioenergy supply chain. For sustainable developments to be achieved, the environmental benefits should be maximized, while concerns and potential negative impacts should be minimized, which can be obtained through research, advanced analysis, technical development, and stakeholders' participation and inputs. McBride et al. [70] developed a suite of 19 indicators as a practical toolset for capturing key environmental effects in six categories namely soil quality, water quality and quantity, GHG, biodiversity, air quality, and biomass productivity to measure the environmental sustainability of bioenergy systems.

Cradle-to-grave life-cycle analysis (LCA) studies [60] assessed and indicated the impacts of biomass-based biofuels on the environment and human health, which included raw materials through production, utilization, and disposal compared with those of fossil fuels. A saving of CO_2 emissions of 10,000–11,000 kg ha^{-1} yr^{-1} was found for *Miscanthus*, wood chips (from short rotation poplar) and winter wheat whole plant. Also, approximately 70 kg CO_2 equivalents (calculated from CO_2, CH_4 and N_2O emissions) was prevented per GJ of energy saved by the biomass tested. Another U.S. National Renewable Energy Laboratory LCA study also indicated a positive energy balance of 11:1 to 16:1 (biomass energy generated:fossil energy consumed) for dedicated wood energy crops biomass gasification system [69].

Notwithstanding the reported benefits, mixed LCA results were found in literature as feedstock-processing technology advanced, new data made available, and additional constraints were considered in advanced and more realistic LCA calculations. A recent review on LCA of second generation bioethanol based on lignocellulosic biomass indicated that 14 studies (64%–86%) concluded a positive net-energy output, while only two studies otherwise; and 28 studies an increase in GHG saving (11%–145%), while only three studies otherwise compared to the gasoline system [126].

Several factors (direct or indirect) of modern LCA, such as the choice of product and technology, system boundary and calculation methodology, the choice of allocation method, land use change (LUC), economic value and market-mediated effects, inclusion of coproduct, efficiency of technologies, percent of biofuel blend used, type of land used for feedstock production, set of impact categories analyzed (e.g., global warming potential, eutrophication, acidification, toxicity), quality of data, and other factors affect the final result [62, 126]. Of these factors, the choice LCA methodology, the inclusion of coproducts, technical design of production system, and LUC have a significant impact on GHG balances and eutrophication for all biofuels. As LCA of any project is unique and specific to local and/or regional conditions, there is no "right" or "wrong" calculation methodology; however, setting strong constraints with respect to energy and environmental consideration instead of indirect effects (e.g., LUC) will ensure the most sustainable biofuel production system in a practical sense. Acknowledging the indirect effects of LUC, while expanding biofuel feedstock production, through the development of practical complementary tools to certification schemes and standardization will avoid potential negative displacement effects [11].

Biomass tends to displace fossil energy systems. This will conserve finite fossil energy resources and reduce the impact on the global climate as they show favorable energy and GHG balances [8]. The significant impact of the CO_2 reduction of biomass can be readily seen from the CO_2 emission per GWh from coal estimated at 1142 Mg, and natural gas at 505–846 Mg, while for biomass this was about 66–107 Mg [68]. However, for the production and transportation of biomass feedstock, fossil fuels are mainly used and this leads to CO_2 and other GHG emission [10]. In a study by Kaltschmitt et al. [60], biomass systems were found to be more destructive than conventional fossil fuels due to higher emissions of N_2O in combustion and cultivation, causing ozone depletion and other non-GHG emissions (SO_2 and NO_x). Overall, energy crops are preferable to fossil fuels for energy, and annual or perennial crops for electricity and heat are preferable to liquid fuel routes [45]. Recent developments with innovative cropping systems (with multiple species) indicate substantial scope and opportunities for bioenergy crops to provide multiple ecosystem services such as soil carbon storage, reductions in GHG emissions, and diverse landscapes for wildlife, pollinators and other habitat [91] (Figure 2.8).

2.3.4 MODERN PROCESSING, SUSTAINABILITY, AND ENERGY SECURITY

2.3.4.1 Concept of Biorefinery

The main driver of the concept of a biorefinery is the call for sustainability [23]. The following definition of biorefinery was developed by the International Energy Agency (IEA) Bioenergy Task 42 [22] "Biorefinery is the sustainable processing of biomass into a spectrum of marketable products (food, feed, materials, chemicals) and energy (fuels, power, heat)." The biorefineries should be designed for sustainability along the entire value chain covering the whole lifecycle including consequences on environmental, economic, and social sustainability.

The modern biorefinery concept, analogous to oil and petrochemical refineries producing a range of fuels and products, represents a biorefinery as a large industrial facility that processes a flexible range of biomass feedstocks into component streams and transforms them into an array of products (fuels, power, renewable chemicals, and biomaterials) using integrated processing units [101]. Biorefineries, in contrast to petrochemical refineries, will fully use the state-of-the-art bioprocessing and biochemical technologies, along with conventional mechanical, thermal, and thermochemical processing platforms at a scale to realize the scale-of-economy and efficiency, and with no waste (Figure 2.9). Several countries throughout the world are now actively developing and coordinating multifaceted action plans through biorefinery deployment to deliver their environmental and economic long-term goals [101].

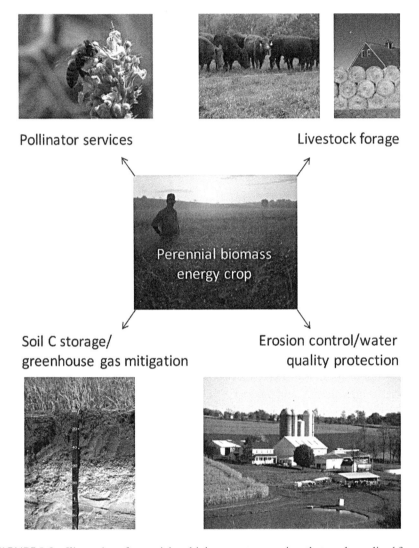

FIGURE 2.8   Illustration of potential multiple ecosystem services that can be realized from perennial biomass energy crops.

2.3.4.2   Advanced Feedstock Supply Systems

Biomass feedstocks are highly variable in type, quality, and physicochemical properties. Furthermore, biomass in the raw form has low mass and energy densities because of its high moisture content, which also affects its storage properties. For a biorefinery to operate efficiently, a steady stream of uniform feedstock is necessary, similar to grain or coal storage

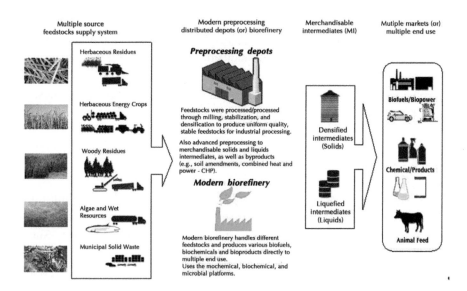

FIGURE 2.9 Concept of modern biorefinery with end use and advanced feedstock supply system with modularized preprocessing distributed depots producing merchandisable intermediates. Logistics of feedstocks in raw or preprocessed form are performed using trucks or rail cars (Adapted from Refs. [64, 96], cliparts from https://openclipart.org).

and processing facilities. To address this issue, advanced feedstock supply systems were designed to deliver infrastructure compatible feedstocks that facilitate economic transport over long distances with known physical and chemical characteristics, and that are stable when stored, have a high bulk density, and better material handling characteristics [96].

2.3.4.3 Modern Modularized Distributed Preprocessing

The modern concept of modularized depots (distributed preprocessing centers), an improvement of the advanced feedstock supply system that is capable of incorporating advanced preprocessing or modular conversion systems (e.g., ammonia fiber expansion or pyrolysis), has been developed [96]. These depots are envisaged to produce salable intermediates, while providing uniform and stable densified feedstock, and removing the complete dependency on a single industry/biorefinery (Figure 2.9). The modularized depot concept can be seen as a component of the modern biorefinery system, where the depots feed preprocessed intermediates into the biorefinery generating various product streams. For the nascent bioenergy industry, the availability of merchandisable intermediate products for multiple markets would greatly increase the customer base for depots and remove the total dependency on a single major industry/ biorefinery. The modern concept of modularized preprocessing was developed based on stakeholder input to address sustainability issues. The concept continues to evolve and will require time to mature and eventually realize at an industry scale [96].

2.3.4.4   Energy Security

The IEA defines energy security as "the uninterrupted availability of energy sources at an affordable price" [51]. Efficient modern bioenergy technologies that are viable can contribute to energy security. Such technologies tend to improve and enhance our management and stewardship of security/development/ economic considerations such as water, food, and the environment [104]. Efficient production, conversion, and end-use technologies must also be appropriately managed to mitigate risks. Economically efficient markets provide security for the bioenergy products trade. The challenge, however, is that many biomass or bioenergy-related markets are strongly influenced by the domestic or international policies that affect long-term investment in bioenergy and other alternative energy ventures. Creating a long-term investment environment for sustainable bioenergy to contribute to the transition to sustainable energy systems may require assistance via fiscal policies and interest from all concerned in the supply chain [104]. To stimulate investment on the scale required to realize the deployment of sustainable biofuels, concerted action by all stakeholders is critical. Furthermore, governments must take the lead role in creating a favorable climate for industry investments by creating a stable, long-term biofuel policy framework to enhance investor confidence and allow for the sustainable expansion of biofuel production, among other measures, such as common sustainability criteria, incentives for using waste, feedstock availability mapping, reduction of trade barriers, international collaboration, among others [52].

2.3.4.5   Sustainability and Energy Security Through Perennial Crops

Growing perennial crops for renewable fuel production is assumed to be more environmentally sustainable than conventional farming of ethanol grain crops. Sustainability measures have productivity, economic, environmental, and social components. There are very few, if any, long-term case studies or formal research projects at the farm scale that verify this, however. The nearest analog of perennial bioenergy cropping is grassland farming for hay, grazing, and conservation purposes [92]. There are many examples of hay and grazing lands in the U.S. and worldwide sustainably managed for decades under low to moderate inputs [88, 106]. Management of perennial bioenergy crop production is envisioned to be similar to that of hay and grazing lands [87].

Modeling at national scales indicates that *Miscanthus* and switchgrass managed as bioenergy crops have limited effects on water quantity and quality [103]. Nitrogen leaching under switchgrass and *Miscanthus* is relatively low [71]. In a comprehensive assessment of 35 sustainability indicators of bioenergy crop production in Tennessee, switchgrass production was ranked more environmentally sustainable than corn for ethanol or unmanaged pasture [79]. Corn production, however, was ranked more economically sustainable than switchgrass (mainly because a biomass market for switchgrass and other energy crops does not exist yet) or pasture.

Producing bioenergy from locally grown biomass feedstocks could increase the energy security of communities and countries. It should be noted, however, that the use of agricultural land for food and fuel raises issues of food security in addition to energy security. The production of perennial crops on either marginal or degraded lands is seen as one solution to the food-fuel issue [61]. Enhancing the productivity and efficiency of these crops on lower quality lands along with fully exploiting the potential of coproducts from biomass feedstocks can also contribute to solving food-fuel issues and ultimately contribute to both energy and food security [61].

2.4 CONCLUSIONS AND FUTURE DIRECTIONS

The benefits and challenges of bio-based feedstocks for biofuels are well-recognized, and a definite interest in the utilization of these feedstocks exists worldwide. Biofuel feedstock is unique from other forms of renewable energies in its ability to generate solid, liquid and gaseous fuels that can be stored and transported. Green technologies such as green chemistry use biofuel feedstocks, among other renewable sources, to work towards a sustainable supply of bioenergy demands as well as to address the climate change issues and mitigate greenhouse gas emissions. For transitioning from petroleum-based economy to bio-based economy (bio-economy), several nations set and continuously revise mandates on the usage of renewable energy from biofuel feedstocks. These mandates translate into great opportunities to the entire supply chain including production, processing, research and development, local job creation, logistics, and export activities.

Substantial progress has been made in developing sustainable bioenergy crops, especially perennial grasses. New varieties of highly productive grasses, such as switchgrass, have been released and are ready for wider deployment as the bioenergy industry comes into its own. Challenges remain, however, such as how to balance both feedstock production and environmental quality goals. Realistically, tradeoffs will be required in production system practices and ecosystem service expectations. Land availability to produce both food and fuel continues to be a challenge. Potential solutions include using marginal or degraded lands for perennial grass production and sustainably intensifying production practices on higher quality land.

A steady increase in biofuel feedstock production and consumption are observed globally. Even though studies indicate uncertainties, a sustainable biomass availability has demonstrated to displace a significant amount of petroleum consumption (e.g., U.S. DOE 2016 Billion-Ton Report). Dealing with biomass feedstocks, being biological in nature, encounter various challenges associated with production, logistics, conversion, and economics; however, technological advances based on sound scientific research help address the challenges. Among biomass feedstocks, energy crops are found to be preferable to fossil fuels for energy, and annual or perennial crops for electricity and heat are preferable to liquid fuels.

Expansion of the biofuel sector into other products such as advanced biofuels, biopower, and bioproducts, much beyond the present bioethanol, could be a powerful jobs stimulus and create new categories of jobs. Governmental programs also incentivize the bio-economy development.

Available state-of-the-art green chemistry strategies for the valorization of waste biomass to platform chemicals were available that can create specialty high-value chemicals based on feedstocks' unique biochemical structure. From the biomass feedstocks, U.S. researchers identified a list of 12 building block chemicals, as well as other second-tier group chemicals, which can be subsequently processed into a suite of high-value bio-based chemicals, derivatives or products catering to various industrial applications.

Life-cycle analysis results of biomass utilization demonstrated a significant CO_2 emissions savings compared to fossil fuels, but also resulted in higher emissions of N_2O from biomass feedstocks. A highly positive energy balance (generation:consumption) of 11:1 to 16:1 in biomass gasification system shows the suitability of biomass feedstock for energy applications.

The concept of the "biorefinery" should be considered while developing new biofuel industries where a sustainable processing of various biomass feedstocks into a spectrum of marketable products are produced using all applicable processing platforms. To develop the nascent bioenergy industry and address sustainability issues, the modern concept of 'modularized preprocessing depots' to produce merchantable intermediates while providing uniform and stable feedstock was proposed. This would increase the customer base for depots and eliminate complete dependency on a single industry/biorefinery.

Future directions of biofuel feedstock utilization might address the whole gamut of "energy security" activities that aim at providing the uninterrupted availability of energy sources at an affordable price. These activities may include efficient modern production, conversion, and end-use technologies through research and development; favorable climate for industry development; long-term investment environment at an appropriate scale for sustainable bioenergy creation; and governmental actions leading to common sustainability criteria development, incentives for waste usage, feedstock availability mapping, trade barriers reduction, and international collaboration.

KEYWORDS

- **biomass**
- **bioproducts**
- **energy crops**
- **green chemistry**
- **renewable energy**

REFERENCES

1. Adler, P., Sanderson, M. A., Weimer, P. J., & Vogel, K. P. (2009). Plant species composition and biofuel yields of conservation grasslands. *Ecol. Appl., 19*, 2202–2209.

2. Alexopoulou, E., Zanetti, F., Scordia, D., Zegada-Lizarazu, W., Christou, M., Testa, G., Cosentino, S. L., & Monti, A. (2015). Long-term yields of switchgrass giant reed, and Miscanthus in the Mediterranean basin. *Bioenerg. Res.* 2015, 8, 1492-1499.

3. Anastas, P., & Eghbali, N. (2010). Green chemistry: Principles and practice. *Chem. Soc. Rev., 39*, 301-312.

4. Anderson, W. F., Sarath, G., Edme, S., Casler, M. D., Mitchell, R. B., Tobias, C. M., Hale, A. L., Sattler, S. E., & Knoll, J. E. (2016). Dedicated herbaceous biomass feedstock genetics and development. *Bioenerg. Res.*, DOI: 10.1007/s12155-015-9709-9708.

5. Arnoult, S., & Brancort-Hulmel, M. (2015). A review on Miscanthus biomass production and composition for bioenergy use: Genotypic and environmental variability and implications for breeding. *Bioenerg. Res., 8*, 502–526.

6. Balan, V. (2014). Current challenges in commercially producing biofuels from lignocellulosic biomass. Review Article. Article ID 463074. *ISRN Biotech.*, 1-31.

7. Bennett, A. B., Meehan, T. D., Gratton, C., & Isaacs, R. (2015). Modelling pollinator community response to contrasting bioenergy scenarios. *PLOS One 9*, e110676. Doi:101371/journal.pone.0110676.

8. Biewinga, E. E., & van der Bijl, G., (1996), Sustainability of energy crops in Europe: A methodology developed and applied, Centre for Agriculture and Environment (CLM), Utrecht.

9. Boe, A., Owens, V., Gonzalez, H. J., Stein, J., Lee, D. K., & Koo, B. C. (2009). Morphology and biomass production of prairie cordgrass on marginal lands. *GCB Bioenergy., 1*, 240–250.

10. Boman, U. R., & Turnbull, J. H. (1997). Integrated biomass energy systems and emissions of carbon dioxide. *Biomass Bioenerg., 13*, 333–343.

11. Börjesson, P., & Tufvesson, L. M. (2011). Agricultural crop-based biofuels–resource efficiency and environmental performance including direct land use changes. *J. Cleaner Prod., 19*, 108–120.

12. Brown, C., Griggs, T., Keene, T., Marra, M., & Skousen, J., (2016). Switchgrass biofuel production on reclaimed surface mines: I. soil quality and dry matter yield. *Bioenerg. Res., 9*, 31–39.

13. Burns, J. C., Godschalk, E. B., & Timothy, D. H. (2008). Registration of 'BoMaster' switchgrass. *J. Plant Reg., 2*, 31–32.

14. Cansino, J. M., Pablo-Romero, M. D. P., Román, R., & Yñiguez, R. (2011). Promoting renewable energy sources for heating and cooling in EU-27 countries. *Energy Policy., 39*, 3803–3812.

15. Campbell, J. E., Lobell, D. B., Genova, R. C., & Field, C. B. (2008). The global potential of bioenergy on abandoned agricultural lands. *Env. Sci. Technol., 42*, 5791–5794.

16. Carlson, I. T., Oram, R. N., & Suprenant, J. (1996). Reed canarygrass and other Phalaris species. Cool-season forage grasses. *Agronomy Monograph 34*, ASA-CSSA-SSSA, Madison, WI, p. 569–604.

17. Christian, D. G., Richie, A. B., & Yates, N. E. (2002). The yield and composition of switchgrass and coastal panic grass grown as a biofuel in southern England. *Bioresource Technol., 83*, 115–124.

18. Chung, J. H., & Kim, D. S. (2012). Miscanthus as a potential bioenergy crop in East Asia. *J. Crop Sci. Biotech., 5*, 65–77.

19. Clifton-Brown, J. C., & Lewandowski, I. (2000). Overwintering problems of newly established Miscanthus plantations can be overcome by identifying genotypes with improved rhizome cold tolerance. *New Phytol., 148*, 287–294.

20. Dale, V. H., Kline, K. L., Wright, L. L., Perlack, R. D., Downing, M., & Graham, R. L. (2011). Interactions among bioenergy feedstock choices, landscape dynamics, and land use. *Ecol. Appl., 21,* 1039–1054.

21. DeHaan, L. R., Weisberg, S., Tilman, D., & Fornara, D. (2009). Agricultural and biofuel implications of a species diversity experiment with native perennial grassland plants. *Agric., Ecosyst., Environ., 137,* 33–38.

22. de Jong, E., Langeveld, H., & Van Ree, R. (2016). IEA Bioenergy Task 42 Biorefinery (2009). Brochure 26 pages. Accessed at http://www.biorefinery.nl/fileadmin/biorefinery/docs/Brochure_Totaal_definitief_HR_opt.pdf, on October 16, 2017).

23. de Jong, E., & Jungmeier, G. (2015). Biorefinery concepts in comparison to petrochemical refineries. Chapter 1. In A. Pandey, R. Höfer, M. Taherzadeh, M. Nampoothiri, C. Larroche (Eds.) *Industrial Biorefineries and White Biotechnology,* Elsevier, Waltham, USA. pp 3-33.

24. Dickmann, D. I. (2006). Silviculture and biology of short-rotation woody crops in temperate regions: Then and now. *Biomass Bioenergy., 30,* 696–705.

25. Dickson, T. L., & Gross, K. L., (2015). Can the results of biodiversity-ecosystem productivity studies be translated to bioenergy production? *PLOS One., 10,* 1-15. e0135253. Doi:10.137/journal.pone.0135253.

26. EIA. (2016). Monthly Energy Review. U.S. Department of Energy, Energy Information Administration, Washington, DC. April (2016). DOE/EIA-0035(2016/4). (Accessed at http://www.eia.gov/totalenergy/data/monthly/pdf/mer.pdf on May 16, 2017).

27. Eisentraut, A., & Brown, A. (2012). Bioenergy status today. p. 10. In *Technology Roadmap, Bioenergy for Heat and Power.* 2nd Ed. Paris, France: International Energy Agency (IEA). (Accessed at https://www.iea.org/publications/freepublications/publication/2012_Bioenergy_Roadmap_2nd_Edition_WEB.pdf on October 16, 2017).

28. Elbersen, H. W., Christian, D. G., El-Bassam, N., Sauerbeck, G., Alexopoulou, E., Sharma, N., & Piscioneri, I. (2004). A management guide for planting and production of switchgrass as a biomass crop in Europe. pp. 140–142. *In Proc. 2nd World Conf. on Biomass for Energy, Industry, and Climate Protection,* 10–14 May. Rome, Italy.

29. Elliott, D. C. (2004). *Biomass, Chemicals from (No. PNNL-SA-36685).* Pacific Northwest National Laboratory (PNNL), Richland, WA (US).

30. EPA. (2016). US *Environmental Protection Agency.* Basis of green chemistry. URL: https://www.epa.gov/greenchemistry/basics-green-chemistry.

31. Eranki, P. L., Bals, B. D., & Dale, B. E. (2011). Advanced regional biomass processing depots: A key to the logistical challenges of the cellulosic biofuel industry. *Biofuels Bioprod. Bioref., 5,* 621–630. doi:10.1002/bbb.318.

32. Eurostat. Statistics Explained, Energy trends. http://ec.europa.eu/eurostat/statistics-explained/index.php/Energy_trends. ISSN 2443-8219, 2015 (Accessed on October 16, 2017).

33. Eurostat. Statistics Explained, Renewable energy statistics. http://ec.europa.eu/eurostat/statistics-explained/index.php/Renewable_energy_statistics. ISSN 2443–8219, 2016 (Accessed on October 16, 2017).

34. Evanylo, G. K., Abaye, A. O., Dundas, C., Zipper, C. E., Lemus, R., Sukkariyah, B., & Rockett, J. (2005). Herbaceous vegetation productivity, persistence, and metals uptake on a biosolids-amended mine soil. *J. Environ. Qual., 34,* 1811–1819.

35. Farrell, A. E., & Sperling, D. (2007). A low-carbon fuel standard for California, Part 1, Technical analysis. Institute of Transportation Studies. URL: *http://escholarship.org/uc/item/6j67z9w6.*

36. FCCC. United Nations Framework Convention on Climate Change, Paris, France, 30 November to 11 December 2015. URL: https://unfccc.int/resource/docs/2015/cop21/eng/l09.pdf, 2015.

37. FSA. (2016). United States Department of Agriculture, Farm Service Agency. Conservation Reserve Program Statistics. CRP Enrollment and Rental Payments by State, 1986-2016. (Accessed at https://www.fsa.usda.gov/programs-and-services/conservation-programs/reports-and-statistics/conservation-reserve-program-statistics/index on October 16, 2017).

38. Galatowitsch, S. M., Anderson, N. O., & Ascher, P. D. (1999). Invasiveness in wetland plants in temperate North America. *Wetlands., 19*, 733–755.

39. Gelfland, I. (2011). Carbon debt of Conservation Reserve Program (CRP) grasslands converted to bioenergy production. *Proc. Natl. Acad. Sci. USA., 108*, 13864–13869.

40. Gelfland, I., Sahajpal, R., Zhang, X., Izaurralde, R. C., Gross, K. L., & Robertson, G. P. (2013). Sustainable bioenergy production from marginal lands in the US Midwest. *Nature, 493*, 514–517.

41. Gill, J. R., Burks, P. S., Staggenborg, S. A., Odvody, G. N., Heiniger, R. W., Macoon, B., Moore, K. J., Barrett, M., & Rooney, W. L. (2014). Yield results and stability analysis from the sorghum regional biomass feedstock trial. *Bioenerg. Res., 7*, 1016–1034.

42. Golden, J. S., Handfield, R. B., Daystar, J., T. E. & McConnell. (2016). *An Economic Impact Analysis of the U.S. Bio-based Products Industry*: A Report to the Congress of the USA. A Joint Publication of the Duke Center for Sustainability & Commerce and the Supply Chain Resource Cooperative at North Carolina State University.

43. Griffith, A. P., Epplin, F. M., Fuhlendorf, S. D., & Gillen, R. (2011). A comparison of perennial polycultures and monocultures for producing biomass for biorefinery feedstock. *Agron. J., 103*, 617–627.

44. Guintoli, J., Caserini, S., Marelli, L., Baxter, D., & Agostini, (2015). A. Domestic heating from forest logging residues: Environmental risks and benefits. *J. Cleaner Prod., 99*, 206–2016.

45. Guretzky, J. A., Biermacher, J. T., Cook, B. J., Kering, M. K., & Mosali, J. (2011). Switchgrass for forage and bioenergy: Harvest and nutrient rate effects on biomass yields and nutrient composition. *Plant Soil., 339*, 69–81.

46. Hall, D. O., & Scrase, J. I. (1998). Will biomass be the environmentally friendly fuel of the future? *Biomass Bioenerg., 15*, 357–367.

47. Heaton, E. A., Dohleman, F. G., & Long, S. P. (2008). Meeting US biofuel goals with less land: The potential of Miscanthus. *Glob. Change Biol., 14*, 200–2014.

48. Heinsoo, K., Hein, K., Melts, I., Holm, B., & Ivask, M. (2011). Reed canary grass yield and fuel quality in Estonian farmers' fields. *Biomass Bioenerg., 35*, 616–625.

49. Hinchee, M., Rottmann, W., Mullinax, L., Zhang, C., Chang, S., Cunningham, M., Pearson, L., & Nehra, N. (2011). Short-rotation woody crops for bioenergy and biofuels applications. In: D. Tomes, P. Lakshmanan, & D. Songstad (eds). *Biofuels,* Springer: New York, pp. 139–156.

50. Hong, C. O., Owens, V. N., Bransby, D., Farris, R., Fike, J., Heaton, E., Kim, S., Mayton, H., Mitchell, R., & Viands, D. (2014). Switchgrass response to nitrogen fertilizer across diverse environments in the USA: A regional feedstock partnership report. *Bioenerg. Res., 7*, 777–788.

51. Huber, G. W. (2007). *Breaking the Chemical and Engineering Barriers to Lignocellulosic Biofuels*: Next Generation Hydrocarbon Biorefineries, U. Massachusetts Amherst.

52. IEA. (2014). *Energy Supply Security - Emergency Response of IEA Countries*. OECD/ IEA, France.

53. IEA. (2011). *Technology Roadmap - Biofuels for Transport*. OECD/IEA, France.

54. Igathinathane, C., Archer, D., Gustafson, C., Schmer, M., Hendrickson, J., Kronberg, S., Keshwani, D., Backer, L., Hellevang, K., Faller, T. (2014). Biomass round bales infield aggregation logistics scenarios. *Biomass Bioenerg., 66*, 12–26.

55. Igathinathane, C., Tumurulu, J. S., Keshwani, D., Schmer, M., Archer, D., Liebig, M., Hendrickson, J., & Kronberg, S. (2016). Biomass bale stack and field outlet locations assessment for efficient infield logistics. *Biomass Bioenerg., 91*, 217–226.

56. Jakubowski, A. R., Casler, M. D., & Jackson, R. D. (2011). Has selection for improved agronomic traits made reed canarygrass invasive? *PLOS One* 6, e25757 doi:10.1371/ journal.pone.0025757.

57. Jensen, N. (2006). Plant Guide for prairie cordgrass (*Spartina pectinata* Bosc ex Link). USDA-NRCS, Bismark Plant Materials Center, Bismarck, North Dakota 58404.

58. Johnson, G. A., Wyse, D. L., & Sheaffer, C. C. (2013). Yield of perennial herbaceous and woody biomass crops over time across three locations. *Biomass Bioenerg., 58*, 267–274.

59. Jungers, J. M., Clark, A. T., Betts, K., Mangan, M. E., Sheaffer, C. C., & Wyse, D. L. (2015). Long-term biomass yield and species composition in native perennial bioenergy cropping systems. *Agron. J., 107*, 1627–1640.

60. Jungers, J. M., Fargione, J. E., Sheaffer, C. C., Wyse, D. L., & Lehman, C. (2013). Energy potential of biomass form conservation grasslands in Minnesota, USA. *PLOS One* 8, e61209.

61. Kaltschmitt, M., Reinhardt, G. A., & Stelzer, T. (1997). Life cycle analysis of biofuels under different environmental aspects, *Biomass Bioenerg., 12*, 121–134.

62. Kapr, A., & Richter, G. M. (2011). Meeting the challenge of food and energy security. *J. Exp. Bot., 62*, 3263–3271.

63. Kendall, A., & Yuan, J. (2013). Comparing life cycle assessments of different biofuel options. *Curr. Opin. Chem. Biol., 17*, 439–443.

64. Kim, S. M., Guo, J., Kwak, S., Jin, Y. S., Lee, D. K., & Singh, V. (2015). Effects of genetic variation and growing condition of prairie cordgrass on feedstock composition and ethanol yield. *Bioresource Technol., 183*, 70–77.

65. Kurian, J. K., Nair, G. R., Hussain, A., & Raghavan, G. V. (2013). Feedstocks, logistics and pretreatment processes for sustainable lignocellulosic biorefineries: A comprehensive review. *Renewable Sustainable Energy Rev., 25*, 205–219.

66. Landström, S., Lomakka, L., & Andersson, S. (1996). Harvest in spring improves yield and quality of reed canary grass as a bioenergy crop. *Biomass Bioenerg., 11*, 333–341.

67. Leduc, S. D., Zhang, X., & Izauralde, R. C. (2016). Cellulosic feedstock production on Conservation Reserve Program land: Potential yields and environmental effects. *Global Change Biol. Bioenerg.,* Online. doi: *10*.1111/gcbb.12352.

68. Madakadze, I. C., Coulman, B. E., Mcelroy, A. R., Stewart, K. A., & Smith, D. L. (1998). Evaluation of selected warm-season grasses for biomass production in areas with a short growing season. *Bioresource Technol., 65*, 1–12.

69. Martin, J. A. (1997). A total fuel cycle approach to reducing greenhouse gas emissions: Solar generation technologies as greenhouse gas o sets in U.S. utility systems. *Solar Energy,* 59, 195–203.

70. Mann, M. K., & Spath, P. L. (1997). Life cycle assessment of a biomass gasification combined-cycle power system, US National Renewable Energy Laboratory report, NREL/TP-430-23076.

71. McBride, A. C., Dale, V. H., Baskaran, L. M., Downing, M. E., Eaton, L. M., Efroymson, R. A., Garten, C. T., Kline, K. L., Jager, H. I., Mulholland, P. J., & Parish, E. S. (2011). Indicators to support environmental sustainability of bioenergy systems. *Ecol. Indic., 11*, 1277–1289.

72. McIsaac, G. F., David, M. B., & Mitchell, C. A. (2010). Miscanthus and switchgrass production in Central Illinois: Impacts on hydrology and inorganic nitrogen leaching. *J. Environ. Qual., 39*, 1790–1799.

73. Monti, A., Venturi, P., & Elbersen, H. W. (2001). Evaluation of the establishment of lowland and upland switchgrass (*Panicum virgatum* L.) varieties under different tillage and seedbed conditions in northern Italy. *Soil Till. Res., 63*, 75–83.

74. Monti, A., & Zegada-Lizarazu, W. (2016). Sixteen-year yield and soil carbon storage of giant reed (*Arundo donax* L.) grown under variable nitrogen fertilization rates. *Bioenerg. Res., 9*, 248–256.

75. Mulkey, V. R., Owens, V. N., & Lee, D. K. (2006). Management of switchgrass-dominated Conservation Reserve Program lands for biomass production in South Dakota. *Crop Sci., 46*, 712–720.

76. Mullett, J., Morishige, D., McCormick, R., Truong, S., Hilley, J., McKinley, B., Anderson, R., Olson, S. N., & Rooney, W. (2014). Energy *Sorghum* - a genetic model for the design of C$_4$ grass bioenergy crops. *J. Exp. Bot., 65*, 3479–3489.

77. Muth, D. J., Bryden, K. M., & Nelson, R. G. (2013). Sustainable agricultural residue removal for bioenergy: A spatially comprehensive US national assessment. *Appl. Energy, 102*, 403–417.

78. NRCS. (2002). Indiangrass Plant Fact Sheet. USDA NRCS Plant Materials Program. URL: http://plants.usda.gov/factsheet/pdf/fs_sonu2.pdf.

79. Osgood, R. V., Dudley, N. S., & Jakeway, L. A. (1996). A demonstration of grass biomass production on Molokai. Hawaii Agriculture Research Center, Kunia.

80. Parish, E. S., Dale, V. H., English, B. C., Jackson, S. L., & Tyler, D. D. (2016). Assessing multimetric aspects of sustainability: Application to a bioenergy crop production system in East Tennessee. *Ecosphere 7*, e01206.

81. Pavanan, K. C., Bosch, R. A., Cornelissen, R., & Philp, J. C. (2013). Biomass sustainability and certification. *Trends Biotechnol. 31*, 385–387.

82. R&M. (2013). Research and Markets. Biomass Industry in Brazil. Dublin, Ireland. (Accessed at http://www.researchandmarkets.com/reports/2142425/ on October 16, 2017).

83. RFA. (2015). *Renewable Fuels Association.* Going Global 2015 Ethanol Industry Outlook, Washington, DC. www.EthanolRFA.org.

84. Robertson, G. P., Hamilton, S. K., Del Grosso, S. J., & Parton, W. J. (2011). The biogeochemistry of bioenergy landscapes: Carbon, nitrogen, and water considerations. *Ecol. Appl., 21*, 1055–1067.

85. Ros, J., Olivier, J., Notenboom, J., Croezen, H., & Bergsma, G. (2012). Sustainability of biomass in a bio-based economy: A quick-scan analysis of the biomass demand of a bio-based economy in 2030 compared to the sustainable supply.

86. Rosillo-Calle F. (2006). Biomass energy–An overview. *Landolt-Börnstein Numerical Data and Functional Relationships in Science and Technology,* pp. 334–373.

87. Sanderson, M. A., Archer, D., Hendrickson, J., Kronberg, S., Liebig, M., Nichols, K., Schmer, M., Tanaka, D., & Aguilar, J. (2013). Pastures and integrated crop-livestock systems for multiple ecosystem services. *Renew. Agr. Food Syst., 28*, 129–144.

88. Sanderson, M. A., & Cannayen, I. (2013). Growing perennial forages for biomass. pp. 17–23. In: S. Bittman and D. Hunt (eds.) Cool forages: Advanced management of temperate forages. Pacific Field Corn Association, Agassiz, BC, Canada.

89. Sanderson, M. A., Jolley, L., & Dobrowolski, J. (2012a). Pastureland and hayland in the U.S.: Conservation practices and ecosystem services. pp. 25–40. In: C. J. Nelson (ed) Environmental Outcomes of Conservation Practices Applied to Pasture and Hayland in the U.S: *The Pastureland Conservation Effects Assessment Project* (CEAP). Allen Press, Lawrence, KS.

90. Sanderson, M. A., Schmer, M., Owens, V., Keyser, P., & Elbersen, W. (2012b). Crop management of switchgrass. *Green Energy and Technology*, 87–112. Chap 4. Spring-Verlag. A. Monti (Ed.).

91. Sanderson, M. A., Skinner, R. H., Barker, D. J., Edwards, G. R., Tracy, B. F., & Wedin, D. A. (2004). Plant species diversity and management of temperate forage and grazing land ecosystems. *Crop Sci., 44*, 1132–1144.

92. Sanderson, M. A., & Wätzold, F. (2010). Balancing tradeoffs in ecosystem functions and services in grassland management. *Grassl. Sci. Eur., 15*, 639–648.

93. Sanderson, M. A., Wedin, D. A., & Tracy, B. F. (2009). Grasslands: Definitions, origins, extent, and future. p. 57–74. *In*: W. F. Wedin and S. L. *Fales (ed.). Grass*: Quietness and Strength for a New American Agriculture. American Society of Agronomy, Madison, WI.

94. Sarath, G., Baird, L. M., & Mitchell, R. B. (2014). Senescence, dormancy and tillering in perennial C_4 grasses. *Plant Sci., 217*, 140–151.

95. Scarlat, N., Martinov, M., & Dallemand, J. F. (2010). Assessment of the availability of agricultural crop residues in the European Union: potential limitations for bioenergy use. *Waste Manage, 30*, 1889–1897.

96. Scordia, D., Zanetti, F., Varga, S. S., Alexopoulou, E., Cavallaro, V., Monti, A., Copani, V., & Cosentino, S. L. (2015). New insights into the propagation methods of switchgrass, Miscanthus, and giant reed. *Bioenerg. Res., 8*, 1480–1491.

97. Searcy, E., Lamers, P., Hansen, J., Jacobson, J., & Webb, E. (2015). *Advanced feedstock supply system validation workshop,* Golden, Colorado. Vol. INL/EXT-10–18930.

98. Sheldon, R. A., Arends, I. W. C. E., & Hanefeld, U. (2007). *Green Chemistry and Catalysis*, Wiley-VCH, Weinheim.

99. Sheldon, R. A. (2014). Green and sustainable manufacture of chemicals from biomass: State-of-the-art. *Green Chem., 16*, 950–963.

100. Sikkema, R., Steiner, M., Junginger, M., Hiegl, W., Hansen, M. T., & Faaij, A. (2011). The European wood pellet markets: Current status and prospects for 2020. *Biofuels, Bioprod. Biorefin., 5*, 250–278.

101. Sissine, F. (2007). Energy Independence and Security Act of 2007: *A Summary of Major Provisions*. Library of Congress Washington DC Congressional Research Service. pp CRS-1.

102. Skeel, V. A., & Gibson, D. J. (1996). Physiological performance of *Andropogon gerardii, Panicum virgatum*, and *Sorghastrum nutans* on reclaimed mine spoil. *Restor. Ecol., 4*, 355–367.

103. Smith, W. (2007). Mapping the development of UK biorefinery complexes (NFC 07/008). *Tamutech Consultancy*, National Non Food Crops Centre Report.

104. Somerville, C., Youngs, H., Taylor, C., Davis, S. C., & Long, S. P. (2010). Feedstocks for lignocellulosic biofuels. *Science, 329*, 790–792.

105. Song, Y., Cervarich, M., Jain, A. K., Khechgi, H. S., Landuyt, W., & Cai, X. (2016). The interplay between bioenergy grass production and water resources in the United States of America. *Environ. Sci. Technol., 50*, 3010–3019.

106. Souza, G. M., Victoria, R. L., Joly, C. A., & Verdade, L. M. (2015) eds. Bioenergy & sustainability: bridging the gaps. *Scientific Committee on Problems of the Environment (SCOPE) 72.*

107. Stupak, I., Asikainen, A., Jonsell, M., Karltun, E., Lunnan, A., Mizaraitė, D., Pasanen, K., Pärn, H., Raulund-Rasmussen, K., Röser, D., & Schroeder, M. (2007). Sustainable utilization of forest biomass for energy—possibilities and problems: Policy, legislation, certification, and recommendations and guidelines in the Nordic, Baltic, and other European countries. *Biomass Bioenerg., 31*, 666–684.

108. Suttie, J. M., & Reynolds, S. G. (2005).Batello, Grasslands of the world. *Plant Production and Protection Series,* No. 34. FAO, Rome.

109. Tahir, M. H. N., Casler, M. D., Moore, K. J., & Brummer, E. C. (2011). Biomass yield and quality of reed canarygrass under five harvest management systems for bioenergy production. *Bioenerg. Res., 4*, 111–119.

110. Takara, D., & Khanal, S. K. (2015). Characterizing compositional changes of Napier grass at different stages of growth for biofuel and bio-based products potential. *Bioresource Technol., 188*, 103–108.

111. Taube, F., Gierus, M., Hermann, A., Loges, R., & Schönbach, P. (2014). Grassland and globalization – challenges for north-west European grass and forage research. *Grass Forage Sci., 69*, 2–16.

112. Tilman, D., Hill, J., & Lehman, C. (2006). Carbon-negative biofuels from low-input high-diversity grassland biomass. *Science, 314*, 1598–1600.

113. Tubeileh, A., Rennie, T. J., & Goss, M. J. (2016). A review on biomass production from C_4 grasses: Yield and quality for end-use. *Curr. Opin. Plant Biol., 31*, 172–180.

114. Tubeileh, A., Rennie, T. J., Kerr, A., Saita, A. A., & Patanè, C. (2014). Biomass production by warm-season grasses as affected by nitrogen application in Ontario. *Agron. J. 106*, 416–422.

115. Urbanchuk, J. M. (2008). *Economic Impact of the Energy Independence and Security Act of 2007.* LECG, LLC, January 2008. U.S. Metro Economies, Green Jobs in the U.S.

116. Urbanchuk, J. M. (2013). Contribution of the Ethanol Industry to the Economy of the United States, *Renewable Fuel Association*, 2 Feb.

117. U.S. DOE. U.S. Department of Energy. (2011). U.S. Billion-Ton Update: *Biomass Supply for a Bioenergy and Bioproducts Industry.* R. D. Perlack and B. J. Stokes (Leads), ORNL/TM-2011/224. Oak Ridge National Laboratory, Oak Ridge, TN, 2011.

118. U.S. DOE. U.S. Department of Energy. (2016). 2016 Billion-Ton Report: *Advancing Domestic Resources for a Thriving Bioeconomy*, Vol. *1,* Economic Availability of Feedstocks. M. H. Langholtz, B. J. Stokes, and L. M. Eaton (Leads), ORNL/TM-2016/160. Oak Ridge National Laboratory, Oak Ridge, TN.

119. U.S. DOE. Bioenergy green jobs factsheet (2013). U.S. Department of Energy, Energy Efficiency & Renewable Energy. Bioenergy Technology Office, 2013.

120. Vogel, K. P. (2004). Switchgrass. In: Moser, L. E., Burson, B. L., Sollenberger, L. E. (ed.) Warm-season (C_4) grasses. ASA-CSSA-SSSA, Madison, WI.

121. Vogel, K. P., Mitchell, R. B., Casler, M. D., & Sarath, G. (2014). Registration of 'Liberty' switchgrass. *J. Plant Reg., 8,* 242–247.

122. Wachendorf, M., Richter, F., Fricke, T., Graß, R., & Neff, R. (2009). Utilization of seminatural grassland through integrated generation of solid fuel and biogas from biomass.

I. effects of hydrothermal conditioning and mechanical dehydration on mass flows of organic and mineral plant compounds, and nutrient balances. *Grass Forage Sci., 64*, 132–143.

123. Walter, A., Dolzan, P., & Piacente, E. (2006). *Biomass Energy and Bioenergy Trade*: Historic developments in Brazil and current opportunities – country report for IEA Bioenergy Task 40. Unicamp. Campinas, Brazil. 35 p. (Accessed at http://www.globalbioenergy.org/uploads/media/0604_Biomass_Energy_and_Bio-energy_Trade_Historic_Developments_in_Brazil_and_Current_Opportunities_IEA_T40.pdf on October 16, 2017).

124. Wennerberg, S. (2004). Big Bluestem Plant Guide. USDA NRCS National Plant Data Center, Baton Rouge, Louisiana. (Accessed at http://plants.usda.gov/plantguide/pdf/pg_ange.pdf on October 16, 2017)

125. Werling, B. P., Dickson, T. L., Isaacs, R., Gaines, H., Gratton, C., Gross, K. L., Liere, H., Malmstrom, C. M., Meehan, T., Ruan, L., Robertson, B. A., Robertson, G. P., Schmidt, T. M., Schrotenboer, A. C., Teal, T. K., Wilson, J. K., & Landis, D. A. (2014). Perennial grasslands enhance biodiversity and multiple ecosystem services in bioenergy landscapes. *Proc. Natl. Acad. Sci., 111*, 1652–1657.

126. Werpy, T., Petersen, G., Aden, A., Bozell, J., Holladay, J., White, J., Manheim, A., Eliot, D., Lasure, L., & Jones, S. (2004). *Top value added chemicals from biomass. Volume 1-Results of screening for potential candidates from sugars and synthesis gas* (No. DOE/GO-102004-1992). DOE, Washington DC.

127. Wilhelm, W. W., Hess, J. R., Karlen, D. L., Johnson, J. M. F., Muth, D. J., Baker, J. M., Gollany, H. T., Novak, J. M., Stott, D. E., & Varvel, G. E. (2010). Balancing limiting factors and economic drivers for sustainable Midwestern US agricultural residue feedstock supplies. *Ind. Biotechnol., 6*, 271–287.

128. Wiloso, E. I., Heijungs, R., & De Snoo, G. R. (2012). LCA of second generation bioethanol: A review and some issues to be resolved for good LCA practice. *Renew. Sustainable Energy Rev., 16*, 5295–5308.

129. Wright, C. K., & Wimberly, M. C. (2013). Recent land use change in western corn belt threatens grasslands and wetlands. *Proc. Natl. Acad. Sci.*, 4134–4139.

130. Wrobel, C., Coulman, B. E., & Smith, D. L. (2009). The potential use of reed canarygrass (*Phalaris arundinacea* L.) as a biofuel crop. *Acta Agriculturae Scandinavica, Section B – Soil&Plant Science., 59*, 1–18.

131. Wullschleger, S. D., Davis, E. B., Borsuk, M. E., Gunderson, C. A., & Lynd, L. R. (2010). Biomass production in switchgrass across the United States: Database description and determinants of yield. *Agron. J., 102*, 1158–1168.

132. Zhao, G., Bryan, B. A., King, D., Luo, Z., Wang, E., & Yu, Q. (2015). Sustainable limits to crop residue harvest for bioenergy: Maintaining soil carbon in Australia's agricultural lands. *GCB Bioenergy, 7*, 479–487.

133. Zilverberg, C. J., Johnson, W. C., Owens, V., Boe, A., Schumacher, T., Reitsma, K., Hong, C. O., Novotny, C., Volke, M., & Werner, B. (2014). Biomass yield from planted mixtures and monocultures of native prairie vegetation across a heterogeneous farm landscape. *Agric. Ecozyst. Environ., 186*, 148–159.

CHAPTER 3

FUELS FROM RECYCLED CARBON

MICHELE ARESTA[1,2] and ANGELA DIBENEDETTO[3,4]

[1]Department of Chemical and Biomolecular Engineering, NUS, 117858 Singapore, SG

[2]Department of Chemical Engineering, University of Bath, BA27AY Bath, UK

[3]Department of Chemistry, University of Bari, 70126 Bari, IT

[4]CIRCC, via Celso Ulpiani 27, 70126 Bari, IT

CONTENTS

ABSTRACT

"Recycling carbon" is necessary for stepping from the *linear-* to the *circular C-economy*. Either the direct conversion of captured CO_2 from concentrated sources or the use of biomass, which uses atmospheric CO_2, can be the winning strategies, better if combined. The integration of biotechnology and catalysis may fasten the large-scale conversion of CO_2 in a *man-made C-cycle,* which may complement the *natural* one and save fossil-C for future generations.

3.1 INTRODUCTION

Fossil carbon is the major source of energy and chemicals since over two centuries now. Coal, oil and gas are exploited at an ever-increasing rate and our life will largely depend on them in the future 40–50 years or so. Nevertheless, they are not an infinite resource and, what is more dramatic, their expanding use is causing, directly or indirectly, huge problems to the environment and life on Earth. Measures must be urgently taken to limit their use through the exploitation of perennial energy sources "SWHG" (sun, wind, hydropower, and geothermal-) and renewables (terrestrial and aquatic biomass).

3.1.1 EFFECTS OF THE LINEAR CARBON-ECONOMY

The intensive *linear* use of fossil carbon (Figure 3.1) during the last two centuries has caused the accumulation of CO_2 into the atmosphere causing its concentration to rise from 275 ppm of the preindustrial era to actual 400 ppm. Even today, 85% of the energy used in anthropic activities is derived from fossil carbon. The parallel trend of growing of world population, energy consumption, CO_2 emission and atmospheric CO_2 concentration is causing serious worries about the effect that the continuous use of fossil carbon may have on climate change.

As a matter of fact, we use fossil carbon in a very inefficient way as only an average 32% of its chemical energy is converted into other forms of energy (Figure 3.1), the rest being lost as heat transferred to the atmosphere causing its thermal destabilization. In such framework, CO_2 is suited for underground disposal-CCS (carbon capture and storage). It is worth to note, that release of heat to the atmosphere causes a high water vapor pressure and, in turn, heavy precipitations.

To such direct perturbation, adds the increasing CO_2 emission (20 Gt at 1990 *vs ca.* 35 Gt today) that causes accumulation of CO_2 in the atmosphere, thus enhancing with water vapor the natural greenhouse effect that may eventually

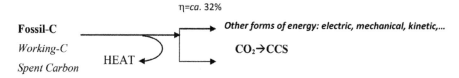

FIGURE 3.1   The Linear C-Economy

influence the climate change. Although fluctuation of the temperature is constant in the history of our planet, it is a fact that peaks cause dramatic events. Therefore, it is imperative to avoid large increases of temperature, decreasing the release of thermal energy to the atmosphere and stopping CO_2 accumul

3.1.2   CIRCULAR CARBON-ECONOMY AND CARBON RECYCLING

The need to reduce the emission of CO_2 into the atmosphere is pushing towards the adoptions of measures for increasing the efficiency of energy production from fossil carbon and its usage, the use of alternative energy sources, such as SWHG perennial sources and renewables (biomass). *Recycling carbon* [1] is expected to play a key role in the future for avoiding CO_2 accumulation in the atmosphere (COP21 Report, Conference of the Parties, Paris 2015). As a matter of fact, it would be possible to develop man-made industrial processes for "carbon recycling" [2], converting, thus, *spent carbon* as CO_2 into *working carbon* [3], as that present in valuable chemicals or fuels, mimicking Nature. The use of *recycled carbon*, may help to avoid as much as possible burning "fossil carbon." Such practice would fall again into the utilization of "renewable carbon" [4–7], as the man-made process would perfectly mimic the natural process. A "close to zero emission" cycle can in principle be implemented that effectively reduces the emission of CO_2 and complements the natural carbon-cycle (C-cycle).

In this chapter, we make the state-of-the-art of CO_2 conversion and give a perspective view of its integration with biomass conversion into fuels and, in part, chemicals, merging chemical catalysis and biotechnology.

Each atom of carbon we can recycle is an atom of fossil carbon left in the ground for next generations that will not reach the atmosphere today.

3.2 USE OF RENEWABLE CARBON

3.2.1 NATURAL AND MAN-MADE C-CYCLING

It is now clear that there is no natural remedy to the anthropogenic emission of CO_2 (Figure 3.2). Nature cannot buffer the *ca.* 35 Gt/y produced in human activities, despite it cycles some 720 Gt_{CO2}/y. Otherwise, one should not have observed its continuous accumulation in the atmosphere.

Therefore we must find a counterbalance that may reduce the CO_2 atmospheric level. There are two possible strategies: (i) to reduce the consumption of fossil-C, and (ii) to avoid that produced CO_2 may reach the atmosphere. The recent history tells that, despite the urgent need to preserve natural resources, there is an expansion of use of fossil-C due to the growing demand of energy and goods by our society, especially from developing economies (mainly China and India, which use increasing amounts of coal, the worst CO_2-emitter among the fossil-C fuels). Therefore, the urgent reduction of emission of CO_2 must take place in a frame of expansion of use of energy and raw materials, until equilibrium can be reached that will include the control of the growth of the planetary population. The

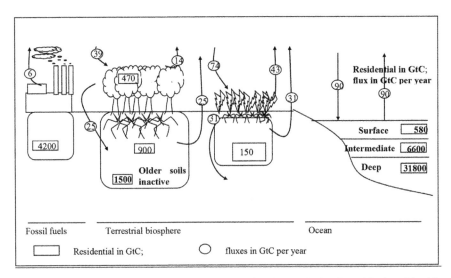

FIGURE 3.2   The natural carbon-cycle. (Reprinted with permission from "Carbon Dioxide Utilization: Greening Both the Energy and Chemical Industry: An Overview", in Utilization of Greenhouse Gases, Chapter 1, pp 2–39, DOI: 10.1021/bk-2003-0852.ch001, ACS Symposium Series, Vol. 852, ISBN13: 9780841238275. eISBN: 9780841219564. Copyright (2003) American Chemical Society.)

time being, we need to reduce the use of fossil carbon as energy source by exploiting SWHG perennial energies and try to complement the natural C-cycle by reusing carbon through the conversion of CO_2 coupled to a better use of biomass. The ideal would be to decarbonize energy and use fossil-C only for making chemicals and materials, which cannot be decarbonized. Waiting for really exploitable hydrogen economy, as an intermediate solution, recycling carbon (through natural and man-made cycles) is mandatory. On the other hand, this solution would be the less demanding from the economic point of view as the existing assets in energy distribution, transportations and industry would be used, avoiding large investment in infrastructure changes. In this chapter, we will discuss how to implement such strategy, keeping on front line the production of fuels, due to their larger market with respect to chemicals, but still paying due attention to chemicals and materials, which even if are roughly sized to be 1/14 of fuels, nevertheless have a higher E factor (ratio of waste to product mass) than fuels (E=10–100 for chemicals with respect to <1–3 for fuels), that means that they emit 10–30 times more CO_2 per unit mass than fuels. Therefore, although fuels and chemical markets differ by more than one order of magnitude, their emissions are closer.

3.2.2 BIOMASS AND ITS USES

Biomass is a complex system used as source of materials and food since ever in the human history, and as source of energy since Lower Paleolytic (*Homo Erectus*) when the control of fire was firstly managed. With the discovery of coal, oil, and gas, biomass has continued to play a role as energy source, but at a much lower level. Biomass is a complex substance, which may be used for the extraction or production of various chemicals and materials, or for the production of heat and fuels (solid, liquid, gaseous). Burning biomass, as said, is a most primitive use and the less economically rewarding. The use of biomass for producing heat is still today practiced, but more and more frequently residual refractory biomass, more than primary biomass, is used to this end. In fact, biomass is an extremely rich raw substance, which can be used as source of many different molecular compounds and polymeric materials, increasing the profit and reducing the environmental burden of its use. Recently, the conversion of primary biomass into Syngas ($CO+H_2$) has been pursued as an objective, which is affected by a drawback: complex matter is converted into a C1 molecule (CO) which is then used to build more complex Cn molecules. Such huge change in entropy (Figure 3.3) in using biomass is energetically inefficient. The direct use of the complexity of biomass is a much wiser approach to its exploitation.

Biorefinery is a recently implemented concept for making the most economically profitable and environmentally friendly use of biomass.

Today, biomass is regaining consideration because it is renewable and its use can play a key role in a C-circular economy.

3.2.2.1   Applying the Biorefinery Concept

In recent years, the approach to the use of biomass has shifted from *one technology for all biom*ass to *several technologies for a single biomass,* implementing the *biorefinery* concept. According to such view, biomass is converted into a wide spectrum of bio-based products including biofuels, biochemicals, biomaterials, feed, heat and power. Ideally, full-scale, highly efficient and integrated biorefineries allow manufacture of bio-based products, which are fully competitive with their conventional fossil-C derived equivalents (Scheme 1).

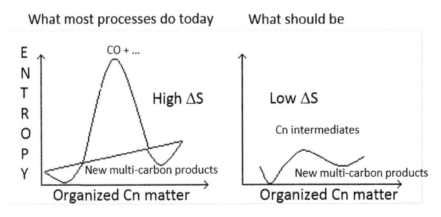

FIGURE 3.3   Change in entropy during the conversion of biomass into chemicals based on gasification (*left*) and innovative technologies (*right*).

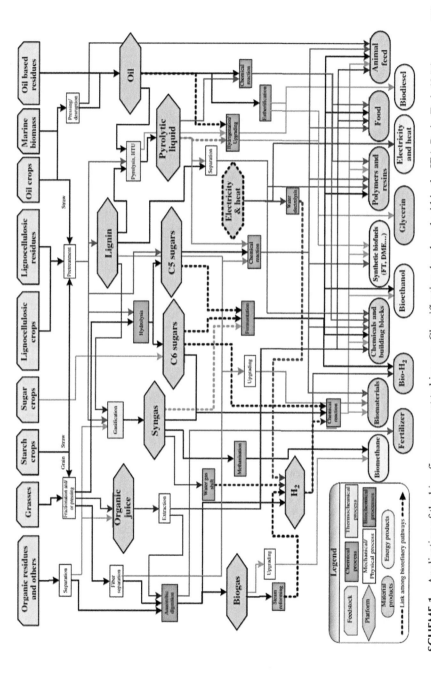

SCHEME 1 Application of the biorefinery concept to biomass. Classification developed within the IEA-Paris, Task 42 Bioenergy [8]. (From: http://www.ieabioenergy.com/wp-content/uploads/2013/10/Task-42-Booklet.pdf)

A diverse and flexible biomass production should be in place to continuously and cost-effectively supply biorefineries with biomass such as dedicated lignocellulosic crops including agricultural and forestry, residual biomass from agriculture, forestry, agri-food and urban organic waste, and immobilized biomass, together with aquatic biomass. A combination of several processes in an integrated way, provides optimal processing solutions to multiple and valuable marketable products. Economic constraints and sustainability criteria such as low cost operation and efficient use of resources, sustainable production throughout the full product life cycle are the critical requirements for the biorefineries viability. Product sustainability implies that it is used to generate bioenergy at the end of its life (biofuels, bioheat, biopower) or it is recyclable, and biodegradable (biochemicals and biomaterials). According such guidelines, biorefineries should implement the ideal equilibrium by delivering to end-users environmentally friendly products with low carbon and water footprint, matching or even improving the properties of their fossil equivalents, at a competitive price.

Several challenges are still there to be win along the entire value-chain, including biomass cultivation, harvesting, storage, transport, pretreatment, conversion, product separation, (new) product specifications. Several bottlenecks are still on the whole chain, from land requisites (marginal lands should be used), to avoiding food-energy/chemicals competition (second and third generation bio-fuels/chemicals), developing of efficient logistics and full process engineering for reducing costs (both economic and energetic), optimization of added value extraction *via* low-entropy processes which avoid destructuring of complex molecular structures and take advantage of them, improving conversion processes increasing selectivity, integrating biochemical and chemocatalytic processes for enhancing the most efficient aspect of each, among others.

The concept of biorefinery is quite recent with respect to conventional oil-refineries and biorefineries need to grow achieving high degree of integration at various levels, from process, to use of existing assets, to market and business. The potential impact on the job market is high, but its full deployment depends on how competitive will be the new products with respect to those on the market and derived from fossil fuels, which benefit of the low price of fossil-C such as oil and, even more, shale-gas, and the efficiency of well established technologies such as Fisher-Tropsch for Syngas conversion into fuels. The introduction of new bio-based products maybe even more difficult. The education of end-users and environmental friendliness of biorefineries will play a fundamental role for winning such competition.

3.2.2.2 Terrestrial Lignocellulosic Biomass

There is a huge potential for agriculture and managed forestry to support bio-industries in a "bio-based economy." Climatic factors, such as air temperature, rainfall and insulation time, and soil quality play a key role in determining which plant species is optimal for a given environment. The most important driving forces for the selection of the plant species to be grown are the demand and supply for certain crops and the local (national or Communitary) rules of the *Agricultural Policy and Renewable Energy Directives*. The recent specific policy targets for biofuels proved to have an important impact on land use in view of implementation of sustainable agricultural biomass chains for biorefinery [9]. Key parameters are: the geographic specificities in terms of ecosystems, climate variation, land use patterns as well as resource types, crop management, culture rotation, productivity, feedstock (lignocellulosic or oily crops) handling and associated logistics (harvesting and storage, transport).

The identification of areas in a region suitable for the cultivation of the selected crops is based on spatial distribution of parameters influencing conditions for cultivation (e.g., germination, growing, flowering, seed production, etc.). For that purpose, available climatic datasets, land use – land cover datasets and elevation datasets are necessary. Terrestrial biomass can be categorized as lignocellulosic biomass, fresh vegetables and oily biomass: each has its own properties which make it suitable for a particular treatment/conversion.

Lignocellulosic are composed of three polymeric materials (cellulose, hemicellulose, lignin) having quite different properties and behaviors. Long-term (>10 y) crops (mainly trees) may afford yields >15 t/ha of dry matter, while willow, which have a good potential to efficiently exploit less favorable lands, may produce around 9 t/ha of dry matter. Other grass-like cellulose rich plants can also be exploited. Non-food cellulosic crops must be used in order to avoid any food-energy/chemicals conflict (second-third generation fuels) or residual cellulosic materials from food-plants (straws, husky, cellulosic cakes, bones, prunings, etc.) can be used.

Fresh vegetables are quite suited for biogas generation through anaerobic fermentation as they have a high amount of water and lower amount of polymeric materials as with respect to plants mentioned above.

Non-food annual and perennial oil crops (crambe, castor, safflower, etc.) can be used for the sustainable production of various chemicals and fuels. Averaged yields over 3–5 years range from 1.3 t/ha.y (crambe) to 2.4–2.5 (safflower-castor).

3.2.2.2.1 *Pretreatment and Conversion Technologies*

Terrestrial lignocellulosic biomass is characterized by its composition made of three polymeric materials: cellulose, hemicellulose and lignin, each playing a functional and/or structural role. Such polymeric materials must be converted first into depolymerized or monomeric species (Figure 3.4), easier to use as commodities and platform-molecules in chemical and biotechnological processes for eventually produce fuels, chemicals, goods, by using "catalytic technologies" (chemocatalysis and enzymatic catalysis) or physical treatments. The complete exploitation of biomass is today achieved through the implementation of the concept of "biorefinery" (*vide infra*).

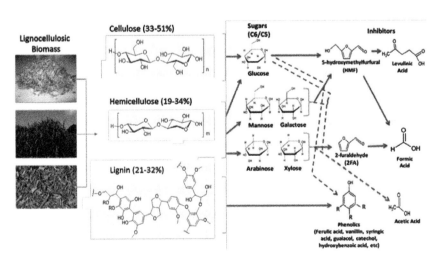

FIGURE 3.4 Separation of lignocellulosic biomass into components and depolymerized materials.

Heterogeneous and homogeneous catalysis ('chemo-catalysis') play a role of the upmost importance in the establishment of biorefineries. Together with controlled thermal processes (physical processes) and biotechnological transformations (bio-catalysis), chemo-catalysis enables exploitation of raw materials to produce a variety of chemicals, such as materials, intermediates or fine chemicals of high commercial value, and fuels. Oleaginous plants produce other families of commodities, such as triglycerides (Scheme 2) and fatty compounds (acids and esters), which allow the production of different products and fuels.

Hereafter, the most important pretreatment technologies will be discussed for biomass conversion into commodities and platform-monomeric species, while in Chapter 4 the production of target compounds will be discussed. Biomass can be processed using various technologies to obtain hydrolysates, liquid and gaseous fuels and chemicals. Some technologies are better labeled as pretreatment as they convert biomass into an intermediate complex system which is then further worked up to afford final products. The various conversion processes can be grouped into three main categories: therm(ochemic)al, biochemical and chemical processes. A pretreatment often used for deconstructing lignocellulosic materials is Steam-Explosion (SE). In SE the biomass is heated with high-pressure steam to temperatures >450 K; rapidly dropping the pressure in a blow tank, causes biomass opening and separation of the three main components (cellulose, hemicellulose and lignin).

3.2.2.2.1.1   Controlled fast pyrolysis

Fast pyrolysis consists of heating organic materials at 700–875 K in absence of oxygen. Under these conditions, biomass is converted into a gas phase,

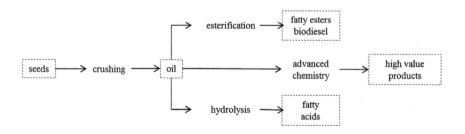

SCHEME 2   Value-chain based on the treatment of oleaginous seeds.

a liquid (bio-oil) and char. Typically, 60–75 wt.% of the feedstock is converted into oil, with 15–25% char and 10–20% gasses. Pyrolysis offers the possibility of concentrating energy and represents a most interesting intermediate step between small and diffused scale of residual biomass (agricultural) and large-scale plants for biooil treatment.

The process is characterized by high heating rates and rapid quenching of the liquid products to terminate the secondary conversion of the products. The main advantages of the fast pyrolysis are the high yields of liquid biooil and the relatively low production cost [10]. The process has been demonstrated at a demo scale employing several different reactor types ranging from entrained flow to ablative and fluidized bed, with capacities between 1 and 50 t/h [11].

Pyrolysis-oils are a very complex mixture (>300) of oxygenated hydrocarbons [12] such as acids, aldehydes, ketones, alcohols, glycols, esters, ethers, phenols and phenol derivatives, as well as carbohydrates and derivatives, and a large proportion (20–30 wt.%) of lignin-derived oligomers [13] (Table 3.1).

Such complex mixture is characterized by high content of oxygen, low heating value, immiscibility with hydrocarbon fuels, low chemical stability,

TABLE 3.1   Typical Properties of Wood Pyrolysis Bio-Oil

Physical property	Bio-oil
Moisture content (wt%)	15–30
pH	2.5–3.5
Specific gravity	1.2
Elemental composition (wt%)	
C	55.3–63.5
H	5.2–7.0
O	30–40
N	0–0.4
Ash	0–0.3
HHV (MJ/kg)	16–19
Viscosity, at 773K (cP)	40–100
Density (kg/m^3)	1110–1250
Solids (wt%)	0.2–1.0
Distillation residue (wt%)	Up to 50

high viscosity and high corrosiveness that do not make it recommended for a direct use as fuel. The reduction of the content of oxygen may improve the quality of bio-oil, converting it into a liquid fuel that can compete with mineral oil refinery fuels [10, 14–17].

In this direction, catalytic pyrolysis of biomass constitutes a very attractive route for the in-situ upgrading of bio-oil as the heavy oxygenated compounds are converted into lighter fuels and chemicals. The catalysts selectively favor decarboxylation and decarbonylation reactions, thus reducing the aggressivity of bio-oil. Zeolites, mesoporous materials with uniform pore size distribution (MCM-41, MSU and SBA-15), microporous/mesoporous hybrid materials doped with noble and transition metals, and base catalysts have been used in catalytic biomass pyrolysis [19]. Typically, hydrodeoxygenation (HDO) is used to remove most of the oxygen groups contained in the bio-oil under high pressure (up to 20 MPa) and temperatures in the range 570–670 K affording naphtha-like and diesel streams that can be blended in refineries with conventional transportation fuels, with yields ranging between 0.3–0.5 L of product per L of bio-oil depending on the extent of deoxygenation [18, 20–25]. The used catalysts are traditional hydrodesulphurization catalysts, such as NiMo and CoMo catalysts on alumina or silica alumina supports, or metal catalysts, such as Pd/C, which need improvement for their lifetime. A strategy to minimize hydrogen consumption in HDO is to operate a series of cascade catalytic transformations so to obtain second-generation liquid biofuels from lignocellulosic biomass in a cost-efficient way through the use of tailored nano-catalysts.

In addition to biomass itself, even starch and sugars originated from cellulosic biomass can be processed by HDO-related technologies bearing to intermediates such as alcohols, ketones, furans, paraffins and other oxygenated hydrocarbons depending on operating parameters, the catalytic system and the starting biomass-derived feed. These compounds further undergo transformations *via* different reaction pathways (condensation, hydrodeoxygenation, dehydration, oligomerization, etc.) to afford longer chain hydrocarbons used as fuels (BioForming Technology commercialized by Virent), that are reported may be competitive at crude oil prices higher than 60$/bbl [26].

3.2.2.2.1.2   Gasification

Gasification is a thermal process that converts solid fuels into a gaseous fuel mixture of low or medium calorific value using air or oxygen as oxidant or water vapor (H_2O). The difference between air driven gasification and combustion lays practically in the air ratio, which in the former case is substoichiometric ($\lambda < 1$) while in the latter is overstoichiometric ($\lambda > 1$) with respect to the amount of oxygen required for complete combustion. The gasification of biomass can be performed in fixed, moving or fluidized bed reactors at temperatures >973 K, much higher than pyrolysis. Many of the reactions occurring during gasification are endothermic: the required thermal energy can be provided by partial/total oxidation of biomass itself (if the gasification agent is oxygen or air); conversely, heat can be provided from an external source in case of steam driven gasification. In the first case the process is called autothermal, in the second allothermal. Overall the solid raw material is converted mainly into gases (CO, H_2, CO_2, H_2O, and CH_4), and other inorganic-organic compounds having concentration in the range from ppm to a few units% (H_2S, COS, HCl, NH_3, HCN, etc.). Small quantity of heavy hydrocarbons (tars) is formed, with some residual fraction of the original biomass together in addition to ash (mainly metal-oxides).

Fixed bed gasifiers are used as small-scale reactors (<1 MWth), while fluidized bed gasifiers (silica sand is the fluidizer) are used for large-scale applications. The gasification occurs at temperature of max. 1125 K.

The composition of the produced gas, its quality, and its calorific capacity vary depending on the gasification system and the process reagent (air or steam) [27–29] (Table 3.2).

In general, the gas must be further cleaned for eliminating particles, heavy hydrocarbons and inorganics to allow its use in gas boilers, internal combustion engines gas turbines, and chemical syntheses as bio-Syngas [28] (See Subsection 3.4.1.2).

TABLE 3.2   Quality of the Gas Produced in a Gasification Process

Process	H_2	CO	CO_2	CH_4	N_2	HHV (MJ/m³)
Fluidized bed*/air	9–17	14–24	9–20	3–7	48–53	5.4–5.7
Fluid bed/oxygen	30–33	46–48	14–16	1.5–3	1–3	9.8–10.4
Pyrolysis	38–40	19–22	18–21	20–23	0.5–1.5	11.2–13.4

* Updraft or downdraft.

3.2.2.2.1.3   Hydrolysis

Hydrolysis of cellulose produces sugars from which second generation ethanol is produced. Ethanol is currently the most important renewable fuel in terms of volume and market value. In 2010 worldwide bioethanol production reached 113 BL, with the United States and Brazil as the world's top producers accounting together for 80% of global production. By 2022, world ethanol production is projected to increase by almost 70% compared to the average of 2010–12 and reaching some 168 BL [30]. Ethanol has been and still is industrially produced from sweet juice (e.g., sugarcane, sugar beet juice, or molasses) and starch (e.g., corn, wheat, barley, cassava). The major drawbacks of such first-generation biofuel are:

- Competition with crops for land that could be used for food production;
- Rising cost of food due to increased demand of grain crops for first-generation biofuel production. Such crops represent in fact the staple grains in the diets of many people, especially in less developed countries;
- Necessity to irrigate crops, which in some regions adds more stress on groundwater sources.
- High input of fertilizers and pesticides necessary for putting poor quality land into production.

Second-generation ethanol can be produced from lignocellulosic biomass such as agricultural and forestry residues, weeds and waste paper, some municipal and industrial wastes, etc., avoiding any competition between feeding and fueling.

For the production of ethanol, sugars must be released from cellulose and hemicellulose (Figure 3.4). The close association of cellulose fibrills with hemicellulose and lignin makes lignocellulosic biomass highly stable and recalcitrant to enzymatic or chemical hydrolysis. Pretreatment is required to alter the biomass structure and chemical composition in order to facilitate the release of the carbohydrate fraction, decrystalyzing and partially depolymerizing cellulose [31, 32]. Pretreatment can be carried out by mechanical, physical, chemical, physicochemical and biological actions or a combination of them. In some pretreatment processes, lignin can be separated from hemicellulose and cellulose. After pretreatment, two main processes can be used to hydrolyze cellulose and hemicellulose into monomeric sugar for their fermentation into ethanol, namely: enzymatic or chemical acid (diluted or concentrated) processes.

Enzymatic hydrolysis of cellulose and hemicellulose is carried out by cellulase and hemicellulase enzymes. The hydrolysis takes place under mild conditions (e.g., pH 4.5–5.0 and temperature 313–323 K). Main advantages of this process, compared to acid hydrolysis, are lower corrosion problems, low utility consumption, and absence of fermentation inhibitors release [33].

Novel lignocellulolytic enzymes are under study, which may be able to hydrolyze pretreated cellulose and hemicellulose more rapidly, withstanding extreme pHs, different temperatures and inhibitory agents which can be found in the pretreated biomass. The cost of enzymes is still high and its reduction is a high priority topic addressed by large international enzyme companies such as Novozymes, Genencor, DSM, Iogen and several others. In a batch process, the pretreated solid biomass 10–20% dry weight (dw) is used. After a few hours, the digested material starts to release partially degraded cellulose and hemicellulose making a slurry. Increased loadings in hydrolysis are a topic of great interest, as it also is the separation of lignin that can bind enzymes and inhibit them. Enzymatic hydrolysis is often combined with steam explosion (SE) pretreatment. Under such conditions, hemicellulose will split off acetate groups, which will form acetic acid with pH reduction, and will produce fermentation inhibitors such as furfural, 5-hydroxymethyl-furfural (5-HMF). Furthermore, the lignins are condensed and degraded to low MW creating a higly polydispersed lignin with lower O-content and with very low reactivity and low solubility in water or other solvents. This process is implemented into the Inbicon's demonstration plant in Denmark, and Borregard process in Norway [9].

In acid hydrolysis processes, both diluted and concentrated strong acids are employed. Diluted acids typically are mineral acids such as sulfuric acid or hydrochloric acid used at elevated temperature (around 400 K) and pressure. The acid hydrolysis will produce large amounts of furfural (from xylose), 5-HMF (from glucose), acetic acid (from hemicellulose) and other inhibitors of the fermentation microorganisms.

The concentrated acid processes is old and employed already in first half of the 20th century in Europe, Soviet Union and USA to produce ethanol from wood. The process consumes large amounts of mineral acids (hydrochloric or sulfuric acid). First the raw material is softened with concentrated acid, then the acid is diluted with water to start the hydrolysis process since the concentrated acid does not hydrolyze cellulose. Modern processes using concentrated acid pretreatment include a step for separation and recirculation of the acid either by solvent extraction (Weyland), ion exchange resins (BlueFire) or membrane technology (TNO).

3.2.2.3   Terrestrial Oily Biomass

Several plants produce oleaginous seeds from which oil can be obtained using mechanical and chemical technologies. The most popular, but old, technology is the discontinuous one and consists of crushing seeds, loading the resulting pulp on discs piled in a hydraulic press and application of pressure (40–60 MPa) at room temperature. In this way, oil and water are released, which are separated by centrifugation that facilitates the separation of the two immiscible liquid phases. Alternatively, a continuous process (Figure 3.5) can be applied which crushes and presses seeds in a endless screw apparatus.

The liquid stream is separated into oil and water by centrifugation. In this way, on the basis of the pressure applied it is possible to extract up to 90% of the oil present in seeds. For a more complete extraction, a solvent (hexane) extraction is carried out on the residual solid that will allow producing some more 8+% oil. The extraction can also be assisted by ultrasounds (US) or microwave (MV), which promote the release of liquid from the solid. Using only pressure or pressure plus extraction is dictated by the value of the oil. A high value oil would suggest to extract most of it from the solid (complementing the pressure extraction with the solvent extraction) as the additional units % extracted can pay for the extra energy spent and other investment and operational costs.

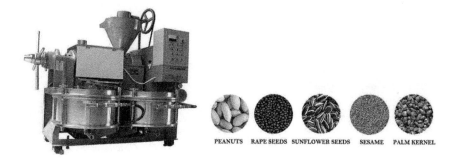

PEANUTS   RAPE SEEDS   SUNFLOWER SEEDS   SESAME   PALM KERNEL

FIGURE 3.5   Continuous screw-press process for oil extraction from seeds and drupes.

3.2.2.4 Aquatic Biomass

Aquatic biomass can be classifed into: Macroalgae, Microalge and Plants. They have different properties and uses.

Macro-algae (Figure 3.6) are classified as *Phaeophyta* or brown algae, *Rhodophyta* or red algae, and *Chlorophyta* or green algae based on the composition of photosynthetic pigments. Green macroalgae have evolutionary and biochemical affinity with higher plants. The life cycles of macroalgae are complex and diverse, with different species displaying variations of annual and perennial life histories, combinations of sexual and asexual reproductive strategies, and alternation of generations.

The distribution of macroalgae is worldwide. They are abundant in coastal environments, primarily in near shore coastal waters with suitable substrate for attachment. Macro-algae also occur as floating forms in the open ocean, and floating seaweeds are considered one of the most important components of natural materials on the sea surface [34]. The use of macroalgae for energy production has received attention only very recently [35]. The great advantage of macroalgae with respect to terrestrial biomass is their high biomass productivity (faster growth in dry weight ha^{-1} y^{-1} than for most terrestrial crops). The productivity of natural basins is in the range 1–20 kg m^{-2} y^{-1} dw (10–150 t$_{dw}$ ha^{-1} y^{-1}) for a 7–8 month culture. Interestingly, macroalgae are very effective in nutrients (N, P) uptake from sewage and industrial wastewater.

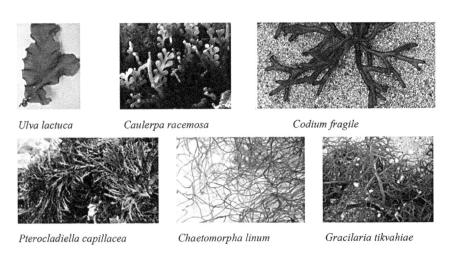

| *Ulva lactuca* | *Caulerpa racemosa* | *Codium fragile* |

| *Pterocladiella capillacea* | *Chaetomorpha linum* | *Gracilaria tikvahiae* |

FIGURE 3.6 Different types of macroalgae.

The estimated recovery capacity is 16 kg ha^{-1} d^{-1} [36]. To this end macroalgae have been used for cleaning municipal wastewater [37] (essentially in Europe), for recycling nutrients and for the treatment of fishery effluents [38, 39] (either in Europe or in Japan). Macroalgae are suitable for biogas (*vide infra*) production as they have low content of lipids (ca. 20%).

Micro-algae are microscopic organisms and are currently cultivated commercially as feed for fish around the world in several dozen small- to medium-scale production systems, producing from a few tens to several hundred tons of biomass annually. The main algae genera currently cultivated photo-synthetically (e.g., with light) for various nutritional products are *Botryococcus braunii, Arthrospira platensis, Haematococcus pluvialis, Dunaliella sp* (Figure 3.7).

Micro-algae can be grown in open ponds or in photo-bioreactors (PBR). The culture in open ponds is more economically favorable with respect to PBR [40]. The production cost may vary from \$8 to \$15/kg dry algae biomass in open ponds, to 50–200\$/kg in closed photobioreactors due to larger operating and investment costs [41]. Microalgae can present a large content of lipids up to 70%. The application of the biorefinery concept to microalgae may play a key role for their full valorization [42].

Aquatic plants (Figure 3.8), also known as hydrophytes, grow in all ponds, shallow lakes, marshes, ditches, reservoirs, swamps, canals, and sewage lagoons. Less frequently, they also live in flowing water, in streams, rivers and springs. They can be divided into four categories according to the habitat of growth: *floating unattached, floating attached, submersed,* and *emergent.* Plants are often used for water phytodepuration as they efficiently use N and P compounds present in wastewater; some species can also concentrate heavy metals [43].

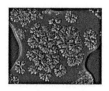 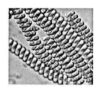 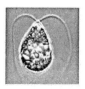

Botryococcus braunii   *Arthrospira platensis*   *Haematococcus pluvialis*   *Dunaliella sp*

FIGURE 3.7   Different types of microalgae.

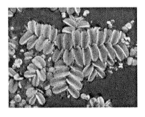 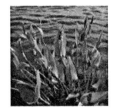 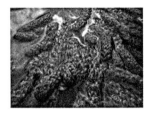

Salvinia natans   ***Pontederia cordata***   *Lagarosiphon major*

FIGURE 3.8   Different type of plants.

With respect to micro and macroalgae, hydrophytes may contain a larger amount of cellulosic materials and require different technologies for their treatment. They can be used for thermal energy production.

Aquatic biomass has a different composition than terrestrial plants. Macro- and microalgae have a quite low content of cellulose and hemicellulose, while lignin is absent. Therefore, their treatment is in a sense easier than lignocellulosic plants, but made complex by the high product-entropy that makes energetically intensive their separation.

3.2.3   MAN-MADE CONVERSION OF CO₂

The chemical utilization of CO_2 is not a new attitude. Industrial processes were developed as early as in the 1880–1893s, namely: the synthesis of urea [44], the soda Solvay process and the synthesis of hydrogen carbonates [45], the production of salycilic acid [46]. Interestingly, in the former process CO_2 recovered from the synthesis of NH_3 is used, reducing the environmental impact of the latter process. In the 1900s there was not a great interest in developing new applications of CO_2. As a matter of fact, since the late 1800s the chemistry of CO (derived from fossil carbon) has been developed for the synthesis of chemicals and fuels and had its golden era in the 1900–1970s, and still today plays a key role in the production of chemicals and fuels.

Only in the 1970s there was a revival in the exploitation of CO_2 as additive to CO in the synthesis of methanol [47] and as comonomer in the pioneering production of organic carbonates from epoxides [48], *via* direct carboxylation. Figure 3.9 gives the actual use of carbon dioxide in the synthesis of chemicals and the perspective use at 2030 [49], calculated considering the expected

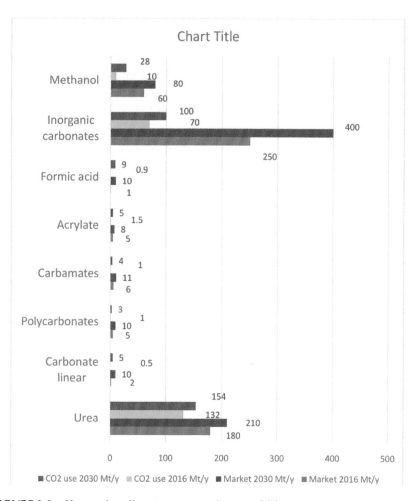

FIGURE 3.9 Short and medium term perspective use of CO_2.

market growth for the listed chemicals and assuming that new technologies will be developed that ensure a large conversion of CO_2. Data reported in Figure 3.9 show that in the best of cases the utilization of CO_2 will grow from 180 Mt/y in 2014 to 207 Mt/y in 2016 and 332 Mt/y in 2030: a great performance *per se*, but still a drop in the ocean of the over 35 000 Mt/y emitted today. If one considers the amount of *avoided CO_2* more than the amount of *used CO_2*, then one may have a better result as, being the ratio avoided/used spanning over a range 2–5, with a good average around 3, *ca.* 1000 Mt_{CO_2}/y would be avoided.

The oxidation state of the carbon-atom in the various compounds produced from carbon dioxide is a key point relevant to the energetics of any
CO_2-conversion reaction, which depends on the variation of the C-oxidation
state in the reaction. Figure 3.10 shows the Gibbs free-energy of formation
of several C1 species. It is quite evident that when the oxidation state of the
carbon atom is reduced from +4 in CO_2 to 2 or lower, a significant amount
of energy is needed for the conversion to occur, while when the oxidation state remains +4 (i.e., synthesis of organic carbonates and carbamates,
located in the circle around CO_2) or close to it (+3 in C2 species such as
oxalic acid, HO_2C-CO_2H) the reaction is quasi-neutral or even exothermic,
as can be found in the synthesis of inorganic carbonates, which lay well
below CO_2.

On such basis, in the middle 1980s we have classified the CO_2 reactions
in two classes [50], according to the fact that CO_2 is incorporated such as
in a given product (Class A) or it is converted into one of its reduced forms
(Class B).

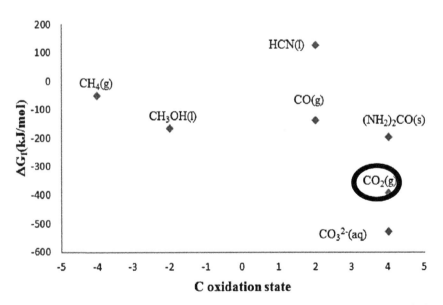

FIGURE 3.10   Gibbs free energy of formation of C1 species. (Adapted with permission
from Aresta, M.; Dibenedetto, A.; Angelini, A. Catalysis for the valorization of exhaust
carbon: from CO2 to chemicals, materials and fuels. Technological use of CO2. Chem Rev.
2014, 114, 1709-1742. Copyright (2013) American Chemical Society.)

Class A: CO_2 fixation into inorganic carbonates-M_2CO_3, organic carbonates-$(RO)_2CO$, carbamates-$RR'N-CO_2R$, polycarbonates, polyurethanes, isocyanates-NCO^-.

Class B: CO_2 reduction to CO or hydrogenated products such as methanol, methane, higher hydrocarbons.

Noticeably, the two classes are characterized by a distinct use of the products and a quite different size of their market. *Class A* species fall into the chemicals category, while *Class B* are fuels with a market that is some 12–14 times that of chemicals, as aid above. Therefore, if one targets to convert large volumes of CO_2 must pursue its conversion into fuels. But if the target is to avoid CO_2, then chemicals should also be taken into due consideration: both classes of compounds must be targeted for maximizing the reduction of CO_2 emission in the atmosphere. Moreover, if one deals with fuels a new issue comes out: where to get the necessary energy for the conversion (see Figure 3.10) and the hydrogen for the production of hydrocarbons. It is obvious that H_2 cannot be derived from fossil-C, but must come from water or organic waste, while energy must be supplied by perennial SWHG sources. A new approach must be developed for H_2 production with respect to the actual one based on reforming (of coke or methane) at high temperature, a strongly endergonic process (Eq. 1–3).

$$C + H_2O \rightarrow CO + H_2 \text{(Water Gas Reaction-WGR)} \qquad \Delta H^0_{298K} = 131.3 \text{ kJ/mol}$$

$$(1)$$

$$CH_4 + H_2O \rightarrow CO + 3H_2 \text{(Methane Wet Reforming)} \qquad \Delta H^0_{298K} = 206 \text{ kJ/mol}$$

$$(2)$$

$$CO + H_2O \rightarrow CO_2 + H_2 \text{(Water Gas Shift-WGS)} \qquad \Delta H^0_{298K} = -41 \text{ kJ/mol}$$

$$(3)$$

3.2.3.1   Key Issues in the Conversion of CO_2

The conversion of CO_2 is a quite complex issue [51], complicated by the fact that if it targets carbon mitigation, the carbon balance must be kept under strict control, with the concept of "*avoided*" CO_2 being prevalent on that of "*used*" CO_2. As a matter of fact, the use of CO_2 in new chemical processes can be quite interesting as it avoids the emission of large volumes of CO_2 (with respect to processes on stream), much larger than the amount of converted CO_2. Correct values of "*used*" and "*avoided*" CO_2 may be obtained by applying the LCA methodology.

However, the key point is: synthetic routes based on CO_2 *must* respond to a stringent requisite, namely: *the new process must minimize the CO_2 emission with respect to processes on stream.* In order to satisfy such condition, an immediate subcondition is: *the CO_2-based process must be a consumer and not a producer of CO_2.*

3.2.3.2   Performance Indicators in CO_2 Conversion

Indicators which may help to assess a CO_2-based process are:

- (a) the carbon utilization fraction (the percentage of reagent-C fixed into the products);
- (b) the carbon-footprint (the CO_2 emission in the process per unit of product);
- (c) the energy consumption factor (ratio of the input- to output-energy);
- (d) the waste production factor (waste produced per unit of product, w/w);
- (e) the "avoided" to "used" ratio.

The above indicators heavily depend on the reaction conditions. The reaction "*parameter space*" is defined by the following factors: (i) solvent; (ii) co-reagents; (iii) catalysts; (iv) temperature; (v) pressure; (vi) overall energy expenditure-time of reaction; (vii) conversion of reagents; (viii) formation of coproducts/selectivity of the process; (ix) waste generation; and (x) end of process separation energy. A life cycle assessment (LCA) study can give a reliable answer to the question whether a particular use of CO_2 is avoiding CO_2 emission or increasing it.

3.3   BIOMASS AS SOURCE OF FUELS

As reported above, biomass has been itself used as fuel since man discovered fire. This is not the most efficient way to use it. Biomass can be converted either into liquid or gaseous fuels, easy to transport and use in existing infrastructures and transportation means. Ethanol, biodiesel, gasoline and methane can be derived from biomass. The available technologies will be discussed in the following subsections.

3.3.1   FUELS FROM CELLULOSIC BIOMASS

3.3.1.1   Production of Ethanol

The production of lignocellulosic ethanol can be divided in four main steps: (i) pretreatment, (ii) hydrolysis, (iii) fermentation, and (iv) distillation. Based on the integration of the above-mentioned steps, four process schemes, characterized by a different level of process integration, can be identified:

(i)   separate hydrolysis and fermentation (SHF);
(ii) simultaneous saccharification and fermentation (SSF);
(iii) simultaneous saccharification-and co-fermentation (SSCF); and
(iv) consolidated bioprocessing (CBP).

Currently, integrated processes are privileged for economic reasons. However, a reduction of the costs can also be obtained optimizing the individual steps. In addition, hybrid processes are under development, which allow individual steps taking place under their optimal conditions. For example, cellulose can be only partially hydrolyzed under optimal conditions, then the operational conditions are changed, and fermentation starts upon addition of the suited agents [52].

CBP is in general considered the best possible option for a profitable second-generation ethanol production. For the development of an efficient CBP, microbial catalysts should show the following features:

(i)   excellent ethanol-producing capability;
(ii) efficient (hemi) cellulase production;
(iii) tolerance to ethanol, to fermentation inhibitors and other stresses commonly found in the ethanol production;

(iv) since the most efficient cellulases to date have an optimal operative temperature of 323 K, the ideal microorganisms have also to be thermostable. At industrial level high temperatures are beneficial as they allow the reduction of cooling costs and decrease the contamination risk by mesophiles.

Currently, no organism combines all the above properties, although many match most of them [53]. Consequently, metabolic and genetic engineering are used to generate a recombinant biocatalyst, which can be employed in CBP. The two engineering strategies that are being pursued:

1. Converting a cellulolytic microorganism into an efficient ethanol producer. To make a cellulolytic microorganism ethanologenic, the introduction of heterologous ethanol synthetic pathways has been attempted. Most research has been focused on thermophilic Gram-positive bacteria. Many of such bacteria are strict anaerobes and produce mixtures of fermentation products. Generally they display a low tolerance to ethanol and to fermentation inhibitors. Metabolic engineers have sought to eliminate fermentation byproducts and increase the ethanol tolerance. One of the most studied microorganisms in this regard is *Clostridium thermocellum*. It is a thermophilic anaerobic bacterium, which can grow at temperatures as high as 333 K and is capable of naturally producing ethanol albeit at low concentrations (< 3 g/L). As many *Clostridia*, it expresses a high number of different cellulases and hemicellulase on its cell surface. These enzymes are linked to a scaffold protein and constitute a complex known as cellulosome. *C. thermocellum* cellulosome has been proved to be more efficient than free hemicellulases since the multienzymatic complex provides a synergistic mechanism of action. Several engineered strains have been developed using directed evolution to improve ethanol or inhibitor tolerance. Despite all that, the utilization of cellulolytic microorganisms in a economically feasible CBP is still far from being achieved [54, 55].

2. Developing an ethanologenic microorganism, which expresses and secretes heterologous cellulases. The expression of cellulases and hemicellulase in an ethanologenic microorganism is a difficult task since the hydrolysis of the lignocellulosic biomass requires the simultaneous presence of many different enzymatic

activities. Two expression strategies have been pursued: (a) secretion of cellulolytic enzymes by recombinant ethanologens; (b) expression and display of these enzymes on the cell surface. The latter approach appears to be superior since the activity of the enzymes displayed on the cell surface are retained as long as the expressing cells keep their viability. Moreover in this way it is possible to produce a large amount of biomass prior to add it to the pretreated lignocellulosic material that has to be fermented. A number of ethanologenic hosts have been chosen for the expression but much research has been focused on *S. cerevisiae* for its known properties as ethanol producer. However as outlined before, thermostability is an important feature in CBP; hence other thermotolerant yeasts such as *Kluyveromyces marxianus* and *Hansenula polymorpha* have also been employed. Promising results have been achieved but research is still needed in the direction of identifying an industrial (hemi)cellulose-producing ethanologenic microorganism capable of converting pretreated raw lignocellulosic biomass into ethanol in an economically acceptable process [53, 54].

3.3.1.2   Microbial Production of Long Chain Hydrocarbons from Bio-Syngas

Bio-syngas is a syngas ($CO+xH_2$) produced from biomass more than from fossil C. bio-syngas can supplant syngas in the many mature technologies known for producing several of the most important chemicals, and even fuels. In a few cases, such technologies may find application in biorefineries to exploit the whole biomass value. However, in most cases the viability, from both the energetic and the economic point of view, of using biomass to feed large-scale plants is still an open question. Considering the feedstock versatility of the gasification technology, and the development of chemical and biotechnological routes for chemicals production either from syngas or, directly, from industrial flue gases to exploit waste biomass as feedstock. Such approach would afford valuable products starting from raw materials with nearly zero (or even negative) cost, at the same time providing routes for carbon recycling and, more generally, to mitigate the environmental impact of several human activities.

Not surprisingly, Syngas can be exploited by few microorganisms able to grow autotrophically on CO/H_2O or on H_2/CO_2 rather than on sugars, as in traditional fermentations. In fact, microbes grow on gas emissions from hydrothermal vents and volcanoes, which, most likely, have been the only, carbon and energy source for the first life forms. Interestingly, gas from hydrothermal vents have quite similar composition as several industrial emissions (e.g., steel manufacturing), being formed by CO, CO_2, H_2S, H_2, and CH_4. Therefore, industrial flue gases can be exploited as both nutrient and energy source to feed fermentations and to produce a number of chemicals, providing a new route to carbon capture and reuse. The best-developed fermentations mostly afford ethanol, along with some acetic acid or acetate anion, according to the fermentation conditions. The overall transformations are:

Ethanol production:

$$6 \text{ CO} + 3 \text{ H}_2\text{O} \rightarrow \text{C}_2\text{H}_5\text{OH} + 4 \text{ CO}_2 \tag{4}$$

$$2 \text{ CO}_2 + 6 \text{ H}_2 \rightarrow \text{C}_2\text{H}_5\text{OH} + 3 \text{ H}_2\text{O} \tag{5}$$

Acetic acid production:

$$4 \text{ CO} + 2 \text{ H}_2\text{O} \rightarrow \text{CH}_3\text{CO}_2\text{H} + 2 \text{ CO}_2 \tag{6}$$

$$2 \text{ CO}_2 + 4 \text{ H}_2 \rightarrow \text{CH}_3\text{CO}_2\text{H} + 2 \text{ H}_2\text{O} \tag{7}$$

Carbon monoxide-water is the preferred substrate with respect to the CO_2/H_2 mixture: typical CO conversions for laboratory-scale fermentations are about 90%, while hydrogen conversions are around 70%.

The ratio of ethanol to acetic acid depends upon the strain and the fermentation conditions. The microorganisms are inhibited by low pH and high concentrations of acetate ion. When acetic acid is formed and the pH drops or when the acetate concentration rises, microorganisms switch to ethanol production to alleviate further stress. Typically, pH is kept around 4.5 in ethanol production.

Many of the microorganisms are mesophiles or even thermophiles, with temperature optimum in the range between room temperature and 363 K. A fairly rich medium is required, with possible contamination problems. However, contamination risks are greatly reduced by the harsh fermentation conditions: high temperatures, low nutrients levels, and low pH. Furthermore, the high level of carbon monoxide inhibits the growth of methanogenic bacteria, while some tolerance to S-compounds might be possible. All the above issue requires further research for full exploitation.

Simple gas-sparged tank reactors, operating either in batch or in continuous mode, can be used. Ethanol can be recovered by distillation as head fraction ethanol/water azeotropic mixture, and water separated using known technologies such as pervaporation membranes.

The energy efficiency (heat of combustion of products /heat of combustion of feed) is 0.80–0.81 for reactions (4) and (5) and 0.77 for reactions (6) and (7) compared to 0.98 or better for an anaerobic fermentation.

At the lab scale, a number of organic compounds are produced, including propanols, butanols, *iso*-butene, 2,3-butanediol, acetic acid, etc. Only ethanol production has been scaled up to precommercial stage by LanzaTech that has put into operation two plants built in partnership with Chinese steel producers, each plant producing 300 t/y of ethanol.

CO_2 can be converted into long-chain hydrocarbon ($C_{15}H_{24}$) using cyanobacteria modified genetically (*Anabaena* sp. PCC 7120) that exhibit an higher activity with respect to wild type [56].

3.3.1.3 *Production of Fuels from C4-C5-C6 Platform Molecules*

Heavier alcohols, mainly butanols, easily transported by pipeline, have been used as gasoline additives for over 40 years. Recently, they have attracted attention as raw materials for the production of jet fuel. Therefore, efforts are directed towards the development of processes for the production of *renewable butanols,* using biomass derived sugars, even converting existing cornstarch ethanol plants into isobutanol plants [57]. Isobutanol's properties (low reid vapor pressure, above average octane, good energy content, low water solubility and low oxygen content) allow blending with gasoline. They can also undergo transformation to other valuable products providing in such a way great flexibility in industry. Isobutanol serves as a platform molecule, as it can be converted to isobutene, a precursor for a variety of transportation fuel products such as iso-octene (gasoline blendstock), iso-octane (alkylate-high-quality gasoline blendstock and/or aviation gasoline blendstock), iso-paraffinic kerosene (jet fuel) and diesel. The strategy to convert isobutanol to jet fuel includes dehydration followed by oligomerization, hydrogenation and distillation (Figure 3.11).

Gevo of Englewood, CO. claim the following properties of the renewable jet fuel: high blend rate, very low freeze point (193 K), high thermal oxidation stability, meeting the ASTM distillation curve requirements. Renewable bio-butanols production has been targeted for developing a process for the production of jet and diesel fuels [58]. Specific research goals include optimization of the dehydration chemistry for the conversion of bio-n-butanol to -butene, followed by oligomerization of the latter into jet fuel. Additional focus is on converting biobutanol into butyl ether, which will be mixed with n-butanol and other compounds targeted to a viable drop-in diesel fuel replacement.

A key issue in such C4 conversion is improving the reaction control of steps occurring on acid zeolites [59–62], including the first step of dehydration of butanol to butenes, as the latter may undergo conversion into gasoline hydrocarbons *via* dimerization, isomerization, aromatization, and alkylation reactions. In the presence a H-ZSM-5, a gasoline yield of 50–55 wt.% at 573–623 K has been reported [62]. The liquid stream is composed of aliphatic, olefinic and aromatic hydrocarbons and the product distribution strongly depends on the temperature and zeolites used. The dehydration of a mixture containing 62.9 wt % n-butanol, 29.3 wt % acetone, and 7.8 wt % ethanol [63] on either alumina (γ-Al_2O_3) or zeolite (ZSM-5) affords a mixture of unsaturated hydrocarbons in the range of C_2–C_{16}. Three phases were formed consisting of gas products (light hydrocarbons and carbon dioxide), organic liquid phase (heavy hydrocarbons) and an aqueous phase (dissolved oxygenated hydrocarbons). Interestingly the catalytic dehydration of the mixture revealed a synergy of the reacting components, resulting in a product with high heating value. Dehydration on γ-Al_2O_3 at 673 K produces the

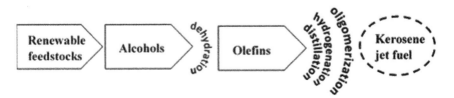

FIGURE 3.11   Isobutanol conversion to jet fuel

highest amount of liquids with high heating value. An alternative strategy for the production of fuels and fuel additives based on alcohols is represented in Scheme 3 [64]: the heavy alcohols/branched paraffins can be blended as components of aviation gasoline and jet fuel. The feasibility of this approach is supported by integrated tests at demo scale and the complete technology development shows the potential for industrial implementation.

Besides C4, C5 and C6 polyols derived from hemicellulosic- and cellulosic-biomass, respectively, can be used as source of liquid fuels. The catalytic upgrading pathway has great potential in converting sugars such as sorbitol, glucose, fructose, xylose into drop-in fuel blendstocks over the range of C_5–C_{12} for gasoline, C_9–C_{16} for jet fuel, and C_{10}–C_{20} for diesel applications. Low temperatures (typically less than 600 K) and moderate pressure (around 3 MPa) processes in a liquid phase are targeted [65]. The concept includes controlled conversion of sugars to platform compounds and subsequent transformation to hydrocarbons *via* dehydration, reforming, hydrogenation, hydrogenolysis (for oxygen removal), aldol condensation and oligomerization (Scheme 4) [26]. Interestingly, the hydrophilic starting materials are converted into hydrophobic hydrocarbons with spontaneous separation that decreases the processing costs. The fuels so produced are fully compatible with fossil-C derived fuels [66].

The concept above is the basis of the Virent's bioforming process which combines aqueous phase reforming (APR) for the production of the necessary hydrogen and several dehydration, hydrogenation and base-catalyzed condensation reactions. The above type of processing is flexible and can use

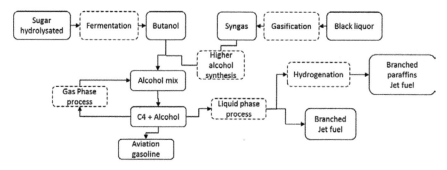

SCHEME 3 C4 alcohols as source of fuels and chemicals [64]. (From: http://www.virent. com/technology/bioforming/)

C5-C6 sugars
C3-C4 polyols
Starches

Reforming
↓
Processing

Chemicals
Gasoline
Diesel
Jet fuel

SCHEME 4   Concept scheme for sugars conversion into liquid transportation fuels and chemicals [26].

a wide range of biomass-derived compounds as illustrated in Figure 3.12 [67]. Catalysts used must be able to perform several reactions and require specific functionalities.

Levulinic acid is formed from 5-HMF in the transformation of C6-sugars into hydrocarbons and can be upgraded to hydrocarbon fuels (gasoline, jet fuel and diesel) [68]. Transformation of levulinic acid involves dehydration/hydrogenation so as to minimize the oxygen content and ketonization in order to

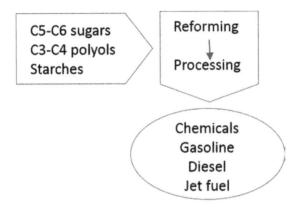

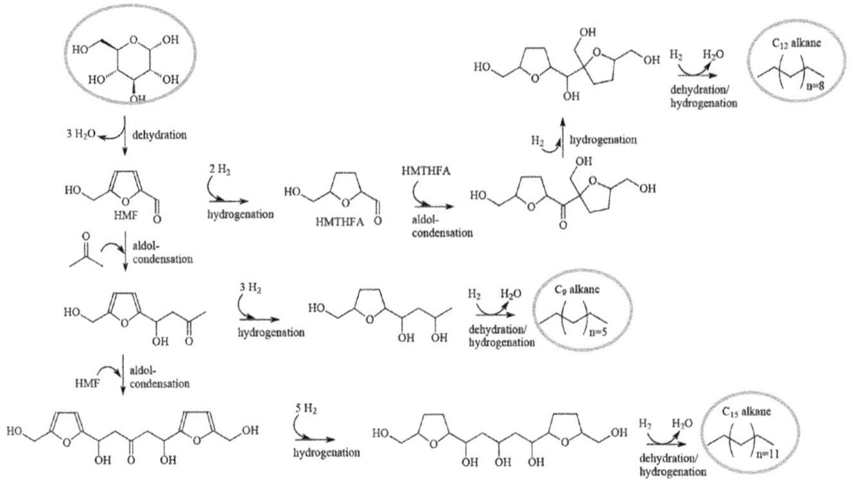

FIGURE 3.12   Conversion of biomass-derived glucose acid to liquid hydrocarbons.

increase the molecular mass. Pd/Nb_2O_5 catalyst allows this reaction sequence to be performed in a cascade manner with minimum steps. γ-Valerolactone formed from levulinic acid can be converted into liquid hydrocarbon fuels without the need of an external source of hydrogen [68]. The routes described here make use of structured components of only partially deconstructed biomass for producing hydrocarbon fuels, avoiding the gasification, a strongly endothermic process. Lignocellulose is the cheapest and most abundant form of biomass in some cases cost-competitive with crude oil on an energy basis. However, its complexity and scarce reactivity are main hurdles to its large-scale utilization as a source of liquid fuels, either alcohols or hydrocarbons. Due to the large presence of oxygen in the raw material, hydrogen is needed for its conversion into hydrocarbons. This is a key issue as the source of hydrogen and the energy necessary for its production may strongly affect the processes and the cost of fuels. Processes described above are characterized by technology readiness level (TRL) in the range 6–9: some are on the market others need further development to reach exploitation. Due to the complexity of the matrix, reaction mechanisms are not fully understood in some cases, and this needs investment in research for the design of active and robust catalysts. Even reactor design requires research for a correct exploitation of the potential of this chemistry. The integration into a full biorefinery plan may make economically viable the polyols to hydrocarbons conversion.

3.3.2 BIODIESEL FROM OILY BIOMASS

Oils can be derived from seeds and drupes produced from terrestrial plants or can be extracted from algae; even animal fats can be used as source of oils. Oils are derived from glycerides or fatty acid (long chain saturated-monounsaturated-polyunsaturated) esters with glycerol, the form they exist in nature (Figure 3.13)

Oils have a different composition according to their source (Table 3.3) for what concerns the presence of saturated, monounsaturated, di-, and poly-unsaturated FAs [42, 69] and the chain length (Cn).

In order to clarify the potential of vegetal or animal oils for biodiesel production, one has to consider that biodiesel must have properties as much as close to the fossil-C derived diesel which is made of saturated hydrocarbons. Therefore, strictly speaking, looking at Figure 3.13, only the saturated chains of lipids would be suited for biodiesel production. Unsaturated hydrocarbons

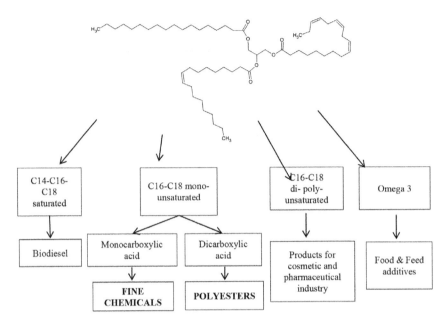

FIGURE 3.13   Triglycerides and the nature of fatty acids (FAs).

are allowed to be present in the biodiesel blend, but the number of unsatura-
tions should be not higher than one. Polyunsaturated hydrocarbons may cause
the formation of gums at high temperature with damage to engines. Therefore,
mixtures of oils containing polyunsaturated Fas should preferably undergo
hydrogenation and be converted into saturated species. Similarly, free acids
are not wished components of biodiesel as they are corrosive: Fatty Acids
Methyl Esters-FAMEs are better candidates. Glycerol present in triglycerides
may also cause problems for its viscosity. As a matter of fact, glycerides are not
directly used as biodiesel, but the linear saturated hydrocarbons derived from
them upon hydrolysis, transesterification with methanol (FAMEs) and partial
controlled hydrogenation of (poly)unsaturated species. As shown in Table 3.3,
palm oil among seed-derived oils is the most suited for biodiesel production
due to its high content of saturated C16 and C18 acids. Palm oil is by far the oil
with the largest production worldwide (> 30 Mt/y). The main producing countries are located in Asia (Indonesia, Malaysia, China, India) with about 50%
of the market (Figure 3.14). It must be emphasized that still today the most
widely used oils are edible oils such as palm, soybean, canola and sunflower
oils, which account for about 70% of total production. Non-edible oils such

TABLE 3.3 Composition of various oils from terrestrial and *aquatic* biomass

Oil Fatty acid (%)	C14:0 Myristic	C16:0 Palmitic	C16:1 Palmitoleic	C16:2 Hexadecadienoic	C16:3 Hexadecatrienoic	C18:0 Stearic	C18:1 Oleic	C18:2 Linoleic	C18:3 Linolenic	C20:1 Eicosenoic	C22:1 Erucic	C18:1-OH Ricinoleic	C20:5 Eicosapentaenoic
Palm	–	45	–	–	–	5	39	9	–	–	–	–	–
Soybean	–	7	–	–	–	5	19	68	1	–	–	–	–
Rapeseed	–	3	–	–	–	1	22	14	7	–	–	–	–
Sunflower	–	7	–	–	–	5	19	68	1	–	–	–	–
Sunflower (high oleic)	–	3	–	–	–	5	82	8	. <1	–	–	–	–
Linseed	–	7	–	–	–	4	39	15	35	–	–	–	–
Castor	–	1	–	–	–	1	3	4	–	–	–	89	–
Safflower	–	6	–	–	–	3	11	78	–	–	–	–	–
Safflower (high oleic)	–	5	–	–	–	1	87	9	1	–	–	–	–
Crambe	–	2	–	–	–	1	17	9	5	–	62	–	–
Tobacco	<1	8	0.2	–	–	1	14	75	1	–	–	–	–
Cardoon	<1	11	0.1	–	–	4	27	58		–	–	–	–
Rapeseed (high oleic)	<1	4	0.3	–	–	2	62	20	9	1	<1	–	–
Rapeseed (high erucic)	<1	3	0.2	–	–	1	8	17	15	5	44	–	–
Sunflower (high oleic)	<1	4	0.2	–	–	0.2	84	10	<1	–	–	–	–
Nannochloropsisgaditana	4	40	36	–	–	1.4	9	<1	<1	–	–	–	8
Scenedesmusobliquus	–	28	8	3	5	2	36	7	10	–	–	–	–
Phaeodactylum tricornutum	6	19	42	–	–	2	5	1	3	–	–	–	13

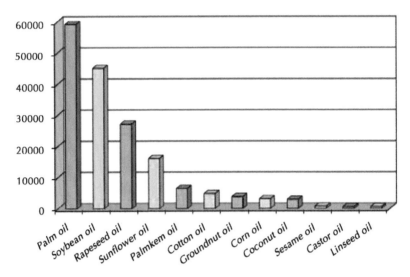

FIGURE 3.14A   Oils supply (2014) by type [70]. (From: http://www.fediol.eu/web/
world%20production%20data/1011306087/list1187970075/f1.html)

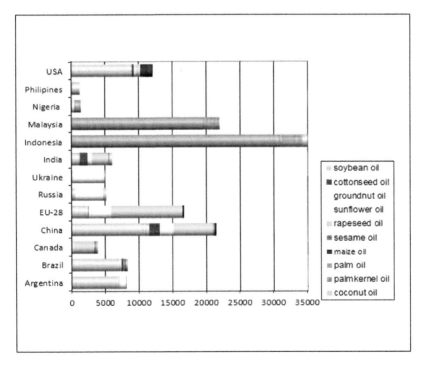

FIGURE 3.14B   Production of oil by Country (2014).
(From: http://www.fediol.eu/web/world%20production%20data/1011306087/list1187970075/f1.html)

as castor, linseed or tall oils are limited to about 1% of the global oils production. This is a point of attention as even in this area the conflict food-energy/chemistry must be solved. This means that new cultures of nonedible oils must be developed. Typical nonedible oils are castor oil and the algal oils, which show a much larger complexity that the terrestrial plant derived oils (Table 3.3, lower part). Algal oil composition may vary with strains, but even with the culture conditions of the same strain. Some oils are quite rich in saturated and monounsaturated C16-C18 Fas, suitable for direct FAMEs production for use as biodiesel. As an example, strain *N. gaditana* has a content of >41% of saturated Fas (C16+C18). However, algal oils are produced at higher costs than seed-oils and this is an issue for their economically convenient use as biodiesel source.

Vegetable oils are since long time an important renewable feedstock for the chemical industry, offering several advantages as low toxicity, inherent biodegradability, unique molecular structures usable for further modification (especially in the case of chemicals and materials), and in some cases, affordable costs. Nowadays, about 15% of oils production is consumed for chemicals, polymers and biofuels [71] and the chemical industry is paying a great attention to nonedible oils to avoid the food competition. The key interest is the development of cultures using marginal lands and nonedible species, favoring the agricultural biodiversity, an important aspect for the sustainability of renewable feedstocks.

As said above, biodiesel can be produced by hydrolysis/hydrogenation of lipids, that brings to long chain hydrocarbons (C16-C20+). But this is not the only way to go, as there is the possibility of designing new fuels with specific properties by new catalytic routes.

Table 3.4 gives an idea of the large network of reactions that can be carried out on oils for their conversion into chemicals and fuels. The application of any of the listed reactions may open new scenarios bringing to new products/fuels. In Table 3.4, two particular plants are mentioned, namely castor and lesquerella which were largely investigated in the EuroBioref Project funded by the European Union [64].

The application of the concept of biorefinery opens new potentialities, as one process residues can be used as raw material for another one and waste can be converted into valuable molecules.

The reactions listed in Table 3.4 can be networked in many ways and used in cascade so that the key features of the molecular structure of the biomass are used in an intelligent way, bringing to a more complex picture of

TABLE 3.4 Network of Reactions that May Convert Oils/Lipids into Chemicals and Fuels

Ester/Acid reactions	Double bonds reactions	Hydroxyl group reaction (castor in Table 3.5)
• Hydrolysis	• Oxidation	• Dehydration
• Esterification	• Epoxidation	• Caustic fusion
• Saponification	• Polymerisation	• Pyrolysis
• Reduction/hydrogenation	• Hydrogenation	• Alkoxylation
• Amidation	• Halogenation	• Esterification
• Halogenation	• Addition reaction	• Halogenation
• Nitrilation/ammoniation	• Sulfonation/Sulfurisation	• Urethane formation
	• Metathesis	• Sulfatation
	• Oxidative cleavage	
	• Hydroformylation	

opportunities for specific applications. An example is given in Figure 3.15, where the use of the various fatty acids is shown.

After this excursus on oleo-biomass, let us go back to biodiesel production. Fatty acids (FAs) had a worldwide production of 7.2 Mt in 2014 [72]. As said above, saturated FAs are ideal candidates for biodiesel, which is produced by a double acid-base esterification process (the acid process uses sulfuric acid and converts free-FAs into FAMEs: conversely, the basic process uses sodium methylate and converts glycerided into FAMEs and aqueous glycerol. A great improvement here is the use of heterogeneous bifunctional catalysts, which convert at the same time FFAs, and glycerides into FAMEs [73]. In order to eliminate excess unsaturated C=C bonds, polyunsaturated fatty acid esters can be hydrogenated into monounsaturated or saturated molecules. Also fatty alcohols can be produced by carbon-oxygen double bond hydrogenation. Furthermore, complete hydrogenation of unsaturated fatty acids derivatives or fatty alcohols can lead to the complete removal of oxygen and the formation of saturated hydrocarbons. Homogeneous or heterogeneous catalysts based on Group 8 -10 metals, such as Ni, Co, Pd, Pt ,and Rh, Cu are generally used to perform the partial hydrogenation of the carbon-carbon double bond under moderate operating conditions. During hydrogenation, isomerization (regio-isomerization and cis-trans isomerization) must be taken under control as trans isomers are undesired species as they do not undergo hydrogenation.

Catalytic hydrogenation of carbon-oxygen double bond requires more drastic conditions and can be achieved by using homogeneous or

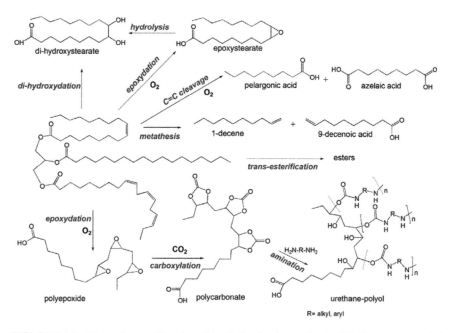

FIGURE 3.15 Uses of properties of the FAs chains for the synthesis of fuels and chemicals/materials.

heterogeneous catalysts. For heterogeneous catalysts, it is well recognized that the best catalysts have two different adsorption sites, a metallic center for H_2 adsorption and an electron deficient center like SnO_x for carbon-oxygen activation. Most of the current catalytic processes are based on copper-chromite, cobalt, and nickel catalysts. It is obvious that extensive hydrogenation will increase the biodiesel manufacture cost and make it less competitive with respect to fossil-C derived fuels. Also, the source of hydrogen is a key issue: it cannot be produced using fossil-C.

3.3.3 BIOGAS FROM ANAEROBIC DIGESTION OF LOW-LIGNOCELLULOSIC BIOMASS

Non-cellulosic fresh vegetal materials (the so called Fruit-Vegetal-Garden-FVG residues), animal manure, water treatment sludge, some residues of the food industry and other like materials are characterized by a high water content that does make their thermal treatment economically and energetically disadvantageous. Conversely, such humid biomass (HB) is suitable for the generation of energy products like methane *via* an anaerobic digestion process, a technology that during last years has found a renewed interest for the benefits it generates. Anaerobic digestion is an interesting route to the valorization of waste and contributes to: (i) reducing landfilling, that is under strict limitation in many countries, (ii) reduce water and soil pollution, (iii) water recovery and reutilization, while producing usable energy that would otherwise be lost.

An important aspect of anaerobic digestion is that the energy input factor (Energy in/Energy out) is less than one making the overall energetic balance positive (at least for medium-high concentrated waste and well designed and managed plants) giving to such technology a premium over other biological or nonbiological treatments.

It is worth to remind that the conversion of HB can also take place in presence of oxygen (aerobic treatment or composting), not discussed here.

As said, the anaerobic digestion converts organic carbon into "biogas," i.e., a mixture of methane and CO_2, from which the energy rich methane can be separated. The process takes place in a closed and controlled bioreactor and its cost is determined by capital investment (CAPEX) and operative costs (OPEX). In general, bioreactors are quite simple with not high CAPEX and OPEX, and can have various geometries (vertical, inclined, horizontal). The overall conversion efficiency is quite variable (30–55%) and depends on the amount of low biodegradable solid fraction (see below) present in the raw biomass (cellulose, lignin, hemicellulose are not easily biodegraded). The process has long retention times (20–30 days) [74]. Biogas technology is being continuously improved by optimizing the process parameters and reactor geometry [75] and with process integration. The methane separation technology is mature and continuously improved for its efficiency [76]. The produced gas can be locally used for thermal or electric energy production or else emitted into methanoducts.

Humid Biomass treatment must take place close to the area where it is produced for two main reasons:

- the low energy/volume density makes the transportation quite expensive;
- HB is a good substrate for bacterial growth and, therefore, is easily attacked by microorganisms with partial conversion that would occur in the containers during long-term transport.

The main theoretical bottlenecks to the application of an anaerobic process are:

- incomplete conversion of the substrate: often more than 50% of the organic material (the polymeric fraction) is not degraded, making the cellulosic biomass scarcely suited for biogas production;
- medium-or long-retention time;
- formation and persistence of some acids that may be polluting agents;
- Bacteria may need some nutrients that are not available in the original substrate. Their growth may be slow because of the scarce energy available;
- Permanence of ammonia (NH3) and other N-compounds.

A preliminary question to answer is whether or not a given HB is suited for biogas production. An answer to such question can be given either by laboratory scale test or by simple calculations.

The transformation of an organic molecule into methane and carbon dioxide during the anaerobic digestion process can be described by Eq. (8) in which a, b, c, d represent either the stoichiometric indexes of the elements in a well-defined compound or the elemental composition of a mixture of compounds, and α, β, γ, δ are the stoichiometric coefficients of species in the equation that represents the conversion of the compound/mixture into CH_4, CO_2, NH_3.

$$C_aH_bO_cN_d + \alpha H_2O \rightarrow \beta CH_4 + \gamma CO_2 + \delta NH_3 \qquad (8)$$

By applying a mass balance to Eq. (8), one can obtain Eq. (9)(i–iv).

i) $a = \beta + \gamma$ $\qquad\qquad\qquad\qquad\qquad\qquad\qquad\qquad (9)$
ii) $b + 2\alpha = 4\beta + 3\delta$
iii) $c + \alpha = 2\gamma$
iv) $d = \delta$

Solving the system of Eqs. (8) and (9), one obtains Eq. (10) that represents a molar ratio of the species CH_4, H_2O, NH_3 obtained from the raw material:

$$C_aH_bO_cN_d + \left(a - \frac{b}{4} - \frac{c}{2} + \frac{3d}{4}\right)H_2O \rightarrow \left(\frac{4a+b-2c-3d}{8}\right)CH_4 + \left(\frac{4a-b+2c+3d}{8}\right)CO_2 + dNH_3$$

$$(10)$$

The volume of methane will be given by Eq. (11) where 22.415 is the molar volume of gases at standard conditions, while methane abundance in the gas phase (P_{CH4}) will be given by Eq. (12).

$$B_0 - methane \left[\frac{m_n^3}{kg_{VS}} \right] = \frac{\dfrac{4a+b-2c-3d}{8}.22.415}{12a+b+16c+14d} \tag{11}$$

$$p_{CH_4} \left[\frac{m_{n-CH_4}^3}{m_{n-biogas}^3} \right] = \frac{B_{0-methane}}{B_{0-biogas}} = \frac{4a+b-2c-3d}{8} \tag{12}$$

From Eqs. (11) and (12) one can deduce that the methane content in the biogas will increase with the increase of the ratio H/C in the raw material.

The equations above allow to check in a quick mode whether a given biomass is suited for biogas production or not. Biogas that contains low percentage of methane (<40%) is not interesting, as the energy expenditure may not be compensated by the energy produced.

3.4 USE OF CO_2 FOR THE SYNTHESIS OF HIGH-ENERGY PRODUCTS

CO_2 can be used as source of carbon for the production of a variety of high-energy hydrogenated products, such as CH_4, CH_3OH, DME, Cn hydrocarbons. Their synthesis will be singularly discussed below.

3.4.1 DRY REFORMING OF METHANE

CO_2 (dry) reforming of methane (DRM) is becoming an attractive alternative to Steam Reforming in view of the fact that the latter produces large volumes of CO_2 while the former is a CO_2 consumer. DRM produces Syngas (1:1 mixture of CO and H_2 in the specific case, eq. 13) that can be used as feedstock for industrial processes such as Fischer–Tropsch, methanol synthesis or hydrocarbonylations [77]. Interestingly, DRM can use as feedstock either natural gas or biogas (produced from anaerobic fermentation of fresh biomass, see § 3.3.2.1.1.4): both contain large amount (40%+) of CO_2.

DRM (Eq. 14) is a strongly endothermic reaction, which has similar thermodynamics and equilibrium characteristics with steam reforming of methane (Eq. 13), which produces Syngas with higher H_2/CO ratio [51].

$$CH_4 + H_2O \rightarrow CO + 3H_2 \qquad \Delta H°_{298} = 228 \text{ kJ mol}^{-1} \qquad (13)$$

$$CO_2 + CH_4 \rightarrow 2CO + 2H_2 \qquad \Delta H°_{298} = 247 \text{ kJ mol}^{-1} \qquad (14)$$

The CO: H_2 ratio is affected by simultaneous occurrence of RWGS reactions (Eq. 15) that consumes H_2 and produces CO and steam, which enables the steam/carbon gasification (Eq. 16).

$$CO_2 + H_2 \rightarrow CO + H_2O \qquad \Delta H°_{298} = 41 \text{ kJ mol}^{-1} \qquad (15)$$

$$C + H_2O \text{ (g)} \rightarrow CO + H_2 \qquad \Delta H°_{298} = 131 \text{ kJ mol}^{-1} \qquad (16)$$

As a matter of fact, carbon deposition originated from methane decomposition (Eq. 17) and Boudouard reaction (Eq. 18) is a cause of catalyst deactivation and may damage the reactor [78].

$$CH_4 \rightarrow C_{ads}+2H_2 \qquad \Delta H°_{298} = 75 \text{ kJ mol}^{-1} \qquad (17)$$

$$2CO \rightarrow C_{ads}+CO_2 \qquad \Delta H°_{298} = -173 \text{ kJ mol}^{-1} \qquad (18)$$

Based on Boudouard equilibrium [79], coke formation by CO disproportionation is less favored at high temperatures (973 K and above). In general, the dissociation of methane occurs on metal surface to generate highly reactive C_α, which can be further gasified by reactions with H_2O, CO_2 or H_2 [79]. The encapsulation of metal atoms (e.g., Ni atoms) by carbon favors the rapid growth of carbon nanotubes (CNT), which can block the catalyst and plug the reactor system [80]. Therefore, in DMR the design of a highly active, stable and economically viable catalyst is a key issue, as the catalyst will both kinetically inhibit the coke formation, and improve the conversion in the DRM reaction. Interestingly, metals deposited on CNT (M@CNT) are used as catalysts (*vide infra*).

Throughout the past decades, the integration of DRM, SRM and partial oxidation of methane (POM) has been investigated in order to mitigate the negative thermodynamics of DRM and SRM: the concept of 'tri-reforming" was introduced by Song et al. [81]. Variable H_2/CO ratio can be obtained by adjusting the amount of CO_2, H_2O and O_2 in the feedstock, and carbon formation on the catalyst can be suppressed [82]. Also, the exothermic nature of POM provides energy for the reforming process, hence increasing the energy efficiency.

In DRM, noble metals such as Rh, Pt, Pd (resistant to corrosion and oxidation, good carbon resistance [83]) and some other transition metals such as Ru and Ni are used as catalysts. Rh, Pd, Pt and Ru are known to reduce carbon deposition. Due to their high cost and scarce availability, low loadings (e.g., *ca.* 0.5–1 wt% Pt on zirconia) of precious metal have been investigated [84, 85]. The size of the Pt particles and the stability of the carbonates formed from CO_2 on the support are crucial factors in determining the rate of carbon formation. Smaller Pt particles and supports such as zirconia with high affinity for carbonate promote the catalyst stability in DRM. The concentration of accessible surface atoms can also be a key factor [82]. As higher loadings of active metals can favor the conversion, cheaper metals have been used (Group 8 transition metals), Ni being the one that has comparable activity to noble metals [86], but, as aforementioned, nickel catalysts are prone to catalyst deactivation due to carbon formation. Nickel based catalysts of most suitable form for providing high activity and better carbon resistance, have been investigated such as bimetallic catalyst, oxide supported Ni catalyst, Ni based perovskite, and Ni core-shell structure catalysts which show interesting properties. DRM is even enhanced by addition of various promoters onto the catalyst surface [87], which promote CO_2 activation, improve metal dispersion [88, 89] and decrease coke formation [90]: they include oxides of Group 2 elements and La, such as La_2O_3, MgO, BaO and CaO. Promoters even contribute to a high catalytic activity and stability, strong metal-support interaction, as well as lattice oxygen mobility, factors of paramount importance in this reaction. Several other additives have been used or Ni has been structured in peculiar habitats, as summarized in Table 3.5, which improve the catalyst stability and improve DRM efficiency.

Therefore, the key to optimize the carbon resistance and promotion of activity of catalysts in DRM lies in good catalyst dispersion and promotion with adequate additives to enhance CO_2 adsorption and C-H activation. However, design and synthesis of novel nano-structured Ni catalysts will pave the way to future exploitation of DRM processes and coimplementation in existing industrial systems.

TABLE 3.5 Effect on Ni Activity/Stability in DRM upon: (i) Addition of Additives, (ii) Structuring Ni

Additive	Role	Effects	Notes
Ga_2O_3 on SiO_2	Form surface carbonate and hydrogencarbonate species	More facile reaction with the Deposited carbon than the h1-O linked CO_2 or physically adsorbed CO2 which leads to higher coke resistance	
Sr on La_2O_3	High mobility of O-surface	C-H activation and lower operational temperature (873 K)	
Group 1 metals on borated alumina	Highly active surface −OH groups	Easy oxidation of surface carbon species derived from methane decomposition	
Second metal (Pd on Ni)	Alloying causes catalyst modification	"Synergistic" effect between the two metals in using α-oxygen on Y_2O_3 surface fostering dissociation of CH_4	
Multimetal such as Ni-Co-Al-Mg-O	Higher stability and activity	Low deactivation of the catalyst in 2000 h operation	
Perovskite-type Ni $ANiO_3$ (A=lanthanide)	High thermal stability		
Spinel oxide Ni-based ABO_4 or A_2BO_4	High dispersion of NiO into the spinel, stability of the structure at low temperature formation of Ni phase in the same temperature region than the catalytic reaction and presence of Ni oxide.	Limit the growing of particles (7 nm). High conversion rate (85% for CH_4 and 93% for CO_2) with no carbon deposition after 160 h of operation [92]	Enhanced reaction between $La_2O_2CO_3$ and the Ni–CHx species
$LaSrNiO_3$	Lattice oxygen species highly active in C-H activation, low carbon formation	Increased efficiency, high stability	Formation of $La_2O_2CO_3$
Lanthanum-zirconate pyrochlores ($La_2Zr_2O_7$)	High thermal stability	Longer life and higher activity	
Nanocatalysts	High dispersion, minimization of surface energy, increasing the interaction with the support	Prevent agglomeration, longer life, higher activity	
Core-shell Ni@SiO_2	Metal@metal oxide nanoreactor	Resist sintering under high temperature (>1070 K) operations	Ni-phyllosilicate formation
NI in porous silica	Nano-ensembles of Ni	Lower temperature operation (<820K)	
Ni-silicide (Ni_3-Si_2)	Small Ni nanoparticles	High Syngas formation	
NiLaSi-OA + 1% La_2O_3	Good dispersion, no carbon deposition	>80% Syngas (near equilibrium)	OA is oleic acid

The reaction mechanisms for the DRM reaction have been widely studied and a variety of differing opinions expressed based on the type of active metal and nature of support. Most of the proposed mechanisms are based on the Langmuir-Hinshelwood-Hougen-Watson (LHHW) kinetic model, where one reaction step is assumed to be slow and rate determining, while the others are at thermodynamic equilibrium [93].

The major steps involved in the DRM reaction are dissociation of CH_4 and CO_2 followed by adsorption of intermediates on the active sites leading to formation of products, i.e., CO, H_2 and H_2O, which are eventually desorbed. Among these steps, activation of both CH_4 and CO_2 play the dominant role in the DRM reaction.

3.4.1.1 CH_4 Activation

The most kinetically significant step in the DRM reaction is the adsorption and subsequent activation of CH_4 which dissociates directly on the active metal, forming carbon, CH_x radicals or formyl intermediates and hydrogen adatoms as follows [88, 94, 95] (Eq. 19–22):

$$CH_{4(g)} \rightarrow CH_{3(a)} + H_{(a)} \tag{19}$$

$$CH_{3(a)} \rightarrow CH_{2(a)} + H_{(a)} \tag{20}$$

$$CH_{2(a)} \rightarrow CH_{(a)} + H_{(a)} \tag{21}$$

$$CH_{(a)} \rightarrow C_{(a)} + H_{(a)} \tag{22}$$

According to Rostrup Nielsen and Bak Hansen [83], during the reforming process, there exists the possibility for the formation of three types of carbon species, namely:

i)   Whisker-type carbon (formation temperature above 723 K).
ii) Encapsulating amorphous carbon formed *via* polymerization at temperatures less than 773 K.
iii) Pyrolytic carbon nanotubes formed by methane cracking at temperatures above 873 K.

The type of carbon formed depends on the reaction conditions, whereby higher reaction temperatures favor the formation of the more inert-graphitic carbon nanotubes. Based on kinetic and isotopic investigations on the mechanism of DRM reaction over Ni/MgO catalysts, Wei and Iglesia [96] observed a similarity in turnover rates and first order rate constants with CH_4 decomposition. Hence, they concluded that such dissociation is the kinetically relevant step for the DRM reaction and that the Ni behavior resembles that of supported noble metal catalysts (Rh, Pt, Ir, Ru). Several other studies have contributed specific knowledge to the role of the support and metal particles. A summary can be found in Ref. [89].

3.4.2 HYDROGENATION OF CO_2

A common issue for all processes discussed in this subchapter is the availability of hydrogen produced from nonfossil-C based sources. If large volumes of CO_2 must be converted, water and other cheap and abundant sources such as cultivated or residual biomass must be used as source of H_2 and H_2 must be obtained using perennial SWHG energy sources. The moment being, electrochemical generation of H_2 is the most suited route. In the medium-long-term, high temperature water splitting using Concentrators of Solar Power-CSP may become an alternative solution, or, even better, coprocessing of CO_2 and H_2O in photochemical devices at room temperature can become a practical solution. The thermodynamic stability of CO_2 requires high-energy coreagents or electroreductive processes for its transformation into valuable chemicals in which the carbon atom has a lower oxidation state than 4 [5, 97–100] and a H/C ratio >0. Catalytic hydrogenation of carbon dioxide has been acknowledged as one of the major technologies for CO_2 valorization to fuels, or other C1-molecules (e.g., HCOOH, CH_3OH, H_2CO) usable as either potential hydrogen carriers or useful chemicals [5, 97, 101].

Catalytic conversion of CO_2 to high-energy products such as light olefins and liquid hydrocarbons can generally proceed *via* either (i) conversion of CO_2 into CO that will be used in Fischer-Tropsch processes (a combination of CO_2 hydrogenation by RWGS and further hydrogenation of CO to hydrocarbons), or (ii) direct (without CO formation) hydrogenation of CO_2 to methanol, dimethyl ether (DME), higher alcohols, methane and higher hydrocarbons. Due to the stability of the CO_2 molecule, a nonfavorable thermodynamics and high kinetic barriers are expected. Hence, it is highly crucial to employ suitable catalysts, which can decrease the energy barriers, thus resulting in lower energy states of the system. Exploring the mechanistic pathways of such reactions may help to make the CO_2 conversion feasible at lower temperatures.

3.4.2.1   RWGS and Synthesis of C2+ Hydrocarbons

CO_2 hydrogenation may occur either *via* Reverse Water Gas Shift-(RWGS) (7.058) that produces CO [102], or via the formation of a formate species, $HC(O)O^-$, subsequently reduced to other C1 species (*vide infra*). RWGS [103], shown in Eq. [23], is an endothermic reaction occurring at high temperatures (>973 K).

$$CO_2 + H_2 = CO + H_2O \ \Delta H°_{298K} = 41.2 \text{ kJ mol}^{-1} \tag{23}$$

Several undesired parallel and side reactions tend to occur as well (Eqs. 24–26):

$$\text{Sabatier Reaction: } CO_2 + 4H_2 = CH_4 + 2H_2O \ \Delta H°_{298K} = -165 \text{ kJ mol}^{-1} \tag{24}$$

$$\text{Boudouard Reaction: } 2CO = C + CO_2 \ \Delta H°_{298K} = -172.6 \text{ kJ mol}^{-1} \tag{25}$$

$$\text{Methanation Reaction: } CO + 3H_2 = CH_4 + H_2O \ \Delta H°_{298K} = -206 \text{ kJ mol}^{-1} \tag{26}$$

All such reactions occur simultaneously any time H_2O, CO, CO_2, H_2, C are present in the reaction medium. Their control is of crucial importance in order to maximize the yield towards a target product. It has generally been assumed that most of the reaction mechanisms that occur for Water Gas Shift-WGS are also applicable for RWGS.

The two main mechanisms for WGS reactions proposed are: (i) surface redox mechanism; (ii) dissociative mechanism of water to afford OH and H species, with subsequent formation of formate species (HCO_2-M, obtained by an attack of OH groups on M-CO moieties) or metalla carboxyl species (M-CO_2H, which might result from the reaction of M-H moieties with CO_2 or even by protonation of metal-bound CO_2) as intermediates [102]. The catalysts used are common to the methanol synthesis (Table 3.6) and are based on the quaternary $CuO/ZnO/Al_2O_3$ system, added with various species for increasing the activity and stability [104–106].

3.4.2.2 Synthesis of Methanol and Dimethylether

3.4.2.2.1 Methanol

Methanol is a fuel or a building block in the chemical industry due its versatility in the synthesis of several important chemicals such as chloromethane and other chlorinated C-1 species, acetic acid, methyl tert-butyl ether (MTBE), and formaldehyde [47, 107–108]. The relevant dimethyl ether (DME) is attracting a lot of attention as it can be used in fuel cells and diesel engines [109]. Methanol is also used for the production of higher hydrocarbons (through the methanol-to-gasoline route [110–112]) or of unsaturated hydrocarbons (through the methanol to olefins-MTO or

TABLE 3.6 Catalysts Used in the Synthesis of methanol and DME, Also Active in RWGS, and the Properties of Additives

Catalyst	Conditions	Notes
ZnO Cr_2O_3	20 MPa 573 K	Original BASF process (1923)
$CuO/ZnO/Al_2O_3$		ZnO favors Cu particles dispersion
CuO/ZrO_2		ZrO_2 produces higher surface area and higher selectivity
$CuO/ZnO/Ga_2O_3$	523–543 K	Ga_2O_3 promotes dispersion ans stabilization of Cu-centers
$CuO/ZnO/CeO_2$		CeO_2 enhances the hydrogenation rate of intermediates
$CuO/ZnO/Al2O_3/ZrO_2/$ HSMZ-5		HSMZ-5 favors water elimination and DME formation
$CuO/ZnO/CNT$-Pd		CNT disperses the Cu centers, Pd fosters the CO_2 hydrogenation
$CuO/ZnO/FeOx$		Fe prevents Cu-aggregation and oxidation
CuO-$Fe_2O_3/HZSM$-5/Zr		Zr improves DME selectivity
$CuO/ZnO/Al_2O_3/ZrO_2/$ HSMZ-5/Pd		Pd enhances DME production and retards the CO formation due to spillover of H
Co and Co/Fe		Increase the formation of methane
Ni/Al_2O_3		Favours methanation

methanol to propene-MTP routes). It is currently produced from Syngas as feedstock with some CO_2 left in for a better use of H_2 (ICI process).

In general, CO_2 is gaining prominency as substitute of toxic CO, derived from fossil carbon [113], in several processes. Even though hydrogenation of CO_2 to methanol has favorable thermodynamics (Eq. 27) high activation energy barriers must be overcome and this requires the use of appropriate catalysts.

$$CO_2 + 3H_2 \; CH_3OH + H_2O \quad \Delta H^\circ_{298K} = -49.5 \; kJ \; mol^{-1} \tag{27}$$

Formation of other by-products during the CO_2 hydrogenation, such as CO, hydrocarbons and higher alcohols [99] requires highly selective heterogeneous catalysts with the important function of improving the process sustainability. CuO-ZnO is the most used catalyst, added with several other oxides having peculiar roles (Table 3.6).

Despite the numerous theories on the mechanistic pathways thesis, and the extensive investigation, there is still uncertainty on the definition of the role of Cu°, Cu^+, Cu-Zn alloy and the carrier sites [114]. In the past, it has been assumed that CO hydrogenation is the main pathway for methanol synthesis. However, isotopic labeling experiments conducted by Chinchen et al. [115] have revealed that methanol is formed directly from CO_2, while CO scavenges the oxygen atoms, which hinder the active metal sites [116, 117].

According to earlier proposed mechanisms, formate hydrogenation on CuO/ZnO catalysts is the rate-limiting steps-RDS. This is based on data reported by Fujitani et al. [118] who found that the formate coverage on CuO/ZnO catalysts is proportional to the turn over frequency for methanol formation. The proposed reaction pathway is shown in Eqs. (28)–(30).

$$CO_2 + \tfrac{1}{2}H_2 \leftrightarrow HCOO_{(a)} \tag{28}$$

$$HCOO_{(a)} + 2H_{(a)} \leftrightarrow CH_3O_{(a)} + O_{(a)} \, (RDS) \tag{29}$$

$$CH_3O_{(a)} + H_{(a)} \leftrightarrow CH_3OH \tag{30}$$

Recent kinetic studies claim that the RDS is the formation and hydrogenation of a dioxo-methylene reactive intermediate (M-O-C(H₂)-O-M') on ZnO and ZrO_2 surface sites in the interface with Cu. Noteworthy, such dioxomethylene intermediate, is only rarely mentioned in general and has not been identified neither *via* experimental nor theoretical studies in most systems. Its formation may be linked to the nature of the support that also may play a key role in driving the mechanism in different directions.

Thermodynamically, a decrease of the reaction temperature or an increase of the reaction pressure can favor the synthesis of methanol. A reaction temperature higher than 513 K facilitates the CO_2 activation and, consequently, the methanol formation [99, 100, 119].

3.4.2.2.2 Dimethyl Ether

Dimethyl ether (DME, CH_3OCH_3) is generally produced *via* methanol dehydration (Eq. 32). It can even be directly produced by CO_2 hydrogenation. DME is an efficient alternative to petroleum based transportation fuels (due to its high cetane number, 40% higher than diesel and much better than methanol itself) and liquefied natural gas and has been found to lead to a low environmental impact since it does not generate sulfur oxide or soot [120, 121]. In the chemical industry, DME is a useful intermediate for the synthesis of chemicals such as methyl acetate, dimethyl acetate and light olefins [122, 123]. Two main pathways bring to DME from CO_2: (i) a two-step process, i.e., methanol is synthesized on a suitable metal catalyst, which is then dehydrated on an acid catalyst (Eq. 31), and (ii) a single-step process, using a bifunctional catalyst that produces methanol and causes its dehydration [124].

Eqs. (31)–(33) summarizes the thermodynamic properties of the conventional (CO based) synthesis of DME *via* the 2-step process [122, 125, 126] as compared to the one step synthesis based on CO_2.

Conventional 2-step synthesis based on CO
(i) Methanol synthesis

$$CO + 2H_2 \rightarrow CH_3OH \quad \Delta H°_{298K} = -90.6 \text{ kJ mol}^{-1} \qquad (31)$$

(ii) Methanol dehydration (in the presence of solid acid catalyst)

$$2CH_3OH \rightarrow CH_3OCH_3 + H_2O \quad \Delta H°_{298K} = -23.4 \text{ kJ mol}^{-1} \qquad (32)$$

One-step reaction for the synthesis of DME from CO_2

$$2CO_2 + 6H_2 \rightarrow CH_3OCH_3 + 3H_2O \quad \Delta H°_{298K} = -122.2 \text{ kJ mol}^{-1} \quad (33)$$

The one step process, which integrates the methanol synthesis and its dehydration to DME, reduces the investment and operational cost since only one reactor is required [127]. However, for the one step process, catalyst selection is extremely crucial in order to minimize CO formation *via* RWGS reaction [126]. The study of the mechanism for the one step reaction still needs investigation and much work is necessary for developing active bifunctional catalysts. The studies carried out so far [122] indicate that the DME formation is driven by two factors, which are temperature dependent. Below 498 K the reaction is dominated by kinetics, while above 498 K thermodynamics predominates. A multisite mechanism has been proposed, in which methanol is formed on metal sites while H-ZMS provides the dehydration. $Cu°$ is implied in H_2 activation, $ZnO\text{-}ZrO_2$ in CO_2 activation. Spillover of H onto CO_2 produces formate, which undergoes reduction to the methoxo group $M\text{-}OCH_3$ via dioxomethylene/methoxy species [128, 129]. The dehydration is a fast reaction that reaches the equilibrium [126].

3.4.2.3   Hydrogenation to Methane and Superior Hydrocarbons

The hydrogenation of CO_2 to methane is known since very long time [130] and well advanced in application. It is a proof of concept of the fact that storing SW perennial energies into a chemical bond (chemical energy) is much more advantageous from the point of view of the *capacity* than storing it into batteries as electrons. The reaction (Eq. 34) occurs in a wide range of temperature (473–830 K) depending on the catalyst used. The pressure is generally around 2.5 MPa.

$$CO_2 + 4H_2 \rightarrow CH_4 + 2H_2O \quad \Delta H = -165 \text{ kJ/mol} \quad (34)$$

The reaction is strongly exothermic, and this implies the necessity of a strict control of the temperature in the reactor. Besides CH_4, ethane is formed and some coke.

The formation of methane is favored up to maximum 873 K, temperature at which ΔG is equal to zero. At a temperature of 823 K and pressure of 0.1 MPa the conversion into methane is 78%, while at 2 MPa a conversion of

93% can be achieved. Under such conditions ethane concentration is very low, as C2 formation is not favored above 680 K [131].

The catalyst used is based on Ni and must be accurately formulated in order to resist the thermal changes and be stable under the operative conditions. Co,Fe-catalysts have also been used [131] The reactor design has a crucial importance for eliminating heat and assuring good isothermal conditions [132]. In general two stages-fixed bed reactors are used, even with special geometries for easy heat exchange. An interesting review has been recently published [133] which makes an analysis of reaction conditions.

Interestingly, the catalytic (Ni-zeolite pellets, 10% loading) low-temperature plasma technology has been used for the methanation of CO_2, [134] showing a very beneficial influence of nonthermal plasma on CO_2 (or CO) conversion that reaches an interesting 93% value. It has been deduced that the use of plasma radiations speeds-up the rate-determining-step of the reaction. Plasma even influences the size of the Ni-particles, which under plasma conditions are smaller and better distributed than in thermal conditions (633 K max).

More recently, it has been shown that Fe@CNT has an interesting reduction capacity of CO_2 with H_2, and the product distribution (C1-Cn) can be controlled with additives (alkali metals and others) [135]. The authors have optimized the reaction temperature, pressure and feed gas flow rate to maximize conversion and selectivity towards (valuable) long chain HCs and/or short olefins. The addition of promoters (particularly alkali metals) further improves both, particularly shifting selectivity away from CH_4 and significantly increasing the olefin/paraffin ratio up to C7 HCs.

CO_2 can be, thus, hydrogenated to afford high-energy products such as CO, methanol (or DME) and CH_4 or HCs. Such reactions make a complex network and are interrelated, not only in terms of reaction pathways (Scheme 5), but also in terms of the catalysts used.

The reaction pathways are mainly determined by the nature and properties of the catalyst, i.e., redox properties or acid-base properties, and supports. Recent advances in the synthesis of highly dispersed nano-catalysts appear to be promising in terms of carbon resistance.

The simplest CO_2 hydrogenation reaction is the RWGS reaction which converts CO_2 into CO. CO_2 can be used for methanol production *via* formate: instead of going through the Syngas route, methanol and DME can directly be produced *via* CO_2 hydrogenation. The most widely used catalysts for CO_2 hydrogenation are Cu-based. Evidence of the formate route has recently been gained that changes the belief that CO_2 is first converted into CO through RWGS and then the Syngas route is followed. Catalysts which are good for RWGS can also be modified and used for direct methanol synthesis from CO_2. Methanol molecules can further undergo dehydration to produce DME in a separate process, but the direct conversion of CO_2 to DME in a single reactor is now being considered. Such approach requires the modification of the methanol synthesis catalysts so to have acid functions to promote DME formation.

As a conclusion, the use of CO_2 as a carbon source for the synthesis of various energy rich molecules *via* the high temperature reactions discussed in this section shows a great potential for industrial exploitation on a large scale. Rational designs of active catalysts play a key role in terms of improvement towards reaction activity and selectivity. The use of solar energy *via* solar power concentrators would be highly beneficial in this field that deals with endergonic reactions carried out at high temperature, despite its discontinuity than can be buffered using heat storage systems such as molten salts.

Co-processing of CO_2 and water under solar irradiation at room temperature to afford chemicals and fuels, would represent a great achievement: but this is a long-term objective.

3.5   HYBRID TECHNOLOGIES: INTEGRATION OF BIOTECHNOLOGY AND CHEMICAL CATALYSIS

Biotechnology, which provides new opportunities for sustainable production of existing and new products and services, can be applied to the conversion of CO_2 into useful products under optimized conditions by using (modified) organisms. Possible applications include:

1. Aquatic biomass production from which specialty chemicals, food and feed, and materials are produced by using chemical technologies.
2. Advanced biotechnological processes, where the ability of cyanobacteria (a branch of microalgae) to use CO_2 as a *carbon source* and sunlight for energy are merged with the metabolic pathways of known microorganisms.
3. CO_2 fermentation, where CO_2 is fermented to a desired molecule using hydrogen produced in situ as energy carrier.

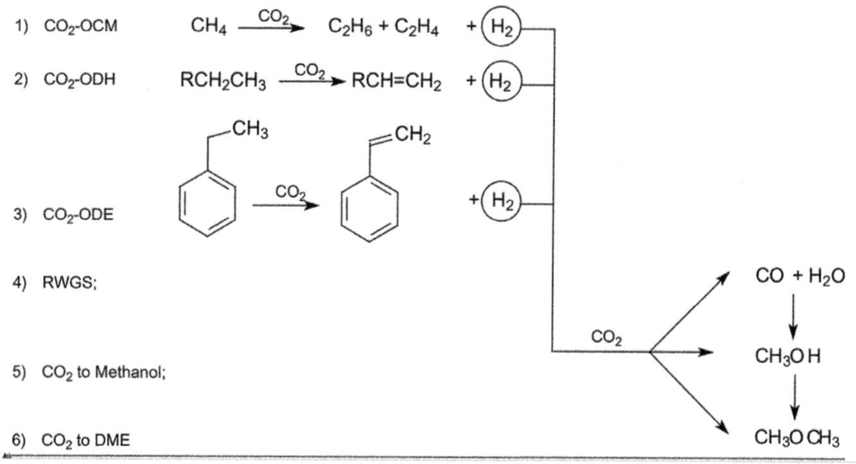

1) CO$_2$-OCM CH$_4$ $\xrightarrow{CO_2}$ C$_2$H$_6$ + C$_2$H$_4$ + (H$_2$)

2) CO$_2$-ODH RCH$_2$CH$_3$ $\xrightarrow{CO_2}$ RCH=CH$_2$ + (H$_2$)

3) CO$_2$-ODE   (benzene with CH$_3$) $\xrightarrow{CO_2}$ (benzene with CH$_2$) + (H$_2$)

4) RWGS;

5) CO$_2$ to Methanol;

6) CO$_2$ to DME

CO$_2$ → CO + H$_2$O → CH$_3$OH → CH$_3$OCH$_3$

SCHEME 5 Network of reactions showing the role of CO$_2$ in dehydrogenation or hydrogenation reactions.

4. Bioelectrochemical systems, where enzymes or microorganisms use CO$_2$ as a carbon source and PV-electricity as energy source;

5. Man-made photosynthesis, where CO$_2$ is converted to desired chemicals with a (bio)catalyst reacting with water, under conditions mimicking natural processes.

3.5.1 AQUATIC BIOMASS TECHNOLOGIES

The production of aquatic biomass (micro and macroalgae) is quite attractive for CO$_2$ enhanced fixation as it has a very high photosynthetic efficiency (6–8% solar energy utilization) higher than terrestrial biomass (1.5–2.2%). To date, microalgae [136] have been intensively studied, but now interest has been extended also to marine macroalgae [137]. CO$_2$ derived from power plants or recovered from Industrial flue gases could be pumped into a photobioreactor or into ponds under controlled conditions as a source of carbon [138], supposed that the content of NOx (max 150 ppm) and SOy (max 200 ppm) is kept under control. Strains have been cultivated with ambient air containing 10% CO$_2$ [139].

Algal biomass contains three main components (Figure 3.16): carbohydrates, proteins and lipids.

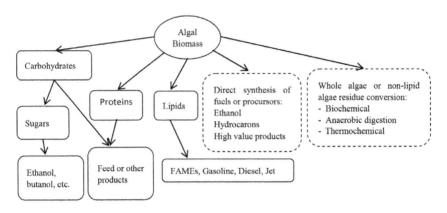

FIGURE 3.16 Production and conversion to fuels and products.

Although microalgae are not the main target of this paper, nevertheless it is useful to summarize the products obtainable from algal biomass (Table 3.7).

Several microalgae are industrially produced for different uses (Table 3.8).

Fuels such as biodiesel, biogas, bioethanol or bio-hydrogen can be produced from aquatic biomass. The quality and composition of the biomass will suggest the best option for the biofuel to be produced. A biomass rich in lipids (40–70%) will be suitable for the production of bio-oil and biodiesel, while a biomass rich in sugars will be better suited for the production of bioethanol. The anaerobic fermentation of the aquatic biomass (sugars, proteins, organic acids) will produce biogas. Noteworthy,

TABLE 3.7 Useful Substances Contained in Algal Biomass

Pigments/carotenoids	ε-carotene, lycopene, γ-carotene and β-carotene, xanthophylls astaxanthin, canthaxanthin, β-cryptoxanthin, echinenone, myxoxanthophyll and oscillaxanthin
Poly unsaturated fatty acids (PUFAs)	γ-linolenic acid (GLA-C18:3), arachidonic acid (AA-C20:4), eicosapentaenoic acid (EPA-C20:5) and docosahexaenoic acid (DHA-C22:6)
Antioxidants	Catalases, poluphenols, superoxide, dismutase, tocopherols
Vitamins	A, B1, B6, B12, C, E, Biotin, riboflavin, nicotinic acid, pantothenate, folic acid
Others	Antigungal, antimicrobial and antiviral agents, toxins, aminoacids, proteins, sterols

TABLE 3.8 Producers of Microalgae and Products

Microalgae species	Application/product	Company	Country
Nannochloropsis	Cosmetics and aquaculture	Astaxa	Germany
Tetraselmis			
Phaeodactylum			
Nannochloropsis	PUFA, omega 3, EPA astaxantin	Bluebiotech	Germany
Haematococcus pluvialis			
Spirulina			
Chlorella			
Haematococcus pluvialis	Astaxantin/human, fish and animal consumption	Alga technologies	Israel
Nannochloropsis Sp	Food additives, animal and fish feed, biofuel	Seambiotic	Israel
Phaeodactylum tricornutum			
Amphora sp			
Navicula sp			
Dunaliella sp			
Chlorococcum sp			
Tetraselmis sp			
Nannochloris sp			
Haematococcus pluvialis	Astaxantin	Biogenic Co. Ltd	Japan
Haematococcus pluvialis	Astaxantin	Cyanotech	USA
Spirulina			

TABLE 3.8 (Continued)

Microalgae species	Application/product	Company	Country
Chlorella	Biofuels, nutritional, health sciences, chemicals	Solazyme	USA
Spirulina	DHA/dietary supplements, acquaculture feeds, cosmetics	Femico	Taiwan
Chlorella			
Crypthecodinium Cohnii			
Dunaliella salina	Nutraceuticals, pharmaceuticals, health, and agricultural	Micoperi Blue Growth	Italy
Chlorella vulgaris			
Haematococcus pluvialis			
Arthrosphira platensgarisis			
Phaeodactylum tricornutum			

algae contain a limited amount of cellulosic materials and do not contain lignin.

Conditions for an extensive use of such approach is the use of process water that may contain nutrients for the growth of the biomass: the addition of nutrients (micro and macro) out-balances both the economics and carbon balance, making this technology not useful for CO_2 reduction.

Of particular interest is the utilization of synthetic biology and genomics to enhance the productivity and increase the utility of algae to produce advanced plastics and chemicals from biomass generated from CO_2. Genetic engineering of the (micro)organism or inclusion of bacterial genes into the algal strains are considered as an alternative to produce plastic materials with new properties meeting economic standards. The production of copolymers using a mix of fossil fuel derived and biomass-derived monomers are also a quite interesting approach. Several polymers have been produced and they include: collagen, gelatine, alginates, casein, elastin, and zein, used in the production of medical textiles.

3.5.2 OTHER BIOTECHNOLOGICAL APPLICATIONS

3.5.2.1   Advanced Biotechnological Processes

Many cyanobacterial species are easier to genetically manipulate than eukaryotic algae and other photosynthetic organisms and are being engineered for the production of chemicals directly from CO_2 [140].

Polyhydroxyalkanoate (PHA), a type of biodegradable polymer for potential application in biomedical or pharmaceutical field, is produced by several cyanobacteria such as *Aphanothece* sp. [141], *Oscillatoria limosa* [142], some species of the genus *Spirulina* [143, 144], and the thermophilic strain *Synechococcus* sp. MA19 [145] Genetic modification has been used [146]. The highest PHA production obtained from photosynthetic cultures of genetically *Synechocystis* sp. was 14 wt%. High PHA accumulation of up to 52% dry cell weight was demonstrated in marine cyanobacterium *Synechococcus* sp. PCC 7002 [147].

The modified *Synechococcus elongatus* PCC 7942 has been used for direct photosynthetic conversion of CO_2 to 3-hydroxypropionic acid (3HP) [148] and also used to produce 1-butanol from CO_2 [149]. Cyanobacterium *Synechocystis sp.* has been also engineered to produce isoprene (120 mg g^{-1}) and/or ethylene.

3.5.2.2 Bioelectrochemical Systems

Bioelectrochemical systems (BES) have recently been proposed as a new and sustainable technology for generation of energy and useful products from wastes: in a BES, bacteria interact with solid-state electrodes by exchanging electrons with them, either directly or via redox mediators [150].

A possible application is the electrochemical reduction of carbon dioxide to methane according to the following reaction:

$$CO_2 + 8\,H^+ + 8e^- \rightarrow CH_4 + 2H_2O \qquad (35)$$

$$CO_2 + 4H_2 \rightarrow CH_4 + 2H_2O \qquad (36)$$

Indeed, both the electrons and the carbon dioxide released at the anode during the microbial oxidation of the organic matter contained in a waste stream can be in principle exploited for the cathodic generation of methane, according to the schematic drawing reported in Figure 3.17. At

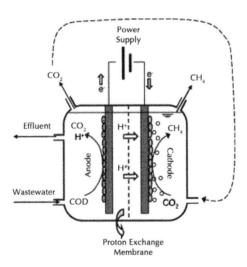

FIGURE 3.17 Schematic drawing of a bioelectrochemical system for wastewater treatment and simultaneous CH_4 production based on bioelectrochemical CO_2 reduction [151]. (Reprinted with permission from Villano, M., Aulenta, F., Ciucci, F. A. C., Ferri, T., Giuliano, A., & Majone, M. (2010). Bioelectrochemical reduction of CO_2 to CH_4 via direct and indirect extracellular electron transfer by a hydrogenophilic methanogenic culture *Biores. Technol., 101*(9), 3085–3090. © 2010 Elsevier.)

standard conditions, this reaction requires a theoretical voltage of -0.244 V (vs. SHE) at pH 7, but it is usually affected by quite large overpotentials that, however, could be possibly reduced by using a microbial biocathode.

Although some enzymatic reaction systems have been reported that can interconvert CO_2 to formate electrochemically [152], these enzymes originate from strictly anaerobic microbes with extremely weak stability in the presence of oxygen, which could be a severe obstacle for the application of enzymatic CO_2 reduction. Although one example of oxygen-tolerant formate dehydrogenase has been reported, this enzyme requires an expensive NADH cofactor with hydrogen gas as an electron donor [153]. In addition, the use of separated enzymes requires extra purification steps that may increase the cost of the reaction system.

Interestingly, in order to facilitate the process microbial whole cell system has been used that can be applied in aerobic conditions without use of cofactors, such as NAD(P)H, for electro-biocatalytic reduction of CO_2. *Methylobacterium* microbial were found to produce formate from CO_2 by using electrons supplied from cathode electrode [154, 155].

Bioelectrochemical systems have been used also for the microbial electrosynthesis (MES) to generate acetate from the biocathodic reduction of carbon dioxide. Bicarbonates (dissolved form of carbon dioxide) has been used as the substrate for the bioelectrochemical production of acetate under mild applied cathodic potential of -400 mV (vs SHE) in single chamber electrochemical cells [156].

3.5.2.3 CO_2 Fermentation

Work on gas fermentation started in the late 1980s at the University of Kansas. The microorganisms are obligate anaerobes and the best known among them are Clostridia, e.g., *Clostridium ljungdahlii* or *C. autoethanogenum*. They are able to exploit carbon monoxide, with or without hydrogen, or carbon dioxide/hydrogen mixtures. The idea to convert CO_2 and H_2 to biomethane (Eq. 37) through a chemoautotrophic conversion mediated by methanogenic *archaea* is still undeveloped because most of the H_2 production worldwide came so far from steam reforming of CH_4 [157].

However, if one consider the implementation of renewable energies and produce H_2 from wind and solar power through water electrolysis can consider the transformation of carbon dioxide to biomethane, which can be injected into natural gas (NG) grids or employed as fuel for vehicles, very attractive [158].

CO_2 can be selectively fermented to specialty, commodity chemicals, food components or fuels using metabolically engineered biocatalysts with high product selectivity [159] in contrast with chemical syngas catalysis characterized by low selectivity. CO_2-rich syngas or captured CO_2 with added hydrogen can be completely fermented by engineered biocatalyst with zero CO_2 process emissions to target product with inexpensive H_2 source available (sea water hydrolysis using electricity produced by the DOE approved high efficiency solar panels in situ) [159].

Acetogenic bacteria are used to produce alcohols and organic acids directly from CO_2 and H_2. In particular *Clostridium carboxidivorans* and *Clostridium ragsdalei* can metabolize syngas components to produce ethanol and acetic acid [160–163].

3.5.2.4 Man-Made Photosynthesis

Nature—that generates up to 115 billion metric tons of biomass annually from the reduction of CO_2 using solar energy—provides inspiration to develop artificial systems able to capture solar energy to convert CO_2 and H_2O to value-added chemicals. Two classes of enzyme, carbon monoxide dehydrogenases (CODH) and formate dehydrogenases (FDH), catalyze two-electron reduction of CO_2, the first and crucial stage of its entry into organic chemistry. The enzymes avoid radical intermediates such as CO_2^- or COOH (-1.9 V *vs.* SHE at pH 7 [164]) proceeding instead *via* proton-coupled electron transfers (PCET) in single concerted steps to CO or HCOOH. Both CODH and FDH are reversible electrocatalysts when attached to graphite electrodes [165, 166], suggesting their potential as CO_2 reduction catalysts in (bench-scale) man made photosynthesis systems.

Interesting is also the hybrid bioinspired systems used for the enzymatic reduction of CO_2 to CH_3OH in water [167] that combines two processes: the enzymatic reduction of CO_2 to CH_3OH promoted by the reduced form of coenzyme NADH with the *in situ* photocatalytic reduction of NAD^+ to afford NADH, using semiconductors. The objective is to reach a highly efficient and selective reduction of NAD^+ upon visible-light irradiation to 1,4-NADH or other equally active isomers. To this end a number of semiconducting materials that behave as photocatalysts and absorb visible-light, such as: Cu_2O, $InVO_4$, TiO_2 modified either with the organic compound rutin, or with the inorganic complex $[CrF_5(H_2O)]^{2-}$) [168] and the doped sulfide Fe/ZnS have been prepared and used for the reduction of NAD^+ to NADH.

Regeneration of the cofactor NADH from NAD^+ has been achieved by using visible light-active heterogeneous TiO_2-based photocatalysts. The efficiency of the regeneration process is enhanced by using a Rh^{III}-complex for facilitating the electron and hydride transfer from the H-donor (water or a water-glycerol solution) to NAD^+. In this way one mol of NADH was used for producing from 100 to 1000 mol of CH_3OH, opening the way to a practical application using as mediator a Rh-complex [167].

Interesting is also the system were a newly developed graphene-based photocatalyst is integrated sequentially with enzymes formate dehydrogenase, formaldehyde dehydrogenase, and alcohol dehydrogenase as depicted in Figure 3.18 [169].

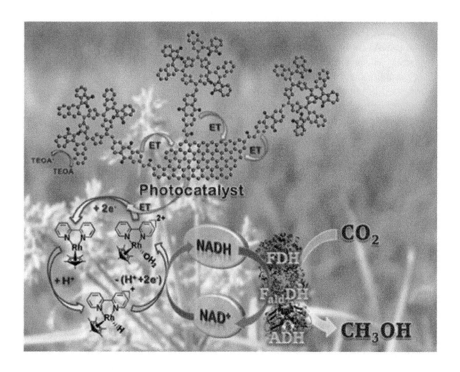

FIGURE 3.18 Schematic illustration of photocatalyst/biocatalyst integrated system to reduce CO_2 to methanol. (Adapted with permission from Yadav, R. K., Oh, G. H., Park, N.-J., Kumar, A., Kong, K-J., & Baeg, J.-O. (2014). Highly Selective Solar-Driven Methanol from CO_2 by a Photocatalyst/Biocatalyst Integrated System. J. Am. Chem. Soc., 136, 16728–16731. © 2014 American Chemical Society.)

KEYWORDS

- **biomass**
- **carbon dioxide**
- **carbon-economy**
- **high-energy products**
- **hybrid technologies**

REFERENCES

1 Aresta, M., Forti, G., (Eds.), *Carbon dioxide as Carbon Source*, Biochemical and Chemical Uses, NATO ASI Series C206, D. Reidel Publ, Dordrecht, Holland (1987).

2. Aresta, M., (Ed.), *Carbon Dioxide Recovery and Utilization*, Kluwer Acad Publ., Dordrecht, The Netherlands (2003).

3. Aresta, M., (Ed.), *Carbon Dioxide as Chemical Feedstock*, Wiley VCH, Verlag GmbH& Co. KGaA, Weinheim (2010).

4. Aresta, M., & Dibenedetto, A. (2007). Utilization of CO_2 as a chemical feedstock: opportunities and challenges. *Dalton Trans* 2975–2992.

5. Aresta, M., Dibenedetto, A., & Angelini, A. (2014). Catalysis for the valorization of exhaust carbon: from CO_2 to chemicals, materials and fuels. Technological use of CO_2. *Chem Rev., 114*, 1709–1742.

6. Aresta, M., Dibenedetto, A., & Dutta, A. (2016). Energy issues in the utilization of CO_2 in the synthesis of chemicals: The case of the direct carboxylation of alcohols to dialkyl-carbonates. *Catal. Today* http://dx.doi.org/10.1016/j.cattod.2016.02.046 2016.

7. Aresta, M., Dibenedetto, A., & Quaranta, E. (2016). State-of-the-art and perspectives in catalytic processes for CO_2 conversion into chemicals and fuels: the distinctive contribution of chemical catalysis and biotechnology *J. Catal.*, http://dx.doi.org/10.1016/j.jcat.2016.04.003.

8. *https://iea-bioenergy-task42biorefineries.com.*, Introduction IEA Bioenergy Task42 "Biorefining in a Future BioEconomy" in new triennium (2016-2018) Newsletter Number 1., May 2016.

9. Aresta, M., Dibenedetto, A., Dumeignil, F., (Eds.), *Biorefinery: from biomass to chemicals and fuels,* De Gruyter, Germany (2012).

10. Mohan, D., Pittman, C. U. Jr., & Steele, P. H. (2006). Pyrolysis of wood/biomass for bio-oil: a critical review. *Energy Fuel, 20*, 848–889.

11. Venderbosch, R. H., & Prins, W. (2010). Fast pyrolysis technology development. *Biofuel Bioprod Bioref., 4*, 178–208.

12. Marsman, J. H., Wildschut, J., Mahfud, F., & Heeres, H. J. (2006). Identification of components in fast pyrolysis oil and upgraded products by comprehensive two-dimensional gas chromatography and flame ionization detection. *J. Chromatogr A., (1150).* 21–27.

13. Samolada, M. C., Baldauf, W., & Vasalos, I. A. (1998). Production of a bio-gasoline by upgrading biomass flash pyrolysis liquids via hydrogen processing and catalytic cracking. *Fuel, 7*, 1667–1675.

14. Oasma, A., & Czernik, S. (1999). Fuel oil quality of biomass pyrolysis oils - State-of-the-art for the end users. *Energ Fuel., 13*, 914–921.

15. Czernik, S., & Bridgwater, A. V. (2004). Overview of applications of biomass fast pyrolysis oil. *Energy Fuel, 18*, 590–598.

16. Yaman, S. (2004). Pyrolysis of biomass to produce fuels and chemical feedstocks. *Energ. Convers. Manage, 45*, 651–671.

17. Adjaye, J. D., Sharma, R. K., & Bakhshi, N. N. (1992). Characterization and stability analysis of wood-derived bio-oil. *Fuel Process Technol., 3*, 1241–1256.

18. Zhang, Q., Chang, J., Wang, T., & Xu, Y. (2007). Review of biomass pyrolysis oil properties and upgrading Research. *Energ. Convers. Manage, 48*, 87–92.

19. Lappas, A. A., Kalogiannis, K. G., Iliopoulou, E. F., Triantafyllidis, K. S., & Stefanidis, S. D. (2012). Catalytic pyrolysis of biomass for transportation fuels. *WIREs: Energy and Environment, 1*, 285–297.

20. Huber, G. W., Iborra, S., & Corma, A. (2006). Synthesis of transportation fuels from biomass: chemistry, catalysts, and engineering. *Chem. Rev., 10*, 64044–4098.

21. Elliott, D. (2007). Historical developments in hydroprocessing bio-oils. *Energ. Fuel, 21*, 1792–1815.

22. Furimsky, E. (2000). Catalytic hydrodeoxygenation. *App. Cat. A: Gen, 199*, 147–190.

23. Demirbas, A. (2007). Progress and recent trends in biofuels. *Progr. Energy Combust. Sci, 33*, 1–18.

24. Demirbas, M. F. (2009). Biorefineries for biofuel upgrading: A critical review. *Appl. Energy, 86*, S151-S161.

25. Bulushev, D. A., & Ross, J. R. H. (2011). Catalysis for conversion of biomass to fuels via pyrolysis and gasification. *Catal. Today, 171*, 1–13.

26. Melero, J. A., Iglesias, J., & Garcia, A. (2012). Biomass as renewable feedstock in standard refinery units. Feasibility, opportunities and challenges. *Energy Environ. Sci., 5*, 7393–7420.

27. Bridgwater, A. V. (2002). The future for biomass pyrolysis and gasification: status, opportunities and policies for Europe, ALTENER Contract No: 4.1030/S/01–009/2001, *Bio-Energy Research Group*, Aston University, Birmingham B4 7ET, UK,

28. Faaij, A. P. C. (2006). Bio-energy in Europe: changing technology choices. *Energy Policy, 34*(3), 322–342.

29. Bridgwater, A. V. (1995). The technical and economic feasibility of biomass gasification for power generation. *Fuel, 74*, 631–653.

30. OECD-FAO Agricultural Outlook (2014).

31. Sun, Y., & Cheng, J. (2002). Hydrolysis of lignocellulosic materials for ethanol production: a review. *Bioresour. Technol., 83*, 1–11.

32. Mosier, N., Wyman, C., Dale, B., Elander, R., Lee, Y. Y., Holtzapple, M., & Ladisch, M. (2005). Features of promising technologies for pretreatment of lignocellulosic biomass. *Bioresour. Technol., 96*, 673–686.

33. Chandel, A. K., Chan, E. S., Rudravaram, R., Narasu, M. L., Rao, L. V., & Ravindra, P. (2007). Economics and environmental impact of bioethanol production technologies: an appraisal. *Biotechnology and Molecular Biology Reviews., 2*, 14–32.

34. Vandendriessche, S., Vincx, M., & Degraer, S. (2006). Floating seaweed in the neustonic environment: A case study from Belgian coastal waters. *J. Sea Research., 55,* 103–112.

35. Aresta, M., Dibenedetto, A., Tommasi, I., Cecere, E., Narracci, M., Petrocelli, A., & Perrone, C. (2002). The use of marine biomass as renewable energy source for reducing CO_2 emissions. Elsevier, Special Issue Dedicated to GHGT-6, Kyoto.

36. Ryther, J. H., DeBoer, J. A., & Lapointe, B. E. (1979). Cultivation of seaweeds for hydrocolloids, waste treatment and biomass for energy conversion. *Proceedings International Seaweed Symposium, 9,* 1–16.

37. Schramm, W. (1991). Seaweed for wastewater treatment and recycling of nutrients in Guiry, M. D., Blunden, G. Eds *Seaweed Resources in Europe: Uses and Potential,* John Wiley & Sons, Chichester, 149–168.

38. Cohen, I., & Neori, A. (1991). *Ulva lactuca* biofilters for marine fishpond effluents I. Ammonia uptake kinetics and nitrogen content. *Bot. Mar., 34,* 977–984.

39. Hirata, H., & Xu, B. (1990). Effects of feed addictive *Ulva* produced in feedback culture system on the growth and color of Red Sea Bream. *Pagure major Suisanzoshoku, 38,* 177–182.

40. Oilgae. *Comprehensive Oilgae Report.* Oilgae: Tamilnadu, India. (2010).

41. Ozkan, A., Kinney, K., Katz, L., & Berberoglu, H. (2012). Reduction of water and energy requirement of algae cultivation using an algae biofilm photobioreactor. *Bioresource Technol., 114,* 542–548.

42. Dibenedetto, A., Colucci, A., & Aresta, M. (2016). The need to implement an efficient biomass fractionation and full utilization based on the concept of "biorefinery" for a viable economic utilization of microalgae *Environmental Science and Pollution Research,* 1–10.

43. Dhote, S., & Dixit, S. (2009). Water Quality Improvement through Macrophytes - A Review. *Environ. Monit. Asses. 152,* 149–153.

44. Bazarov, A. I. (1870). Obtaining urea directly from Carbon Dioxide and Ammonia. *J. Prakt. Chem., 2,* 283–312.

45. Steinhauser, G. (2008). Cleaner production in the Solvay Process: general strategies and recent developments. *J. Cleaner Prod., 16,* 833–841.

46. Kolbe, H. (1875). Ueber eine neue Darstellungsmethode und einige bemerkenswerte Eigenschaften der Salicylsäure. *J. Prakt. Chem., 10,* 89–120.

47. Liu, X. M., Lu, G. Q., Yan, Z. F., & Beltramini, J. (2003) Recent advances in catalysts for methanol synthesis *via* hydrogenation of CO and CO_2, *Ind. Eng. Chem. Res., 42,* 6518–6530.

48. Tsuda, T., Chujo, Y., & Saegusa, T. (1976). Copper(I) cyanoacetate as a carrier of activated carbon dioxide. *J. Chem Soc. Chem. Commun.* 415–416.

49. Aresta, M., Dibenedetto, A., & He, L. N. (2013). Analysis of demand for captured CO_2 and products from CO_2 conversion, *TCGR report.*

50. Aresta, M., Quaranta, E., Tommasi, I., Giannoccaro, P., & Ciccarese, A. (1995). Enzymatic *versus* Chemical Carbon Dioxide Utilization. Part I. The Role of Metal Centres in Carboxylation Reactions. *Gazz. Chim. Ital., 125,* 509–538.

51. Aresta, M., Dibenedetto, A., & Quaranta, E., *Reaction Mechanisms in the Conversion of CO_2,* Springer-Verlag: Berlin Heidelberg, (2015).

52. Jäger, G., & Büchs, J. (2012). Biocatalytic conversion of lignocellulose to platform chemicals. *J. Biotechnol., 7,* 1122–1136.

53. Teixeira, L. C., Linden, J. C., & Schroeder, H. A. (2000). Simultaneous saccharification and cofermentation of peracetic acid-pretreated biomass. *Appl. Biochem. Biotechnol.,* 84–86, 111–127.

54. Ask, M., Mapelli, V., Hock, H., Olsson, L., & Bettiga, M. (2013). Engineering gluta-thione biosynthesis of Saccharomyces cerevisiae increases robustness to inhibitors in pretreated lignocellulosic materials. *Microb. Cell. Fact., 12*, 87–97.

55. Akinosho. H., Yee, K., Close, D., & Ragauskas, A. (2014). The emergence of Clos-tridium thermocellum as a high utility candidate for consolidated bioprocessing appli-cations. *Front. Chem., 2*, 66–74.

56. Halfmann, C., Gu, L., Gibbons, W., & Zhou R. (2014). Genetically engineering cya-nobacteria to convert CO_2, water, and light into the long-chain hydrocarbon farnesene. *Applied Microbiology and Biotechnology*, *98*(23), 9869–9877.

57. http://www.gevo.com/our-markets/isobutanol/.

58. www.cobalttech.com.

59. Gayubo, A. G., Aguayo, A. T., Atutxa, A., Aguado, A., & Bilbao, J. (2004). Transforma-tion of oxygenate components of biomass pyrolysis oil on H-ZSM-5 zeolite. Alcohols and phenols. *Ind. Eng. Chem. Res., 43*, 2610–2618.

60. Fuhse, J., & Bandermann, F. (1987). Conversion of organic oxygen compounds and their mixtures on H-ZSM-5. *Chem. Eng. Technol. 10*, 323–329.

61. Le Van Mao, R., & McLaughlin, GP. (1989). Conversion of light alcohols to hydrocar-bons over ZSM-5 zeolite and asbestos-derived zeolite catalysts. *Energ. Fuel, 3*, 620–624.

62. Varvarin, A. M., Khomenko, K. M., & Brei, V. V. (2013). Conversion of n-butanol to hydrocarbons over H-ZSM-5, H-ZSM-11, H-L and H-Y zeolites. *Fuel, 106*, 617–620.

63. Nahreen, S., & Gupta, R. B. (2013). Conversion of the Acetone–Butanol–Ethanol (ABE) Mixture to hydrocarbons by catalytic dehydration. *Energ. Fuel, 27*, 2116–2125.

64. www.eurobioref.org.

65. Chheda, J. N., Huber, G. W., & Dumesic, J. A. (2006). Liquid-phase catalytic process-ing of biomass-derived oxygenated hydrocarbons to fuels and chemicals. *Angew. Chem. Int. Ed., 46*, 7164–7183.

66. Kim, Y. T., Dumesic, J. A., & Huber, G. W. (2013). Aqueous-phase hydrodeoxygen-ation of sorbitol: A comparative study of Pt/Zr phosphate and PtReOx/C. *J. Catal., 304*, 72–85.

67. http://www.virent.com/technology/bioforming/.

68. Bond, J. Q., Martin-Alonso, D., Wang, D., West, R. M., & Dumesic, J. A. (2010). Inte-grated catalytic conversion of g-valerolactone to liquid alkenes for transportation fuels. *Science, 327*, 1110–1114.

69. Buono, S., Colucci, A., Angelini, A., Langelotti, A. L., Massa, M., Martello, A., Fogliano, V., & Dibenedetto, A. (2016). Productivity, biochemical composition and CO_2 fixation ability of *Scenedesmus obliquus* and *Phaeodactylum tricornutum*: effects of different cultivation approaches. *J. Appl Phycol*, DOI 10.1007/s10811–016–0876–6.

70. www.fediol.eu.

71. Chikkali, S., & Mecking, S. (2012). Refining of plant oils to chemicals by olefin metathesis. *Angew. Chem. Int. Ed, 5*, 5802–5808.

72. Malveda, M., Blagoev, M., & Funada, C. (2015). Natural fatty acids. *CEH Marketing research report*, HIS,

73. Aresta, M., Dibenedetto, A., Angelini, A., Pastore, C., & di Bitonto, L. (2013). Catalysts for the production of biodiesel from bio-oils, MI2013A001730,

74. Weemaes, M., Grootaerd, H., Simoens, F., & Verstraete W. (2000). Anaerobic digestion of ozonized biosolids. *Water Res., 34*(8), 2330–2336.
75. International Energy Agency (IEA). Bioenergy Annual Report (1994).
76. Farina, R., & Spagni, A. (2012). From lab-scale to full-scale biogas plants, in Aresta, M., Dibenedetto, A., Dumeignil, F. Eds. *Biorefinery: from biomass to chemicals and fuels.* Walter de Gruyter, 405–435.
77. Vasant, R. C., & Kartick, C. M. (2006). CO_2 reforming of methane combined with steam reforming or partial oxidation of methane to syngas over $NdCoO_3$ perovskite-type mixed metal-oxide catalyst. *Appl. En., 83*, 1024–1032.
78. Zhu, X., Huo, P., Zhang, Y., Cheng, D., & Liu, C. (2008). Structure and reactivity of plasma treated Ni/Al_2O_3 catalyst for CO_2 reforming of methane. *Appl. Catal. B: Env., 81*, 132–140.
79. Liu, C. J., Ye, J., Jiang, J., & Pan, Y. (2011). Progresses in the preparation of coke resistant Ni-based catalyst for steam and CO_2 reforming of methane. *Chem. Cat. Chem., 3*, 529–541.
80. Rostrup-Nielsen, J., & Trimm, D. L. (1977). Mechanisms of carbon formation on nickel-containing catalysts. *J. Catal. 48*, 155–165.
81. Song, C., & Pan, W. (2004) Tri-reforming of methane: a novel concept for catalytic production of industrially useful synthesis gas with desired H_2/CO ratios. *Catal. Tod.. 98*, 463–484.
82. Jiang, H. T., Li, H. Q., & Zhang, Y. (2007). Tri-reforming of methane to syngas over Ni/Al_2O_3 thermal distribution in the catalyst bed. *J. Fuel Chem. Technol., 35*, 72–78.
83. Rostrup-Nielsen, J., & Bak-Hansen, J. H. (1993). CO_2-reforming of methane over transition metals. *J. Catal., 144*, 38–49.
84. Bitter, J. H., Seshan, K., & Lercher, J. A. (1999) Deactivation and coke accumulation during CO_2/CH_4 *Reforming over Pt. Catal., 183*, 336–343.
85. Nagaoka, K., Seshan, K., Aika, K., & Lercher, J. A. (2001). Carbon deposition during carbon dioxide reforming of methane—comparison between Pt/Al_2O_3 and Pt/ZrO_2. *J. Catal., 197*, 34–42.
86. Gao, J., Hou, Z., Lou, H., & Zheng, X. (2011). Dry (CO_2) reforming. *Fuel Cells, 7*, 191–221.
87. Ruckenstein, E., & Hu, Y. H. (1996). Role of support in CO_2 reforming of CH_4 to syngas over Ni catalysts. *J. Catal., 162*, 230–238.
88. Pakhare, D., & Spivey, J. (2014). A review of dry (CO_2) reforming of methane over noble metal catalysts. *Chem. Soc. Rev., 43*, 7813–7837.
89. Hu, Y. Y., & Ruckenstein, E. (2004). Catalytic conversion of methane to synthesis gas by partial oxidation and CO_2 reforming. *Adv. Catal., 48*, 297–345.
90. Pakhare, D., Schwartz, V., Abdelsayed, V., Haynes, D., Shekhawat, D., Poston, J., & Spivey, J. (2014). Kinetic and mechanistic study of dry (CO_2) reforming of methane over Rh-substituted $La_2Zr_2O_7$ pyrochlores. *J. Catal., 316*, 78–92.
91. Aresta, M., Dibenedetto, A., & Quaranta, E. (2015). *Reaction Mechanisms in the Conversion of CO_2*, Springer-Verlag Berlin Heidelberg, 7, 237–310.
92. Gallego, G. S., Mondragón, F., Tatibouët, J. M., Barrault, J., & Batiot-Dupeyrat, C. (2008). Carbon dioxide reforming of methane over La_2NiO_4 as catalyst precursor—Characterization of carbon deposition. *Catal. Tod., 133–135*, 200–209.
93. Mark, M. F., Maier, W. F., & Mark, F. (1997). Reaction kinetics of the CO_2 reforming of methane. *Chem. Eng. Technol., 20*, 361–370.

94. Tsipouriari, V. A., & Verykios, X. E. (2001). Kinetic study of the catalytic reforming of methane with carbon dioxide to synthesis gas over Ni/La_2O_3 catalyst. *Cat. Tod., 64*, 83–90.

95. Ferreira-Aparicio, P., Rodriguez-Ramos, I., Anderson, J. A., & Guerrero-Ruiz, A. (2000). Mechanistic aspects of the dry reforming of methane over ruthenium catalysts. *Appl. Catal. A. Gen., 202*, 183–196.

96. Wei, J., & Iglesia, E. (2004). Isotopic and kinetic assessment of the mechanism of reactions of CH_4 with CO_2 or H_2O to form synthesis gas and carbon on nickel catalysts. *J. Catal., 24*, 370–383.

97. Moret, S., Dyson, P. J., & Laurenczy, G. (2014). Direct synthesis of formic acid from carbon dioxide by hydrogenation in acidic media. *Nat. Commun., 5*, 1–7.

98. Chueh, W. C., Falter, C., Abbott, M., Scipio, D., Furler, P., Haile, S. M., & Steinfeld, A. (2010). High-flux solar-driven thermochemical dissociation of CO_2 and H_2O using nonstoichiometric ceria. *Science, 330*, 1797–1801.

99. Wang, W., Wang, S., Ma, X., & Gong, J. (2011). Recent advances in catalytic hydrogenation of carbon dioxide. *Chem. Soc. Rev. 40*, 3703–3727.

100. Ma, J., Sun, N. N., Zhang, X. L., Zhao, N., Mao, F. K., Wei, W., & Sun, Y. H. (2009). A short review of catalysis for CO_2 conversion. *Catal. Tod., 148*, 221–231.

101. Inui, T. (1966). Highly effective conversion of carbon dioxide to valuable compounds on composite catalysts. *Catal. Tod., 29*, 329–337.

102. Chen, C. S., Wu, J. H., & Lai, T. W. (2010). Carbon dioxide hydrogenation on Cu nanoparticles. *J. Phys. Chem. C., 114*, 15021–15028.

103. Pekridis, G., Kalimeri, K., Kaklidis, N., Vakouftsi, E., Iliopoulou, E. F., Athanasiou, C., & Marnellos, G. E. (2007). Study of the reverse water gas shift (RWGS) reaction over Pt in a solid oxide fuel cell (SOFC) operating under open and closed-circuit conditions. *Catal. Tod., 127*, 337–346.

104. Gines, M. J. L., Marchi, A. J., & Apesteguia, C. R. (1997). Kinetic study of the reverse water-gas shift reaction over $CuO/ZnO/Al_2O_3$ catalysts. *Appl. Catal. A: Gen., 154*, 155–171.

105. Behrens, M., Kisner, S., Girsgdies, F., Kasatkin, I., Hermerschmidt, F., Mette, K., Ruland, H., Muhler, M., & Schlogl, R. (2011). Knowledge-based development of a nitrate-free synthesis route for Cu/ZnO methanol synthesis catalysts *via* formate precursors. *Chem. Commun., 47*, 1701–1703.

106. Kaluza, S., Behrens, M., Schiefenhovel, N., Kniep, B., Fischer, R., Schlogl, R., & Muhler, M. (2011). A novel synthesis route for $Cu/ZnO/Al_2O_3$ catalysts used in methanol synthesis: combining continuous consecutive precipitation with continuous aging of the precipitate. *Chem. Cat. Chem., 3*, 189–199.

107. Zuo, Z.-J., Wang, L., Han, P.-D., & Huang, W. (2014). Methanol synthesis by CO and CO_2 hydrogenation on Cu/γ-Al_2O_3 surface in liquid paraffin solution. *Appl. Surf. Sci., 290*, 398–404.

108. Mei, D. H., Xu, L. J., & Henkelman, G. (2008). Dimer saddle point searches to determine the reactivity of formate on $Cu(111)$. *J. Catal., 258*, 44–51.

109. Olah, G. A. (2013) Towards oil independence through renewable methanol chemistry. *Angew. Chem. Internl. Ed., 52*, 104–107.

110. Fujiwara, M., Kieffer, R., Ando, H., & Souma, Y. (1995). Development of composite catalysts made of Cu-Zn-Cr oxide/zeolite for the hydrogenation of carbon dioxide. *Appl Catal A: Gen., 121*, 113–124.

111. Fujiwara, M., Kieffer, R., Ando, H., Xu, Q., & Souma, Y. (1997). Change of catalytic properties of Fe/ZnO/zeolite composite catalyst in the hydrogenation of carbon dioxide. *Appl. Catal. A: Gen., 154*, 87–101.

112. Lunev, N. K., Shmyrko, Y. I., Pavlenko, N. V., & Norton, B. (2001). Synthesis of iso-hydrocarbons mixture from CO_2 and H_2 on hybrid catalysts. *Appl. Organomet. Chem., 15*, 99–104.

113. Zhang, R., Wang, B., Liu, H., & Ling, L. (2011). Effect of surface hydroxyls on CO_2 hydrogenation Over Cu/γ-Al_2O_3 catalyst: A theoretical study. *J. Phys. Chem. C., 115*, 19811–19818.

114. Gnanamani, M. K., Jacobs, G. Pendyala, V. R. R., Ma, W., & Davis, B. H. (2014). Hydrogenation of carbon dioxide to liquid fuels, In: *Green Carbon Dioxide: Advances in CO_2 Utilization*, First Edition, Centi, G., Perathonen, S. (Eds.) John Wiley & Sons, *Inc.* 99–118.

115. Chinchen, G. C., Waugh, K. C., & Whan, D. A. (1986). The activity and state of the copper surface in methanol synthesis catalysts. *Appl. Catal., 25*, 101–107.

116. Arena, F., Mezzatesta, G., Zafarana, G., Trunfio, G., Frusteri, F., & Spadaro, L. (2013). Effects of oxide carriers on surface functionality and process performance of the Cu–ZnO system in the synthesis of methanol *via* CO_2 hydrogenation. *J. Catal., 300*, 141–151.

117. Melian-Cabrera, I., Granados, M. L., & Fierro, J. L. G. (2002). Reverse topotactic transformation of a Cu-Zn-Al catalyst during wet Pd impregnation: Relevance for the performance in methanol synthesis from CO_2/H_2 mixtures. *J. Catal., 210*, 273–284.

118. Fujitani, T., Nakamura, I., Uchijima, T., & Nakamura, J. (1997). The kinetics and mechanism of methanol synthesis by hydrogenation of CO_2 over a Zn-deposited Cu(111) *Surface. Surf. Sci., 383*, 285–298.

119. Zou, J. J., & Liu, C. J. (2010). Utilization of Carbon Dioxide through nonthermal plasma approaches. In *Carbon Dioxide as Chemical Feedstock, Aresta, M. Ed.,* 267–289.

120. Olah, G. A., Goeppert, A., & Surya Prakash, G. K. (2009). Chemical recycling of carbon dioxide to methanol and dimethyl ether: from greenhouse gas to renewable, environmentally carbon neutral fuels and synthetic hydrocarbons. *J. Org. Chem., 74*, 487–498.

121. Kim, I. H., Kim, S., Cho, W., & Yoon, E. S. (2010). Simulation of commercial dimethyl ether production plant. *Computer Aided Chem. Eng., 28*, 799–804.

122. Chen, W. H., Lin, B. J., Lee, H. W., & Huang, M. N. (2012). One-step synthesis of dimethyl ether from the gas mixture containing CO_2 with high space velocity. *Appl. Energy., 98*, 92–101.

123. Kang, S. W., Bae, J. W., Jun, K. W., & Potdar, H. S. (2008). Dimethyl ether synthesis from syngas over the composite catalysts of Cu–ZnO–Al_2O_3/Zr-modified zeolites. *Catal. Commun., 9*, 2035–2039.

124. Wang, S., Mao, D., Guo, X., Wu, G., & Lu, G. (2009). Dimethyl ether synthesis *via* CO_2 hydrogenation over CuO–TiO_2–ZrO_2/HZSM-5 bifunctional catalysts. *Catal. Commun., 10*, 1367–1370.

125. Pellegrini, L. A., Soave, G., Gamba, S., & Lange, S. (2011). Economic analysis of a combined energy–methanol production plant. *Appl. Energy., 88*, 4891–4897.

126. Bonura, G., Cordaro, M., Spadaro, L., Cannilla, C., Arena, F., & Frusteri, F. (2013). Hybrid Cu–ZnO–ZrO_2/H-ZSM5 system for the direct synthesis of DME by CO_2 hydrogenation. *Appl. Catal. B: Environ., 140–141*, 16–24.

127. Frusteri, F., Cordaro, M., Cannilla, C., & Bonura, G. (2015). Multifunctionality of Cu–ZnO–ZrO$_2$/H-ZSM5 catalysts for the one-step CO$_2$-to-DME hydrogenation reaction. *Appl. Catal. B: Environ.*, *162*, 57–65.

128. Arena, F., Italiano, G., Barbera, K., Bonura, G., Spadaro, L., & Frusteri, F. (2009). Basic evidences for methanol-synthesis catalyst design. *Catal. Tod.*, *143*, 80–85.

129. Bonura, G., Cordaro, M., Cannilla, C., & Frusteri, F. (2014). The changing nature of the active site of Cu-Zn-Zr catalysts for the CO$_2$ hydrogenation reaction to methanol. *Appl. Catal. B: Environ.*, 152–153, 152–161.

130. Sabatier, P., & Senderens, J. B. (1902). Hydrogénation directe des oxides de charbon, *Acad Sci.*, *134*, 689–691.

131. Schaaf, T., Gunig, J., Schuster, M. R., Rothenfluh, T., & Orth, A. (2014). Methanation of CO$_2$ - storage of renewable energy in a gas distribution system *Energy, Sustainability and Society*, *4*, *2*, 1–14.

132. Visconti, C. G., Tronconi, E., Groppi, G., & Zennano, R. (2011). Monolytic catalysts with high thermalconductivity for the Fischer Tropsch synthesis in tubular reactors. *The Chem. Eng. J.*, *171*, 1294–1307.

133. Stowe, R. A., & Russel, W. W. (1954). Co, Fe and some of their alloys as catalysts for the hydrogenation of CO$_2$. *J. Am. Chem. Soc. 76*, 319–323.

134. Jwa, E., Lee, S., Lee, H. W., & Mok, Y. S. (2013). Plasma-assisted catalytic methanation of CO and CO$_2$ over Ni–zeolite catalysts *Fuel Proc. Technol.*, *108*, 89–93.

135. Mattia, D., Jones, M. D., O'Byrne, J. P., Griffiths, O. G., Owen, R. E., Sackville, E., McManus, M., & Plucinski, P. (2016). Towards carbon neutral CO$_2$ conversion to hydrocarbons, *Chem. Sus. Chem.*, *8*(23), 4064–4072.

136. Gao, K., & McKinley, K. R. (1994). Use of macroalgae for marine biomass production and CO$_2$ remediation: a review *J. Appl. Phycol. 6*, 45–60.

137. Buono, S., Dibenedetto, A., Colucci, A., Langellotti, A. L., Morana, M., Fogliano, V., Aresta, M. XIII *International Conference on Carbon Dioxide Utilization*, July, 5-9, 2015, Singapore.

138. Yoo, C., Jun, S.-Y., Lee, J.-Y., Ahn, C.-Y., & Oh, H.-M. (2010). Selection of microalgae for lipid production under high levels carbon dioxide *Biores. Technol.*, *101*, S71–S74.

139. Zeiler, K. G., Heacox, D. A., Toon, S. T., Kadam, K. L., & Brown, L. M. (1995). The use of microalgae for assimilation and utilization of carbon dioxide from fossil fuel fired power plant flue gas. *Energy Convers. Mgmt.*, *36*, 707–712.

140. Xue, Y., Zhang, Y., Cheng, D., Daddy, S., & He, Q. (2014). Genetically engineering *Synechocystis* sp. Pasteur Culture Collection 6803 for the sustainable production of the plant secondary metabolite *p*-coumaric acid *Proc. Natl. Acad. Sci.*, U.S.A. *111*, 9449–9454.

141. Capon, R. J., Dunlop, R. W., Ghisalberti, E. L., & Jefferies, P. R. (1983). Poly 3-hydroxy-alkanoates from marine and freshwater cyanobacteria. *Phytochem.*, *22*(5), 1181–1184.

142. Stal, L. J., Heyer, H., & Jacobs, G. (1990). Occurrence and Role of Poly Hydroxy-Alkanoate in the Cyanobacterium *Oscillatoria Limosa* In Dawes, E. A. Ed. *Novel Biodegradable Microbial Polymers.* NATO ASI Series, *186*, 435–438.

143. Campbell III, J., Stevens Jr., S. E., & Balkwill, D. L. (1982). Accumulation of poly beta-hydroxybutyrate in *Spirulina platensis*. *J. Bacteriol.*, *149*(1), 361–363.

144. Vincenzini, M., Sili, C., de Philippis, R., Ena, A., & Materassi, R. (1990). Occurrence of poly beta-hydroxybutyrate in *Spirulina* species. *J. Bacteriol.*, *172*(5), 2791–2792.

145. Miyake, M., Erata, M., & Asada, Y. (1996). A thermophilic cyanobacterium, *Synechococcus* sp. MA19, capable of accumulating poly β-hydroxybutyrate *J. Fermentation and Bioengineering.*, *82*(5), 512–514.

146. Lau, N.-S., Foong, C. P., Kurihara, Y., Sudesh, K., & Matsui, M. (2014). RNA-Seq Analysis Provides Insights for Understanding Photoautotrophic Polyhydroxyalkanoate Production in Recombinant *Synechocystis Sp. PLoS ONE*, *9*(1), 1–11.

147. Akiyama, H., Okuhata, H., Onizuka, T., Kanai, S., Hirano, M., Tanaka, S., Sasaki, K., & Miyasaka, H. (2011). Antibiotics-free stable polyhydroxyalkanoate (PHA) production from carbon dioxide by recombinant cyanobacteria. *Biores. Technol.*, *102*(23), 11039–11042.

148. Lan, E. I., Chuang, D. S., Shen, C. R., Lee, A. M., Ro, S. Y., & Liao, J. C. (2015). Metabolic engineering of cyanobacteria for photosynthetic 3-hydroxypropionic acid production from CO_2 using *Synechococcus elongatus* PCC 7942. *Metab. Eng.*, *31*, 163–170.

149. Lan, E. I., & Liao, J. C. (2011). Metabolic engineering of cyanobacteria for 1-butanol production from carbon dioxide *Metab. Eng. 13*, 353–363.

150. Rabaey, K., & Rozendal, R. A. (2010). Microbial electrosynthesis - Revisiting the electrical route for microbial production *Nature Reviews Microbiology.*, *8*, 706–716.

151. Villano, M., Aulenta, F., Ciucci, F. A. C., Ferri, T., Giuliano, A., & Majone, M. (2010). Bioelectrochemical reduction of CO_2 to CH_4 via direct and indirect extracellular electron transfer by a hydrogenophilic methanogenic culture *Biores. Technol.*, *101*(9), 3085–3090.

152. Armstrong, F. A., & Hirst J. (2011). Reversibility and efficiency in electrocatalytic energy conversion and lessons from enzymes *Proc. Natl. Acad. Sci.* U.S.A., *108*, 14049–14054.

153. Hartmann, T., & Leimkühler S. (2013). The oxygen-tolerant and NAD^+-dependent formate dehydrogenase from *Rhodobacter capsulatus* is able to catalyze the reduction of CO_2 to formate. *The FEBS J.*, *280*, 6083–6096.

154. Hwang, H., Yeon, Y. J., Lee, S., Choe, H., Jang, M. G., Cho, D. H., Park, S., & Kim, Y. H. (2015). Electro-biocatalytic production of formate from carbon dioxide using an oxygen-stable whole cell biocatalyst. *Biores. Technol.*, *185*, 35–39.

155. Alissandratos, A., Kim, H.-K., & Easton, C. J. (2014). Formate production through carbon dioxide hydrogenation with recombinant whole cell biocatalysts. *Biores. Technol.*, *164*, 7–11.

156. Gunda, M., Seelam, J. S., Vanbroekhoven, K., & Pant, D. Paper ID: 170, XIII *International Conference on Carbon Dioxide Utilization*, July, 5-9, 2015, Singapore Singapore.

157. Ullmann, F. (2000). Ullmann's Encyclopedia of Industrial Chemistry, (seventh ed.) Wiley-VCH, Weinheim.

158. Deublein, D. (2011), *Biogas from Waste and Renewable Resources: An Introduction*, Steinhauser A. Wiley.

159. Berzin, V., Kiriukhin, M., & Tyurin, M. (2012). Selective production of acetone during continuous synthesis gas fermentation by engineered biocatalyst *Clostridium sp. MAceT113. Lett. Appl. Microbiol.*, *55*, 149–154.

160. Ukpong, M. N., Atiyeh, H. K., De Lorme, M. J. M., Liu, K., Zhu, X., Tanner, R. S., Wilkins, M. R., & Stevenson, B. S. (2012). Physiological response of *Clostridium carboxidivorans* during conversion of synthesis gas to solvents in a gas-fed bioreactor. *Biotechnol. Bioeng.*, *109*, 2720–2728.

161. Datar, R. P., Shenkman, R. M., Cateni, B. G., Huhnke, R. L., & Lewis, R. S. (2004). Fermentation of biomass-generated producer gas to ethanol *Biotechnol. Bioeng.*, *86*, 587–594.

162. Ramachandriya, K. D., Wilkins, M. R., De Lorme, M. J. M., Zhu, X. G., Kundiyana, D. K., Atiyeh, H. K., & Huhnke, R. L. (2011). Reduction of acetone to isopropanol using producer gas fermenting microbes *Biotechnol. Bioeng.*, *108*, 2330–2338.

163. Ramachandriya, K. D., Kundiyana, D. K., Wilkins, M. R., Terrill, J. B., Atiyeh, H. K., & Huhnke, R. L. (2013). Carbon dioxide conversion to fuels and chemicals using a hybrid green process. Original *Appl. Ener.*, *112*, 289–299.

164. Kumar, B., Llorente, M., Froehlich, J., Dang, T., Sathrum, A., & Kubiak, C. P. (2012). *Annu. Rev. Phys. Chem.*, *63*, 541.

165. Reda, T., Plugge, C. M., Abram, N. J., & Hirst, J. (2008). Reversible interconversion of carbon dioxide and formate by an electroactive enzyme. *Proc Natl Acad Sci* USA , *105*, 10654–10658.

166. Parkin, A., Seravalli, J., Vincent, K. A., Ragsdale, S. W., & Armstrong, F. A. (2007). Rapid and Efficient Electrocatalytic CO_2/CO Interconversions by *Carboxydothermus hydrogenoformans* CO Dehydrogenase I on an Electrode. *J. Am. Chem. Soc.*, *129*, 10328–10329.

167. Aresta, M., Dibenedetto, A., Baran, T., Angelini, A., Łabuz, P., & Macyk, W. An (2014). Integrated Photocatalytic-Enzymatic System for the Reduction of CO_2 to Methanol in Bio-Glycerol-Water. *Beilstein J. Org. Chem.*, *10*, 2556–2565.

168. Aresta, M., Dibenedetto, A., Macyk, W., & Baran T. (2013). *Photocatalysts working in the visible region for the reduction of NAD^+ to NADH within an hybrid chemo-enzymatic process of CO_2 reduction to methanol* MI2013A001135.

169. Yadav, R. K., Oh, G. H., Park, N.-J., Kumar, A., Kong, K-J., & Baeg, J.-O. (2014). Highly Selective Solar-Driven Methanol from CO_2 by a Photocatalyst/Biocatalyst Integrated System. *J. Am. Chem. Soc.*, *136*, 16728–16731.

CHAPTER 4

GREEN CATALYSTS AND CATALYTIC PROCESSES FOR BIOFUEL PRODUCTION

ATAL SHIVHARE, KAREN WILSON, and ADAM F. LEE

European Bioenergy Research Institute, Aston University, Birmingham B4 7ET, UK

CONTENTS

ABSTRACT

Global population growth and rapid urbanization drive the quest for alternative, sustainable energy sources, especially for the transportation sector, which alone contributed to 21% of worldwide anthropogenic CO_2 emissions from fossil fuels in 2013. The natural abundance and potential carbon neutrality of plant and algal biomass render it ideal feedstocks for production of sustainable liquid transportation fuels. A variety of catalytic technologies have been developed for the energy efficient conversion of lignocellulosic biomass to bio-derived fuels and chemicals. Here we review a range of such heterogeneously catalyzed processes, including esterification, transesterification, Fischer-Tropsch synthesis and hydrodeoxygenation, and associated inorganic nanocatalysts, for transformation of lignin, carbohydrate and oil feedstocks. Design of robust catalytic materials, with mass transport properties tailored for the rapid diffusion of bulky molecules, high selectivity and minimal deactivation, is a particular focus of discussions.

4.1   BIOMASS PROPERTIES AND PRETREATMENTS FOR BIOFUELS AND CHEMICALS

Dwindling supplies of easily accessible fossil fuels due to a sharp rise in their consumption associated with an increasing global population and urbanization, in conjunction with anthropogenic climate change due to emitted CO_2 and other greenhouse gases, are driving the quest for alternative sustainable energy resources [1]. According to 2015 report by the International Energy Agency, atmospheric CO_2 concentrations reached 397 ppm in 2014, 40% higher than that in the mid-1800s, and increasing at a rate of 2 ppm per annum over the past ten years [2]; continued human reliance on fossil fuels as a primary energy resource will undoubtedly exacerbate severe climate events. Of the possible renewable energy solutions explored thus far, biomass is the only one suitable as a readily implementable substitute to fossil fuels in the transportation sector, and a feedstock for chemicals production [3–5]. Biomass refers to biogenic sources of carbon containing materials, with the most abundant sources being lignocellulose which are major constituents of plants and trees, and also prevalent in agricultural wastes, industrial and municipal waste streams, which collectively are view as viable short- to mid-term alternates to fossil fuels [6, 7]. Biomass transformation to fuels and chemicals offer the possibility of significantly reduced net CO_2 emissions associated with their production and use, although the early premise of a carbon neutral economy now appears overly optimistic [8].

Lignocellulose is the most abundant renewable biomass available on earth [9], and is primarily composed of cellulose, hemicellulose, and lignin [10]. Cellulose is a polymer of D-glucose, wherein individual glucose units are linked to each other through β-(1,4)-glycosidic bonds to form long, linear polymeric chains. These cellulose polymer chains are linked by hydrogen and Van der Waals bonds to form rigid crystalline structures. Hemicellulose comprises shorter branched chains of different monosaccharides, including pentoses (xylose, rhamnose, and arabinose), hexoses (glucose, mannose, and galactose) and uronic acids (4-O-methylglucuronic, D-glucuronic, and D-galactouronic acids), resulting in an amorphous, less tightly bound structure which is more easily hydrolysed than cellulose. Lignin is a complex, three-dimensional polymer of cross-linked phenolic monomers, guaiacyl propanol, p-hydroxyphenyl propanol, and syringyl alcohol. Lignin is an amorphous polymer, which forms the outer part of cell walls imparting impermeability, structural support, and protection against microbial attack. Cellulose is the main structural component of the cell wall, which is embedded within hemicellulose and lignin [10]. The composition of cellulose, hemicellulose, and lignin vary with plant species, stage of growth, and environment (Table 4.1) [11].

Polysaccharides present in lignocellulosic biomass can be deconstructed into sugar monomers (precursors to both bio-fuels and high value platform chemicals) through hydrolysis by acids or enzymes. However, the impermeability of lignin and structural rigidity of cellulose renders lignocellulose recalcitrant towards such hydrolysis, necessitating its mechanical, chemical or biological pretreatment (Figure 4.1). Mechanical pretreatments include reducing the physical size of biomass to increase its surface area through chipping, grinding and/or milling. However, in most of the cases the energy used in mechanical pretreatments are higher than the energy content of the parent biomass [12]. Physiochemical pretreatments include steam explosion [13], ammonia explosion [14], and CO_2 explosion [15]. Here, biomass is treated with steam, NH_3, or CO_2 under high pressure, and the pressure suddenly released to allow explosive decompression of the biomass; this approach disrupts the structure of lignin and polysaccharides making the biomass more porous and enhancing the efficiency of subsequent hydrolysis.

Physiochemical pretreatments have low energy requirements compared to mechanical comminution. Chemical pretreatments include ozonolysis, acid or alkaline hydrolysis, oxidative delignification, and organosolv processes [10]. Ozonolysis involves biomass pretreatment with ozone at room temperature, inducing lignin degradation and hence improved access to hemicellulose and cellulose during subsequent acid/enzyme hydrolysis [16]. The mild conditions and absence of toxic residues are significant advantages to ozonolysis, however the large quantities of ozone required negatively

TABLE 4.1 Composition of Cellulose, Hemicellulose, and Lignin in Common Agricultural and Industrial Waste Streams [11]

Lignocellulosic material	Cellulose (%)	Hemicellulose (%)	Lignin (%)
Hardwood stems	40–55	24–40	18–25
Softwood stems	45–50	25–35	25–35
Nut shells	25–30	25–30	30–40
Corn cobs	45	35	15
Grasses	25–40	35–50	10–30
Paper	85–99	0	0–15
Wheat straw	30	50	15
Sorted refuse	60	20	20
Leaves	15–20	80–85	0
Cotton seed hairs	80–95	5–20	0
Newspaper	40–55	25–40	18–30
Waste papers from chemical pulps	60–70	10–20	5–10
Primary wastewater solids	8–15		
Solid cattle manure	1.6–4.7	1.4–3.3	2.7–5.7
Coastal Bermuda grass	25	35.7	6.4
Switchgrass	45	31.4	12
Swine waste	6.0	28	N/A

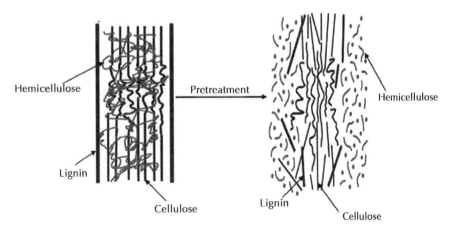

FIGURE 4.1 Cartoon of lignocellulosic biomass pretreatment [10].

impact on the process economics. Concentrated mineral acids such as H_2SO_4 and HCl are widely reported for the pretreatment of lignocellulosic materials [17]. Such concentrated acid hydrolysis releases fermentable sugar from lignocellulosic biomass, however such acids tend to be toxic and hazardous, requiring corrosion-resistant reactors which increases associated process costs [18], and requires acid recovery from the reaction mixture to mitigate the economics [18]. Dilute acid hydrolysis of lignocellulosic biomass has also been performed successfully [17]. Dilute sulfuric acid (<4 wt%) can hydrolyse hemicellulose to xylose and other sugars, and subsequently decompose xylose to furfural [17]. Use of dilute acids recovers most of the hemicellulose in the form of aqueous sugars aiding subsequent cellulose digestion. Alkaline hydrolysis involves the treatment of biomass with bases such as sodium, potassium, calcium and ammonium hydroxides [10]. Of these, calcium hydroxide is the least expensive soluble base, and can be recovered from aqueous reaction mixtures as insoluble calcium carbonate [19]. In comparison with acid hydrolysis, alkaline hydrolysis is slower and results in less sugar degradation. Oxidative delignification uses an oxidant such as H_2O_2 to strip out the lignin, enhancing the susceptibility of biomass to enzymatic hydrolysis [10]. Organosolv processes treat biomass with organic solvents such as methanol, ethanol, acetone, ethylene glycol, triethylene glycol, and tetrahydrofurfuryl alcohol, in the presence of organic/inorganic acids [20], and achieves the simultaneous hydrolysis and delignification of biomass. Residual solvents must be removed from the reactor prior to prevent enzyme inhibition in any additional hydrolysis steps. Biological pretreatments include the use of diverse microorganisms and fungi [10], and are advantageous in terms of their low energy consumption compared to mechanical or chemical processes; however, hydrolysis rates in biological pretreatments are often very low. The preferred pretreatment method will therefore depend on the composition of biomass, its energy content, and the value of the resulting reaction products which all influence the overall process cost.

4.2 LIQUID TRANSPORTATION BIOFUELS

The International Energy Agency reports that 31.7% of global primary energy needs in 2015 were met by oil [21], representing a 53.5% rise in oil consumption since 1973 (Figure 4.2a). Of the total oil consumed in

2015, 49.7% arose from the transportation sector, which also contributed to 17.2% of global CO_2 emissions from fossil fuels (Figure 4.2b). Energy consumption in the transportation sector is expected to continue rising due to increased population growth and urbanization, and hence there is a pressing need to identify alternative low carbon fuel sources for transportation.

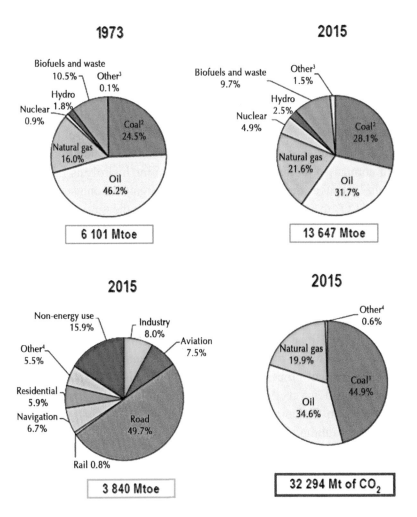

FIGURE 4.2 (a) 1973 and 2013 fuel shares of total primary energy supply; and (b) 2013 share of world oil consumption and CO_2 emission form fuel consumption [21]. [Note: [1]Includes international aviation and international marine bunkers. [2]In these graphs peat and oil shale are aggregated with coal. [3]Includes geothermal, solar, wind, heat, etc. [4]Includes industrial waste and non-renewable municipal waste].

Liquid fuels produced from biomass are termed biofuels, and commonly categorized into three categories based on the type of biomass feedstock they derive from. First generation biofuels are typically obtained from edible starch and sugar containing food crops, vegetable oils and animal fats [22]. The former, prevalent in sugarcane, corn, sweet sorghum and cassava can be converted into ethanol through hydrolysis and subsequent fermentation. Such bioethanol produced is already widely available in many countries as a blend with gasoline for use in spark-ignition engines, or in pure form within flexible-fuel vehicles, notably in Brazil. Triglycerides present in oil and animal fats are widely converted into fatty acid methyl ester (FAME) by catalytic transesterification, with the resulting FAMEs, colloquially termed biodiesel, widespread as diesel substitutes, particularly in blends. First generation biofuels have drawn severe criticism due to their competition for food crops, leading to a heated 'food vs. fuel' debate in the academic and public media [23]. Rapid deforestation and land use changes in Malaysia and Indonesia have also highlighted the problems facing large-scale energy crop production and their negative impact on biodiversity [24].

Second generation biofuels are derived from lignocellulosic biomass, usually in the form of forestry, agricultural, municipal and industrial wastes [22]. The abundance of nonedible lignocellulosic biomass has resulted in it being viewed as viable raw material for liquid biofuel production. Lignocellulose conversion into liquid fuels mainly occurs through hydrolysis, gasification and pyrolysis (Figure 4.3) [25]. As discussed in the previous section, hydrolytic pretreatments facilitate the depolymerisation of polysaccharides present in lignocellulose into their constituent monosaccharides. These monosaccharides may subsequently be converted into ethanol (biofuel) through fermentation, or into liquid hydrocarbon fuels through catalytic thermochemical processing or aqueous phase reforming [25]. Gasification is a thermochemical process whereby lignocellulosic biomass undergoes high temperature oxidative degradation into syngas (CO and H_2), water, carbon dioxide, and short-chain hydrocarbons. Syngas may be further converted into liquid biofuels (diesel, gasoline, and kerosene) through Fischer-Tropsch (F-T) catalysis [26]. Pyrolysis involves the anaerobic decomposition of lignocellulosic biomass at lower temperatures than employed in gasification, which favors biomass decomposition into noncondensable gases, liquid pyrolysis oil and biochar. Pyrolysis oils retain up to 70% of the parent biomass energy value [27], but are highly acidic and typically possess high oxygen contents of 30–40 wt% [28], and consequently must be upgraded through additional low temperature

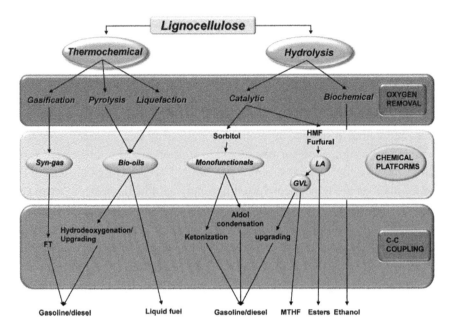

FIGURE 4.3 Conversion of lignocellulosic biomass to liquid biofuels through various routes [81]. (Reprinted with permission from Alonso, D. M., Bond, J. Q. (2010). Catalytic conversion of biomass to biofuels. *Green Chem.*, 2010, 12, 1493-1513. © 2010 Royal Chemical Society.)

pretreatments such as esterification [29], aldol condensation [30] and ketonization [30] prior to hydrodeoxygenation [27] (HDO) reactions over bifunctional metal/solid acid catalysts, to ensure engine compatibility [28].

Third generation biofuels are considered those derived from microorganisms such as microalgae, yeast, fungi etc. Microalgae, the most common example of third generation biofuel, under stress produce triglycerides (TAGs), which can be converted into FAMEs (biodiesel) through heterogeneous or homogeneous transesterification [31]. In contrast to first and second-generation biofuels feedstocks, which require considerable land use, microalgae can be cultivated in aquatic environments or with small land footprints, resulting in far higher biodiesel yields. For example, high oil content microalgae can produce up to 121,104 kg of biodiesel per hectare per year, 50–350 times that possible through existing first generation biofuel feedstocks (Table 4.2) [31]. Unfortunately microalgae suffer high growth and processing costs, which has to date restricted their commercial production. First generation biofuel production has been limited to a handful of

TABLE 4.2   Biodiesel Productivity of Some Feedstocks [31]

Crop	Oil yield (L/ha/year)	Biodiesel productivity (Kg/ha/year)	Crop	Oil yield (L/ha/year)	Biodiesel productivity (Kg/ha/year)
Rapeseed	1190	862	Sunflower	952	946
Oil palm	5950	4747	Jatropha	1892	656
Corn	172	152	Microalgaea	58700	51927
Soybean	446	562	Microalgaeb	136900	121104

[a]Algae contain 30 wt% oil in biomass.
[b]Algae contain 70 wt% oil in biomass.

countries (notably the USA) due to sociopolitical concerns over the diversion of edible crops for fuel production. While second generation biofuels are more attractive, the high cost of lignocellulose pretreatment and the upgrading of pyrolysis bio-oils, or gasification coupled with F-T, still presents major challenges for scale-up but are the basis of commercial ventures. Third generation biofuels based on microalgae have great potential, however the development of new reactor designs and robust strains is require in order to reduce the cost of microalgae derived biofuels.

4.3   HETEROGENEOUS CATALYSTS FOR BIOFUELS SYNTHESIS

Porous inorganic solids with good mass transfer properties have shown recent promise for applications in the synthesis of liquid biofuels [32], as either catalysts themselves or as catalyst supports, through F-T synthesis conversion of bio-syngas from biomass pyrolysis or gasification, or the transesterification and esterification of TAGs and free fatty acids (FFAs).

F-T synthesis yields a variety of hydrocarbons from CO and H_2 mixtures, with selectivity to specific chain lengths, CH_4 formation, and the extent of competing water gas shift reaction dependent on the choice of support, metal, and metal dispersion [26]. In particular, hierarchically porous supports offer superior dispersion of metal nanoparticles and improved reactant/product diffusion in-pore, and hence deliver improved conversion and selectivity to longer chain hydrocarbons. Cobalt nanoparticles supported over hierarchically macroporous-mesoporous silica have been prepared by introducing silica gel into the macropores of silica sols, and their subsequent impregnation by Co, resulting in high CO conversion and reduced CH_4 formation.

This was attributed to improved alkane diffusion through the macropores, which prevented secondary cracking reactions [33]. Hierarchically meso-macroporous hematite Fe_2O_3, prepared by infiltrating iron nitrate, ethylene glycol, and methanol into the voids of polymethyl methacrylate (PMMA) as a macropore-directing template followed by calcination, also proved an excellent F-T catalyst [34]. Here, the selectivity to CH_4 and the propensity for water gas shift reaction were lower for the hierarchically macromeso-porous Fe_2O_3 catalyst compared to mesoporous Fe_2O_3. The hierarchically macroporous-mesoporous Fe_2O_3 catalyst offered a higher chain growth probability (0.83) compared to mesoporous Fe_2O_3 (0.80), again attributed to enhanced diffusion of hydrocarbon products and hence more pronounced chain growth. Investigation of Co over mesoporous SBA-15 and MCM-41 silica supports with various pore sizes for F-T synthesis revealed that pore dimensions influenced the size and reducibility of Co nanoparticles;[35] smaller pores stabilized small, essentially irreducible Co particles while larger pores favored larger and readily reducible Co particles. The degree of Co reducibility correlated with selectivity to methane and hydrocarbon chain growth probability.

Biodiesel is conventionally synthesized from triglycerides through their transesterification with low molecular weight (typically methanol or etha-nol) alcohols in the presence of soluble base catalysts [29]. While soluble bases such as sodium or potassium hydroxide and methoxide offer high rates of transesterifications, they require aqueous quench and energy intensive separation steps to isolate the desired FAME and high purity glycerol by-product, and are susceptible to saponification in the presence of FFA impu-rities, which vary between 2–20 wt% (the latter for waste cooking oils). Removal of FFAs by catalytic pretreatments such as esterification with light alcohols is possible, although of greater interest would be catalysts able to simultaneously esterify fatty acids and transesterify triglycerides in a single process. In any event, the use of homogeneous catalysts for biodiesel pro-duction remains problematic due to the difficulty of their separation from the reaction mixture.

Solid acid and base catalysts such as zeolites, resins, alkali earth oxides, hydrotalcites, and dolomitic rocks potentially offer facile biodiesel recov-ery without concomitant soap/emulsion formation, and such materials have been heavily investigated for esterification and transesterification respec-tively [29]. While such materials facilitate separation from biodiesel, they introduce additional issues relating to catalyst stability and leaching of active components, and low reactivity particularly for bulky TAGs or FFAs compared to their homogeneous counterparts due to diffusion limitations. Much research in this field has therefore focused on the development of solid catalysts with tailored porosity and good long-term stability, and novel reactors to e.g. achieve efficient mixing or continuous biodiesel production. Heterogeneous catalysts with tunable pore sizes and interconnectivity, and amenable to functionalization by acid or base functions have shown promise for bulky substrates common in real plant oils. Mesoporous SBA-15 silica, possessing ordered hexagonal arrays of cylindrical pores, was functionalized by postsynthetic grafting with poly (styrene sulfonic-acid) for the esterification of oleic acid, an FFA common to most plant oils [36]. The resulting $PrSO_3H$/SBA-15 catalyst was superior to commercially available Amberlyst-15, despite the latter possessing a higher acid site density, attributed to the superior accessibility of acid sites within the silica catalyst. In a related study on the effect of poor diameter on the esterification of palmitic acid with methanol over $PrSO_3H$/SBA-15, expanding the mesopores by incorporating a poragen during the silica sol-gel synthesis enhanced the rate of esterification, again implicating the mass transport limitations as rate-determining in this reaction [37]. The influence of pore connectivity was also explored in the esterification of a range of FFAs over mesoporous propylsulfonic acid functionalized silicas [38]. Comparison of $PrSO_3H$/SBA-15, comprising parallel and notionally noninterconnected pore channels, with a mesoporous $PrSO_3H$/KIT-6 catalyst possessing a gyroidal network of interconnected mesopores revealed significantly higher activity for the interconnected pore network, particularly for longer chain fatty acids. A subsequent study explored the benefits of incorporating macropores into the SBA-15 mesopore network to form hierarchically macroporous-mesoporous SBA-15 propylsulfonic acid catalysts for the transesterification of tricaprylin with methanol. Rates of TAG conversion to FAME increased with the proportion of macropore template introduced, again indicating that in-pore mass transport was rate-limiting but can be mitigated through tailored porous architectures [39].

4.4 ESTERIFICATION OF FREE FATTY ACIDS AND BIO-OILS

Oils feedstocks extracted from both edible and nonedible plants contain a mix of TAGs and FFAs. As discussed, liquid base catalysts are currently the commercial catalyst of choice for biodiesel production through oil transesterification due to their high activities [29], but are prone to soap/emulsion in the presence of FFAs [40]. While, the use of liquid acid catalysts offer an avenue to circumvent this problem, being able to catalyze both FFA esterification and TAG transesterification with light alcohols, acid catalyzed transesterifications are typically one order of magnitude less active than liquid bases [41], and still present challenges in their separation from biodiesel product. Solid acid catalysts offer a more attractive prospect, being able to esterify FFAs under mild reaction conditions, albeit still exhibiting poor transesterification performance [29]. Solid acid catalyzed esterification is also an important approach to stabilizing bio-oils obtained from biomass pyrolysis [42], which typically contain 2–10 wt% acetic acid, which renders such bio-oils corrosive to engines and prone to polymerization with an attendant increase in viscosity and poor combustion properties. The reaction mechanism in the case of solid acid catalysts involves the formation of protonated intermediate, followed by nucleophilic attack by alcohol (rate limiting step) to yield a protonated carbonyl precursor to the desired ester (Scheme 4.1) [43].

The most common solid acid catalysts for esterification of FFAs and other carboxylate-containing components of bio-oils are sulfated/sulfonated metal oxides, ion exchange resins, and zeolites [29]. Wilson and co-workers used propylsulfonic acid functionalized silica as catalyst for the esterification of acetic acid with benzyl alcohol [44], with good activity obtained

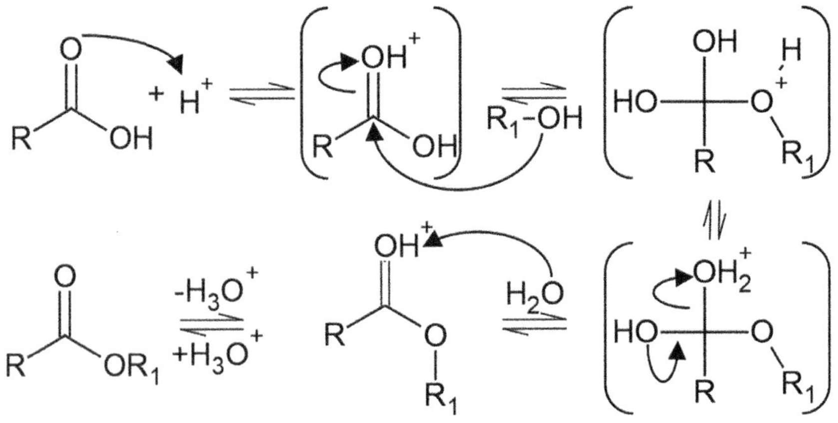

SCHEME 4.1   Proposed reaction mechanism for solid acid catalyzed esterification [43].

even in the presence of toluene to simulate a model pyrolysis bio-oil, and proportional to sulfonic acid surface density. Shanks and co-workers also employed propylsulfonic acid functionalized SBA-15 for acetic acid the esterification with methanol [45], reporting similar activity to H_2SO_4, and again scaling with sulfonic acid loading. Water tolerance tests showed that their $PrSO_3H/SBA$-15 catalyst was less sensitive to reactively formed water than H_2SO_4, attributed to hydrophobic propyl groups in the solid acid. Dacquin and co-workers also investigated the effect of surface hydrophobicity through cografting of alkyl and sulfonic acid groups onto a mesoporous MCM-41 silica surface [46]. Water adsorption over surfaces is strongly dependent upon their polarity, and by controlling the relative coverage of sulfonic acid versus octyl grafted functions, surface hydrophobicity could be readily tuned as shown in Figure 4.4a. Monte-Carlo dynamic simulations of a single pore, combined with ammonia flow-calorimetry, revealed that in the absence of cografted octyl functions, sulfonic acid moieties were able to strongly associate with free silanols on the silica surface, lowering their acid strength and directing them away from the pore interior, resulting in lower turnover frequencies (TOFs) for butanol esterification with acetic acid. In contrast, octyl cofunctionalization helped to direct sulfonic acid groups into the pore, increasing their acidity and reactivity (Figure 4.4b).

Sulphated zirconia (SZ) has gained significant attention due to its superacidic properties ($pK_{H+} > 12$) and tunable Brönsted/Lewis character [47]. The strong inductive effect of S=O groups at the surface of SZs can increase the Lewis acidity of exposed Zr^{4+} sites (Figure 4.5) [43], although debate remains as to whether such Lewis sites are converted into Brönsted acid sites in the presence of water [47]. Despite their versatile acidic properties conventional, bulk SZs possess low surface area and pore volume, and hence there is interest in the development of nanostructured analogs with ordered porosity.

Deveulapelli et al. investigated the performance of a mesoporous SZ prepared using cetyltrimethylammonium bromide as template under hydrothermal conditions on the esterification of 4-methoxyphenylacetic acid with dimethyl carbonate at 403–443 K [48], wherein they observed significant rate enhancements compared with conventional SZ, attributed to an increased surface acid site density and improved mass-transport due to mesopore incorporation. Yu and co-workers explored acetic acid esterification with ethanol (2:1 molar ratio of alcohol:acid) over rare earth oxide and alumina promoted SZ at 340 K [49], noting that pyridine adsorption studies indicated the total Brönsted and Lewis acid sites on the oxide promoted SZ was lower than the parent SZ, although the proportion of superacid sites was increased; greatest superacidity being observed for doubly promoted Yb_2O_3-Al_2O_3 SZ catalysts (SZYA). The number and strength of acid sites correlated well with ethyl acetate yield, with the SZYA material, which possessed the highest surface area offering 60% ester.

The porous nature of many ion exchange resins, coupled with their hydrophobic character, strong acidity, and recyclability, have been considered promising catalysts for bio-oil upgrading by esterification. A copolymer of acidic ionic liquid oligomers and divinylbenzene (PIL) was used as a catalyst for the simultaneous esterification and transesterification of FFA-containing triglyceride mixtures (waste cooking oil). This copolymer exhibited a high acid density of 4.4 mmol.g^{-1}, large pore volume and a surface area of 323 $m^2.g^{-1}$, coupled with wide (35 nm) mesopores [29], permitting efficient reactant diffusion through the pore network. The PIL copolymer was more active than the acidic ionic liquid alone, giving >99% conversion of oleic acid with MeOH at only 1 wt% catalyst loading. PIL also achieved >99% yield in rapeseed transesterification with MeOH under the same reaction conditions, and efficiently converted high FFA content waste cooking oil into biodiesel with 99% yield in 12 h; albeit recyclability, cost and toxicity was not considered in detail.

Zeolites are naturally occurring alumina-silicates possessing both Brönsted and Lewis acid sites arising from framework-substituted aluminum [41]. Zeolites have been widely studied for bio-oil upgrading through

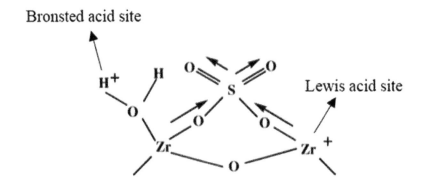

FIGURE 4.5 A simplified structure of sulfated zirconia showing Brönsted and Lewis acid sites [43].

esterification. Milina and co-workers investigated the esterification of acetic acid with o-cresol over various zeolite framework types (FER, MFI, MOR, BEA and FAU) and hierarchical mesoporous-microporous architectures [50]. Large pore Beta and Faujasite zeolites catalyzed efficient ester formation at 453 K, with yields up to 25%, whereas smaller pore frameworks such as mordenite, ZSM-5 and ferrierite were only active at 473 K, with the reactively formed cresol acetate apparently retained within the pore network due to its relatively large molecular size which in turn contributed to subsequent carbon laydown over strong Brönsted acid sites. Hierarchical Faujasite and MFI zeolites, synthesized through alkaline-mediated desilication, exhibited significantly improved acid conversion and ester yields over their conventional microporous counterparts (Figure 4.6). This was attributed to superior mass-transport through intracrystalline mesopores, and lower coking, notably for the narrow micropore ZSM-5. While such simple postsynthetic modification of commercially available zeolites can enhance acetic acid esterification, it also lowered the Brönsted acid site densities, and hence resulted in relatively poor recycling performance.

The influence of Pd doping upon Brönsted acidity and concomitant acetic acid esterification with methanol was studied by Koo et al. at 373 K over H-ZSM-5 and H-ferrierite zeolites [51]. Both parent protonated zeolites exhibited modest acetic acid conversion, but excellent selectivity to methyl acetate (~15% and 90%, respectively), with palladium addition increasing conversion to ~25% and methyl acetate yields to ~95%. DRIFTS vibrational studies revealed that strong Brönsted sites (prevalent in the lower Si:Al ratio ferrierite) facilitated strong methanol adsorption and the production of undesired alcohol dimers, in competition with acid esterification. Ammonia TPD studies suggested that palladium doping resulted in Pd^{2+} cations which preferentially bound to stronger Brönsted acid sites, thus preventing alcohol dimerization, consistent with the smaller observed promotion of the H-ZSM-5 zeolite (which possessed fewer strong Brönsted sites).

4.5 TRANSESTERIFICATION OF TRIGLYCERIDES

Triglycerides present in oils extracted from edible/nonedible plants, microalgae and fungi [29] can be converted into biodiesel through

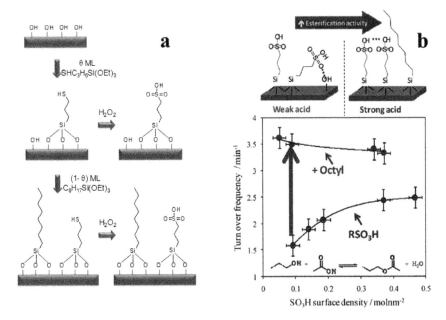

FIGURE 4.4 (a) Sulfonic acid and alkyl silane grafted onto an MCM-41 surface, (b) Catalytic activity of sulfonic acid functionalized MCM-41 in the esterification of butanol with acetic acid. Increased acid site density and hydrophobicity increases the turnover frequencies of the catalysts [46].

transesterification with low molecular weight alcohols to deliver a low carbon fuel (Scheme 4.2) [29].

The past decade has seen significant advances in the development of solid acid and base catalysts for TAG transterification [29]. Solid bases include metal oxides, alkali-doped metal oxides, and layered double hydroxides

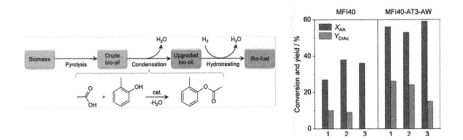

FIGURE 4.6 (Left) Potential application of acetic acid esterification with o-cresol in bio-oil upgrading; (Right) superior performance of hierarchical versus conventional MFI zeolites in cresol acetate production [50].

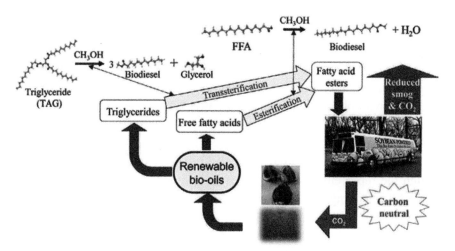

SCHEME 4.2 Biodiesel production cycle from renewable bio-oils via catalytic transesterification and esterification [29].

(notably hydrotalcites). CaO, MgO [52], and transition metal oxides such as MnO, TiO$_2$, and ZrO$_2$ are the most common basic oxides for transesterification, wherein active sites are proposed to comprise low coordination number M-O ionic pairs, particularly those present at corners and edges of nanoparticles, or high Miller index kinked/stepped surfaces (Figure 4.7) [53, 54].

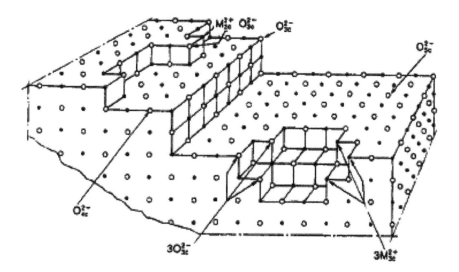

FIGURE 4.7 Mg-O ion pairs of different coordination numbers on the surface of MgO [53, 54].

Pretreatment of basic metal oxides at high temperature is generally required in order to remove carbonates formed either during their synthesis (as in the case precipitation as a metal hydroxycarbonate) [55] or via reaction with atmospheric CO_2 during storage. Varying the activation temperature can generate different base sites corresponding to ion pairs of different coordination numbers, although a quantitative relation between the nature of the active site specific ion-pairs combinations has yet to be established [53].

Alkali-doped metal oxides have been investigated for transesterification with varying success. In general, alkali dopants enhanced base strength through the replacement of M^{2+} by M^+ cations and associated defect generation [29]. Doping by Li, Na, K, Cs on MgO, CaO, and Al_2O_3 have been explored for the transesterification of rapeseed oil to biodiesel [56]. All alkali dopants increased the activity of the alkaline earth metal oxides, attributed to enhanced basicity due to the formation of O^- centers through the substitution of M^+ ions into the alkaline earth oxide lattice. Although alkali metal doping can enhance transesterification rates, such materials are prone to leaching, and since the rates of homogeneously catalyzed transesterification by alkali hydroxides are exceptionally high, much of the literature in this area is likely compromised by artifacts due to solution phase base catalysis [57, 58]. Synchrotron X-ray absorption spectroscopy of Cs-doped MgO nanoparticles, prepared via a supercritical sol-gel route, has identified $Cs_2Mg(CO_3)_2(H_2O)_4$ as the active phase responsible for the low temperature transesterification of tricaprylin, trilaurin and olive oil, with highly electron-deficient Cs atoms inducing strong charge transfer to oxygen vacancy traps, thereby generating superoxide anion superbasic sites [59].

Hydrotalcites are layered double hydroxides with brucite-like $Mg(OH)_2$ sheets containing octahedrally coordinated M^{2+} and M^{3+} cations, separated by interlayer A^{n-} anions to balance the net charge [29]. Mg-Al hydrotalcites have been widely applied to TAG transesterification for poor and high quality oil feeds, such as refined and acidic cottonseed oil and animal fat, delivering 99% conversion within 3 h at 473 K [60]. Conventional hydrotalcites are microporous, and hence ill-suited to the transesterification of bulky C_{16}-C_{18} triglycerides common in plant and algal oils. They are also typically prepared via coprecipitation of the metal nitrates through reaction with alkali hydroxides/carbonates, resulting in artifacts due to alkali leaching as discussed above [61]. The former problem has been addressed through the incorporation of secondary porosity (meso or macro) porosity [55]. Macropores introduced via hard-templating by colloidal nanospheres, act as rapid access conduits for the transport of long chain TAGs to active base sites present on the external surface of nanocrystalline alkali-free hydrotalcites conferring a ten-fold rate-enhancement in triolein transesterification with methanol over that attainable over a conventional microporous alkali-free Mg-Al hydrotalcite of identical composition (Figure 4.8). Spiking experiments confirmed that triolein transesterification by the hierarchical macroporous hydrotalcite was less susceptible to poisoning by reactively formed glycerol than a microporous hydrotalcite (wherein glycerol completely suppressed biodiesel production).

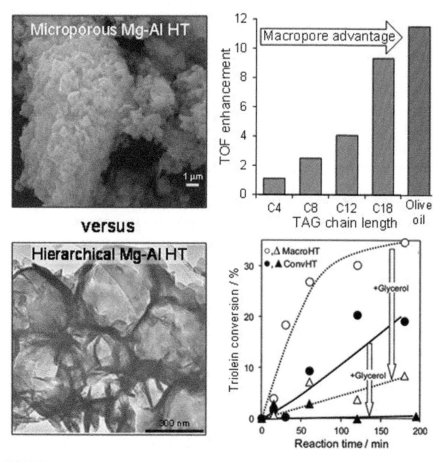

FIGURE 4.8 Superior catalytic performance of a hierarchical macroporous-microporous Mg-Al hydrotalcite solid base catalyst for TAG transesterification to biodiesel versus a conventional microporous analog [55].

Solid acid catalysts have also been evaluated in transesterification, including functionalized mesoporous silicas, heteropolyacids, and acidic polymeric resins [29]. Sulfonic acid functionalized SBA silicas are particularly attractive materials and exhibit activities comparable to commercial Nafion and Amberlyst resins in palmitic acid esterification [62], however they typically possess pore diameters <6 nm, and hence in-pore diffusion is slow and corresponding TOFs low. This problem has been examined through the use of poragens such as trimethylbenzene [63], triethylbenzene, and triisopropylebenzene[64] during synthesis of the mesoporous silica, which can induce swelling of the P123 surfactant micelles, resulting in silica nanostructures with pore diameters spanning 5–30 nm. $PrSO_3$/SBA-15 with expanded pores was used for tricaprylin and triolein transesterification with methanol under mild conditions [55]. TOFs for both reactions significantly increased with mesopore diameter, highlighting the recurring theme of poor mass-transport. Ordered macroporous-mesoporous $PrSO_3$/SBA-15 with tunable mesopores and macropores spanning 5–20 nm and 200–500 nm respectively have been prepared using microemulsion or cosurfactant routes for transesterification of bulky tricaprylin [39]. The propylsulfonic acid functionalized macromesoporous SBA-15 conferred significant rate-enhancements due to ready access of the TAG to $PrSO_3H$ active sites located within mesopores. Ti-doped SBA-15 was recently used for the esterification and transesterification of vegetable oils (soybean, rapeseed, crude palm, crude jatropha oil) and waste cooking oil [65]. Here, mesoporous structure of SBA-15 afforded improved accessibility to weakly Lewis acidic Ti^{4+} centers, resulting in higher activity compared to microporous titanosilicate and pure TiO_2 supports.

Heteropolyacids (HPAs) are an interesting class of coordination clusters exhibiting superacidity and with flexible compositions and supramolecular structures [29]. However, their use as heterogeneous catalysts for biodiesel synthesis has received less attention due to their high solubility in polar media, although ion-exchange of larger cations into phospho- and silicotungstic acids can increase their chemical stability. Cesium substituted phosphotungstic acid, $Cs_xH_{(3-x)}PW_{12}O_{40}$ and $Cs_yH_{(4-y)}SiW_{12}O_{40}$ are almost insoluble in water and catalytically active for tributyrin transesterification [66]. Absolute TOFs for tributyrin transesterification was higher for $Cs_xSiW_{12}O_{40}$ salt compared to homogeneous $H_4SiW_{12}O_{40}$ polyoxometalate clusters. Essayem et al. investigated the transesterification of rapeseed oil with ethanol over $H_3PW_{12}O_{40}$, $H_4SiW_{12}O_{40}$, $H_3PMo_{12}O_{40}$, $H_4SiMo_{12}O_{40}$, H_2SO_4, and phosphoric acid catalysts. Heteropolyacids achieved higher transesterification than mineral acids due to their higher acid strengths. However, the activity of HPAs did not correlate directly with acid strength, with proton solvation by water uncovered as a crucial parameter. Mo-containing HPAs exhibited the highest activities due to their ability to release crystalline water at lower temperatures compared to W-containing HPAs [67].

Acidic polymers and resins are advantageous for the diffusion of bulky TAGs and FFAs due to the ease of tuning their hydrophobicity. Sulfonated, mesoporous polydivinylbenzene (PDVB) exhibits higher absorption capacities for sunflower oil compared to $H_3PO_{40}W_{12}$, SZ, $PrSO_3H/SBA$-15, and Amberlyst 15, which is attributed to their superior performance in tripalmitin transesterification, affording an 80% methyl palmitate yield after 12 h reaction [68]. SO_3H-PDVB proved easily recyclable, showing only a modest drop in FAME yield after three recycles, ascribed to a combination of its high surface area, large pore volume, high acid site density, and hydrophobic/oleophilic pore network. Liu et al. used an aminophosphonic acid resin, built on a polystyrene backbone, in the microwave-assisted esterification of stearic acid with ethanol [69], obtaining FAME yields of 90% after microwave heating to (notionally) 353 K for 7 h with a high catalyst loading of 9 wt%, compared to 88% from conventional heating, albeit at longer reaction times. XRD, TGA and SEM measurements indicated this resin was stable structurally, and also proved recyclable negligible loss in acid conversion after five reaction cycles (Figure 4.9).

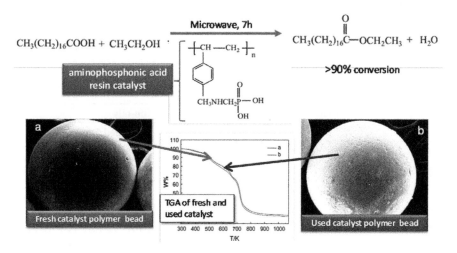

FIGURE 4.9   Stability of a solid acid resin catalyst for stearic acid esterification [69].

4.6   CATALYTIC HYDRODEOXYGENATION OF PYROLYSIS BIO-OILS

Hydrotreating is a widely used approach in petroleum refining to remove sulfur, nitrogen, metals, and oxygen to produce high performance and environmentally friendly liquid fuels suitable for modern internal combustion engines [27]. Hydrotreating methods include hydrodesulfurisation, hydrodenitrogenation, hydrodemetallation (removal of metal impurities), and hydrodeoxygenation (HDO), which are usually carried out under high hydrogen pressures in the presence of a heterogeneous catalyst. Since fossil fuels contain comparatively little oxygen, the petrochemical industry has traditionally focused on hydrotreating technologies for sulfur and nitrogen, with HDO neglected historically (Table 4.3).

The shift towards biomass feedstocks, which comprise significant proportions of carbohydrates, is driving the search for new HDO catalysts and processes which can remove oxygen without significantly lowering the energy density of the resulting biofuel. Pyrolysis bio-oils typically contain oxygenates present as carboxylic acids, carbonyls, hydroxyls, and ethers. Sulphided Mo/Al_2O_3 catalysts, promoted by Ni or Co, have shown promise in HDO of oxygen containing compounds [27], however such catalysts require a constant supply of H_2S in order stabilize them in sulfided form against deactivation by reactively formed water [30]. Transition metal promoters are believed to help weaken Mo-S bonds, resulting in the creation of catalytically active sites by creating sulfur vacancies at the edge MoS_2 crystallites. Studies of phenol and cresol HDO over a CoMo catalyst identified two independent reaction pathways, hydrogenation and deoxygenation. Similar observations were made for 4-methyl phenol HDO: direct

TABLE 4.3   Composition of Some Feeds for HDO [27]

	Conventional crude	Coal-derived naphtha	Oil shale crude	Bio-oils	
				Liquefied	Pyrolyzed
Carbon	85.2	85.2	85.90	74.8	45.3
Hydrogen	12.8	9.6	11.0	8.0	7.5
H/C	1.8	1.4	1.5	1.3	2.0
Sulphur	1.8	0.1	0.5	<0.1	<0.1
Nitrogen	0.1	0.5	1.4	<0.1	<0.1
Oxygen	0.1	4.7	1.2	16.6	46.9

deoxygenation (C-O cleavage) to toluene (DDO route); and hydrogenation to 4-methyl cyclohexanol (HYD) route (Scheme 4.3) [27].

Laurent and Delmon proposed that DDO and HDO require different active sites on MoS$_2$ catalysts. Romero et al. suggested that vertical η_1 adsorption of 2-ethyl phenol through the hydroxyl oxygen to sulfur vacancies favored DDO, whereas η_5 adsorption of 2-ethyl phenol through the aromatic ring, involving neighboring sulfur vacancies, favored HYD (Scheme 4.4) [70].

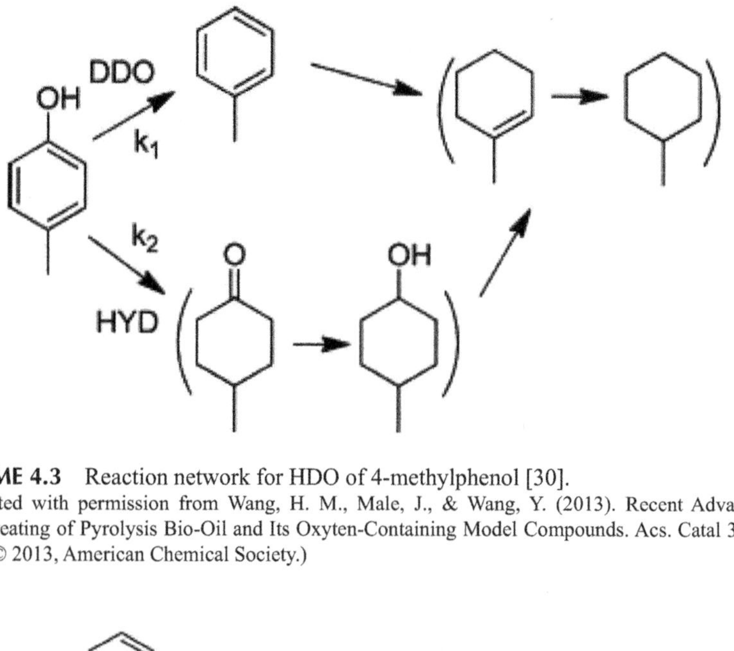

SCHEME 4.3 Reaction network for HDO of 4-methylphenol [30].
(Reprinted with permission from Wang, H. M., Male, J., & Wang, Y. (2013). Recent Advances in Hydrotreating of Pyrolysis Bio-Oil and Its Oxyten-Containing Model Compounds. Acs. Catal 3, 1047-1070. © 2013, American Chemical Society.)

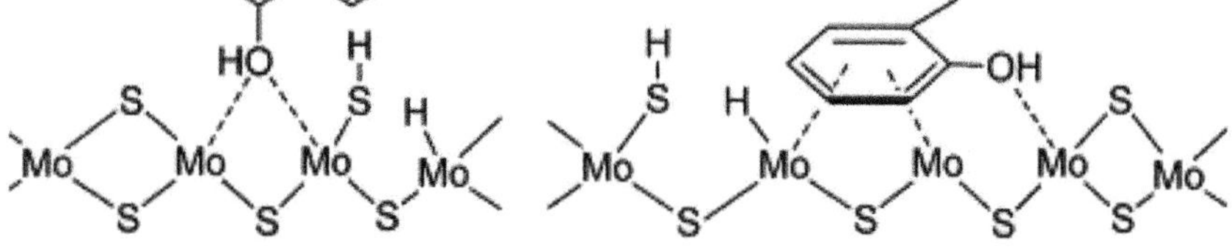

SCHEME 4.4 Possible adsorption modes of 2-ethyl phenol over MoS$_2$: (A) vertical η_1 adsorption through oxygen and (B) η_5 adsorption through aromatic ring and oxygen [30].
(Reprinted with permission from Wang, H. M., Male, J., & Wang, Y. (2013). Recent Advances in Hydrotreating of Pyrolysis Bio-Oil and Its Oxyten-Containing Model Compounds. Acs. Catal 3, 1047-1070. © 2013, American Chemical Society.)

Despite a rich history of sulfided Mo/Al_2O_3 catalysts in oil refineries for hydrotreating processes, other HDO catalysts have been explored for pyrolysis oil upgrading in an effort to circumvent the toxic H_2S requirement [27, 71] Acidic Al_2O_3 supports are also reported as unstable in the presence of water (present in large quantities in pyrolysis oil) being responsible for coke formation and catalyst deactivation [72]. Supported noble metal nanoparticles such as Pt, Pd, Rh, and Ru exhibit much higher hydrogenation activities than conventional sulfided Mo/Al_2O_3 catalysts, under more milder conditions, with the added benefit that noble metals also catalyze gasification of carbonaceous deposits suppressing coking [73]. Most studies of supported noble metals have been performed on pure phenolic compounds as model substrates common in pyrolysis bio-oils, such as phenol, catechol, anisole, and guaiacol, enabling elucidation of key reaction pathways [30]. Lercher and co-workers studied HDO of phenol, anisole, catechol, and guaiacol over Pd/C in the presence of liquid phosphoric acid, demonstrating that Pd was responsible for ring hydrogenation, while solution phase protons catalyzed deoxygenation (Scheme 4.5) [74].

Jensen and co-workers studied phenol HDO using Pd/C, Pt/C, and Ru/C catalysts at 100 bar H_2 and 548K in the absence of acid [75], reporting 100% alcohol conversion in all cases. The Pt/C catalyst proved the most active overall, with the Ru/C catalyst slowest, however the latter exhibited the highest activity for the deoxygenation step (despite the absence of acid) for which the Pt/C was inactive (Figure 4.10). DFT calculations showed that binding energies of oxygen relative to water (ΔE_0) were -0.01, 1.53, and 1.57 eV over Ru, Pd, and Pt respectively, with the strong affinity of Ru oxygen underpinning its deoxygenation activity.

The tendency of supported noble metals to hydrogenate aromatic rings does raise a concern regarding additional H_2 consumption, which may be economically undesirable. Recent studies using supported Pt and Pd nanoparticles show that this can be ameliorated under lower H_2 pressure and higher temperature [76], under which direct deoxygenation of phenol to benzene was

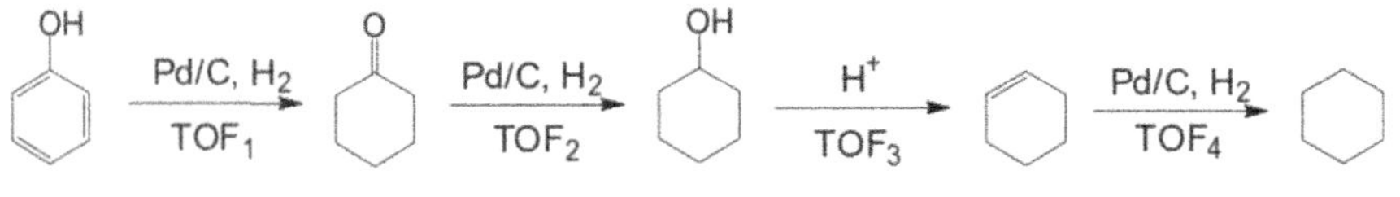

SCHEME 4.5 Reaction pathway for aqueous-phase HDO of phenol in a bifunctional catalyst system of Pd/C and H_3PO_4 at 473 K and 5 MPa hydrogen pressure [74].

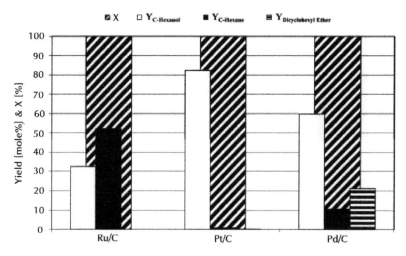

FIGURE 4.10 Conversion of phenol (x) and yields of cyclohexanol, cyclohexane, and dicyclohexyl ether with different types of reduced noble metal catalysts (Reprinted with permission from "Screening of Catalysts for Hydrodeoxygenation of Phenol as a Model Compound for Bio-oil" in ACS Catalysis 3 (2013), 10.1021/cs400266e. © 2013 American Chemical Society.)

preferred over phenol hydrogenation to cyclohexanol; lower H_2 pressures being insufficient to drive ring hydrogenation. The consensus is that HDO occurs through H_2 activation over metal surfaces, with oxygenates and the adsorbed/activated either at the metal-support interface or metal surface alone. Interactions between oxygenates and the (oxide) supports is usually driven by oxygen vacancies generated under hydrogen atmospheres, and/or the support Lewis acidity [77], with the choice of support the dominant factor in coke formation [77]. The incorporation of mesopores into ZSM-5 was also shown to enhance the dispersion of Pd nanoparticles throughout the hierarchical mesoporous-microporous framework, significantly accelerating m-cresol HDO relative to a conventional microporous ZSM-5, and boosting selectivity towards the desired methylcyclohexane deoxygenated product. High acid site densities enhanced m-cresol conversion and selectivity to methylcyclohexane, through rapid dehydration of the methylcyclohexanol intermediate (Figure 4.11) [78].

In light of the high cost of noble metals, inexpensive base metals such as Ni, NiCu bimetallics, and metal phosphides such as Ni_2P, MoP, NiMoP, CoMoP, Fe_2P, WP, and RuP have also been explored for HDO [30]. Supported Ni and NiCu bimetallic nanoparticles were active anisole HDO, giving superior conversions to sulfided Mo/Al_2O_3 [75]. In terms of support selection, CeO_2

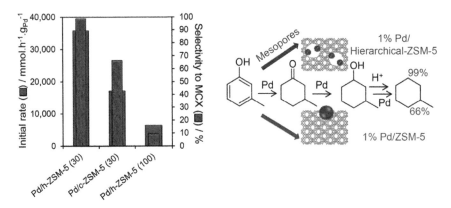

FIGURE 4.11 (Left) Activity and selectivity to methylcyclohexanol (MCX) of Pd catalyzed HDO over conventional (c) and hierarchical (h) ZSM-5 catalysts in m-cresol HDO; and (Right) stepwise ring hydrogenation and deoxygenation of m-cresol to methylcyclohexanol [78].

and ZrO_2 were optimal in terms of activity, attributed to their propensity for activating oxy-compounds. Transition metal phosphides have also been used for anisole and guaiacol HDO, with Ni_2P the most active [79]. However, there is evidence that metal phosphides deactivate in the presence of water [80].

4.7 CONCLUSIONS

Biomass has many attractive qualities as an alternative and renewable feedstock for bio-fuels (and bio-derived chemicals) production, although careful biomass selection is essential to avoid competing human or animal food use and/or land use changes. Lignocellulose, particularly that derived from nonedible forestry and agricultural wastes and triglycerides derived from microalgae represent the most promising biomass feedstocks for advanced biofuels, but are currently beset by energy intensive pretreatments due to their thermochemical stability or costly growth environments. Heterogeneous catalysis is a key enabling technology for the conversion of both lignocellulosic and lipid biomass into high-energy density liquid biofuels for the transportation sector. Nanoporous solid acid catalysts such as zeolites, sulfonic acid functionalized mesoporous silicas and polymeric resins show promise in the low temperature esterification of free fatty acids to biodiesel, albeit typically with requirements for high alcohol:acid ratios, and the intermediate upgrading of pyrolysis bio-oils containing high levels of acetic acid. Solid acids also offer a route to the simultaneous esterification and transesterification of oil (triglyceride) feedstocks containing high levels of free fatty acid impurities to biodiesel, albeit with modest rates of transesterification. Solid acids, particularly alkali-promoted alkaline earth and transition metal oxides, and microporous hydrotalcites exhibit high rates for triglyceride transesterification under mild conditions. Mass-transport limitations are an important consideration for both esterification and transesterification over porous solid acid/base catalysts, with hierarchical porous architectures offering significant rate-enhancements through the duel soft-hard pore templating strategies.

While metal oxide acid/base catalysts are well-suited to low temperature bio-fuels production and intermediate upgrading of bio-oils, deoxygenation of pyrolytic bio-oils to drop-in hydrocarbon fuels requires bifunctional metal/acid catalysts operating under high hydrogen pressures and reaction temperatures. Optimization of the balance of metal and acid sites is important to control selectivity in such bio-oil hydrodeoxygenation due to competing hydrogenation and deoxygenation pathways. Despite the significant advances made in the past two decades towards sustainable biofuels, important challenges remain for catalytic scientists and engineers. Future developments must address the important issues of long-term catalyst stability, use of precious metals, slow reaction kinetics due to poor mass-transport of bulky molecules, and process intensification through a transition from batch to continuous biofuels production.

KEYWORDS

- **biodiesel**
- **biomass**
- **heterogeneous catalysis**
- **nanomaterials**
- **porous solid**

REFERENCES

1. Asif, M., & Muneer, T. (2007). Energy supply, its demand and security issues for developed and emerging economies. *Renew Sust Energ Rev.*, *11*, 1388–1413.

2. International Energy Agency. CO_2 emissions from fuel combustion. http://www.iea. org/publications/freepublications/publication/CO2EmissionsTrends.pdf, 2015; Paris, France.

3. Cherubini, F. (2010). The biorefinery concept: Using biomass instead of oil for producing energy and chemicals. *Energ Convers Manage, 51*, 1412–1421.

4. Huber, G. W., Iborra, S., & Corma, A. (2006). Synthesis of transportation fuels from biomass: Chemistry, catalysts, and engineering. *Chem Rev., 106*, 4044–4098.

5. Besson, M., Gallezot, P., & Pinel, C. (2014). Conversion of Biomass into Chemicals over Metal Catalysts. *Chem. Rev., 114*, 1827–1870.

6. Duku, M. H., Gu, S., & Ben Hagan, E. (2011). A comprehensive review of biomass resources and biofuels potential in Ghana. *Renew. Sust. Energ. Rev., 15*, 404–415.

7. Demirbas, A. (2001). Biomass resource facilities and biomass conversion processing for fuels and chemicals. *Energ. Convers. Manage, 42*, 1357–1378.

8. Ragauskas, A. J., Williams, C. K., Davison, B. H., Britovsek, G., Cairney, J., Eckert, C. A., Frederick, W. J., Hallett, J. P., Leak, D. J., Liotta, C. L., Mielenz, J. R., Murphy, R., Templer, R., & Tschaplinski, T. (2006). The path forward for biofuels and biomaterials. *Science, 311*, 484–489.

9. Isikgor, F. H., & Becer, C. R. (2006). Lignocellulosic biomass: a sustainable platform for the production of bio-based chemicals and polymers. *Polym Chem-Uk z., 6*, 4497–4559.

10. Kumar, P., Barrett, D. M., Delwiche, M. J., & Stroeve, P. (2009). Methods for Pretreatment of Lignocellulosic Biomass for Efficient Hydrolysis and Biofuel Production. *Ind. Eng. Chem. Res., 48*, 3713–3729.

11. Jorgensen, H., Kristensen, J. B., & Felby, C. (2007). Enzymatic conversion of lignocellulose into fermenfigure sugars: challenges and opportunities. *Biofuel Bioprod Bior., 1*, 119–134.

12. Cadoche, L., & Lopez, G. D. (1989). Assessment of Size-Reduction as a Preliminary Step in the Production of Ethanol from Lignocellulosic Wastes. *Biol Waste, 30*, 153–157.

13. Sun, Y., & Cheng, J. Y. (2002).Hydrolysis of lignocellulosic materials for ethanol production: a review. *Bioresource Technol, 83*, 1–11.

14. Alizadeh, H., Teymouri, F., Gilbert, T. I., & Dale, B. E. (2005). Pretreatment of switchgrass by ammonia fiber explosion (AFEX). *Appl Biochem Biotech, 121*, 1133–1141.

15. Zheng, Y. Z., Lin, H. M., & Tsao, G. T. (1998). Pretreatment for cellulose hydrolysis by carbon dioxide explosion. *Biotechnol Progr, 14*, 890–896.

16. Quesada, J., Rubio, M., & Gomez, D. (1999). Ozonation of lignin rich solid fractions from corn stalks. *J Wood Chem Technol, 19*, 115–137.

17. Mosier, N., Wyman, C., Dale, B., Elander, R., Lee, Y. Y., Holtzapple, M., & Ladisch, M. (2005). Features of promising technologies for pretreatment of lignocellulosic biomass. *Bioresource Technol., 96*, 673–686.

18. Vonsivers, M., & Zacchi, G. A (1995). Technoeconomic Comparison of 3 Processes for the Production of Ethanol from Pine. *Bioresource Technol., 51*, 43–52.

19. Kim, S., & Holtzapple, M. T. (2006). Effect of structural features on enzyme digestibility of corn stover. *Bioresource Technol., 97*, 583–591.

20. Pan, X. J., Arato, C., Gilkes, N., Gregg, D., Mabee, W., Pye, K., Xiao, Z. Z., Zhang, X., & Saddler, J. (2005). Biorefining of softwoods using ethanol organosolv pulping: Preliminary evaluation of process streams for manufacture of fuel-grade ethanol and coproducts. *Biotechnol Bioeng., 90*, 473–481.

21. International Energy Agency. Key world energy statistics. *https://www.iea.org/publica-tions/freepublications/publication/KeyWorld_2017.pdf* , Paris, France.

22. Naik, S. N., Goud, V. V., Rout, P. K., & Dalai, A. K. (2010). Production of first and second generation biofuels: A comprehensive review. *Renew Sust Energ. Rev.*, *14*, 578–597.

23. Srinivasan, S. (2009). The food v. fuel debate: A nuanced view of incentive structures. *Renew. Energ.*, *34*, 950–954.

24. Wicke, B., Sikkema, R., Dornburg, V., & Faaij, A. (2011). Exploring land use changes and the role of palm oil production in Indonesia and Malaysia. *Land Use Policy.*, *28*, 193–206.

25. Serrano-Ruiz, J. C., & Dumesic, J. A. (2011). Catalytic routes for the conversion of biomass into liquid hydrocarbon transportation fuels. *Energ. Environ. Sci.*, *4*, 83–99.

26. Dry, M. E. (2002). The Fischer-Tropsch process: 1950–2000. *Catal Today*, *71*, 227–241.

27. Furimsky, E. (2000). Catalytic hydrodeoxygenation. *Appl Catal a-Gen. 199*, 147–190.

28. Mohan, D., Pittman, C. U., & Steele, P. H. (2006). Pyrolysis of wood/biomass for bio-oil: A critical review. *Energ Fuel. 20*, 848–889.

29. Lee, A. F., Bennett, J. A., Manayil, J. C., & Wilson, K. (2014). Heterogeneous catalysis for sustainable biodiesel production via esterification and transesterification. *Chem. Soc. Rev. 43*, 7887–7916.

30. Wang, H. M., Male, J., & Wang, Y. (2013). Recent Advances in Hydrotreating of Pyrolysis Bio-Oil and Its Oxygen-Containing Model Compounds. *Acs. Catal 3*, 1047–1070.

31. Deng, X. D., Li, Y. J., & Fei, X. W. (2009). Microalgae: A promising feedstock for biodiesel. *Afr. J. Microbiol Res. 3*, 1008–1014.

32. Stocker, M. (2008). Biofuels and Biomass-To-Liquid Fuels in the Biorefinery: Catalytic Conversion of Lignocellulosic Biomass using Porous Materials. *Angew. Chem Int. Edit 47*, 9200–9211.

33. Parlett, C. M. A., Wilson, K., & Lee, A. F. (2013). Hierarchical porous materials: catalytic applications. *Chem Soc. Rev. 42*, 3876–3893.

34. Zhang, X. J., Hirota, R., Kubota, T., Yoneyama, Y., & Tsubaki, N. (2011). Preparation of hierarchically meso-macroporous hematite Fe2O3 using PMMA as imprint template and its reaction performance for Fischer-Tropsch synthesis. *Catal Commun.*, *13*, 44–48.

35. Lu, Y. W., Zhou, P., Han, J., & Yu, F. (2015). Fischer-Tropsch synthesis of liquid hydrocarbons over mesoporous SBA-15 supported cobalt catalysts. *Rsc. Adv.*, *5*, 59792–59803.

36. Martin, A., Morales, G., Martinez, F., van Grieken, R., Cao, L., & Kruk, M. (2010). Acid hybrid catalysts from poly(styrenesulfonic acid) grafted onto ultra-large-pore SBA-15 silica using atom transfer radical polymerization. *J. Mater Chem.*, *20*, 8026–8035.

37. Dacquin, J. P., Lee, A. F., Pirez, C., & Wilson, K. (2012) Pore-expanded SBA-15 sulfonic acid silicas for biodiesel synthesis. *Chem Commun. 48*, 212–214.

38. Pirez, C., Caderon, J. M., Dacquin, J. P., Lee, A. F., & Wilson, K. (2012). Tunable KIT-6 Mesoporous Sulfonic Acid Catalysts for Fatty Acid Esterification. *Acs Catal.*, *2*, 1607–1614.

39. Dhainaut, J., Dacquin, J. P., Lee, A. F., & Wilson, K. (2010). Hierarchical macroporous-mesoporous SBA-15 sulfonic acid catalysts for biodiesel synthesis. *Green Chem.*, *12*, 296–303.

40. Kulkarni, M. G., & Dalai, A. K. (2006). Waste cooking oil-an economical source for biodiesel: A review. *Ind Eng Chem Res.*, *45*, 2901–2913.

41. Canakci, M., & Van Gerpen, J. (1999). Biodiesel production via acid catalysis. *T Asae.*, *42*, 1203–1210.
42. Moens, L., Black, S. K., Myers, M. D., & Czernik, S. (2009). Study of the Neutralization and Stabilization of a Mixed Hardwood Bio-Oil. *Energ. Fuel.*, *23*, 2695–2699.
43. Ciddor, L., Bennett, J. A., Hunns, J. A., Wilson, K., & Lee, A. F. (2015). Catalytic upgrading of bio-oils by esterification. *J. Chem. Technol. Biot.*, *90*, 780–795.
44. Manayil, J. C., Inocencio, C. V. M., Lee, A. F., & Wilson, K. (2016). Mesoporous sulfonic acid silicas for pyrolysis bio-oil upgrading via acetic acid esterification. *Green Chem.*, *18*, 1387–1394.
45. Miao, S. J., & Shanks, B. H. (2011). Mechanism of acetic acid esterification over sulfonic acid-functionalized mesoporous silica. *J. Catal.*, *279*, 136–143.
46. Dacquin, J. P., Cross, H. E., Brown, D. R., Duren, T., Williams, J. J., Lee, A. F., & Wilson, K. (2010). Interdependent lateral interactions, hydrophobicity and acid strength and their influence on the catalytic activity of nanoporous sulfonic acid silicas. *Green Chem.*, *12*, 1383–1391.
47. Chen, F. R., Coudurier, G., Joly, J. F., & Vedrine, J. C. (1993). Superacid and Catalytic Properties of Sulfated Zirconia. *J. Catal.*, *143*, 616–626.
48. Devulapelli, V. G., & Weng, H. S. (2009). Esterification of 4-methoxyphenylacetic acid with dimethyl carbonate over mesoporous sulfated zirconia. *Catal. Commun.*, *10*, 1711–1717.
49. Yu, G. X., Zhou, X. L., Li, C. L., Chen, L. F., & Wang, J. A. (2009). Esterification over rare earth oxide and alumina promoted SO42-/ZrO2. *Catal Today*, *148*, 169–173.
50. Milina, M., Mitchell, S., & Perez-Ramirez, J. (2014). Prospectives for bio-oil upgrading via esterification over zeolite catalysts. *Catal Today*, *235*, 176–183.
51. Koo, H. M., Lee, J. H., Chang, T. S., Suh, Y. W., Lee, D. H., & Bae, J. W. (2014). Esterification of acetic acid with methanol to methyl acetate on Pd-modified zeolites: effect of Bronsted acid site strength on activity. *React Kinet. Mech. Cat.*, *112*, 499–510.
52. Montero, J. M., Gai, P., Wilson, K., & Lee, A. F. (2009). Structure-sensitive biodiesel synthesis over MgO nanocrystals. *Green Chem. 11*, 265–268.
53. Hattori, H. (1995). Heterogeneous Basic Catalysis. *Chem. Rev.*, *95*, 537–558.
54. Fujita, T., Guan, P. F., McKenna, K., Lang, X. Y., Hirata, A., Zhang, L., Tokunaga, T., Arai, S., Yamamoto, Y., Tanaka, N., Ishikawa, Y., Asao, N., Yamamoto, Y., Erlebacher, J., & Chen, M. W. (2012). Atomic origins of the high catalytic activity of nanoporous gold. *Nat. Mater*, *11*, 775–780.
55. Woodford, J. J., Dacquin, J. P., Wilson, K., & Lee, A. F. (2012). Better by design: nanoengineered macroporous hydrotalcites for enhanced catalytic biodiesel production. *Energ. Environ. Sci.*, *5*, 6145–6150.
56. MacLeod, C. S., Harvey, A. P., Lee, A. F., & Wilson, K. (2008). Evaluation of the activity and stability of alkali-doped metal oxide catalysts for application to an intensified method of biodiesel production. *Chem. Eng. J.*, *135*, 63–70.
57. Alonso, D. M., Mariscal, R., Granados, M. L., & Maireles-Torres, P. (2009). Biodiesel preparation using Li/CaO catalysts: Activation process and homogeneous contribution. *Catal Today*, *143*, 167–171.
58. Yang, Z. Q., & Xie, W. L. (2007). Soybean oil transesterification over zinc oxide modified with alkali earth metals. *Fuel Process Technol*, *88*, 631–638.
59. Woodford, J. J., Parlett, C. M. A., Dacquin, J. P., Cibin, G., Dent, A., Montero, J., Wilson, K., & Lee, A. F. (2014). Identifying the active phase in Cs-promoted MgO nanocatalysts for triglyceride transesterification. *J Chem Technol. Biot.*, *89*, 73–80.

60. Barakos, N., Pasias, S., & Papayannakos, N. (2008). Transesterification of triglycerides in high and low quality oil feeds over an HT2 hydrotalcite catalyst. *Bioresource Technol.*, *99*, 5037–5042.

61. Cross, H. E., & Brown, D. R. (2010). Entrained sodium in mixed metal oxide catalysts derived from layered double hydroxides. *Catal Commun.* *12*, 243–245.

62. Mbaraka, I. K., Radu, D. R., Lin, V. S. Y., & Shanks, B. H. (2003). Organosulfonic acid-functionalized mesoporous silicas for the esterification of fatty acid. *J. Catal.*, *219*, 329–336.

63. Chen, D. H., Li, Z., Wan, Y., Tu, X. J., Shi, Y. F., Chen, Z. X., Shen, W., Yu, C. Z., Tu, B., & Zhao, D. Y. (2006). Anionic surfactant induced mesophase transformation to synthesize highly ordered large-pore mesoporous silica structures. *J. Mater Chem.*, *16*, 1511–1519.

64. Cao, L., Man, T., & Kruk, M. (2009). Synthesis of Ultra-Large-Pore SBA-15 Silica with Two-Dimensional Hexagonal Structure Using Triisopropylbenzene As Micelle Expander. *Chem. Mater*, *21*, 1144–1153.

65. Chen, S. Y., Mochizuki, T., Abe, Y., Toba, M., & Yoshimura, Y. (2014). Ti-incorporated SBA-15 mesoporous silica as an efficient and robust Lewis solid acid catalyst for the production of high-quality biodiesel fuels. *Appl. Catal. B-Environ.*, *148*, 344–356.

66. Narasimharao, K., Brown, D. R., Lee, A. F., Newman, A. D., Siril, P. F., Tavener, S. J., & Wilson, K. (2007). Structure-activity relations in Cs-doped heteropolyacid catalysts for biodiesel production. *J. Catal.*, *248*, 226–234.

67. Morin, P., Hamad, B., Sapaly, G., Rocha, M. G. C., de Oliveira, P. G. P., Gonzalez, W. A., Sales, E. A., & Essayem, N. (2007). Transesterification of rapeseed oil with ethanol I. Catalysis with homogeneous Keggin heteropolyacids. *Appl. Catal. a-Gen*, *330*, 69–76.

68. Xia, P., Liu, F. J., Wang, C., Zuo, S. F., & Qi, C. Z. (2012). Efficient mesoporous polymer based solid acid with superior catalytic activities towards transesterification to biodiesel. *Catal. Commun.*, *26*, 140–143.

69. Liu, W., Yin, P., Liu, X. G., Chen, W., Chen, H., Liu, C. P., Qu, R. J., & Xu, Q. (2013). Microwave assisted esterification of free fatty acid over a heterogeneous catalyst for biodiesel production. *Energ. Convers Manage*, *76*, 1009–1014.

70. Laurent, E., & Delmon, B. (1994). Influence of Water in the Deactivation of a Sulfided Nimo Gamma-Al2o3 Catalyst during Hydrodeoxygenation. *J. Catal.*, *146*, 281–291.

71. Romero, Y., Richard, F., & Brunet, S. (2010). Hydrodeoxygenation of 2-ethylphenol as a model compound of bio-crude over sulfided Mo-based catalysts: Promoting effect and reaction mechanism. *Appl. Catal. B-Environ*, *98*, 213–223.

72. Furimsky, E., & Massoth, F. E. (1999). Deactivation of hydroprocessing catalysts. *Catal. Today*, *52*, 381–495.

73. Wildschut, J., Mahfud, F. H., Venderbosch, R. H., & Heeres, H. J. (2009). Hydrotreatment of Fast Pyrolysis Oil Using Heterogeneous Noble-Metal Catalysts. *Ind. Eng. Chem. Res.*, *48*, 10324–10334.

74. Zhao, C., He, J. Y., Lemonidou, A. A., Li, X. B., & Lercher, J. A. (2011). Aqueous-phase hydrodeoxygenation of bio-derived phenols to cycloalkanes. *J. Catal.*, *280*, 8–16.

75. Mortensen, P. M., Grunwaldt, J. D., Jensen, P. A., & Jensen, A. D. (2013). Screening of Catalysts for Hydrodeoxygenation of Phenol as a Model Compound for Bio-oil. *Acs. Catal.*, *3*, 1774–1785.

76. Nimmanwudipong, T., Runnebaum, R. C., Block, D. E., & Gates, B. C. (2011). Catalytic Conversion of Guaiacol Catalyzed by Platinum Supported on Alumina: Reaction Network Including Hydrodeoxygenation Reactions. *Energ. Fuel*, *25*, 3417–3427.

77. He, Z., & Wang, X. (2013). Hydrodeoxygenation of model compounds and catalytic systems for pyrolysis bio-oils upgrading. *Catalysis for Sustainable Energy*, 28–52.

78. Hunns, J. A., Arroyo, M., Lee, A. F., Escola, J. M., Serrano, D., & Wilson, K. (2016). Hierarchical mesoporous Pd/ZSM-5 for the selective catalytic hydrodeoxygenation of m-cresol to methylcyclohexane. *Catal. Sci. Technol.*

79. Zhao, H. Y., Li, D., Bui, P., & Oyama, S. T. (2011). Hydrodeoxygenation of guaiacol as model compound for pyrolysis oil on transition metal phosphide hydroprocessing catalysts. *Appl Catal a-Gen.*, *391*, 305–310.

80. Li, K. L., Wang, R. J., & Chen, J. X. (2011). Hydrodeoxygenation of Anisole over Silica-Supported Ni2P, MoP, and NiMoP Catalysts. *Energ Fuel.*, *25*, 854–863.

81. Alonso, D. M., Bond, J. Q. (2010). Catalytic conversion of biomass to biofuels. ***Green Chem.***, 2010, 12, 1493-1513.

PART II

BIOFUEL CHEMISTRY AND PROCESS INTENSIFICATION

CHAPTER 5

PROCESS INTENSIFICATION AND PARAMETRIC OPTIMIZATION IN BIODIESEL SYNTHESIS USING MICROWAVE REACTORS

PRANJALI D. MULEY and DORIN BOLDOR

Department of Biological and Agricultural Engineering, Louisiana State University Agricultural Center, Baton Rouge, LA 70803, United States

CONTENTS

ABSTRACT

Use of advanced microwave technology for organic synthesis offers a number of advantages over conventional methods, such as reduced reaction and processing times, lower oil/solvent ratio, enhanced product selectivity, reduced catalyst consumption, and increased overall process efficiency. Microwave heating enhances the rate of reaction and energy efficiency by intensifying the rate of mass and heat transfer during extraction and transesterification. This chapter discusses the application of advanced microwave technology for biodiesel production through transesterification reaction. The chapter gives an overview of microwave theory and dielectric heating mechanism for biodiesel synthesis. The effect of various process parameters on the yield and quality of biodiesel are discussed with an emphasis on microwave reactor designs, from batch to continuous scale and pilot scale biodiesel production. Advances in the field pertaining to process optimization and numerical modeling are also briefly discussed with an overview of biodiesel production microalgae and *in situ* transesterification. Advantages of microwave heating over conventional heating are discussed along with energy efficiency and effect of microwave irradiation on the reaction kinetics.

5.1 OVERVIEW

An inevitable exhaustion of fossil fuels in the future has drawn researchers around the globe to develop a sustainable carbon neutral source of energy. Among the first generation biofuels, biodiesel has a crucial advantage of being a direct alternative to petroleum diesel. Biodiesel has lower emission compared to petroleum-based diesel. The net greenhouse gases produced by biodiesel are minimal and the amount of sulfur exhaust in the atmosphere is negligible [1]. Most physical and chemical properties of biodiesel are comparable with petroleum diesel. The presence of two oxygen atoms, as well as the presence of one or more unsaturated bonds in the biodiesel molecule separates it from diesel model molecule (Figure 5.1). Biodiesel has a higher cetane number, low sulfur content, and lower emissions compared to diesel; however, biodiesel has higher pour and cloud point which makes it difficult to use in colder temperatures, and the NOx emission is higher with burning biodiesel (Table 5.1). Moreover, the production cost of biodiesel is higher compared to petroleum diesel due to lower process efficiency during biodiesel synthesis and the relatively higher cost of feedstock (Table 5.1).

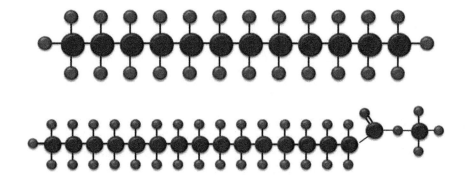

FIGURE 5.1   Diesel and biodiesel molecular structure.

Multiple researchers have tried to address these issues by proposing various alternatives such as low cost reactor design, use of invasive species, increasing reactor efficiency, etc. [2–6]. The use of invasive species such as jatropha [5], and Chinese tallow tree seeds [6] for biodiesel production provide a nonedible source of lipids. Cao et al. studied the effect of a novel semicontinuous membrane reactor to produce biodiesel. They observed that

TABLE 5.1   Comparison of Biodiesel and Diesel Fuel Properties

Fuel property	Biodiesel	Diesel	Standard	Reference
Cetane Number	48–65	40–55	ASTM D613	[12]
High Heating Value Btu/gal	127,042	137,640	ASTM D6751	
High Heating Value Mj/kg	40.168	45.766	ASTM D2015–85	
Kinematic Viscosity @ 40 C	4.0–6.0	1.3–4.1	ASTM D445	
Density lb/gal	7.3	7.1	ASTM D941	
% O	11	0		
% S	0.002	0.04	ASTM D5453–93	
Flash Point (°C)	100–170	60–80	ASTM D93	
Pour Point (°C)	-5 to 10	-35 to -15	ASTM D97–93	
Cloud Point (°C)	-3 to 15	-35 to 5	ASTM D 2500–91	
CO emission (%)	-34.50	0		[13]
NOX emission (%)	+13.54	0		[13]
Production Cost (USD/gal)	2.8	0.75		
Retail Cost (USD/gal) (as on October, 2015)	3.36	2.33		

the methanol loading can be reduced by the use of such reactor and in turn increase the efficiency [2]. He et al. developed a reactive distillation reactor, which decreased the reaction times by 20 to 30 times while increasing the productivity of biodiesel 6–10 times compared to conventional continuous reactors [7]. One of the promising alternatives proposed is the use of microwave technology for the production of biodiesel [8]. Direct volumetric heating, decreased reaction time and reduction of heat losses associated with the heating medium are some of the well-established advantages of microwave heating [9]. The use of microwave technology is expanding from food industry to chemical and pharmaceutical industry, as microwave irradiation is thought to increase the process efficiency. Microwave heating depends on multiple factors such as dielectric and physical properties of the material, operational power and frequency, and system geometry [10].

5.1.1 BIODIESEL OVERVIEW AND CHEMISTRY

Since G. Chavanne (University of Brussels) in 1937 first patented the process for biodiesel synthesis, it has seen multiple advances in terms of technological development and production efficiency. Biodiesel is essentially a fatty acid alkyl ester with chemical and physical properties similar to that of petroleum diesel. Plant oil and animal fat are two main sources of triglycerides. These triglycerides are a mixture of saturated and unsaturated fatty acids with animal source being rich in saturated fatty acids. Biodiesel has been synthesized using edible lipid sources such as soybean oil, rice bran, rapeseed, sunflower oil, etc. while the nonedible sources tested are Chinese tallow seeds, castor oil, jatropha, and microalgae. The triglycerides are converted to glycerol and biodiesel in a three step chemical reaction called transesterification (also known as alcholysis). Each step produces an alkyl ester molecule; their mixture is termed as 'biodiesel" (Eqs. 1 and 2).

$$
\begin{array}{ccccc}
 & O & & O & \\
 & \| & \text{catalyst} & \| & \\
CH_2\text{-}OC\text{-}R_1 & & & R_1\text{-}OC\text{-}R` & CH_2\text{-}OH \\
| & & \Delta & + & | \\
CH\text{-}OOC\text{-}R_2 & + \ 3R`OH \longrightarrow & & R_2\text{-}OOC\text{-}R` & + \ CH\text{-}OH \\
| & \longleftarrow & & + & | \\
CH_2\text{-}OC\text{-}R_3 & & & R_3\text{-}OC\text{-}R` & CH_2\text{-}OH \\
 & \| & & \| & \\
\end{array}
$$

$$\text{O} \qquad\qquad\qquad\qquad\qquad\qquad \text{O}$$

Vegetable oil	Alcohol	Esters Glycerol
(Lipids)	(Biodiesel)	

$$(1)$$

Since the reaction is reversible, excess alcohol is used to shift the equilibrium to the right. The forward reaction becomes a pseudo first order reaction because of the excess alcohol [11].

$$\text{Triglyceride (TG)} + \text{R`OH} \xrightleftharpoons{k} \text{Diglyceride (DG)} + \text{R`COOR}_1$$

$$\text{Diglyceride (DG)} + \text{R`OH} \xrightleftharpoons{k} \text{Monoglyceride (MG)} + \text{R`COOR}_2$$

$$\text{Monoglyceride (MG)} + \text{R`OH} \xrightleftharpoons{k} \text{Glycerol (GL)} + \text{R`COOR}_3$$

$$(2)$$

To date, transesterification is the most commonly employed method for biodiesel production. Some of the common physical and chemical properties of biodiesel and diesel fuel are given in Table 5.1. Fuel standards are defined by ASTM and EN standards. Some important properties that define the quality of the fuel are cetane number, density, specific gravity, kinematic viscosity, flash point, pour point, cloud point, acid number, and oxidative stability.

5.1.1.1 Qualitative Properties: Cetane Number, High Heating Value and Lubricity

Cetane number is one of the most important properties of diesel fuel. It is a measure of the combustion speed of the fuel and can be primarily used to define the quality of diesel. Higher cetane number indicates that the fuel combusts easily in a diesel engine. ASTM D975 sets the minimum value of petroleum diesel at 40. Biodiesel has a higher cetane value compared to petroleum diesel ranging from 48–65. The high heating value of diesel and biodiesel are comparable with HHV for diesel being slightly higher (up to 10%) than that of biodiesel. Lubricity indicates the reduction in friction between the solid surfaces in motion within the engine and affects the fuel injector system in particular. While external lubricants can be added to the fuel, biodiesel in itself has very good lubricity.

5.1.1.2   Physical Properties: Density and Kinematic Viscosity

Density of the fuel significantly affects the air to fuel ratio and the energy content of the fuel volume injected; hence density of fuel is an important property. Biodiesel is slightly denser than petroleum diesel, with density ranging from 7.3–7.5 lb/gal. Kinematic viscosity is a measure of resistance to flow of liquid due to friction. It also affects the lubricity of fuel. Viscosity is an important property as it affects the storage and operational conditions of the fuel. Highly viscous fuel cause poor atomization, causing deposition in the combustion chamber leading to coking which could damage the engine [14]. According to the ASTM specifications, the acceptable range of viscosity is 1.9–6.0 mm^2/sec.

5.1.1.3   Cold Flow Properties: Cloud Point and Pour Point

Cold flow properties are significant in order to insure safe and reliable fuel operation during cold temperatures. While there is no specific method to quantify the cold flow properties, cloud point and pour point are commonly measured. Cloud point is the temperature below which the waxes in the fuel form a cloudy appearance. The solidification of waxes increases the viscosity of the fuel, which may clog the fuel injection line and filters. Pour point is the temperature below which the fuel is semisolid and loses its flow characteristic. The requirement of ASTM standard of the maximum cloud point temperature is 10°C. However, even lower values are desired as this quality is directly associated with the low temperature performance of fuel.

5.1.1.4   Safety and Storage: Acid Number and Oxidative Stability and Flash Point

High acid number reflects presence of high quantity of free and mineral acids in the fuel. High acid number indicates the corrosive nature of the fuel. ASTM standard requires an acid number value for biodiesel to be less than 0.5 mg of KOH/gm of oil. Oxidation stability index of a fuel is determined from the rate of oxidation, which is generally accelerated by the presence of water, acids and metals such as copper. Oxidative stability is an important property that determines the storage life of the fuel. Flash point is defined as the minimum temperature at which the fuel self-ignites. A higher flash point value indicates low fuel volatility and ensures safety in handling, transportation and storage of fuel [14].

5.1.2 MICROWAVE BASICS

The frequency range of microwave is between 300 MHz to 300 GHz. On an electromagnetic spectrum, microwaves fall between infrared and radio waves with wavelengths between 1.0 cm and 1.0 m [15]. Since its application for heating in 1945, microwave technology has been developed and used in numerous industrial applications such as cooking, aseptic sterilization, drying, ceramic and paint industry along with biological and agricultural processing to name a few [16, 17]. In the US, Federal Communications Commission (FCC) has allocated certain microwave frequency bands designated for Industrial, Scientific, and Medical (ISM) applications. Some of these frequency bands are 915, 2450, 5800, 24,125, 61,250, 122,500, and 245,000 MHz [18]. While conventional methods rely on conduction and convection for heat transfer and are slow and inefficient, microwave heating is a direct molecular level heating with high efficiency. A direct molecular level interaction of microwave energy with the reactants eliminates the need for a heat transfer medium, reducing losses, reaction times and operation costs and making microwave reactor a lucrative option.

Microwave field has two active field components; electric field and magnetic field. Dielectric heating, which is dominant for most materials, can be explained by two important mechanisms: dipole polarization and ionic conduction. In dipole polarization, when a polar molecule having an electric dipole moment is exposed to an electromagnetic radiation, it tries to align itself in the direction of the electric field. Since the field is oscillating rapidly, the polar molecules oscillate rotationally along with the changing field. This generates friction between the adjacent molecules resulting in an increased temperature. At the right frequency of operation, which depends on the molecular structure of the individual compound, the dipolar rotation can generate significantly high temperatures. For significantly higher frequencies (>5800 MHz), the electric field component is reversed rapidly, not giving enough time for the molecules to respond to the changing field. Hence even the smallest molecule does not respond to the oscillating field causing a marked decrease in dielectric permittivity.

In case of ionic conduction, the presence of ions or free radicals helps generate heat. These ions when exposed to electromagnetic waves move under the influence of electric field resulting in linear oscillations. As the electric field direction changes, the ions slow down and change direction. In the process, this motion causes collisions resulting in conversion of kinetic energy into heat energy.

Dielectric permittivity is a measure of the interaction of material with the electric field. Dielectric permittivity is denoted by ε and defined by the dielectric constant and dielectric loss of the material [19]. The dielectric constant is the ability of the material to store charge while the dielectric loss factor is defined as the amount of conversion of the stored charge to heat. The equation for the complex dielectric permittivity ε as a function of dielectric constant ε' and dielectric loss factor ε'' is given by the complex equation [20] (Eq. 3):

$$\varepsilon = \varepsilon' - j * \varepsilon'' \tag{3}$$

Where real part is the dielectric constant ε' and the imaginary part is the dielectric loss factor, ε''. In the microwave region, the dielectric properties of material can be measured using a network analyzer. Both dielectric constant and dielectric loss are frequency and temperature dependent. At low frequencies, the electric field components is reversed at a slower pace giving enough time for the molecules to align and to store the applied charge in the dipoles. Thus, the dielectric constant at low frequencies is higher.

5.2 MICROWAVE ASSISTED OIL EXTRACTION

Microwave assisted biodiesel production is generally a two-step process: microwave induced oil extraction followed by transesterification reaction. Multiple researchers have studied microwave assisted oil extraction for biodiesel production on batch, continuous and pilot scale. The efficiency of the process depends on various factors such as frequency of operation, solvent polarity, solubility of meal in solvent, extraction time, and temperature. Microwave heating offers higher product selectivity and yield and lower extraction times and solvent amount compared to conventional extraction.

Extraction efficiency in case of microwave extraction (ME) increases due to direct heating during microwave interaction, and localized superheating. The extent of extraction depends on the interaction between the matrixes (solvent – meal mixture) with the microwaves. Microwave interaction intensifies the mass and heat transfer rates within the sample. As the solvent and meal mixture is irradiated with microwaves, the polar water molecules start rotating under the influence of electric field, whereas the cell structure being transparent to the microwave is unaffected. This causes cell walls to rupture due to pressure built up within the cells, triggering partial or complete disintegration in the cell wall structure [21]. Microwaves penetrating the oilseeds also cause disruption of cell walls triggering migration and diffusion of oil molecules into the extraction solvent. The lipids become more accessible to the solvent, which is also polar. The polarity of solvent increases the rate of collision and chances of interaction between solvent and lipid molecules. As per the microwave heating mechanism, the friction between rotating polar molecules increase the temperature. This phenomenon leads to an overall increase in heat and mass transfer rates.

Solvent based microwave assisted extraction (MAE) is the most efficient and commonly used extraction method. Hexane, isopropanol, acetone, ethanol, methanol and acetonitrile are some commonly used solvents among which hexane, ethanol and isopropanol are the most studied. A typical laboratory scale ME system (batch and continuous) is shown in Figure 5.2. A modified domestic microwave oven or commercially available batch microwave

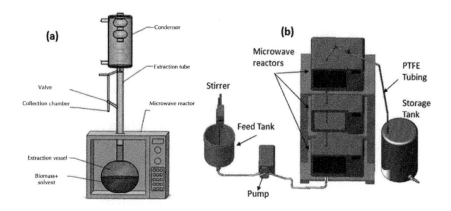

FIGURE 5.2   Microwave-assisted batch extraction system.

ovens are commonly employed for preliminary lab–scale experiments [25]. The reactor has a multimode cavity and the operational frequency is 2450 MHz, as allowed by Federal Communication Commission (FCC). The power output on the microwave oven varied between 900–1100 W. Extraction process is typically carried out at atmospheric pressure in the presence of air. However, some studies have reported use of high-pressure ME that resulted in higher oil yields [26]. The moisture content of the seeds used for extraction is measured; the seeds are sometimes dried to reduce moisture content. They are then milled to flour. The flour is then mixed with appropriate solvent in a known ratio. The solvent to meal ratio depends on the solvent type. Typically, for alcohols such as methanol [27] and ethanol a solvent to meal ratio of 3:1 to 9:1 (w/w) is employed [28], however, other solvents such as n-hexane [29], isopropanol, acetone [27], water or cosolvents can also be used for extraction [30]. The meal and solvent mixture is placed in a microwave transparent flask made from glass or Teflon material. The mixture is continuously stirred using microwave safe magnetic stirrer. The extraction temperature depends on the solvent boiling point and for open extraction, the temperature is maintained slightly below the solvent boiling point temperature. For pressurized systems, higher temperatures ranges have been investigated [31]. Extraction times noted in literature varies from 1–35 min [28, 31]. After extraction, the solvent is separated from the meal. The solvent is recovered typically using rotovap or vacuum centrifuge evaporator and the lipid is collected. The residue lipid is weighed to determine extraction yield. For a continuous lab scale process shown in Figure 5.2, three modified domestic microwave ovens are placed in series with a Teflon tube passing through the reactors. The meal/solvent mixture is continuously pumped through the tube, where it is heated in the microwave heater. The lipid, solvent and meal mixture is collected in a beaker for separation and purification. Other continuous reactor designs include commercial lab-scale oven modified for continuous flow using peristaltic pumps [28]. A pilot scale extraction process was also demonstrated by Terigar et al., where a 915 MHz, 5 kW single mode cavity continuous microwave reactor was used for oil extraction from soybean and ricebran meal [28]. Table 5.2 shows a comparison between conventional and microwave heating. ME yielded higher oil yields as compared to conventional extraction (CE) process for the same extraction time and temperature combinations. In general MAE required lower extraction times (half of that used for conventional extraction methods) as well as lower temperatures. A mixture of two or more solvents have also shown to increase the oil yield for MAE process [22].

TABLE 5.2 Oil Yields From Soybean and Rice Bran Using Different Solvents in Conventional Extraction (CE) and Microwave Extraction (ME) Methods

Solvent	Dielectric constant	% Oil yield – Soybean		Reference	% Oil yield – Rice bran		Reference
		CE	ME		CE	ME	
Hexane	1.88	6.8	9.7	[22]	14	14	[23]
Isopropanol	19.92	6.1	6.9	[22]	12	15	[23]
Ethanol	24.3	11.3	17.3	[24]	12.4	17.2	[24]

5.3 MICROWAVE ASSISTED TRANSESTERIFICATION

The second step in the two-step biodiesel production is the transesterification reaction. Transesterification of various feedstocks have been reported in the literature using both laboratory and industrial scale microwave systems. Since microwave heating takes place at a molecular level, molecular interaction between different reactants increases. This in turn increases the rate of collision between reactant molecules, increasing the rate of reaction. The ions moving in the direction of applied energy field also comes in contact with the reactants, further intensifying reaction rate. Due to this unique feature, microwave heating is one of the highly effective methods for biodiesel production. Lower energy losses are associated with microwave heating due to the absence of heat transfer material. Hence, the energy efficiency of microwave processes is considerably high compared to conventional heating methods [32]. Although there is no direct evidence of the nonthermal effects of microwave, some theoretical evidences exists. The local superheating, increased molecular movement and subsequent molecular level interaction in microwave process increases the rate of reaction [33]. Another explanation is pertaining to the Arrhenius equation (Eq. 4).

$$k = Ae\frac{-Ea}{RT} \tag{4}$$

where, K is the rate constant, Ea is the activation energy, R is the gas constant, T is the temperature, and A is the pre-exponential factor. The frequency factor A represents collision rate or molecular motion and depends on the frequency of vibration. High molecular level interaction during microwave processing could result in an increase in the frequency and rate of collision, affecting the frequency factor A thus, increasing the rate of reaction [34].

Figure 5.3 shows a common microwave assisted 2-step biodiesel production process flow chart. Step one is extraction where the seeds are preconditioned to obtained the right moisture content. The seeds are then ground to a uniform meal size. Lipid from meal is extracted either using solvent or on solvent free basis. The separated and purified oil is then dried to remove any solvent or moisture present. After drying the oil is ready for transesterification. The detailed transesterification procedure is given elsewhere in this chapter.

Typically, three types of reactors employed are: laboratory scale batch reactor, laboratory scale continuous reactor and pilot scale continuous process reactor.

5.3.1 LABORATORY SCALE REACTORS

Laboratory scale microwave reactors used for transesterification are generally domestic ovens or commercial laboratory scale ovens (Figure 5.5) with multimode cavity. A typical domestic oven has a power of 800–1200 W, whereas, commercial microwave ovens offer higher power settings varying from 950–1900 W and a frequency of 2450 MHz. The

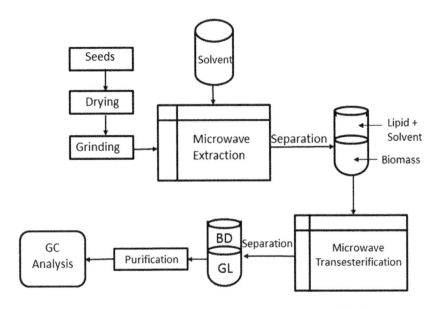

FIGURE 5.3   Flow chart of microwave assisted extraction and transesterification.

difference in the electric field distribution the multimode cavity at 2450 MHz and a single mode focused cavity at 915 MHz modeled in COMSOL Multiphysics is shown in Figure 5.4. In a multimode cavity, microwave radiations interact in a certain manner [35]; whereas in a single mode resonant cavity, the microwave radiations are focused towards the reactor center. While multimode cavity offers flexibility of design, single mode cavity offers high-energy density.

The reactor design for lab scale transesterification reaction is similar to the ME reactors. A typical microwave assisted transesterification process is carried out using polar solvents such as alcohols and in the presence of catalysts. In case of alkaline catalysts, the catalyst is first dissolved in the solvent. Oil is either added to the mixture or pumped separately into the reactor. The oil-alcohol-catalyst mixture is then heated in the microwave reactor. Presence of polar solvents and ionic materials increase the heating efficiency in the microwave reactor. The reaction temperatures noted in literature depend on various factors such as solvent type, catalyst, oil to solvent ratio is discussed elsewhere in this chapter. A typical laboratory scale transesterification reaction employs 100–400 ml oil-alcohol mixture heated at a temperature of 50–100°C and typical reaction times ranging from 1 min to 60 min. Ethanol and methanol are the most commonly used solvents, while NaOH and KOH are the most popular alkaline catalysts [1, 37]. While the stoichiometric requirement for oil to alcohol ratio is 1:1, since the reaction is a reversible one, alcohol is always added in excess to ensure reaction is complete. The

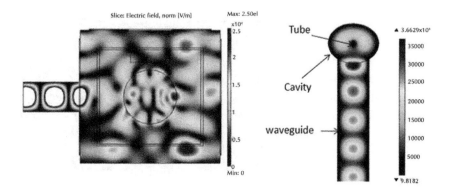

FIGURE 5.4   Electric field distribution inside microwave cavity (a) multimode 2450 MHz (reprinted with permission from Ref. [35] and, (b) single mode focused cavity 915 MHz (reprinted with permission from Ref. [36]).

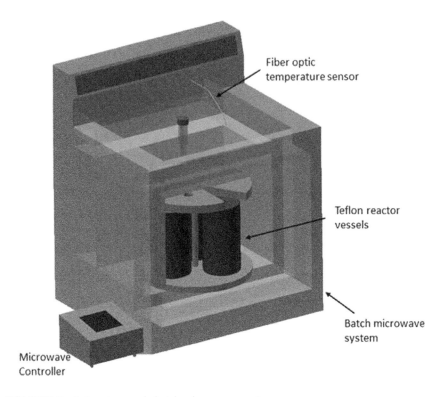

Fiber optic
temperature sensor

Teflon reactor
vessels

Batch microwave
system

Microwave
Controller

· **FIGURE 5.5**   Laboratory scale batch microwave reactor.

products collected from the microwave reactor after reaction is a mixture of alkyl esters (biodiesel), glycerol, excess alcohol, dissolved catalyst, and unreacted lipids. The products are allowed to separate until they form two distinct layers of biodiesel and glycerol. The lower glycerol layer is separated and the biodiesel is washed multiple times with water to remove any impurities. For biodiesel washing, water is sprayed onto the biodiesel at lower velocity. Alcohol, catalyst and other impurities are removed as the water percolated down the biodiesel forming a second layer at the bottom of the separatory funnel [38]. Washed biodiesel is further dried and analyzed for quality check. In a continuous lab scale process, the reactants are either premixed before pumping or are pumped separately to the reaction chamber at a fixed oil-alcohol ratio (Figure 5.7). The products are then filtered and transferred to a separating funnel where biodiesel and glycerol phases separate. The biodiesel obtained is washed with water multiple times to remove any impurities as well as alcohol and catalyst. Washed biodiesel is then dried and stored for quality analysis.

The temperature measurement inside a microwave system poses a challenge, as regular metallic thermocouples cannot be used in microwave environment. Temperature is measured using either an infrared pyrometer or a fiber optic temperature sensor (Figure 5.6) with convertor. An infrared pyrometer measures the IR radiation emitted by the sample and by knowing the emissivity of the sample, determines the actual temperature. A fiber optic thermal sensor on the other hand works by letting a physical disturbance cause a change in the received light through an optical fiber. There are three basic types of fiber optic temperature sensors; a semiconductor absorption type that is based on the temperature dependence of the band gas edge absorption of IR light semiconductor, a Fabry-Perot interferometer and a fluorescence sensor that is based on fluorescence decay [39]. Fiber optic sensors are precise and offer electrical isolation under microwave irradiation, however, they offer lower temperature range (<220°C) and are expensive compared to the less precise IR pyrometers. The reaction chambers used are either Teflon or glass beakers with a stirrer.

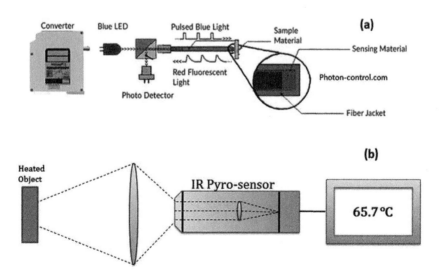

FIGURE 5.6 Temperature measurement inside microwave environment (a) fiber optic thermal sensor (reprinted with permission from photon-control.com) and (b) IR pyro-sensor.

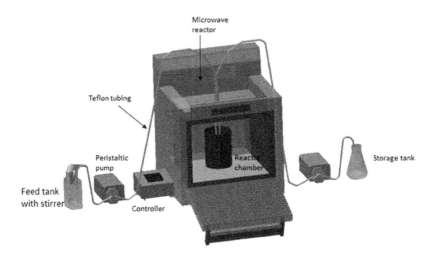

FIGURE 5.7   Laboratory scale continuous microwave reactor.

5.3.2   PILOT SCALE REACTORS

There is limited number of studies reported on the pilot scale microwave assisted biodiesel process. A pilot scale system generally employs an industrial scale microwave system for processing. Both multimode cavities and single mode cavity have been reported to give high conversion rates. While rigorous optimization study has not been studied for scaled up microwave reactor, scale up of continuous flow biodiesel production using microwave technology has been studied by Muley et al. [10] and Kim et al. [40].

The former study used a 915 MHz, 5 kW microwave system. The catalyst (NaOH) was dissolved in ethanol and soybean oil was added to the mixture in the ratio of oil: ethanol = 1:9. According to the study, this ratio was chosen based on the lab scale results reported in Ref. [33]. The mixture was continuously stirred before pumping as oil and alcohol are not miscible. Inline pipe stirrers were installed to ensure no separation occurred during pumping. The mixture was pumped at a flow rate of 840 mL/min. The optimum temperatures reported on batch scale study were 60°C and 73°C [33]. These temperatures were tested for the pilot scale study. The highest microwave power required to reach this desired temperature was 4000 W and 4700 W, respectively (Figure 5.8). The total conversion reported was 99.9%.

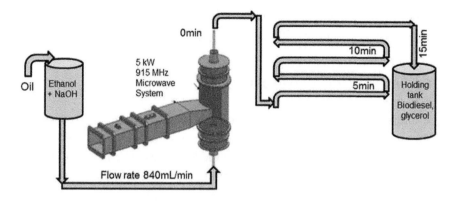

FIGURE 5.8   Pilot scale continuous microwave reactor for biodiesel production (reprinted with permission from Ref. [10]).

Kim et al. [40] demonstrated a scalable microwave unit for biodiesel production. The reactor was a conventional circular reactor modified with a microwave coupler. The modified design ensured that the microwave power was directed to the reactor without any reflection losses. This was done by placing the coupling rod at a distance of 1.2 in from the shorting block. All the power was thus collected at the coupling rod, which effectively transferred the microwave power to the reaction vessel directly. The reactor was a 6 kW, 2450 MHz microwave generator with multimode cavity fixed with a 10 L stainless steel reactor. The soybean oil to methanol ratio was 1:6 and the catalyst used was KOH (1 wt% of oil). The mixture was continuously stirred with 200 rpm and heated at 60°C. The temperature sensor operated at accuracy within ±0.5°C and a feedback control was used to adjust the microwave power. Total conversion reported was 95% with 97% microwave power. Energy efficiency calculations showed that the microwave process displayed higher energy efficiency compared to conventional process.

5.4   EFFECT OF PROCESS VARIABLES ON BIODIESEL PRODUCTION AND QUALITY

Numerous studies reported over the years aimed towards improving and optimizing the biodiesel production process efficiency and reduce operation costs. Some of the crucial parameters affecting the process efficiency are feedstock composition, alcohol type used for reaction, presence and type of catalyst, and temperature of operation.

5.4.1 FEEDSTOCK COMPOSITION

The composition of feedstock used for biodiesel production plays a vital role in the quality of the derived fuel. Triglycerides contribute 90–98% of the total mass of oils and fats derived from the feedstock. The fatty acid radical of the triglyceride molecule have varying C-chain length and degree of saturation. Higher saturated fatty acid content results in higher cloud point of the fuel, which causes plugging problems in the fuel lines during winter.

Cetane number is used to assess the quality of diesel fuel. Cetane number can be directly correlated to the feedstock composition. Longer fatty acid carbon chains and less double bonds (higher degree of saturation) are directly proportional to high cetane number. Higher amounts of linoleic and linolenic acids corresponds to higher degree of unsaturation which leads to production of esters of linoleic and linolenic acids which have lower cetane number [41]. Table 5.3 shows fatty acid profile of common biodiesel feedstock. Biodiesel produced from used frying oil displays low cetane number while palm oil esters have the highest cetane number. These numbers directly correspond to the composition of total saturated compounds. The presence of FFA and moisture also reduces the reaction rate of biodiesel. While unused vegetable oil has lower FFA content, used frying oil and fats from animal source have high amount of FFA, which could prove detrimental to the transesterification reaction.

5.4.2 TYPE OF ALCOHOL AND OIL TO ALCOHOL RATIO

Methanol, ethanol, propanol and butanol can be used to for the transesterification reaction, but the most commonly employed alcohols are methanol and ethanol. Although methanol is preferred over other options due to its availability, lower cost, and other physical and chemical advantages such as polarity and being the shortest chain alcohol [46], ethanol may be sometimes preferred over methanol because it offers better solubility for oil, is less toxic compared to methanol and can be commonly obtained from renewable agricultural resources. Moreover, ethyl esters have higher cetane number compared to methyl esters [10, 33, 47]. Depending on the

TABLE 5.3 Fatty Acid Composition of Some Common Feedstock Used for Biodiesel Production

Oil	Fatty acid (% w/w)						Total saturated	Total unsaturated	Cetane Number	Ref.
	Palmitic (16:0)	Stearic (18:0)	Oleic (18:1)	Linoleic (18:2)	Linolenic (18:3)	Arachidic (20:0)				
Soybean	12.04	1.53	15.06	61.17	9.57	0.81	14.37	85.81	49	[28]
Rice bran	13.00	1.20	36.02	46.27	1.74	1.65	15.06	84.03	51.6 [42]	[28]
Rapeseed	3.49	0.85	64.40	22.30	8.23	N/A	4.34	95.66	55	[43]
Palm oil	36.70	6.6	46.1	8.6	0.3	0.4	35.7	64.3	61	[41]
Used frying oil	12.00	N/A	53.00	33.00	1.00	N/A	12.00	88.00	38.2 [44]	[45]
Sunflower	6.2	3.7	25.2	63.1	0.2	0.3	11.1	88.8	50	[41]

microwave frequency, ethanol may have an advantage over methanol at. The dielectric loss for ethanol is higher at frequencies below 1500 MHz, which would result in better heating of ethanol compared to methanol [9]. However, ethanol has certain disadvantages; being a long chain alcohol, ethanol and other similar alcohols has lower activity compared to methanol. They form stable emulsions during reaction and inhibit the separation and purification process. Ethanol is also highly hygroscopic, forming a 95% azeotrope with water. This significantly impacts the transesterification reaction and special preventive measures have to be employed.

The amount of alcohol used for reaction, in turn the oil: alcohol ratio also plays a vital role in biodiesel synthesis. Although for the reaction to be complete, only three moles of alcohol are needed for one mole of triglyceride to yield three moles of ester and one mole of glycerol, since the reaction is reversible, higher molar ratio is needed for maximum conversion and reaction stability. Using less alcohol could result in lower yields, whereas excessive amount of alcohol increases the solubility of glycerol in the alcohol, thus shifting the reaction equilibrium to left and reducing the ester yields [48] (Figures 5.9 and 5.10). Excessive use of solvent also poses problems with solvent recovery and decrease catalyst concentration [49]. Selecting the appropriate molar ratio depends on other reaction parameters such as feedstock quality and moisture content, catalyst type, heating method and reaction temperature. Higher alcohol to oil ratio is required for acid catalysts (30:1) compared to alkaline catalyst (6–12:1) to achieve higher rate of conversion [50]. Higher alcohol to oil ratio is required for formation of ethyl esters.

5.4.3 CATALYST TYPE

The type of catalyst used affects the performance, reaction rate, and cost of biodiesel production. Homogeneous base catalyst such as NaOH, KOH, and sodium methoxide are the most commonly used catalysts to enhance transesterification process and yield up to 98% conversion (Table 5.4). This catalyst type is cost effective with the reaction rate nearly 4000 times faster than acid catalyst type. Alkaline catalysts do not form water during the transesterification reaction. However, homogenous base catalysts are difficult to separate after reaction and the biodiesel phase requires multiple washings. Moreover, anhydrous reaction conditions should be strictly maintained while using alkali catalyst as presence of moisture could lead to

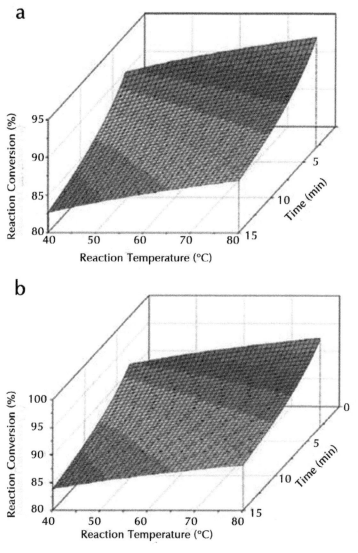

FIGURE 5.9 Reaction conversion versus time and temperature at: (a) alcohol to oil molar ratio of 3 and (b) alcohol to oil molar ratio of 12. Reprinted with permission from Ref. [49].

saponification reaction. The efficiency decreases if the triglycerides used have high FFA content. Heterogeneous base catalyst such as alkaline earth metal oxides are easy to separate after reaction but have low reusability and higher associated costs. While there is some evidence that microwave irradiation increases catalyst activity [51, 52], its effect on biodiesel production has not

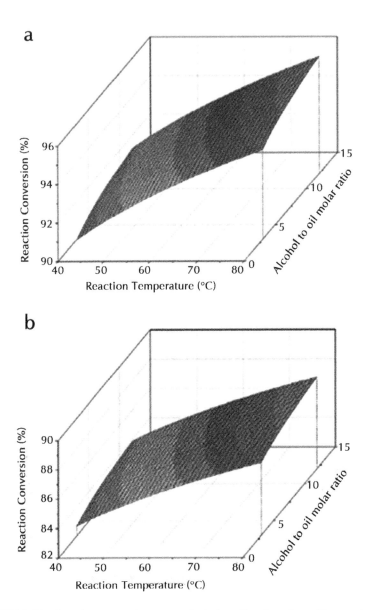

FIGURE 5.10 Reaction conversion versus alcohol to oil molar ratio and temperature at: (a) time of 3 min (b) time of 15 min. Reprinted with permission from Ref. [49].

been definitively established. However, the presence of both polar molecules (solvent) and ionic compounds (catalyst) gives a unique advantage for microwave heating by increasing the heating effects [9].

TABLE 5.4 Optimized Process Parameters for Microwave Assisted Biodiesel Production for Various Feedstocks

Feedstock	Alcohol	Oil:alcohol molar ratio	Catalyst type	Catalyst concentration (% mass of oil)	Reaction temperature (°C)	Reaction time (min)	% Yield	Power (W)	Ref.
Karanja	Methanol	1:9.3	KOH	1.33	N/A	2.5	91.4	180	[55]
Yellow Horn Oil	Methanol	1:12	Heteropoly acid (HPA)	1	60	10.0	96.22	1000 max	[56]
Jatropha crucas L.	Ethanol		KOH	8.15ml	N/A	12.21	90.01	150	[57]
Cotton Seed Oil	Methanol	1:6	KOH	1.50	60	7.0	92.7	N/A	[1]
Soybean Oil	Methanol	1:2	Na K tartrate doped zorconia	10	65	30	93.51	N/A	[58]
Palm Oil	Methanol	1:12	NaOH	1	70	1.75	96.5	400	[59]
Dry Algae	Methanol	1:12	KOH	2	60–64	4.0	71.5	800	[60]
Waste Cooking Oil	Methanol	1:9	KOH	2	80	6.0	92	800	[61]
	Methanol	1:6	CH₃ONa	0.75	N/A	3.0	97.9	750	[62]
Vegetable Oil	Butanol	1:6	KOH	1	120	1.0	93	N/A	[63]
Rapeseed Oil	Methanol	1:6	KOH	1.5	50	5.0	93.7	1200	[64]
FFA	Ethanol	1:11	D-418	9	80	420	90	N/A	[65]

Acid catalysts are efficient for reactants with very high FFA content (> 5%). Commonly used catalysts are sulfuric acid, HCl, and phosphoric acid. The drawback of using acid catalysts is that it requires high operating temperature and pressure conditions, and has low reaction rates compared to the commonly used base catalysts. Acid catalysts are also known to cause environmental problems and pipeline corrosion.

Enzyme catalysts have also been studied for biodiesel production. Enzyme catalysts offer numerous advantages such as absence soap formation, simpler operating conditions such as atmospheric pressure and room temperatures, and easier post processing such as purification, washing and neutralization of biodiesel and higher conversion rate of up to 90% has been reported. Microwave irradiations have been reported to increase the enzyme activity in the presence of ionic liquids for enzyme catalyzed biodiesel process [53]. Yu et al., studied the combined effect of microwave irradiation and ionic liquid on enzyme catalyzed biodiesel production. They observed that the enzyme activity was higher for microwave process compared to conventional process under same processing conditions. Microwave processing also resulted in 92% FAME yield as opposed to 70% for conventional heating [53]. The major drawbacks associated with enzyme catalyst are high cost and longer reaction times compared to acid and base catalysts.

Other studies targeted towards improving the microwave assisted catalytic transesterification have also been conducted. Yuan et al. [54] studied the effect of microwave absorption catalysts on transesterification reaction for FAME synthesis. They observed that the microwave irradiation had an enhanced effect on the transesterification reaction when a microwave absorbing solid catalyst (H_2SO_4/C) was used. The FAME yield reached 94% in 60 min whereas for conventional method the highest yield of 70% was achieved in 180 min reaction time [54].

5.4.4 EFFECT OF TEMPERATURE AND REACTION TIME

Although transesterification can be carried out at room temperature with vigorous mixing of reactants, the reaction time is considerably reduced by increasing the temperature (Figure 5.10). Moreover, longer reaction times could increase formation of by-products and reducing the biodiesel yield and lead to poor product quality [66]. It can be seen from Figure 5.10 that for reaction time of 3.0 min the conversion is 94.5–96.5%; however, when the reaction time is increased to 15 min for the same temperature and alcohol to oil ratio, the conversion reduces to 87–88%. Temperature has the most significant effect on the rate of reaction and total conversion to biodiesel and the quality of product. Microwave processing has the highest advantage over conventional heating in this area. Since microwave irradiation causes a volumetric, molecular level heating, it eliminates the heating medium and the time required to increase the temperature is significantly reduced compared to conventional heating techniques such as heat exchangers, electric heaters etc. Choice of reaction temperature depends on multiple factors including reactant boiling point, pressure conditions, catalyst's sensitivity to temperature, and oil to alcohol ratio. Transesterification reaction is usually carried out at temperatures slightly below the boiling point of alcohol. Most commonly a temperature range of 65–75°C is used for ethanol and 50–65°C for methanol.

The rise in temperature in the microwave environment depends on the dielectric properties of the reactants mixture [9]. Since both dielectric constant and dielectric loss is temperature dependent, the rate of heating changes accordingly [9]. Another advantage of microwave processing is that microwave irradiation causes local superheating, which enhances the rate of reaction. Lower reaction temperatures can lead to slower reaction rates and low yields, similarly very high reaction temperatures have known to reduce product yield. Higher temperatures can lead to the solvent vaporization, which reduces oil and solvent interaction. At high temperatures, the solvent may be in the vapor phase, which reduces oil and solvent interaction. At higher temperatures, methyl esters are also reported to undergo cracking reactions forming aldehydes, ketones and other smaller molecular compounds [49].

Microwave processing not only reduces the time required to attain required temperature but is also known to increase the rate of reaction by having a direct effect on the rate of collision of molecules [34]. Thus, microwave assisted processing significantly reduces the overall biodiesel production time while achieving conversion rate >90%. An average reaction time of 1 to 30 min for microwave processing and 30–120 min for conventional heating has been noted by numerous researchers [8, 10, 21, 33, 59, 64, 67, 68]. Although very long reaction time would give more microwave exposure time, it could also lead to byproducts and intense local superheating causing undesirable results [49].

5.5 MICROWAVE ASSISTED BIODIESEL PRODUCTION FROM MICROALGAE

Microalgae can rapidly grow in harshest of environment because of its simple molecular structure. Microalgae have high lipid content, are easy to cultivate with little or no nutrition. They do not require a dedicated land or water body and hence have gained attention as a viable feedstock for biodiesel production. Microwave heating has been successfully applied for both oil extraction and transesterification of microalgae. Cravatto et al. [25] studied the use of 2450 MHz multimode microwave system for oil extraction from microalgae. They noted that microwave heating greatly improved the extraction efficiency and reduced the time required. Patil et al. [60] demonstrated the use of microwave system for transesterification of dry algal biomass. The optimum conditions based on their study were biomass to methanol ratio of 1:12 with a catalyst concentration of 2 wt% and reaction time of 4 min. Koberg el al. [69] demonstrated the use of ultrasound technology and microwave system for direct transesterification of microalgae. They noted that the microwave assisted system proved to be the simplest and a very effective process for biodiesel production from as-harvested microalgae. While microwave systems improve the process efficiency, one of the major drawbacks with algal biomass is high processing cost associated with harvesting and drying, limiting its use on commercial scale.

5.6 *IN-SITU* TRANSESTERIFICATION

Elimination of oil extraction in the biodiesel production process could decrease the processing cost by up to 70% by reducing the solvent amount and time of operation [30]. For this purpose, in-situ transesterification of seeds has been recently investigated by numerous researchers [30, 70–72] (Figure 5.11). The major challenges for in-situ transesterification are presence of water in the feedstock and lipid solubility. Presence of water in the feedstock precipitates the long chain fatty acids, slowing the reaction rate [72]. It may also interfere with the reaction and, in case of alkaline catalyst, trigger the saponification reaction. In case of microwave assisted process, water being more polar than methanol, could cause high temperatures and hotspots leading to undesirable by-products. Hence drying the feedstock

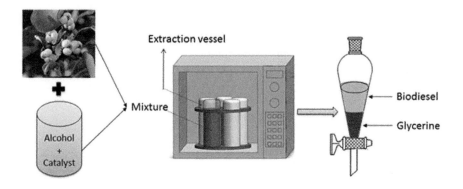

FIGURE 5.11   In-situ transesterification of CTT seeds in a batch microwave reactor.

is recommended before in-situ transesterification to reduce the moisture content under 10%. Barekati et al. [30] studied the in-situ transesterification of Chinese tallow seeds in a batch microwave system and showed that the in-situ transesterification reaction depends on numerous factors such as cosolvents used, ratio of cosolvents, catalyst type, and amount used as well as reaction temperature and time (Figure 5.11). The optimum conditions for this process were 1.74% NaOH catalyst, solvent ratio of 3 (v/w) and reaction time of 20 min at 58°C which resulted in a total biodiesel yield of 84.5%. For microwave-enhanced processes, right ratio of solvents is crucial for optimization. Barekati et al. [30] showed that while hexane has better oil solubility and extraction rate, methanol, being a polar solvent, had better heating rate in microwave system and has a higher transesterification rate. Although lower product yield is achieved with in-situ transesterification, the processing cost could be significantly reduced due to elimination of intermediate steps.

5.7   COMPARISON OF CONVENTIONAL AND MICROWAVE HEATING: ENERGY EFFICIENCY AND REACTION KINETICS

Microwave enhanced reactions show remarkable increase in the product yield and decrease in reaction time at laboratory scale. Quitain et al. [73] showed a considerable increase in the methyl ester yield with microwave processing compared to conventional heating for the same temperature-time combination (Table 5.5). They noted that the bulk temperature in the

TABLE 5.5   Comparison of Conventional and Microwave Parameters for Biodiesel Production

Parameter		Microwave	Conventional	Ref.
Reaction rate constant	Soybean oil	0.0567 (@50°C)	N/A	[33]
		0.0747 (@73°C)	N/A	
	Rice bran oil	0.0684 (@50°C)	N/A	
		0.08 (@73°C)		
	Camelina Sativa	5.195 (catalyst- BaO)	0.0526 (catalyst- BaO)	[77]
		1.584 (catalyst- SrO)	0.0493 (catalyst- SrO)	
Camelina Sativa with KOH	Energy Consumed (kJ)	48	900	[78]
	Reaction Time (s)	60	1800	
	Biodiesel yield (%)	98	98	
Camelina Sativa with NaOH	Energy Consumed (kJ)	19.2	450	
	Reaction Time (s)	60	900	
	Biodiesel yield (%)	80	76	
Soybean oil with KOH	Energy Consumed (kJ/L)	90.1 (4.6 L batch)	94.3	[8, 79]
Palm oil with NaOH	Energy Consumed (kWh/L)	0.1167	0.222	[59]

microwave reactor did not reach the targeted 60°C under 1 min processing time, however the methyl ester yield was higher due to localized superheating effect with the microwave [73]. Leadbeater et al. [8] compared the energy efficiency of the microwave process operating at 1600 W and achieved an energy consumption of 26.0 kJ/L that was approximately a quarter of the energy used by conventional heating methods. Extrapolating these results they concluded that for a large-scale microwave reactor operating at full power, the energy consumed would be approximately 92.3 kJ/L, which is in comparison with the energy data for conventional process that uses 94.3 kJ/L provided by the U.S Department of Energy [8]. Microwave heating also offers an advantage at large-scale reactions. Wall heating in conventional reactors causes corrosion and scaling problems due to high temperatures. Moreover, for heat sensitive reactions, the temperature gradient that exists in conventional reactors can pose a serious problem in terms of product yield and efficiency. Microwave on the other hand, heat the reactants directly, eliminating these issues altogether. At larger scale, as the surface area to volume ratio decreases, with multimode cavity reactors, microwave processes are more energy efficient compared to conventional techniques [74].

Although these results are promising, there are several issues associated with microwave processing. One of the major drawbacks of microwave reactors is that high power densities imparted on low reactant volume results in low energy efficiency as only 20–30% of the total energy imparted is converted to thermal energy [75]. Single mode microwave reactors are less efficient compared to multimode reactors and are energy efficient only under sealed vessel processing [76]. Moreover, single mode reactors are less energy efficient and in some cases highly inefficient compared to conventional methods [74, 76]. In continuous flow processes, the penetration depth of the solution is rather important; as most reactants have a smaller penetration depth (1–3 cm), this poses a problem with wider reaction tubes at large scale [74]. Thus, the energy efficiency and environmental benefits of microwave-assisted processes at a large scale requires further evaluation.

Study of reaction kinetics under microwave heating is a complicated task. The multimode cavity causes nonuniform heating, which causes complications during the reaction and measuring a bulk rate of reaction becomes difficult. While single mode cavities could solve this problem to some extent, the changes in dielectric properties of mixture as the temperature changes also affect the reaction. Some studies have attempted to understand the effect of microwave irradiation on the reaction kinetics [33, 77, 80, 81]. Stuerga et al. [81] studied the effect of microwave irradiation on powder alumina and concluded that the reaction rate in microwave heating is enhanced and can be explained by localized superheating unique to microwave irradiation effect. Raner et al. [80] studied acid catalyzed isomerization of carvone and found no change in the rate of reaction between the two methods. Due to the complexity of the process, it is possible that the increase in rate of reaction could be unique for the given reaction under microwave irradiation. Limited data is available studying the rate of transesterification reaction in microwave environment. One of the reason is because the reaction proceeds so quickly, and the conversion is almost 100%, calculation of reaction kinetics is difficult. [10] Patil et al. studied the reaction kinetics of transesterification of *Camelina Sativa* oil with two different catalysts BaO and SrO [77]. They noted that for microwave assisted heating, the reaction rate constant was two orders of magnitude (98.7 times) higher compared to conventional heating for BaO and one order of magnitude higher with SrO catalyst [77]. Terigar et al. [33] noted higher reaction rate in the first minute of the reaction for both rice bran and soybean oil transesterification. Higher rate of reaction was observed for rice bran oil compared to soybean oil due to the difference in fatty acid composition. Although conflicting conclusions have been noted about the non-thermal effects of microwave processing on reactions, microwave application for biodiesel production is promising in terms of energy efficiency and in turn environmental benefits and should be further evaluated for industrial scale applications.

5.8   ADVANCES IN MICROWAVE BIODIESEL PRODUCTION: NUMERICAL MODELING

Understanding the effect of flow patterns of the fluid, electromagnetic field distribution, temperature profile, heating effects, and reaction kinetics [82] is crucial in developing an optimized process. Numerical analysis is a useful tool for estimating the effects these operating parameters. Microwave heating is a rather complex process and involves solving multiple equations including Maxwell's equations to determine electromagnetic field distribution, Navier-Stokes equation solved for the flow pattern of the liquid, and Fourier's equations of energy balance to calculate the heat transfer in the fluid and the power requirement [83]. A number of studies have documented numerical modeling of microwave heating that have looked at processes involving fluid flow [82, 84–86], while only a few report of studies investigating continuous flow microwave heating [87]. Ratanadecho et al. [88] studied the microwave heating of a liquid in a rectangular waveguide both experimentally and numerically. They proposed a generalized mathematical model to investigate multiple aspects in a microwave reactor. They studied two liquids; water and NaCl-water solution and concluded that the dielectric properties of fluid drive the microwave heating kinetics [75]. Salvi et al. [87] developed a numerical model to understand the effect of microwave power on continuous flowing liquids. Zhang et al. [82] studied the heating of a batch of liquid in a microwave with a three dimensional approach.

Muley et al. [36] developed a model predicting the behavior of biodiesel precursors under microwave irradiation and validating the results experimentally (Figure 5.12). They observed that the maximum electromagnetic power density was 4.7×10^6 W/m^3 and 3.6×10^6 W/m^3 for 4000 W and 4700 W power input respectively [36]. Total power absorbed was 19% (756 W) for 4000 W power input, and 13% (605 W) for 4700 W power input and the temperature ranged from 30°C to 82°C and 45°C to 89°C with an average temperature of 61°C and 73°C for 4000 W and 4700 W power input, respectively [36].

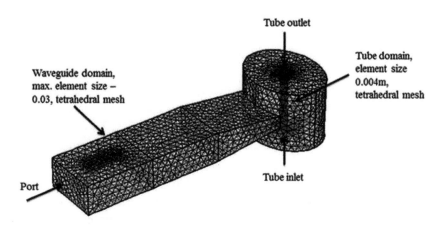

FIGURE 5.12 Mesh generation for microwave system.

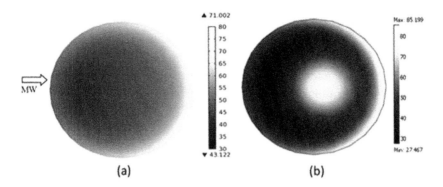

FIGURE 5.13 Temperature distribution (°C) in *xy*-plane for Pin = 4000 W at the center of the tube for (a) oil, ethanol and catalyst mixture (left); (b) water (right). Reprinted with permission from Ref. [36].

Surface heating was dominant unlike center heating for water observed by Salvi et al. [87], mainly due to smaller penetration depth of the mixture (Figure 5.13). Due to limitations of experimental procedures and lack of dielectric data, validation of these models becomes difficult. Numerical modeling helps in predicting the behavior of the systems under certain sets of parameters and can be used for the optimization of the continuous flow microwave heating process.

5.9 FUTURE WORK AND CONCLUSIONS

As the necessity to develop cleaner more reliable fuels increases, more efficient process designs need to be developed. Microwave assisted processes hold a potential to be further developed for energy and cost efficient biofuel synthesis. This chapter gives an overview of the different microwave reactors used for biodiesel synthesis and analyzes the effect of various parameters on the microwave heating process. To overcome the existing limitations related to scale up and uneven heating, more detailed studies need to be performed on a larger scale. Other issues related to the safety, cost of equipment, design related issues of microwave-based processes also need to be addressed. Newer approaches such as numerical modeling, innovative reactor designs help improve the process efficiency and ease of operation.

KEYWORDS

- **biodiesel production**
- **green chemistry**
- **microwave heating**
- **process efficiency**

REFERENCES

1. Azcan, N., & Danisman, A., (2007). Alkali catalyzed transesterification of cottonseed oil by microwave irradiation. *Fuel 86* (17–18), 2639–2644.
2. Cao, P., Tremblay, A. Y., Dubé, M. A., & Morse, K. (2007). Effect of membrane pore size on the performance of a membrane reactor for biodiesel production. *Industrial & engineering chemistry research, 46* (1), 52–58.
3. Yoshida, A., Hama, S., Tamadani, N., Fukuda, H., & Kondo, A. (2012). Improved performance of a packed-bed reactor for biodiesel production through whole-cell biocatalysis employing a high-lipase-expression system. *Biochemical engineering journal, 63*, 76–80.
4. Urban, J., Svec, F., & Fréchet, J. M. (2012). A monolithic lipase reactor for biodiesel production by transesterification of triacylglycerides into fatty acid methyl esters. *Biotechnology and bioengineering, 109* (2), 371–380.
5. Tiwari, A. K., Kumar, A., & Raheman, H. (2007). Biodiesel production from jatropha oil (Jatropha curcas) with high free fatty acids: an optimized process. *Biomass and bioenergy, 31*(8), 569–575.
6. Wen, L., Wang, Y., Lu, D., Hu, S., & Han, H. (2010). Preparation of KF/CaO nanocatalyst and its application in biodiesel production from Chinese tallow seed oil. *Fuel, 89*(9), 2267–2271.
7. He, B., Singh, A. P., & Thompson, J. (2006). A novel continuous-flow reactor using reactive distillation for biodiesel production. *Transactions of the ASABE, 49*(1), 107–112.
8. Barnard, T. M., Leadbeater, N. E., Boucher, M. B., Stencel, L. M., & Wilhite, B. A. (2007). Continuous-Flow Preparation of Biodiesel Using Microwave Heating. *Energy & Fuels, 21*(3), 1777–1781.
9. Muley, P. D., & Boldor, D. (2013). Investigation of microwave dielectric properties of biodiesel components. *Bioresource Technology, 127*, 165–174.
10. Muley, P. D., & Boldor, D. (2013). Scale-up of a continuous microwave-assisted transesterification process of soybean oil for biodiesel production. *Transactions of ASABE, 56*(5), 1847–1854.
11. Zhou, H., Lu, H. F., & Liang, B. (2006). Solubility of multicomponent systems in the biodiesel production by transesterification of Jatropha curcas L. oil with methanol. *Journal of Chemical and Engineering Data, 51*(3), 1130–1135.
12. Tyson, K., (2009) *Biodiesel handling and use guidelines.* DIANE Publishing Third Edition. U.S. department of Energy, Energy Efficiency and Renewable Energy DOE/GO-102006-2358 .

13. Sheehan, J., Camobreco, V., Duffield, J., Shapouri, H., Graboski, M., & Tyson, K. (2000). *An overview of biodiesel and petroleum diesel life cycles*, National Renewable Energy Lab., Golden, CO (US):

14. Demirbas, A. (2009). Progress and recent trends in biodiesel fuels. *Energy Conversion and Management, 50*(1), 14–34.

15. Kappe, C. O. (2008). Microwave dielectric heating in synthetic organic chemistry. *Chemical Society Reviews, 37*(6), 1127–1139.

16. Meredith, R. J. (1998).*Engineers' handbook of industrial microwave heating*. Institution of Electrical Engineers: London.

17. Metaxas, A. C., & Meredith, R. J. (1993). *Industrial microwave heating*. (IEE Power Engineering Series)." Institution of Electrical Engineers Peregrinus: London.

18. Sun, D.-W. (2011). *Handbook of food safety engineering*. John Wiley & Sons, Oxford, UK. ISBM-13: 978-1-4443-3334-3

19. Hippel, A. R. V. (1954). *Dielectric materials and applications: papers by 20-two contributors*. published jointly by the Technology Press of M. I. T. and Wiley.

20. Gabriel, C., Gabriel, S., Grant, E. H., Halstead, B. S. J., & Mingos, D. M. P. (1998). Dielectric parameters relevant to microwave dielectric heating. *Chemical Society Reviews, 27*(3), 213–223.

21. Gude, V. G., Patil, P., Martinez-Guerra, E., Deng, S., & Nirmalakhandan, N. (2013). Microwave energy potential for biodiesel production. *Sustainable Chemical Processes, 1*(1), 5.

22. Li, H., Pordesimo, L. O., Weiss, J., & Wilhelm, L. R. (2004). Microwave and ultrasound assisted extraction of soybean oil. *Transactions of the ASAE, 47*(4), 1187.

23. Zigoneanu, I. G., Williams, L., Xu, Z., & Sabliov, C. M. (2008). Determination of antioxidant components in rice bran oil extracted by microwave-assisted method. *Bioresource Technology, 99*(11), 4910–4918.

24. Kanitkar, A., Sabliov, C., Balasubramanian, S., Lima, M., & Boldor, D. (2011). Microwave-assisted extraction of soybean and rice bran oil: yield and extraction kinetics. *Transactions of the ASABE, 54*(4), 1387–1394.

25. Cravotto, G., Boffa, L., Mantegna, S., Perego, P., Avogadro, M., & Cintas, P. (2008). Improved extraction of vegetable oils under high-intensity ultrasound and/or microwaves. *Ultrasonics Sonochemistry, 15*(5), 898–902.

26. Wang, Y., You, J., Yu, Y., Qu, C., Zhang, H., Ding, L., Zhang, H., & Li, X. (2008). Analysis of ginsenosides in Panax ginseng in high pressure microwave-assisted extraction. *Food Chemistry, 110*(1), 161–167.

27. Pan, X., Niu, G., & Liu, H. (2003). Microwave-assisted extraction of tea polyphenols and tea caffeine from green tea leaves. *Chemical Engineering and Processing: Process Intensification, 42*(2), 129–133.

28. Terigar, B., Balasubramanian, S., Sabliov, C., Lima, M., & Boldor, D. (2011). Soybean and rice bran oil extraction in a continuous microwave system: from laboratory-to pilot-scale. *Journal of Food Engineering, 104*(2), 208–217.

29. Virot, M., Tomao, V., Colnagui, G., Visinoni, F., & Chemat, F. (2007). New microwave-integrated Soxhlet extraction: an advantageous tool for the extraction of lipids from food products. *Journal of chromatography A, 1174*(1), 138–144.

30. Barekati-Goudarzi, M., Boldor, D., & Nde, D. B. (2016). In-situ transesterification of seeds of invasive Chinese tallow trees (Triadica sebifera L.) in a microwave batch system (GREEN3) using hexane as cosolvent: Biodiesel production and process optimization. *Bioresource Technology, 201*, 97–104.

31. Rostagno, M. A., Palma, M., & Barroso, C. G. (2007). Microwave assisted extraction of soy isoflavones. *Analytica Chimica Acta 588* (2), 274–282.

32. Qiu, Z., Zhao, L., & Weatherley, L. (2010). Process intensification technologies in continuous biodiesel production. *Chemical Engineering and Processing: Process Intensification*, *49*(4), 323–330.

33. Terigar, B. G., Balasubramanian, S., Lima, M., & Boldor, D. (2010). Transesterification of Soybean and Rice Bran Oil with Ethanol in a Continuous-Flow Microwave-Assisted System: Yields, Quality, and Reaction Kinetics. *Energy & Fuels*, *24*, 6609–6615.

34. Lidstrom, P., Tierney, J., Wathey, B., & Westman, J. (2001). Microwave assisted organic synthesis - a review. *Tetrahedron*, *57*(45), 9225–9283.

35. Santos, T., Costa, L., Valente, M., Monteiro, J., & Sousa, J. (2010). In *3D electromagnetic field simulation in microwave ovens: a tool to control thermal runaway*, COMSOL Conference, Paris, November 17-19, 2010.

36. Muley, P. D., & Boldor, D. (2012). Multiphysics numerical modeling of the continuous flow microwave-assisted transesterification process. *Journal of Microwave Power and Electromagnetic Energy*, *46*(3).

37. Perin, G., Álvaro, G., Westphal, E., Viana, L. H., Jacob, R. G., Lenardão, E. J., & D'Oca, M. G. M. (2008).Transesterification of castor oil assisted by microwave irradiation. *Fuel*, *87*(12), 2838–2841.

38. Saifuddin, N., & Chua, K. (2004). Production of ethyl ester (biodiesel) from used frying oil: optimization of transesterification process using microwave irradiation. *Malaysian Journal of Chemistry*, *6*(1), 77–82.

39. Berghmans, F., & Decreton, M. (1998). Evaluation of three different optical fiber temperature sensor types for application in gamma radiation environments. *IEEE Transactions on Nuclear Science*, *45*(3), 1537–1542.

40. Kim, D., Seol, S. K., & Chang, W. S. (2015). Energy efficiency of a scaled-up microwave-assisted transesterification for biodiesel production. *Korean Journal of Chemical Engineering*, 1–5.

41. Ramos, M. J., Fernández, C. M., Casas, A., Rodríguez, L., & Pérez, Á. (2009). Influence of fatty acid composition of raw materials on biodiesel properties. *Bioresource Technology*, *100*(1), 261–268.

42. Mohanty, S. K. (2013). A Production of biodiesel from rice bran oil and experimenting on small capacity diesel engine. *International Journal of Modern Engineering Research*, *3*(2), 920–923.

43. Goering, C., Schwab, A., Daugherty, M., Pryde, E., & Heakin, A. (1982). Fuel properties of 11 vegetable oils. *Transactions of the ASAE*, *25*(6), 1472–1477.

44. Encinar, J. M., González, J. F., & Rodríguez-Reinares, A. (2007). Ethanolysis of used frying oil. Biodiesel preparation and characterization. *Fuel Processing Technology*, *88*(5), 513–522.

45. Alcantara, R., Amores, J., Canoira, L. t., Fidalgo, E., Franco, M., & Navarro, A. (2000). Catalytic production of biodiesel from soy-bean oil, used frying oil and tallow. *Biomass and bioenergy*, *18*(6), 515–527.

46. Sanli, H., & Canakci, M. (2008). Effects of Different Alcohol and Catalyst Usage on Biodiesel Production from Different Vegetable Oils. *Energy & Fuels*, *22*(4), 2713–2719.

47. Demirbas, M. F. (2008). Pyrolysis of vegetable oils and animal fats for the production of renewable fuels. *Energy Educ. Sci. Technol.*, *22*(1), 59–67.

48. Meher, L. C., Sagar, D. V., & Naik, S. N. (2006). Technical aspects of biodiesel production by transesterification - a review. *Renewable & Sustainable Energy Reviews*, *10*(3), 248–268.

49. Sajjadi, B., Aziz, A. A., & Ibrahim, S. (2014). Investigation, modeling and reviewing the effective parameters in microwave-assisted transesterification. *Renewable and Sustainable Energy Reviews*, *37*, 762–777.

50. Freedman, B., Butterfield, R. O., & Pryde, E. H. (1986). Transesterification Kinetics of Soybean Oil *Journal of the American Oil Chemists Society 63* (10), 1375–1380.

51. Edmund, S. E. (2013). Microwave-Catalyst Interactions in the Reforming of Hydrocarbons. The University of Michigan.

52. Asahara, H., Kuribayashi, Y., Wang, P., Kobiro, K., & Nishiwaki, N. (2014). An Effect of Microwave Irradiation on Pd/SiC Catalyst for Prolonging the Catalytic Life. *Current Microwave Chemistry*, *1*(2), 142–147.

53. Yu, D., Wang, C., Yin, Y., Zhang, A., Gao, G., & Fang, X. (2011). A synergistic effect of microwave irradiation and ionic liquids on enzyme-catalyzed biodiesel production. *Green Chemistry*, *13*(7), 1869–1875.

54. Yuan, H., Yang, B., & Zhu, G. (2008). Synthesis of biodiesel using microwave absorption catalysts. *Energy & Fuels*, *23*(1), 548–552.

55. Kamath, H. V., Regupathi, I., & Saidutta, M. (2011). Optimization of two step karanja biodiesel synthesis under microwave irradiation. *Fuel Processing Technology*, *92*(1), 100–105.

56. Zhang, S., Zu, Y.-G., Fu, Y.-J., Luo, M., Zhang, D.-Y., & Efferth, T. (2010). Rapid microwave-assisted transesterification of yellow horn oil to biodiesel using a heteropolyacid solid catalyst. *Bioresource technology*, *101*(3), 931–936.

57. Jaliliannosrati, H., Amin, N. A. S., Talebian-Kiakalaieh, A., & Noshadi, I. (2013). Microwave assisted biodiesel production from Jatropha curcas L. seed by two-step in situ process: optimization using response surface methodology. *Bioresource technology*, *136*, 565–573.

58. Li, Y., Ye, B., Shen, J., Tian, Z., Wang, L., Zhu, L., Ma, T., Yang, D., & Qiu, F. (2013). Optimization of biodiesel production process from soybean oil using the sodium potassium tartrate doped zirconia catalyst under Microwave Chemical Reactor. *Bioresource Technology*, *137*, 220–225.

59. Choedkiatsakul, I., Ngaosuwan, K., Assabumrungrat, S., Mantegna, S., & Cravotto, G. (2015). Biodiesel production in a novel continuous flow microwave reactor. *Renewable Energy*, *83*, 25–29.

60. Patil, P. D., Gude, V. G., Mannarswamy, A., Cooke, P., Munson-McGee, S., Nirmalakhandan, N., Lammers, P., & Deng, S. (2011). Optimization of microwave-assisted transesterification of dry algal biomass using response surface methodology. *Bioresource Technology*, *102*(2), 1399–1405.

61. Patil, P. D., Gude, V. G., Reddy, H. K., Muppaneni, T., & Deng, S. (2012). Biodiesel Production from Waste Cooking Oil Using Sulfuric Acid and Microwave Irradiation Processes. *Journal of Environmental Protection*, *Vol.03No.01*, 7.

62. Chen, K.-S., Lin, Y.-C., Hsu, K.-H., & Wang, H.-K. (2012). Improving biodiesel yields from waste cooking oil by using sodium methoxide and a microwave heating system. *Energy*, *38*(1), 151–156.

63. Leadbeater, N. E., Barnard, T. M., & Stencel, L. M. (2008). Batch and continuous-flow preparation of biodiesel derived from butanol and facilitated by microwave heating. *Energy & Fuels*, *22*(3), 2005–2008.

64. Azcan, N., & Danisman, A. (2008). Microwave assisted transesterification of rapeseed oil. *Fuel, 87*(10–11), 1781–1788.
65. Liu, W., Yin, P., Liu, X., Chen, W., Chen, H., Liu, C., Qu, R., & Xu, Q. (2013). Microwave assisted esterification of free fatty acid over a heterogeneous catalyst for biodiesel production. *Energy Conversion and Management, 76,* 1009–1014.
66. Kapilakarn, K., & Peugtong, A. (2007). A comparison of costs of biodiesel production from transesterification. *International Energy Journal, 8*(1), 1–6.
67. Kanitkar, A., Balasubramanian, S., Lima, M., & Boldor, D. (2011). A critical comparison of methyl and ethyl esters production from soybean and rice bran oil in the presence of microwaves. *Bioresource Technology, 102*(17), 7896–7902.
68. Leadbeater, N. E., & Stencel, L. M. (2006).Fast, easy preparation of biodiesel using microwave heating. *Energy & Fuels, 20*(5), 2281–2283.
69. Koberg, M., Cohen, M., Ben-Amotz, A., & Gedanken, A. (2011). Bio-diesel production directly from the microalgae biomass of Nannochloropsis by microwave and ultrasound radiation. *Bioresource Technology, 102*(5), 4265–4269.
70. Velasquez-Orta, S., Lee, J., & Harvey, A. (2012). Alkaline in situ transesterification of Chlorella vulgaris. *Fuel, 94,* 544–550.
71. Patil, P. D., Reddy, H., Muppaneni, T., Mannarswamy, A., Schuab, T., Holguin, F. O., Lammers, P., Nirmalakhandan, N., Cooke, P., & Deng, S. (2012). Power dissipation in microwave-enhanced in situ transesterification of algal biomass to biodiesel. *Green Chemistry, 14*(3), 809–818.
72. Carrapiso, A. I., García, C. (2000)Development in lipid analysis: Some new extraction techniques and in situ transesterification. *Lipids, 35*(11), 1167–1177.
73. Quitain, A. T., Goto, M., Katoh, S. (2011) *Microwave-assisted synthesis of biofuels.* In Biofuel Production-Recent Developments and Prospects. InTech Open Access Publisher.
74. Moseley, J. D., & Kappe, C. O. (2011). A critical assessment of the greenness and energy efficiency of microwave-assisted organic synthesis. *Green Chemistry, 13*(4), 794–806.
75. Hoogenboom, R., Wilms, T. F., Erdmenger, T., & Schubert, U.S. (2009). Microwave-assisted chemistry: a closer look at heating efficiency. *Australian journal of chemistry, 62*(3), 236–243.
76. Razzaq, T., & Kappe, C. O. (2008). On the Energy Efficiency of Microwave Assisted Organic Reactions. *ChemSusChem, 1*(12), 123–132.
77. Patil, P., Gude, V. G., Pinappu, S., & Deng, S. (2011). Transesterification kinetics of Camelina sativa oil on metal oxide catalysts under conventional and microwave heating conditions. *Chemical Engineering Journal, 168*(3), 1296–1300.
78. Patil, P. D., Gude, V. G., Camacho, L. M., & Deng, S. (2009). Microwave assisted catalytic transesterification of Camelina sativa oil. *Energy & Fuels, 24*(2), 1298–1304.
79. Sheehan, J., Camobreco, V., Duffield, J., Graboski, M., & Shapouri, H. (1998).*Life cycle inventory of biodiesel and petroleum diesel for use in an urban bus. Final report,* NREL/SR-580-24089 UC,(available from www. nrel. gov) National Renewable Energy Lab., Golden, CO (US).
80. Raner, K. D., Strauss, C. R., Vyskoc, F., & Mokbel, L. (1993). A comparison of reaction kinetics observed under microwave irradiation and conventional heating. *The Journal of Organic Chemistry, 58*(4), 950–953.
81. Stuerga, D., & Gaillard, P. (1996). Microwave heating as a new way to induce localized enhancements of reaction rate. Non-isothermal and heterogeneous kinetics. *Tetrahedron, 52*(15), 5505–5510.

82. Zhang, Q. O., Jackson, T. H., & Ungan, A. (2000). Numerical modeling of microwave induced natural convection. *International Journal of Heat and Mass Transfer*, *43*(12), 2141–2154.

83. Romano, V. R., Marra, F., & Tammaro, U. (2005). Modelling of microwave heating of foodstuff: study on the influence of sample dimensions with a FEM approach. *Journal of Food Engineering*, *71*(3), 233–241.

84. Patankar, S. V., (1980). *Numerical heat transfer and fluid flow*. Hemisphere Publishing Corporation. ISBN: 0-89116-522-3.

85. Jia, X., & Jolly, P. (1992). *Simulation of microwave field and power distribution in a cavity by a three-dimensional finite element method*. International Microwave Power Institute: Manassas, VA, Vol. 27.

86. Webb J. P, M. G. L., & Ferrari R. L. (1983). Finite element implementation of three dimensional electromagnetic problems. *IEEE Proceedings*, *78*, 5.

87. Salvi, D., Boldor, D., Ortego, J., Aita, G., & Sabliov, C. (2010). Numerical modeling of continuous flow microwave heating: a critical comparison of COMSOL and ANSYS. *Journal of Microwave Power and Electromagnetic Energy*, *44*(4), 187–197.

88. Ratanadecho, P. (2002). In: *Numerical modeling of microwave induced natural convection inside a rectangular wave guide*, Industrial Technology, 2002. IEEE ICIT'02. 2002 IEEE International Conference on, IEEE: pp. 474–479.

CHAPTER 6

PROCESS INTENSIFICATION AND PARAMETRIC OPTIMIZATION IN BIODIESEL SYNTHESIS USING HYDRODYNAMIC CAVITATION REACTORS

PARAG R. GOGATE[1] and ASHISH V. MOHOD[2]

[1]Chemical Engineering Department, Institute of Chemical Technology, Matunga, Mumbai – 400019, India

[2]Chemical Engineering Department, AISSMS College of Engineering, Kennedy Road, Pune – 411001, India

CONTENTS

ABSTRACT

Biodiesel is one of the very important renewable energy sources targeted to meet the ever-growing demands of energy worldwide, though currently the higher costs of production has hampered the potential use at commercial scale. Use of sustainable feedstocks and the process intensification approaches can help in obtaining significant reduction in the costs of production. As the chemical routes for synthesis of biodiesel viz. esterification and transesterification are limited by the severe mass transfer effects, application of hydrodynamic cavitation reactors as process intensification approach holds significant promise. The book chapter covers different aspects including the basic mechanism of expected intensification, fundamentals of hydrodynamic cavitation, different reactor configurations, overview of different applications and important design and operational guidelines for the maximizing the extent of intensification. The focus of the analysis of different studies was on the use of sustainable feedstocks including the nonedible oil and waste cooking oil. Possible combinations of hydrodynamic cavitation reactors with other techniques of intensification have also been discussed. The potential for scale up of hydrodynamic cavitation reactors for biodiesel synthesis has also been analyzed and also the comparison with more conventionally used form of cavitational reactors i.e. ultrasound based reactors has been presented. Overall it appears that hydrodynamic cavitation reactors can give significant process intensification benefits mainly attributed to the intense physical effects of cavitation phenomena and can lead to lower reaction times, requirement of lower excess of reactants as well as reduction in the operating temperature, all pointing towards significant savings in the cost of production.

6.1   INTRODUCTION

Due to ever increasing demand of energy in industries as well as in the domestic sector, it is necessary to develop efficient processes for the production of renewable energy sources/fuels, which can also help in lowering the environmental impact as compared to the conventional sources based on fossil fuels. The renewable source of fuel must be technically feasible, economically competitive, environmentally acceptable and readily available. Renewable sources of energy can be derived from the sun, the wind, water, the Earth's heat and plants. Currently, the major sources meeting the energy requirement of any nation are mostly coal, oil and natural gas but there is limited supply of these sources on the earth. Also, the rate of use of conventional fossil fuels is such that there is a possibility of exhaustion in near future. In view of this, it is rather imperative on the part of researchers and energy planners, to search for alternate and renewable sources of the energy as it is strongly believed that renewable energy has the required potential to fulfill the gap in demand and supply of energy. Use of renewable energy can also lead to a better and greener environment. Mostly, renewable energy technologies have been called "clean" or "green" because they produce few pollutants. There are different forms of renewable energy such as solar energy, wind energy, hydropower and biofuels [1]. The present chapter focuses on the biofuels and among the different forms of biofuels, biodiesel and bioethanol are the two important sources, which have been significantly harnessed for possible use mainly as transport fuel. Biodiesel/bioethanol can be derived from different forms of biomass, both useful and waste. It is known that the use of advanced biomass conversion systems can transform the currently limited sustainable options into significantly utilizable global resources [2]. Among the different forms of biomass or biomass-derived sources, vegetable oils are an interesting source for producing fuels as well as other useful chemicals and new materials [3, 4] based on a variety of chemical and biochemical reactions. In recent years, the food security issues have directed the use of sustainable sources such as nonedible oils or the waste cooking oils or other waste residues as a replacement to the vegetable oils.

The current chapter focuses on biodiesel synthesis highlighting various sustainable feedstocks based on biomass and possible ways of intensified conversion into biodiesel based on the use of hydrodynamic cavitation. The discussion is divided into different sections highlighting the basic governing principles, reactor designs and guidelines for maximizing the intensification with possible reduction in the production costs such the biodiesel cost becomes comparable with more commonly used petroleum based diesel.

6.2   OVERVIEW OF FEEDSTOCK FOR BIODIESEL

The very initial use of alternative form as biodiesel was based on the direct use of vegetable oils in diesel engines. Subsequently, the modern day biodiesel was made by converting vegetable oils into compounds like fatty acid methyl esters using the transesterification of triglycerides (TGs) or the esterification of free fatty acids (FFAs) with low molecular weight alcohols or even in some cases based on the interesterification, where triacetin is obtained as comparatively more valuable side product. Biodiesel is one of the renewable, promising, nontoxic and environment friendly alternative biofuel that can be used with little or no modification in the existing diesel engines. Biodiesel can be produced from a great variety of feedstock including edible oils, nonedible oil, waste oils and animal fats. The choice of feedstock depends largely on geography and it is important to understand that the feedstock properties and the processing conditions affect the physical and chemical properties of the produced biodiesel, which also have direct impact on the performance and emission patterns of the engine [5–11]. It is also important to note here that yield of biodiesel depends on the unsaturated fatty acid content whereas the biodiesel properties such as cetane number, cloud point and cold flow properties depend on the quantity of saturated fatty acid. Vegetable oils such as soybean [12, 13], palm [14], sunflower [15, 16], safflower [17], canola oil [18], rapeseed [19], etc., are the most commonly used feedstock for biodiesel production. Apart from these feedstock, coconut [20] and cottonseed [21] have been also used for biodiesel production. Recently, many sustainable forms of feedstock such as nonedible oils, waste cooking oils, waste greases such as yellow grease and animal fats have also been used as alternative to the vegetable oils for the biodiesel production [18, 22–25] and the interest is growing especially considering the food security issues. The sustainable sources offer advantages because of their easy availability without any concerns and low cost but these feedstock also require some form of pretreatment such as filtration, adsorption, chemical esterification, etc. before they can be used for biodiesel production with desired efficacy. The non edible oils such as nagchampa (*Calophyllum inophyllum*), rubber seed tree (*Hevea brasiliensis*), Mahua (*Madhuca Indica*), Ratan Jyot (*Jatropha curcas*), Karanja (*Pongamia pinnata*), Soapnut (*Sapindus mukorossi*), thumba (*Leucas zeylanica*), and Neem (*Melia azadirachta*) are available in plenty though specific to the geographical regions [7,26–28] and also suffer drawback of higher free fatty acid content. Waste greases and animal fats are also considered low-quality feedstock compared to refined vegetable oils especially in terms of FFA content. The high concentrations of FFAs make all the sustainable sources inappropriate for the conventional direct base-catalyzed transesterification route to biodiesel due to the possibility of soap formation. An alternative multistep process allows the use of feedstocks having high FFA concentrations where the initial steps are based on the acid-catalyzed esterification of the FFAs followed by the base-catalyzed transesterification [23, 24].

Presently, cost of biodiesel mainly based on the use of vegetable oils is almost 10–50% higher than petroleum diesel especially due to the higher raw material costs which accounts a major portion (75–85%) of the total manufacturing cost of biodiesel [29]. The use of sustainable feedstocks though offer as low cost alternative, these also suffer from drawbacks of additional processing so as to remove the impurities present in the feedstock and also to maintain the FFA level below the required values for transesterification, making this approach also cost intensive with production costs still higher than petroleum diesel. Use of multistep approach is also cost intensive based on the additional equipments and processing times. The best option that is required for the production of biodiesel at commercial scale in a cost effective manner is the use of sustainable feedstock coupled with use of intensification approaches such as hydrodynamic cavitation.

6.3   BASICS OF HYDRODYNAMIC CAVITATION

6.3.1   OVERVIEW OF CAVITATION PHENOMENA AND ITS EFFECTS

Cavitation is defined as the generation, subsequent growth, and collapse of cavities resulting in very high but localized energy densities [30]. Cavitation can occur at multiple locations in a reactor simultaneously and generate conditions of very high temperatures and pressures (few thousand atmospheres pressure and few thousand Kelvin temperature) locally [30, 31], with overall ambient operating conditions. Based on mode of generation there are four principal types of cavitation [30]: (i) *Hydrodynamic cavitation,* where cavities are produced by pressure variation in a flowing liquid caused by the velocity variation in the system due to the changes in the flow geometry; (ii) *Acoustic cavitation,* where cavities are generated due to pressure variation introduced in a liquid by passage of ultrasound with typical frequency over the range of 20 kHz to 2 MHz [32]; (iii) *Optic cavitation,* as a result of the rupture of a liquid due to high-intensity light or a laser; and (iv) *Particle cavitation,* where cavities are produced by elementary particle beam (e.g., a proton) rupturing a liquid. Among these four types of cavitation, hydrodynamic and acoustic cavitation are the result of tensions prevailing in the liquid, while optic and particle cavitation are the result of local dissipation of energy. Generally, optic and particle cavitation is useful only for theoretical study of single bubble dynamics and characterization, while acoustic and hydrodynamic cavitation results in generation of required intensity for physical and chemical transformations. The current chapter will focus in details only on hydrodynamic cavitation as it offers higher potential for large-scale application and higher energy efficiencies [33].

Hydrodynamic cavitation can simply be generated using a constriction such as an orifice plate, venturi or throttling valve in a liquid flow. At the constriction, kinetic energy of the liquid increases at the expense of pressure head based on the Bernoulli's principle and if the throttling is sufficient to cause the pressure around the point of vena contracta to fall below the threshold pressure for cavitation (usually vapor pressure of the medium at the operating temperature, e.g., 23.8 mm of Hg (3.2 kPa) for water at an operating temperature of 25°C), cavities are generated. Subsequently, as the liquid jet expands, the pressure recovers and the generaled cavities are subjected to pressure fluctuations before the final collapse in the downstream side of the cavitating device (Figure 6.1). During the passage of the liquid through the constriction, boundary layer separation occurs and a substantial amount(of energy is lost in the form of a permanent pressure drop also generating intense local turbulence. The intensity of turbulence depends on the magnitude of the pressure drop and the rate of pressure recovery, which, in turn, depend on the geometry of the constriction (orifice or circular venturi or slit venturi) and the flow conditions of the liquid (turbulent or laminar flow, viscosity of liquid, temperature, presence of gases/solids etc.). The intensity of turbulence has a profound effect on cavitation intensity. Thus, by controlling the geometric and operating conditions of the reactor, the required intensity of the cavitation for the desired physical or chemical change can be generated wit` maximum energy efficiency [34–37].

6.3.2 REACTOR CONFIGURATIONS

One of the very initial designs used to harness the cavitational effect was based on the prifciple of high-pressure homogenization, where a high-pressure positive displacement pump is coupded with a throttling device and

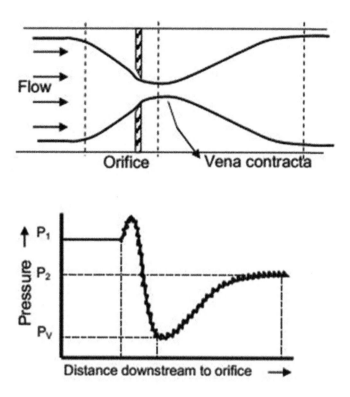

FIGURE 6.1   Fluid flow and pressure variation observed in a hydrodynamic cavitation reactor.

flow loop is introduced for recirculation. The liquid taken in a feed tank is pumped at very high pressure and subjected to sudden constriction (a simple design of throttling valve), where cavities are generated and subsequently subjected to different stages of growth and final violent collapse. The typical range of operating pressures required for generating cavitating conditions are 50 atm (5066 kPa) to 400 atm (40,528 kPa) and generally significant cavitation events are generated only after a critical threshold pressure, which would be dependent on the type of equipment [38]. Shirgaonkar et al. [38] reported a considerable increase in the iodine yield beyond an operating pressure of 5000 psi (34,800 kPa) confirming the occurrence of cavitation.

High-speed homogenizer, mainly based on the use of a stator rotor assembly, can also be used to generate cavitating conditions. This equipment also requires use of a critical speed of rotation for the onset of significant degree of cavitation and the typical operating range is 4000 to 20,000 rpm [38]. The

reactor usually has a cylindrical cross-section and different indentations/sur-
face irregularities are introduced on the rotor to introduce variations in the
cavitational intensity as per the requirement of the specific application. It
is important to note that both high speed and high pressure homogenizers
does not provide significant flexibility in the design parameters to control the
intensity of cavitation. As a result, the typical energy consumption in these
reactors is higher as compared to the low pressure devices based on the use
of orifice or venturi.

The schematic representation of the flow loop for reactor based on the
use of orifice/venturi has been given in Figure 6.2. The set-up essentially
consists of a closed loop circuit including a holding tank of capacity 5–200

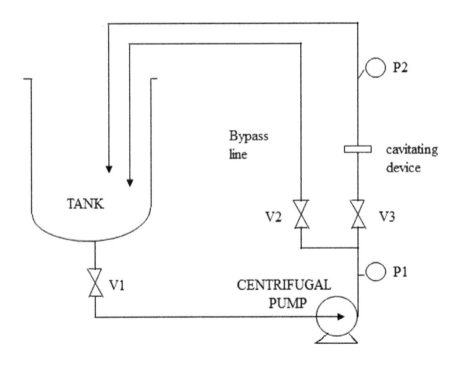

P1, P2 - PRESSURE GAGES

V1,V2,V3 - CONTROL VALVES

FIGURE 6.2   Generalized Schematic representation of flow loop in hydrodynamic cavitation
reactor-based on the orifice/venturi.

liters, a reciprocating pump with varying power rating, piping network (typically main line housing the cavitating device and the bypass lines for controlling the pressure and flow rate) and valves. The suction side of the pump is connected to the bottom of the tank and the discharge line branches into main and bypass lines. Control valves are provided at appropriate locations to suitably control the flow rate through the main line deciding the degree of exposure of the processed liquids to the cavitating conditions. Pressure gauges can also be provided at appropriate locations to quantify the inlet pressure and the fully recovered downstream pressure, which in most of the cases will be equal to 1 atm (101.3 kPa).

Vichare et al. [39] reported the use of various types of multi-hole orifice plates having different combinations of number and diameter of holes (shape can also be a factor though not demonstrated in the work) for hydrodynamic cavitation as shown in Figure 6.3. Each combination of holes in terms of number and diameter as well as shape to some extent allows creating different conditions of cavitational intensity, which can be tailored to meet the requirements of the specific application and increase the overall energy efficiency for the processing. For example, higher number of holes with smaller diameter is typically recommended for applications requiring lower cavitational intensity such as biodiesel synthesis or microbial disinfection whereas smaller number of holes with medium diameter will be useful for applications requiring intense cavitational intensity such as wastewater treatment or chemical synthesis. Also, these reactors offer tremendous flexibility in terms of the operating parameters such as inlet pressure, inlet flow rate and temperature [34, 5].

Sampathkumar and Moholkar [40] reported a modification in the design in terms of provision of a facility for introducing gas bubbles in the flow at the constriction. Due to this modification, additional control over the cavitational intensity can be obtained based on the variations in the type of gas to be introduced, flow rate, pressure at which the gas is introduced and finally the bubble size based on the variation in the gas distributor.

In another recent work, Gogate et al. [41] described a new design of hydrodynamic cavitation reactor based on the use of static mixing elements. The specific geometric arrangement of mixing elements or a mesh of mixing elements within the pipe helps in generating cavitation though the pressure drop required for generation of cavities will be higher as compared to the simple design based on the orifice or venturi. Use

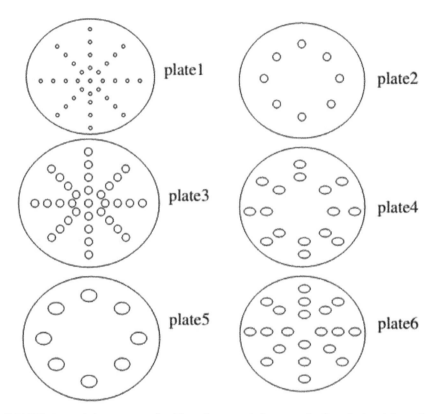

FIGURE 6.3 Various types of orifice plates used for control of cavitational intensity. (Reprinted with permission from N.P. Vichare, P.R. Gogate, A.B. Pandit, Optimization of hydrodynamic cavitation using a model reaction, Chemical Engineering & Technology. 23(2000) 683–691. © 2000 John Wiley and Sons.)

of static mixing elements also helps in efficient mixing which may be a key parameter for application such as biodiesel production, which is dominated mostly by the physical effects of cavitation. The configuration also reports the combined operation of hydrodynamic cavitation and sonochemical reactors in sequential manner where the cavities generated using hydrodynamic manner are made to collapse under the influence of the ultrasonic field. Though the actual application for biodiesel synthesis have not been studied, significantly promising results have been reported for the water recycle in the oil and gas explorations, which works on similar principle of requirement of dominating physical effects. It is important to note that this design based on the use of static mixing elements is the only reported case of hydrodynamic cavitation reactors at commercial scale application [41].

6.4   OVERVIEW OF RECENT APPLICATIONS RELATED TO BIODIESEL SYNTHESIS

The conventional processes for biodiesel production typically need longer reaction time (anywhere between 1 to 12 h depending on the feedstock and catalyst), resulting in requirement of large reactor volume and also large excess of one of the reactants increasing the downstream separation loads. The application of process intensification approaches should aim at reducing both these aspects and can additionally help in reducing the temperature requirement, all of which may drive towards reduction in the production costs. We now discuss some of the recent works describing the use of hydrodynamic cavitation as the process intensification approach for biodiesel synthesis.

Maddikeri et al. [42] investigated the application of hydrodynamic cavitation reactors for the intensification of biodiesel production from waste cooking oil (WCO) based on the use of interesterification reaction. Different cavitating devices such as circular and slit venturi as well as orifice plate were used in the work and effect of different operating parameters such as inlet pressure over the range of 2–5 bar (200 to 500 kPa), molar ratio of oil to methyl acetate over the range of 1:10 to 1:14, and catalyst loading over the range of 0.5 to 1.25% by weight of oil on the yield of biodiesel was investigated. It was reported that maximum yield of biodiesel as 90% was obtained under optimized conditions of catalyst loading of 1.0%, oil to methyl acetate ratio as 1:12, inlet pressure of 3 bar (300 kPa) and using slit venturi as the cavitating device. It was also established that slit venturi resulted in better yield as compared to the other two types of cavitating devices. Comparison of the results with ultrasound based and the conventional route for synthesis [43] also revealed that higher cavitational yield described as the biodiesel produced per unit energy consumed was obtained for the hydrodynamic cavitation based approach. It was reported that the micro level turbulence generated due to the cavitational collapse near the liquid–liquid interface causes the rupture of the interface and results in formation of a fine emulsion, which is also more stable as compared to those obtained using conventional means. The fine emulsions provide enhanced surface area for the reaction, which coupled with turbulence leads to enhanced conversion based on the elimination of mass transfer limitations. It was also demonstrated that the properties of biodiesel match with the ASTM standards as mentioned in Table 6.1 and were superior as compared to the product obtained using conventional route.

TABLE 6.1 Values for the American Society for Testing and Materials (ASTM) Standards, EN Standards of Maximum Allowed Quantities in Diesel and Biodiesel

Property	Biodiesel		Diesel
Standard:	ASTM D6751	EN 14214	ASTM D 975
Composition:		FAME (C12-C22)	Hydrocarbons (C10-C21)
Kinematic Viscosity mm2/s at 40°C	1.9–6.0	3.5–5.0	1.9-4.1
Density at 15°C g/mL	0.87–0.89	0.86–0.90	0.85
Flash Point	100–170	>101	60–80
Cloud Point	–3 to 12	Based on National specification	–15 to 5
Pour Point	–15 to 16		-35 to -15
Water (Vol%)	0.05	500 mg/kg	0.05
Carbon (wt%)	77	0.30%	87
Hydrogen (wt%)	12	—	13
Oxygen (wt%)	11	—	0
Sulphur (wt%)	0.05	—	0.05
Cetane Number	48–60	51	40–55
HFRR micro meter	314	—	685
BOCLE scuff (g)	>7000	—	3600

[a]HFRR-High frequency reciprocating rig.

[b]BOCLE-Ball on cylinder lubricity evaluator.

Pal and Kachhwaha [44] reported the development of test rigs for use of hydrodynamic cavitation for the synthesis of biodiesel from WCO and compared the efficacy with ultrasound based approach as well as the conventional approach. It was demonstrated that hydrodynamic cavitation can be effectively used for the production of biodiesel with more than 90% yield at optimum molar ratio of oil to methanol as 1:4.5 and 0.5% of catalyst loading. The processing capacity of the hydrodynamic cavitation rig was reported to about 10 times higher as compared to the ultrasound based approach which can prompt towards the feasibility for large scale operations. The actual yield obtained in the case of ultrasound-based approach was higher at 95% in 45 min of treatment which can be attributed to much higher power dissipation per unit volume. It would be interesting to compare the trends in terms of actual production per unit power consumption where higher effectiveness for hydrodynamic cavitation can be established, though the authors did not report any such analysis.

Rengasamy et al. [45] investigated the transesterification of sunflower oil to biodiesel using hydrodynamic cavitation with study into effects of operating parameters such as oil to methanol ratio, catalyst load and contact time. The reaction mixture taken in a cylindrical reservoir was circulated through the cavitating device (two plates with varying geometry as 24 holes of 2 mm diameter and 21 holes of 3 mm diameter) using a pump. The preliminary results established that catalyst load of 1 g with oil to methanol ratio of 1:5 and a contact time of 40 min resulted in maximum biodiesel yield as 77%. It was also reported that the plate with higher number of holes resulted in marginally higher biodiesel yield attributed to higher perimeter giving the higher extents of the shear layer effects.

Yusup et al. [46] investigated the use of equal volume mixture of crude palm and rubber seed oil as the feedstock. Use of rubber seed oil offers as a sustainable nonedible feedstock for biodiesel, which can help in reducing the dependency on the crude palm oil. The inlet pressure was kept constant at 3 bar (300 kPa) and an orifice plate having 1 mm hole and 20 mm thickness was used as the cavitating device. It was established that the hydrodynamic cavitation required lower reaction time for the efficient processing of feedstock to methyl esters as compared to the mechanical agitation based conventional approach. It was also reported that the yield of biodiesel per unit supplied energy was 13.5×10^{-4} g/J for the case of hydrodynamic cavitation which was about significantly higher than the conventional process (8×10^{-6} g/J). It was also demonstrated that hydrodynamic cavitation provided final product with desired quality specifications as per the international standards of ASTM D674 and EN 14214.

Chuah et al. [47] reported a new route for intensification of methyl ester synthesis using a hydrodynamic cavitation reactor based on the alkali-catalyzed transesterification reaction of WCO obtained from palm olein. Optimized plate geometry with 21 holes of 1 mm diameter was used in the hydrodynamic cavitation reactor of 50 L capacity. A double diaphragm pump was used for the circulation of the liquid mixture through the cavitating device. The experiments related to understanding the effect of the different parameters such as oil to methanol molar ratio (1:4–1:7), catalyst loading (0.5–1.25 wt%) and reaction temperature (50–65°C) were performed. It was reported that maximum conversion of 98.1% was achieved in 15 min under optimized conditions of 1:6 as the molar ratio of oil to methanol, 1 wt% of catalyst loading and 60°C as the reaction temperature. A significant reduction in the required reaction time (about 6 fold) was demonstrated for transesterification with 90 min being required for mechanical stirring and only 15 min for the hydrodynamic cavitation approach. Calculations of cavitational yield revealed that the optimal yield in the hydrodynamic cavitation was 12.50×10^{-4} g/J which was 8 fold higher than the value obtained in the case of mechanical stirring as 1.5×10^{-4} g/J.

Bokhari et al. [48] reported the use of hydrodynamic cavitation reactor for the pretreatment of the high free fatty acid rubber seed oil (RSO) using esterification reaction. The reactor used in the work had a capacity of 50 L and four different types of orifice plates having different diameter of holes and number of holes were used to investigate the effect of geometry. It was reported that the optimized plate configuration having 21 holes of 1 mm diameter at operating inlet pressure of 3 bar (300 kPa) resulted in a maximum reduction in the acid value from 72.36 to 2.64 mg KOH/g within 30 min of reaction time. The optimum operating parameters established on the basis of response surface methodology were oil to methanol ratio of 6:1, catalyst loading of 8 wt%, and operating temperature of 55°C. It was also demonstrated that use of hydrodynamic cavitation resulted in significant process intensification benefits with the reduction in the reaction time by three fold and increase in the esterification efficiency (product obtained per unit energy consumption) by four fold as compared to the conventional approach involving mechanical stirring.

In another recent work, Chuah et al. [49] investigated the synthesis of biodiesel from a mixture of refined cooking oil and WCO intensified using a hydrodynamic cavitation reactor. Studies were performed using different plate geometries and inlet pressures to establish the interdependency of the results. The optimized conditions were established as oil to methanol molar ratio of 1:6, catalyst loading of 1 wt.% (potassium hydroxide used as the catalyst) and operating temperature of 60°C. It was demonstrated that use of 2 bar (200 kPa) inlet pressure and orifice plate with 21 holes of 1 mm diameter gave best results for biodiesel production and the efficiency was 8 fold higher as compared to the mechanical stirring coupled with 6 fold lower reaction time.

Based on the overview of recent studies, it can be said that hydrodynamic cavitation offers significant benefits of process intensification with reduced processing time (about 50% to 5 times reduction) and higher energy efficiency (about 2 to 10 times) as compared to the conventional approach and in some cases even as compared to the ultrasound based processing. Additional studies related to the use of hydrodynamic cavitation have also been discussed in the later sections related to the effect of design and operational parameters on the yields of biodiesel.

6.5   GUIDELINES FOR DESIGN AND OPERATIONAL PARAMETERS FOR MAXIMIZING THE INTENSIFICATION

6.5.1   UNDERSTANDING HYDRAULIC PROPERTIES

The inlet pressure to the cavitating device and cavitation number, are the two important parameters, which affects the cavitational intensity in the reactor. The number of cavities being generated and the cavitational intensity (magnitude of collapse pressure/energy released during collapse) largely depends on the inlet pressure, which is an indication of energy being supplied into the reactor. Hence, it is important to understand the hydraulic properties for all the cavitating devices such as orifice and venturi. Cavitation number (C_v) is generally used to characterize the cavitational intensity and can be estimated by following equation [35, 36]:

$$C_v = \frac{P_2 - P_v}{(1/2)\rho / v^2} \qquad (1)$$

actual power dissipation into the liquid is important. Maddikeri et al. [42] estimated the actual power dissipation for the supplied power of 1.5 kW to where p_2 is the fully recovered downstream pressure, p_v is the vapor pressure of the liquid, ρ is the liquid density and v is the velocity at the constriction which can be calculated by knowing the main line flow rate and diameter of the orifice. It is important to understand that significant effects of cavitation will be obtained for cavitation number less than 1 (more specifically over the range 0.1 to 0.5). In some cases where dissolved gases are likely to be present, cavitation might occur over cavitation number range of 1 to 2.5 as well but very high intensity is not observed.

Maddikeri et al. [42] studied the variation in the cavitation number as a function of inlet pressure for the intensified synthesis of biodiesel based on the interesterification of waste cooking oil. The details of cavitation device used in the work have been given in Table 6.2. It has been reported that cavitation number decreases with an increase in the pump discharge pressure and the trend can be explained based on an increase in the velocity at the throat of the venturi. It was also reported that cavitation number in the slit venturi was less as compared to circular venturi and orifice plate at similar levels of inlet pressure due to the higher volumetric flow rate obtained in the slit venturi.

Gole et al. [50] reported that the cavitation number was 0.115 and 0.118 (very similar) at the inlet pressures of 10 psi (69 kPa) and 20 psi (138 kPa) respectively and then decreased to 0.055 with an increase in the inlet pressure to 40 psi (276 kPa). It was also reported that too low cavitation number is not beneficial for the desired application as choked cavitation is observed where a large cavity cloud is observed, whose collapse gives much lesser cavitational effects. The onset of choked cavitation which is also described as super cavitation has also been confirmed based on the photographic analysis reported in the work of Saharan et al. [51]. It was recommended to use an optimum cavitation number over the range of 0.1 to 0.2 which can be adjusted with the help of inlet pressure and flow rate through the cavitating device.

Yan and Thorpe [52] reported that for a given size of orifice, the cavitation number remains constant within an experimental error for a specific liquid. The cavitation number does not change with the liquid velocity significantly due to interchange with the inlet pressure but more dominantly increases with an increase in the size of the orifice and also is affected by the dimension of the pipe.

Power dissipation per unit volume is another important parameter that decides the cavitational intensity in the reactor and hence estimation of the

TABLE 6.2 Details of Cavitation Device Used by Maddikeri et al. [42] and Saharan et al. [53]

Dimensions	Maddikeri et al. [42]		Saharan et al. [53]	
	Circular Venturi	Slit Venturi	Circular Venturi	Slit Venturi
Dimensions of throat	Circular hole of 2 mm diameter	$W = 3.7$ mm $H = 0.92$ mm $L = 0.92$ mm	Circular hole of 2 mm diameter	$W = 6.0$ mm $H = 1.9$ mm $L = 1.9$ mm
Venturi Length	106 mm	86 mm	87 mm	87 mm
Length of convergent section	18 mm	18 mm	18 mm	20 mm
Length of divergent section	67 mm	65 mm	67 mm	65 mm
Half angle of convergent section	22.6^0	22.6^0	22.6^0	23.5^0
Half angle of divergent section	6.5^0	6.5^0	6.4^0	5.5^0

the system and confirmed that maximum power was dissipated in the case of slit venturi as compared to the circular venturi and orifice plate. It was also reported that the power dissipated into the system for the slit venturi is almost 1.1 times higher than circular venturi and 1.5 times higher than orifice plate. Similar results were also reported by Saharan et al. [53] confirming that maximum power dissipation was obtained for the slit venturi as compared to the circular venturi though the extent of increase in the power dissipation was different attributed to the differences in the geometry of the cavitating device as outlined in the Table 6.2.

Overall it can be said that it is important to understand the hydraulic properties especially the estimations of cavitation number and the actual power dissipation into the reactor such that the conditions of choked cavitation can be avoided and maximum benefits can be observed under the optimum flow conditions in terms of inlet pressure and the velocity at the vena contracta (position of cavity inception).

6.5.2 EFFECT OF CAVITATING DEVICE

Generally, two types of cavitating devices as orifice and venturi have been used in the hydrodynamic cavitation reactor (low pressure device offering flexibility in control of cavitational intensity as discussed earlier). Various geometries are also possible in the case of orifice plates with variation in the size, shape and number of holes on the plate. The cavitational intensity will be dependent on the geometric parameters such as flow area, diameter of the constriction and also the number of holes in the case of orifice plate. Due to the effect on cavitational intensity, the degree of intensification that can be obtained for biodiesel synthesis will also be affected.

Maddikeri et al. [42] investigated effect of three different cavitating devices as orifice plate, circular and slit venturi on the biodiesel yield and the reported results have been reproduced in Figure 6.4. It can be seen from the figure that maximum yield of biodiesel as 89% is obtained using slit venturi followed by circular venturi (82%) and orifice plate (64%) under a fixed conditions of reactant molar ratio as 1:12, 1% catalyst loading and inlet pressure of 3 bar (300 kPa). The observed results can be explained on the basis of the higher volumetric flow rate for a given pressure drop and lower cavitation number being obtained in slit venturi as compared to orifice plate and circular venturi. The number of cavitational events and the intensity

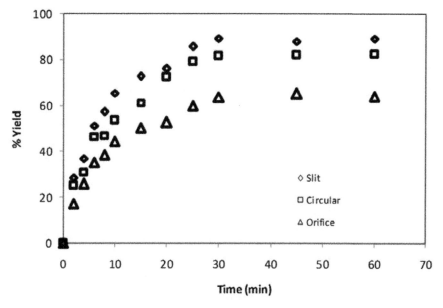

FIGURE 6.4 Effect of geometry on yield of biodiesel under reaction conditions of OMAMR = 1:12; catalyst loading = 1% (by wt% of oil), inlet pressure = 3 bars as per work of Maddikeri et al. [42]. (Reprinted from G. L. Maddikeri, P. R. Gogate, A. B. Pandit, Intensified synthesis of biodiesel using hydrodynamic cavitation reactors based on the interesterification of waste cooking oil, Fuel. 137 (2014) 285–292. © 2014 Elsevier.)

increases with a decrease in cavitation number (avoiding super cavitation) and these cavitational events are responsible for liquid circulation associated with enhanced turbulence and micro scale emulsion (giving higher surface area for reaction) ultimately enhancing the biodiesel yield.

Ghayal et al. [54] investigated the biodiesel production using waste frying oil in a hydrodynamic cavitation reactor with cavitating device as orifice plate (Four different configurations of orifice plates differing in the number and diameter of the circular holes). It was reported that the flow geometry of orifice plate plays a crucial role in deciding the intensification of biodiesel production. Optimized plate geometry of 2 mm hole diameter and 25 holes resulted in maximum of 95% TGs conversion to methyl esters in 10 min of reaction time with cavitational yield of 1.28×10^{-3} g/J (grams of methyl esters produced per joule of energy supplied). The results of control experiment in the absence of orifice plate confirmed that significantly lower extent of conversion (only around 40%) is obtained in the absence of cavitating device. The results can be attributed to existence of only macrolevel mixing in the absence of cavitating device, which is due to the recirculation of the reactants at high flow rate whereas in the case of cavitating device, microscale turbulence is obtained giving microemulsions offering large surface area for the reaction, which helps in achieving significantly higher conversions. The observed results for the effect of geometry was explained in terms of total perimeter of holes for plate 1, plate 2, plate 3, and plate 4 estimated as 31.40, 157, 150.72, and 188.40 mm, respectively. Studies related to understanding the effect of total perimeter at different inlet pressures established that at lower pressure, with an increase in the total perimeter, there was an improvement in the cavitational effect due to enhanced generation of cavities giving higher cavitational intensity. However, at higher pressures, there was an increase in the conversion only till an optimum total perimeter of 157 mm and further increase in total perimeter marginally reduced the conversion. The observed optimum can be explained on the basis of the fact that at higher pressure and higher perimeter, generation of too many cavities reduces the cavitational effect due to possible choked cavitation leading to cushioned collapse of the cavities, which gives lower collapse intensity [51, 55].

Gogate and Pandit [34] studied the effect of diameter of the hole in the orifice plate on the collapse pressure pulse based on bubble dynamics analysis. It was reported that with an increase in diameter of the hole, the collapse pressure generated increases, which can be attributed to the variation in the cavitation inception number with the diameter of the hole. It was also reported that for a larger diameter hole, the cavitation starts at a higher cavitation number, and the extent of the cavitation also increases for the same operating cavitation number in the system, resulting in a higher magnitude of the pressure pulse generated at the time of the collapse, giving beneficial results.

In summary, it can be said that the type of the cavitating device as well as the geometry of the venturi or orifice plays an important role and optimum configuration needs to be selected to maximize the cavitational intensity without leading to the generation of choked cavitation conditions. A summary of the important parameters with likely effects on the cavitational intensity and recommendations for optimum has been illustrated in Table 6.3.

6.5.3   EFFECT OF INLET PRESSURE

Inlet pressure mainly depends on the type of cavitating device used and the capacity of the pump used for recirculation. With an increase in the inlet

TABLE 6.3 Important Geometric Parameters of Cavitating Device Affecting the Cavitational Intensity

S. No.	Parameter	Affects	Observation	Recommendation
1	Type of cavitation device	Flow properties and onset of cavitation (inception and choked)	Venturi offers better characteristics in terms of pressure recovery, slit venturi better as compared to circular and orifice plate	Slit venturi appears to be best design
2	α (ratio of total perimeter of holes to the total flow area on plate)	Level of turbulence and the shear layer effects	Maximum conversion can be obtained with larger value of α though optimum should be established	Increasing number of holes in the case of orifice plate is better. The effect may not be significant at higher inlet pressures due to quick onset of super cavitation.
4	β ratio of hole diameter on orifice to the pipe diameter	Affects the cavity collapse pressure as well as cavitation number	Small size of β gives higher conversion	Smaller size of holes would be useful but the problem of higher pressure drops needs to be suitably tackled based on use of high capacity pump.
5	β_0 ratio of the total flow area on the orifice plate to the cross sectional flow area of pipe	Again affects the cavity collapse pressure as well as pressure drop	Conversion increases with an increasing β_0	Lower flow area would give maximum turbulence with larger shear area but pressure drop issues must be tackled.

pressure, velocity at the throat of cavitating device also increases, which subsequently reduces the cavitation number as per the definition of Cv. As the cavitation number decreases, more number of cavities are formed which result into higher cavitational yield if the conditions of choked cavitation are avoided.

In the case of biodiesel production also, inlet pressure has been found to be an important parameter. Ghayal et al. [54] reported that rate of transesterification reaction increased with an increase in the inlet pressure, though the trend was dependent on the geometry of orifice plate. It was reported that, for the case of orifice plate 1 and plate 3, the reaction time reduced significantly when the pump discharge pressure was increased from 1 to 3 bar (100 to 300 kPa). However, in the case of orifice plate 2 and 4, there was an increase in the rate of transesterification reaction when upstream pressure was increased from 1 to 2 bar, but beyond this optimum pressure of 2 bar (200 kPa), further increase to 3 bar (300 kPa) did not result in any significant increase in the rate of reaction. It should be noted that at lower upstream pressures there was a considerable difference in the reaction rate for all four plates with an increase in the pressure whereas at higher pressures not much difference in the reaction rates have been observed for different geometric configurations of the orifice plates. The observed results were explained on the basis of choked cavitation. It was also established that the interdependency between optimum inlet pressure and geometry depends on the ease of generation of cavitation. If the geometry is favorable to form enhanced cavitation, lower optimum pressure exists as the condition of choked cavitation is reached faster.

Maddikeri et al. [42] also studied the effect of inlet pressure on biodiesel yield over inlet pressure range of 2 to 5 bar (200 to 500 kPa) using slit venturi as the cavitating device under fixed conditions of reactant molar ratio (1:12) and catalyst loading (1% wt). The obtained results have been reproduced in Figure 6.5 and it can be seen from these results that biodiesel yield increases with an increase in the inlet pressure till an optimum value and with further increase in the inlet pressure there was not much increase in biodiesel yield. The reported results are consistent with other studies involving hydrodynamic cavitation [56, 57].

In summary, it can be said that it is important to select an optimum inlet pressure for maximum benefits, the value of which will be dependent on the specific reactor configuration (geometric parameters of the cavitating device and the reactor), which strongly affects the ease of cavitation inception and number of cavities likely to be generated.

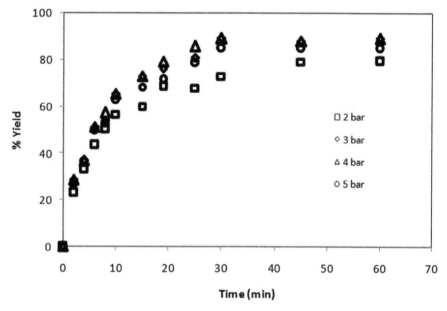

FIGURE 6.5 Effect of inlet pressure on yield of biodiesel under reaction conditions of cavitating device = slit venturi; OMAMR =1:12; Catalyst loading = 1% (by wt% of oil) as per work of Maddikeri et al. [42]. (Reprinted from G. L. Maddikeri, P. R. Gogate, A. B. Pandit, Intensified synthesis of biodiesel using hydrodynamic cavitation reactors based on the interesterification of waste cooking oil, Fuel. 137 (2014) 285–292. © 2014 Elsevier.)

6.5.4 EFFECT OF MOLAR RATIO

One of the most important reaction parameters, which affect the yield of biodiesel as well as the production costs, is the molar ratio of alcohol to triglyceride used in the reaction. As transesterification or esterification is a reversible reaction, generally excess amount of alcohol is used though it is important to optimize the ratio as too much excess of any reactant will lead to higher separation costs in the downstream processing.

Maddikeri et al. [42] studied the effect of oil to methyl acetate molar ratio (OMAMR) over the range of 1:10 to 1:14 on biodiesel yield obtained using interesterification reaction, which is also reversible in nature. It was reported in the study that biodiesel yield increased from 83% to 89% with an increase in the molar ratio from 1:10 to 1:12. With a further increase in the OMAMR from 1:12 to 1:14, significant beneficial effects in terms of the enhanced conversion of oil were not observed. It was mentioned that higher methyl acetate quantity till an optimum favors the forward reaction for the production of desired product resulting in an increase in the equilibrium conversion of WCO to biodiesel. It was also reported that enhanced yield and lower requirement of excess reactants was observed for the hydrodynamic cavitation assisted approach as compared to the conventional approach attributed to the cavitational effects of micro-emulsification and liquid streaming.

Gole et al. [50] investigated the intensified synthesis of methyl esters from Nagchampa oil (having high free fatty acid content as established by the acid value) using hydrodynamic cavitation based on a two step approach where first step was to lower the acid value such that the second step of transesterification can be achieved wathout any problems of soap formation. For esterification reaction, the effect of molar ratio of oil to methanol over the range of 1:2 to 1:5 was investigated at 2% catalyst loading by weight sulfuric acid). The obtained results have been reproduced in Figure 6.6 and it can be seen that the final acid value decreased with an increase in the molar ratio from 1:2 to 1:3, but a further increase in the molar ratio to 1:4 and 1:5 did not yield any significant change in the final acid value. It was reported that the maximum reduction in the acid value was obtained at 1:3 molar ratio within 60 min reaction time. Similar results for the optimum molar ratio were also reported for the second stage of transesterification where the effect of molar ratio of oil to methafol was studied over the range of 1:4–1:8 at constant catalyst (potassium hydroxide) loading of 1% by weight of the oil. It was reported that extent of conversion increases significantly up to oil to methanol ratio of 1:6, and beyond this, only a marginal increase in the extent of conversion is observed when the ratio is further increased to 1:8.

Kelkar et al. [58] used different molar ratios of fatty acids (FA) to methanol as 1:2, 1:5, and 1:10 with the quantity of conc. H_2SO_4 as the catalyst kept constant at 1% by weight of fatty acids. Excess methanol was used since the water formed during the esterification reaction gets dissolved in this excess methanol giving higher conversion due to the shift in equilibrium towards right side of the reaction. The reaction was found to proceed up to 90% conversion (mol%) levels at appreciable rate beyond which the rate of progress of the reaction was substantially slower. The observed trend was attributed to the dilution of the acid catalyst with the water formed in the reaction which reduces its catalytic activity and also attainment of the equilibrium conditions at the given operating temperature. It was also reported that though the final conversion was similar in all the cases of molar ratio, the required time reduced with an increase in the molar ratio. Comparison of the time required for reaching the 90% conversion at different molar ratios

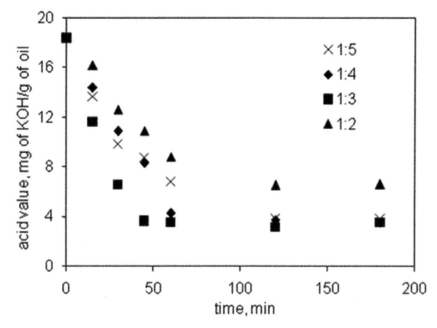

FIGURE 6.6 Effect of molar ratio of methanol to oil on acid value for 2 wt% of H_2SO_4 catalyst as reported in Gole et al. [50]. (Reprinted with permission from V. L. Gole, K. R. Naveen, P. R. Gogate, Hydrodynamic cavitation as an efficient approach for intensification of synthesis of methyl esters from sustainable feedstock, Chemical Engineering and Processing. 71 (2013) 70–76. © 2013 Elsevier.)

confirmed that the time required was the minimum at molar ratio of 1:10 similar to the case of acoustic cavitation.

Chuah et al. [47] investigated intensification of biodiesel synthesis from WCO in hydrodynamic cavitation reactor at different molar ratios over the range of 1:4 to 1:7 with 1 wt% catalyst (KOH) loading and constant reaction temperature of 60°C. It was reported that maximum yield of 98.1% was obtained at optimum molar ratio of 1:6 in 15 min of reaction time. Similar results have also been reported by Ji et al. [59] for the transesterification of soybean oil where a 1:6 molar ratio has been reported as optimum with a reaction time of 30 min for the hydrodynamic cavitation reactor. In another study, Yun et al. [60] investigated the transesterification of rapeseed oil using hydrodynamic cavitation and reported existence of an optimum molar ratio as 1:6.

Overall, it can be said that an optimum molar ratio for maximum benefits exists (for hydrodynamic cavitation, it is lower, say over the range of 1:3 to

1:5 as compared to the conventional approach where it is generally over the range of 1:6 to 1:10 depending on the type of raw material) and the actual value is dependent on the type of raw material. The use of optimum ratio is always recommended to get maximum intensification benefits with reduced separation costs.

6.5.5 EFFECT OF CATALYST LOADING

The objective of using a catalyst is to enhance the reaction rate by providing active ions and suitable path for faster conversion. Catalyst loading plays an important role in deciding the efficacy of biodiesel synthesis especially in the case of heterogeneous catalyst as it affects the cavitational intensity. Maddikeri et al. [42] investigated the effect of potassium methoxide loading on the biodiesel yield over the range of 0.75–1.25%. It was reported that an increase in the catalyst loading from 0.75% to 1% results in a corresponding increase in the biodiesel yield from 79% to 89%. However, a further increase in the catalyst loading from 1 to 1.25 wt% did not show any significant increase in the biodiesel yield. The observed results were attributed to the fact that initially, an increase in the catalyst loading gives enhanced active sites for reaction resulting into higher conversion of triglycerides into the corresponding methyl esters. Beyond the optimum, due to the change in the controlling mechanism and lower cavitational intensity attributed to the scattering of sound waves giving lower energy dissipation, not much improvement in conversion is obtained. Based on these results, it was established that 1% catalyst loading was the optimum, which is important to be determined as the separation costs needs to be weighed against the possible benefits.

Gole et al. [50] investigated esterification and transesterification of nag-champa oil over the catalyst loading range of 0.5–3% and 0.5–1.5% wt% of oil respectively at an optimal molar ratio of 1:6. It was reported that 1% catalyst loading was the optimum loading for both esterification as well as transesterification. It was also established that complete removal of acid catalyst after esterification was essential for avoiding the saponification reaction in the presence of alkali catalyst in the second stage which may lead to lower yield of the fatty acid methyl esters and also give processing issues due to soap formation.

Kelkar et al. [58] studied the effect of catalyst loading (1% and 2% by weight of the reactants) at two different operating molar ratio of FA to methanol (1:5 and 1:10). The reported results confirmed that higher catalyst loading was beneficial in both the cases. The extent of conversion in the case of 1:5 molar ratio increased from 91% in 3 h of reaction time to about 97% in only 90 min of reaction time, when the catalyst loading was increased from 1% to 2%. For the case of operating molar ratio of 1:10, the conversion increased from 98% in 2 h to almost 100% in 90 min of treatment for a similar increase in the catalyst loading from 1% to 2%. Kelkar et al. [58] also investigated the effect of type of the catalyst on the conversion. Heterogeneous catalyst as superacid clay was also used instead of most commonly used catalyst, conc. H_2SO_4. The use of heterogeneous catalyst was with an objective of easier separation and possible reuse, which can reduce the overall production costs. However it was reported that use of heterogeneous clay catalyst significantly slowed down the process and the catalyst was significantly deactivated in the process due to interactions with water and only 41% conversion was obtained with the recycled catalyst.

Chuah et al. [47] studied the effect of KOH loading over the range of 0.5 wt% to 1.25wt% at an optimum molar ratio of 1:6 and reaction temperature of 60 °C. It was reported that conversion increased from 63% to 98.1% with an increase in the catalyst loading from 0.5 wt% to 1.0 wt% in 15 min as the reaction time. With a further increase in the catalyst loading to 1.25 wt%, the conversion decreased marginally from 98.1% at 1% loading to 91.0% obtained at 1.25 wt% loading. It was also reported that beyond the optimum level, soap formation was observed which led to problems in the processing.

Casas et al. [61] investigated the interesterification reaction of sunflower oil and methyl acetate for biodiesel production and reported that a maximum conversion of 76.7% was obtained at an optimized catalyst loading of 1.04% by weight. Similar results have also been reported by Suppalakpanya et al. [62] for the transesterification reaction of crude palm oil with potassium hydroxide as the catalyst and also for transesterification of soybean [59] and rapeseed oil [60] where an optimum loading of catalyst as 1% was reported.

In summary, it can be said that generally sodium hydroxide or potassium hydroxide in the case of transesterification and conc. sulphuric acid in the case of esterification have been reported as the preferred catalyst with existence of the optimum loading of catalyst for maximum benefits which need to be established using laboratory scale studies as it is dependent on the specific raw materials. Use of heterogeneous catalysts does not seem to be a promising option, at least based on the reported studies, due to slower reaction rates and deactivation during the reaction. More studies are indeed required to investigate a wider range of catalysts and intensification approaches which can also provide in-situ activation during the processing.

6.5.6 EFFECT OF OPERATING TEMPERATURE

Operating temperature typically is an important kinetic parameter, which also affects the cavitational intensity in the case of cavitational reactors. The effect of temperature is complex as on one side where it increases the kinetic rate of reaction, it also has a negative effect on the cavitational intensity due to the possibility of cushioned collapse of cavities (presence of vapors) leading to lower intensity and hence reduced degree of intensification. There have not been many studies reporting the effect of temperature in the case of biodiesel synthesis and in general it can be said that using ambient conditions would be the best approach, as this will also avoid the need of heating required in the case of conventional reactions to achieve higher temperatures. Chuah et al. [47] studied the effect of temperature over the range of 50°C to 65°C and reported that with an increase in the temperature from 50°C to 60°C, the conversion increased from 79.0% to 98.1%. The enhanced conversion was attributed to the fast dispersion of methanol in the oil attributed to the reduction in viscosity of waste cooking oil. Enhanced dispersion leads to better contact of the phases giving higher reaction rates. Further increase in the operating temperature to 65°C, however, resulted in a slight reduction in the conversion to 97% in similar reaction time as 15 min, establishing 60°C as the optimum. Bokhari et al. [48] investigated the effect of temperature over the range of 40°C to 60°C and reported that optimum temperature of 55 °C resulted in best results for the esterification of rubber seed (*Hevea brasiliensis*) oil giving the desired reduction in the acid value. Gole et al. [50] did not investigate the effect of temperature but reported that the use of ambient conditions (temperature in the range of 30°C to 35°C) resulted in desirable conversions based on the optimization of other operating parameters. It was also reported that comparison of the results with the conventional method also revealed that hydrodynamic cavitation reactor was effective under ambient conditions, whereas the reflux conditions required higher operating temperature (60°C) for the desired progress of the reaction to yield similar conversions. The effectiveness of hydrodynamic cavitation reactor in giving better results was attributed to the cavitational effects leading to elimination of the mass transfer effects and also to the local hot spots generated in the reactor, which resulted in favorable changes in the liquid physicochemical properties.

Overall it can be said that it is better to operate under ambient conditions without any control on the temperature (a slight increase in the temperature might occur based on the heat dissipation due to cavitating conditions, which also would be beneficial based on the existence of optimum temperature as discussed here), which can also lead to energy savings as no heating or cooling duty will be required. For specific systems based on use of sustainable raw materials, which are very slow even in the presence of hydrodynamic cavitation, higher temperatures till an optimum may be checked as a means to intensify the reaction.

6.6 COMPARISON WITH ULTRASONIC REACTORS AND CONVENTIONAL APPROACHES

It is very important to understand the process intensification benefits obtained by using hydrodynamic cavitation and compare with other approaches so as to evaluate the possibility of using hydrodynamic cavitation in commercial practice. The cavitating effects can also be obtained using the ultrasound-based reactors which have been exhaustively studied in the case of biodiesel production [63, 64]. Thus it becomes even more important to highlight the possible beneficial effects as compared to ultrasonic reactors. We now discuss comparison of the results obtained using hydrodynamic cavitation reactors with ultrasonic and conventional approaches (mechanical stirring and reflux) based on the overview of literature.

Gole et al. [50] compared the results obtained for hydrodynamic cavitation reactors in terms of the optimized parameters, kinetic constants and cavitational yield with ultrasound and conventional reflux based approach [65] and the results have been reproduced in Table 6.4. It can be clearly seen from the results reported in tables that the reaction time required for hydrodynamic cavitation is marginally more as compared to the conventional approach (not considering any preheating time) and ultrasound based approach, which may be attributed to the lower intensity cavitation generated in the case of hydrodynamic cavitation. It is important to understand that significant time (about 120 min) is required for initial preheating to achieve the

TABLE 6.4 Comparison of Results for Hydrodynamic Cavitation, Ultrasound, and Conventional Reflux Approaches [50, 65]

(A) Set of Optimized Parameters

Parameters	Hydrodynamic [50]			Ultrasound [65]		Conventional [65]	
	First Stage E	Second Stage E	T	E	T	E	T
Reaction time, min	60	50	20	15	40	20	90
Molar ratio	1:4	1:1	1:6	1:2	1:6	1:3	1:6
Catalyst Concentration, % w/w	1	1	1	1	1	1	1
Conversion,%	81.9	60.1	92.1	93.6	92.5	92.6	90.6

Note: E – esterification; and T – transesterification.

(B) Kinetic Rate Constants

Rate constant for esterification processing, $k \times 10^{-2}$, lit mole^{-1} min^{-1}

Method	Molar Ratio				Catalyst concentration, w/w			
	1:2	1:3	1.4	1:5	0.5	1	2	3
Hydrodynamic [50]	0.1	1.5	1.5	1.5	0.1	1.0	1.0	1.0
Ultrasound [65]	2.5	2.9	3.0	–	1.2	2.8	–	–
Conventional [65]	0.3	1.7	1.8	–	0.2	1.8	–	–

Rate constant for transesterification processing, $k \times 10^{-1}$, lit mole^{-1} min^{-1}

Method	Molar Ratio			Catalyst concentration, w/w		
	1:4	1:6	1.8	0.5	1	1.5
Hydrodynamic [50]	1.35	4.4	4.5	0.6	4.5	4.7
Ultrasound [65]	0.9	2.1	2.2	1.1	2.2	2.2
Conventional [65]	0.4	0.9	0.9	0.4	0.9	0.9

(C) Cavitational Yield

Reactor	Cavitational yield, g/J $\times 10^{-4}$		
	Esterification	Transesterification	Total
Hydrodynamic [50]	4.8	8.7	13.5
Ultrasound [65]	0.06	0.1	0.16
Conventional [65]	0.03	0.05	0.08

(Reprinted with permission from V. L. Gole, K. R. Naveen, P. R. Gogate, Hydrodynamic cavitation as an efficient approach for intensification of synthesis of methyl esters from sustainable feedstock, Chemical Engineering and Processing. 71 (2013) 70–76. © 2013 Elsevier.)

desired temperature in the case of conventional approach, whereas no pre-treatment is required in the case of hydrodynamic cavitation as only ambient conditions are used for the reaction. Thus, the total time required for processing including the time for pretreatment (heating as applicable) for the case of conventional, ultrasound and hydrodynamic cavitation is 330, 180 and 130 min respectively, which confirms the superiority of hydrodynamic cavitation for synthesis of methyl esters. The obtained results for the kinetic rate constant also confirmed that lower rates are observed in the case of hydrodynamic cavitation as compared to the ultrasound, which again is attributed to intense cavitation generated locally due to high levels of power dissipation in the case of ultrasonic reactors. Calculations of the cavitational yield (yield of product per unit supplied energy to the system) revealed the clear picture as there is variation in the power dissipation as well as volume in different reactors establishing that results obtained only in terms of kinetic rate constants cannot be compared. The cavitational yield (considering both stages of esterification and transesterification) for hydrodynamic cavitation (13.5×10^{-4} g/J) was found to be about 85 times higher as compared to the ultrasound (1.6×10^{-5} g/J) and about 170 times higher as compared to conventional approach (8×10^{-6} g/J). The higher cavitational yield observed in the case of hydrodynamic cavitation is attributed to the fact the major contribution of energy required in preheating the oil is not present and also the actual availability of energy for generation of cavitation events is higher (higher conversion of supplied energy into cavitational energy) as compared to ultrasound. The overall production costs for the biodiesel also depend on the total energy requirement in addition to the cost of raw materials and hence this confirms that hydrodynamic cavitation will be more feasible as compared to the ultrasound-based reactor.

Gole et al. [50] also estimated the capital cost requirement for both hydrodynamic cavitation and conventional approach and reported that the capital cost requirement was about 10% higher in the case of hydrodynamic cavitation as compared to the conventional method. It is important to note that the expected savings in the energy requirements and the processing time during the actual operation should nullify the marginal increase in the capital cost.

Maddikeri et al. [42] also studied the comparison of cavitational yield obtained for hydrodynamic cavitation with the ultrasound-based approach [43] under fixed reaction condition of OMAMR of 1:12 and the catalyst loading of 1% by wt. of WCO. It was reported that though the kinetic rate constants were lower in the case of hydrodynamic cavitation, the cavitational yield (1.22×10^{-3} g/J) was significantly higher than the values obtained in the case of ultrasound based (4.76×10^{-5} g/J) and conventional approaches (3.22×10^{-5} g/J).

Chuah et al. [47] also compared the efficacy of hydrodynamic cavitation with the conventional approach based on mechanical stirring. It was reported that 98.1% conversion was obtained in the case of hydrodynamic cavitation, which was much higher than that obtained in the case of mechanical stirring (only 19%) over similar reaction time of 15 min. Estimations of cavitational yield also confirmed the superiority of hydrodynamic cavitation (12.5×10^{-4} g/J) with 8 times higher value as compared to mechanical stirring (1.5×10^{-4} g/J).

Yu et al. [19] also investigated the comparison of hydrodynamic cavitation and conventional mechanical agitation for the transesterification of rapeseed oil with erucic acid. It was reported that the conversion improved from 94% to 99% with the use of hydrodynamic cavitation at the reaction temperature of 60°C with methanol to oil ratio of 6:1 and KOH loading of 1.0%. More significantly, the reaction time reduced from 60 min to 30 min.

Overall it can be said that hydrodynamic cavitation offers greater promise as compared to the ultrasound based reactors with higher values of cavitational yields and ease of scale up. In addition to these benefits, lower requirement of molar excess and operating temperature are the advantages when compared with the conventional approach based on mechanical agitation and reflux conditions.

6.7   SCALE UP ASPECTS AND COMBINATION WITH OTHER PROCESSES

For successful synthesis of biodiesel using hydrodynamic cavitation at large scale operation, it is important to maximize the cavitational yield which means obtaining maximum product at minimum possible energy consumption. The cavitational yield is dependent on the type of cavitating device, inlet pressure and other reaction parameters such as molar ratio, catalyst loading and temperature. We now provide recommendations for optimum selection of these parameters with a focus on large-scale operations.

It is more beneficial to use a low pressure recirculating type hydrodynamic cavitation reactor consisting of a closed loop with cavitating device such as orifice and venturi. Such a reactor configuration has higher scale up potential due to ease of predictions of flow conditions downstream of the cavitating device based on the numerical simulations and available hydrodynamic simulation codes. Such information on the pressure and flow fields is useful for efficient design and operation of large scale reactors. Also the efficiency of the only energy-consuming device in the configuration (centrifugal or positive displacement pump) typically increases with an increase in the capacity, which can give a cost effective operation even at large scale. The flexibility in selection of the geometry for the cavitating device allows operating with different feedstock as the desired cavitational intensity can be generated so as to suit the requirement for the feedstock. With proper flow geometry and size of constriction or size of pipe, optimized cavitation number can be obtained to give maximum possible cavitational intensity without the onset of choked cavitating conditions. It should be noted here that use of venturi might be more beneficial especially in the case of good quality feedstock and it is recommended rather than orifice plate due to better pressure recovery profiles with generation of desired cavitational intensity. An orifice plate type device would be more beneficial in the case of operation with mixed feedstock or low quality feedstock such as animal fat or grease as the required higher cavitational intensity can be obtained just by using a different combination of holes in terms of number and diameter.

It is important to be note that an increase in the inlet pressure typically yields higher cavitational intensity and desired effects till an optimum value, which depends on the type of cavitating device. With an increase in the pressure till an optimum, cavitational yield is also increased attributed to the efficient formation of fine emulsions and beyond the optimum, marginal decrease in the yield can be obtained attributed to the formation of cavity clouds giving cushioned collapse. Thus it is important to select the optimum inlet pressure so as to give an energy efficient operation.

The reaction parameters such as molar ratio of oil to alcohol, catalyst loading and temperature must also be properly selected so as to maximize the effects at large scale operation. In general, an optimum molar ratio and catalyst loading exists which is dependent on the type of reaction (esterification, transesterification or interesterification) and the feedstock used for the synthesis. The selection of optimum is very important considering significant costs that may be involved in the downstream processing for separation. It is safe to use ambient conditions though in the case of low quality feedstock higher temperature till an optimum may be required to yield the desired degree of process intensification.

The effects obtained using hydrodynamic cavitation can be further intensified based on the combination with other methods such as ultrasound or microwave irradiation. Careful analysis of the literature reveals that combination of hydrodynamic cavitation with ultrasound has only been reported once for the biodiesel production [66]. In the combination reactor, an ultrasonic horn or an ultrasonic flow cell is typically introduced in the recirculation loop just after the cavitating device such that the cavities generated by hydrodynamic cavitation will collapse under the compression cycle of the ultrasound. Franke et al. [66] reported the use of combined hydrodynamic-acoustic cavitation (HAC) reactor for the transesterification of rapeseed oil with methanol. Effect of different parameters such as ultrasound amplitude, molar ratio of methanol to oil, catalyst loading and temperature was investigated using the design of experiments and it was established that the catalyst loading and the ultrasonic amplitude showed the highest effects. Under optimal conditions, it was reported that biodiesel yields of more than 96.5% were achieved in just 10 s of reaction time though significant time as 240 min was required for the subsequent separation to get the final product. Beneficial results for the combined approach have also been reported for other applications such as water disinfection, which is also dominated by the physical effects of cavitation [41, 67, 68]. It is recommended that more studies are required to investigate the combination of reactors in greater details before firm conclusions about the suitability for different types of raw materials especially the sustainable ones can be established.

Though no literature illustration could be obtained for the possible combination of hydrodynamic cavitation with microwave irradiations, possible credence to hypothesis of better results with the combination can be obtained based on the few available reports for combination of ultrasound and microwave. Gole and Gogate [69] investigated the synthesis of biodiesel from the high acid value Nagchampa oil using sequential effect of microwave and ultrasound in a two-step synthesis method. The study also focused on comparison of the sequential operation with individual operation of microwave and ultrasound as well as the conventional method. It was reported that the sequential method was beneficial in intensifying the conversion as well as reducing the requirement of the excess methanol, which can lead to reduction in the separation loads. The optimum molar ratio required for the first step esterification in the case of ultrasound, microwave and sequential approach were 1:4, 1:3 and 1:2, respectively, whereas for the second stage transesterification, the optimum ratio required were 1:6, 1:6 and 1:4 in the same order. The reaction time for the esterification using ultrasound alone was 60 min, which was four times higher as compared to the 15 min for the sequential approach. Similarly, for the transesterification reaction, the use of sequential operation resulted in reduction in the reaction time from 20 min in the case of only ultrasound to only 6 min in the case of combination. It can be said that the results for the combination of cavitation obtained using ultrasound are indeed promising and definitely warrants further studies for the possible combination of hydrodynamic cavitation (similar effects to ultrasound induced cavitation are obtained) and microwave in a sequential mode of operation.

6.8 CONCLUDING REMARKS

The current chapter has provided a detailed analysis into the application of hydrodynamic cavitation for intensification of biodiesel production. It has been clearly established that hydrodynamic cavitation offers advantages in terms of higher energy efficiencies, significant reduction in the reaction time, use of milder operating conditions especially temperature and also lower excess of the reactants, which can immensely help in reducing the separation load in the downstream processing. The selection of geometric (type of cavitating device and distribution of flow area) as well as operating parameters (inlet pressure, molar ratio, and catalyst loading) at optimum level, which depends on the feedstock as well as the degree of cavitational intensity decided by the cavitation chamber, decides the degree of intensification. Guidelines presented in the chapter would be helpful in designing and operating a possible large-scale reactor based on the hydrodynamic cavitation. Comparison of hydrodynamic cavitation with more commonly used ultrasonic reactors revealed that hydrodynamic cavitation offers more promise with higher cavitational yield and ease of scale up. Additional work is recommended for the exploring the application of hybrid methods such as combination of hydrodynamic cavitation and ultrasound or hydrodynamic cavitation and microwave, which can give synergistic results. Overall, it can be said that hydrodynamic cavitation is an efficient process intensification approach with proven benefits as compared to ultrasound and conventional approaches with good potential for scale up and commercial scale applications.

ACKNOWLEDGMENT

Authors would like to acknowledge the support of Department of Science and Technology under the India–Brazil Inter-Governmental Program of Cooperation in Science and Technology entitled *Intensification of Biodiesel Synthesis from Sustainable Raw Materials Using Cavitational Reactors.*

KEYWORDS

- cavitating device
- hydrodynamic cavitation
- operating parameters
- process intensification
- sustainable feedstock

REFERENCES

1. U.S. Department of Energy (DOE) by the National Renewable Energy Laboratory (NREL), a DOE national laboratory Renewable Energy: An Overview, DOE/GO-102001–1102FS175 March (2001).
2. Hall, D. O., Rosillo-Calle, F., Williams, R. H., & Woods, J. (1993). Chapter 3, Biomass for energy, supply prospectus in renewable energy, sources for fuels and electricity, edited by Johansson, T. B., Kelly, H., Reddy, A. K. N., Williams, R. H., Island Press, Washington, D C, USA. pp. 593–651.
3. Biermann, U., Friedt, W., Lang, S., Lühs, W., Machmüller, G., Metzger, J. O., Klaas, M. R., Schäfer, H. J., & Schneider, M. P. (2000). New syntheses with oils and fats as renewable raw materials for the chemical industry, *Angewandte Chemie International Edition., 39*, 2206–2224.
4. Baumann, H., Bühler, M., Fochem, H., Hirsinger, F., Zoebelein, H., & Falbe, J. (1988). Natural fats and oils—renewable raw materials for the chemical industry, *Angewandte Chemie International Edition., 27*, 41–62.
5. Tate, R., Watts, K. C., Allen, C. A., & Wilkie, K. I. (2006). The densities of three bio-diesel fuels at temperature upto $300^{0}C$, *Fuel., 7–8*, 1004–1009.
6. Enweremadu, C. C., & Mbarawa, M. M. (2009). Technical aspects of production and analysis of biodiesel from used cooking oil-A review, *Renewable and Sustainable Energy Reviews., 13*, 2205–2224.
7. Murugesan, A., Umarani, C., Chinnusamy, T. R., Krishnan, M., Subramanian, R., & Neduzchezhain, N. (2009). Production and analysis of bio-diesel from nonedible oils—A review. *Renewable and Sustainable Energy Reviews., 13*, 825–834.

8. Meher, L. C., Vidya Sagar, D., & Naik, S. N. (2006). Technical aspects of biodiesel production by transesterification—a review. *Renewable and Sustainable Energy Reviews., 10*, 248–268.

9. Koh, M. Y., & Mohd. Ghazi, T. I. (2011). A review of biodiesel production from Jatropha curcasL. oil. *Renewable and Sustainable Energy Reviews., 15*, 2240–2251.

10. Sharma, Y. C., Singh, B., & Upadhyay, S. N. (2008). Advancements in development and characterization of biodiesel: a review. *Fuel, 87*, 2355–2373.

11. Zou, L., & Atkinson, S. (2003). Characterising vehicle emissions from the burning of biodiesel made from vegetable oil. *Environmental Technology, 24*, 1253–1260.

12. Freedman, B., Butterfield, R., & Pryde, E. (1986). Transesterification kinetics of soybean oil. *Journal of the American Oil Chemists' Society, 63*, 1375–1380.

13. Noureddini, H., & Zhu, D. (1997). Kinetics of transesterification of soybean oil. *Journal of the American Oil Chemists' Society, 74*, 1457–1463.

14. Darnoko, D., & Cheryan, M. (2000). Kinetics of palm oil transesterification in a batch reactor. *Journal of the American Oil Chemists' Society, 77*, 1263–1267.

15. Antolın, G. Tinaut, F. V., Briceno, Y., Castano, V., Perez, C., & Ramılrez, A. I. (2002). Optimisation of biodiesel production by sunflower oil transesterification. *Bioresource Technology, 83*, 111–114.

16. Soumanou, M. M., & Bornscheuer, U. T. (2003). Improvement in lipase-catalyzed synthesis of fatty acid methyl esters from sunflower oil. *Enzyme and Microbial Technology, 33*, 97–103.

17. Duz, M. Z., Saydut, A., & Ozturk, G. (2011). Alkali catalyzed transesterification of safflower seed oil assisted by microwave irradiation. *Fuel Processing Technology, 92*, 308–313.

18. Cao, P., Dube, M. A., & Tremblay, A. Y. (2008). High-purity fatty acid methyl ester production from canola, soybean, palm, and yellow grease lipids by means of a membrane reactor. *Biomass and Bioenergy, 32*, 1028–1036.

19. Yu, Y., Lu, X., & Wang, Y., Ji, J. (2011). Study on transesterification of rape oil with high erucic acid to prepare biodiesel and erucicacid methyl ester by hydrodynamic cavitation, *Taiyangneng Xuebao/Acta Energiae Solaris Sinica, 32*, 1365–1369.

20. Tan, R. R., & Culaba, A. B., Purvis, M. R. I. (2004). Carbon balance implications of coconut biodiesel utilization in the Philippine automotive transport sector. *Biomass and Bioenergy, 26*, 579–585.

21. Kose, O., Tuter, M., & Aksoy, H. A. (2002). Immobilized Candida antarctica lipase-catalyzed alcoholysis of cotton seed oil in a solvent-free medium. *Bioresource Technology, 83*, 125–129.

22. Parawir, W. (2010). Biodiesel production from Jatropha curcas: A review, *Scientific Research and Essays. 5*, 1796–1808.

23. Canakci, M., & Van Gerpen, J. (2003). A pilot plant to produce biodiesel from high free fatty acid feedstocks, *American Society of Agricultural Engineers meeting paper, 46*, 945–954.

24. Canakci, M., & Van Gerpen, J. (2001). Biodiesel production from oils and fats with high free fatty acids. *American Society of Agricultural Engineers meeting paper, 44*, 1429–1436.

25. Zhang, Y., Dube, M. A., McLean, D. D., & Kates, M. (2003). Biodiesel production from waste cooking oil:2 Economic assessment and sensitivity analysis, *Bioresource Technology, 90*, 229–240.

26. Kumar, A., & Sharma, S. (2011). Potential nonedible oil resources as biodiesel feedstock: An Indian perspective, *Renewable and Sustainable Energy Reviews*, *15*, 1791–1800.

27. Azad, A. K., Rasul, M. G., Khan, M. M. K., Sharma, S. C., Mofijur, M., & Bhuiya, M. M. K. (2016). Prospects, feedstocks and challenges of biodiesel production from beauty leaf oil and castor oil: A nonedible oil sources in Australia, *Renewable and Sustainable Energy Reviews*, *61*, 302–318.

28. Pal, A., Kachhwaha, S. S., Maji, S., & Babu, M. K. G. (2010). Thumba (Citrullus colocyntis) seed oil: A sustainable source of renewable energy for biodiesel production, *Journal of Scientific and Industrial Research*, *69*, 384–389.

29. Haas, M. J., McAloon, A. J., Yee, W. C., & Foglia, T. A. (2006). A process model to costs, *Bioresource Technology*, *97*, 671–678.

30. Gogate, P. R., & Pandit, A. B. (2006). Cavitation: A technology on the horizon, *Current Science*, *91*, 35–46.

31. W. B. McNamara III, Didenko, Y. T., & Suslick, K. S. (1999). Sonoluminescence temperatures during multibubble cavitation, *Nature*, *401*, 772–775.

32. Lorimer, J. P., & Mason, T. J. (1987). Sonochemistry. Part 1 - The physical aspects, *Chemical Society Reviews*, *16*, 239–274.

33. Gogate, P. R., Shirgaonkar, I. Z., Shivkumar, M., Senthilkumar, P., Vichare, N. P., & Pandit, A. B. (2001). Cavitational reactors: efficiency analysis using a model reaction, *American Institute of Chemical Engineers Journal*, *47*, 2526–2538.

34. Gogate, P. R., & Pandit, A. B. (2000). Engineering design methods for cavitation reactors II: hydrodynamic cavitation. *American Institute of Chemical Engineers Journal*, *46*, 1641–1649.

35. Gogate, P. R. (2008). Cavitational reactors for the process intensification of chemical processing applications: a critical review, *Chemical Engineering Processing*, *47*, 515–527.

36. Shah, Y. T., Pandit, A. B., & Moholkar, V. S. (1999).*Cavitation Reactor Engineering*, Springer, USA

37. Kumar, P. S., & Pandit, A. B. (1999). Modelling Hydrodynamic Cavitation, *Chemical Engineering Technology*, *22*, 1017–1027.

38. Shirgaonkar, I. Z., Lothe, R. R., & Pandit, A. B. (1998). Comments on the mechanism of microbial cell disruption in High Pressure and High speed devices, *Biotechnology Progress*, *14*, 657–660.

39. Vichare, N. P., Gogate, P. R., & Pandit, A. B. (2000). Optimization of hydrodynamic cavitation using a model reaction, *Chemical Engineering & Technology*, *23*, 683–691.

40. Sampathkumar, K., & Moholkar, V. S. (2007). Conceptual design of a novel hydrodynamic cavitation reactor, *Chemical Engineering Science*, *62*, 2698–2711.

41. Gogate, P. R., McGuire, D., S. Mededovic Thagard, Cathey, R., Blackmon, J., & Chapas, G. (2014). Hybrid reactor based on combined cavitation and ozonation: from concept to practical reality. *Ultrasonics Sonochemistry*, *21*, 590–598.

42. Maddikeri, G. L., Gogate, P. R., & Pandit, A. B. (2014). Intensified synthesis of biodiesel using hydrodynamic cavitation reactors based on the interesterification of waste cooking oil, *Fuel*, *137*, 285–292.

43. Maddikeri, G. L., Gogate, P. R., & Pandit, A. B. (2013). Ultrasound assisted interesterification of waste cooking oil and methyl acetate for biodiesel and triacetin production. *Fuel Processing Technology*, *116*, 241–249.

44. Pal, A., & Kachhwaha, S. S. (2013). Waste cooking oil: A promising feedstock for bio-diesel production through power ultrasound and hydrodynamic cavitation. *Journal of Scientific and Industrial Research*, *72*, 387–392.

45. Rengasamy, M., Praveen Kumar, E. T., Satheesh, T., Venkadesh, D., & Kumara-guru, K. (2014). Hydrodynamic cavitation for the production of biodiesel from sun-flower oil using NaOH catalyst. *Journal of Chemical and Pharmaceutical Sciences*, *4*, 104–106.

46. Yusup, S., Bokhari, A., Chuah, L. F., & Ahmad, J. (2015). Pre-blended methyl esters production from crude palm and rubber seed oil via hydrodynamic cavitation reactor, *Chemical Engineering Transactions*, *43*, 517–522.

47. Chuah, L. F., Yusup, S., Aziz, A. R. A., Bokhari, A., Klemeš, J. J., & Abdullah, M. Z. (2015). Intensification of biodiesel synthesis from waste cooking oil (Palm Olein) in a Hydrodynamic Cavitation Reactor: Effect of operating parameters on methyl ester conversion. *Chemical Engineering Processing*, *95*, 235–240.

48. Bokhari, A., Chuah, L. F., Yusup, S., Klemeš, J. J., & Kamil, R. N. K., (2016). Optimi-sation on pretreatment of rubber seed (Hevea brasiliensis) oil via esterification reaction in a hydrodynamic cavitation reactor. *Bioresource Technology*, *199*, 414–422.

49. Chuah, L. F., Yusup, S., Aziz, A. R. A., Bokhari, A., & Abdullah, M. Z. (2016). Cleaner production of methyl ester using waste cooking oil derived from palm olein using a hydrodynamic cavitation reactor. *Journal of Cleaner Production*, *112*, 4505–4514.

50. Gole, V. L., Naveen, K. R., & Gogate, P. R. (2013). Hydrodynamic cavitation as an efficient approach for intensification of synthesis of methyl esters from sustainable feedstock, *Chemical Engineering and Processing*, *71*, 70–76.

51. Saharan, V., Badve, M. P., & Pandit, A. B. (2011). Degradation of Reactive Red 120 dye using hydrodynamic cavitation, *Chemical Engineering Journal*, *178*, 100–107.

52. Yan, Y., & Thorpe, R. B. (1990). Flow regime transitions due to cavitation in the flow through an orifice, *International Journal of Multiphase Flow*, *16*, 1023–1045.

53. Saharan, V., Pandit, A. B., Selvam, P., Kumar, S., & Anandan, S. (2012). Hydrodynamic Cavitation as an Advanced Oxidation Technique for the Degradation of Acid Red 88 Dye, *Industrial Engineering Chemistry Research*, *51*, 1981–1198.

54. Ghayal, D., Pandit, A. B., & Rathod, V. K. (2013). Optimization of biodiesel production in a hydrodynamic cavitation reactor using used frying oil, *Ultrasonics Sonochemistry*, *20,* 322–328.

55. Braeutigam, P., franke, M., Wu, Z. L., & Ondruschka, B. (2010). Role of different parameters in the optimization of hydrodynamic cavitation, *Chemical Engineering & Technology*, *33*, 932–940.

56. Mishra, K. P., & Gogate, P. R. (2010). Intensification of degradation of Rhodamine B using hydrodynamic cavitation in the presence of additives, *Separation and Purifica-tion Technology*, *75*, 385–391.

57. Patil, P. N., & Gogate, P. R. (2012). Degradation of methyl parathion using hydrody-namic cavitation: Effect of operating parameters and intensification using additives, *Separation and Purification Technology*, *95*, 172–179.

58. Kelkar, M. A., Gogate, P. R., & Pandit, A. B. (2008). Intensification of esterification of acids for synthesis of biodiesel using acoustic and hydrodynamic cavitation, *Ultrason-ics Sonochemistry*, *15*, 188–194.

59. Ji, J., Wang, J., Li, Y., Yu, Y., & Xu, Z. (2006). Preparation of biodiesel with the help of ultrasonic and hydrodynamic cavitation, *Ultrasonics*, *44*, 411–414.

60. Yun, W., Liang, Y. Y., Hong, L. X., Chao, X. Z., & Bing, J. J. (2008). Intensification of transesterification reaction by hydrodynamic cavitation technique for biodiesel preparation, *Journal of Zhejiang University of Technology*, *36*, 12–15.

61. Casas, A., Ramos, M. J., & Pérez, A. (2011). New trends in biodiesel production: chemical interesterification of sunflower oil with methyl acetate. *Biomass Bioenergy*, *35*, 1702–1709.

62. Suppalakpanya, K., Ratanawilai, S., & Tongurai, C. (2010). Production of ethyl ester from esterified crude palm oil by microwave with dry washing by bleaching earth. *Applied Energy*, *87*, 2356–2359.

63. Veljkovic, V. B., Avramovic, J. M., & Stamenkovic, O. S. (2012). Biodiesel production by ultrasound-assisted transesterification: state-of-the-art and the perspectives, Renewable and *Sustainable Energy Reviews*, *16*, 1193–1209.

64. Badday, A. S., Abdullah, A. Z., Lee, K. T., & Khayoon, M. S. (2012). Intensification of biodiesel production via ultrasonic-assisted process: a critical review on fundamentals and recent development, *Renewable and Sustainable Energy Reviews*, *16*, 4574–4587.

65. Gole, V. L., & Gogate, P. R. (2012). Intensification of synthesis of biodiesel from nonedible oils using sonochemical reactors, *Industrial Engineering Chemistry Research*, *51*, 11866–11874.

66. Franke, M., Ondruschka, B., & Braeutigam, P. (2014). Hydrodynamic-Acoustic-Cavitation for Biodiesel Synthesis. *3rd International Conference on Environment, Chemistry and Biology*, Singapore, IPCBEE vol.78, DOI: 10.7763/IPCBEE. (2014). V78.6.

67. Franke, M., Braeutigam, P., Z-Wu, L., & Ren, Y. (2011). B. Ondruschka. Enhancement of chloroform degradation by the combination of hydrodynamic and acoustic cavitation. *Ultrasonics Sonochemistry*, *18*, 888–894.

68. Braeutigam, P., Franke, M., Schneider, R. J., Lehmann, A., & Stolle, A. (2012). B. Ondruschka. Degradation of carbamazepine in environmentally relevant concentrations in water by Hydrodynamic-Acoustic. Cavitation (HAC). *Water Research*, *46*, 2469–2477.

69. Gole, V. L., & Gogate, P. R. (2013). Intensification of synthesis of biodiesel from nonedible oil using sequential combination of microwave and ultrasound. *Fuel Processing Technology*, *106*, 62–69.

CHAPTER 7

HYDROTHERMAL PROCESSES FOR BIOFUEL AND BIOENERGY PRODUCTION

M. TOUFIQ REZA

Department of Mechanical Engineering, Ohio University, Athens, OH 45701, USA

CONTENTS

ABSTRACT

Hydrothermal processes are considered as green, renewable, and sustainable for biofuel and bioenergy production. Residual moisture in biomass plays dual role both as solvent and as catalyst during hydrothermal processes. Therefore, expensive drying of wet biomass feedstock can be avoided. Thermodynamic properties of sub-and supercritical water vary substantially

---

A part of Section 7.3.1 of this chapter is adapted from M. Toufiq Reza, Janet Andert, Benjamin Wirth, Daniela Busch, Judith Pielert, Joan G. Lynam, and Jan Mumme, (2014). Hydrothermal Carbonization of Biomass for Energy and Crop Production. Applied Bioenergy, 1, 11–28.

with the increase of temperature especially above 180°C. As a result, biomass components follow separate reaction mechanisms and produce different products depending on temperature. Hydrothermal processes, in inert atmosphere, can be categorized into three major methods based on temperature or desired product. Pretreatment of biomass at temperature around 140–200°C is often used to facilitate enzymatic hydrolysis for ethanol production. Biomass pretreatment is covered extensively in the earlier sections of the book. Therefore, hydrothermal processes rather than pretreatment are discussed in this chapter. Hydrothermal carbonization (HTC) is the mildest process, where biomass is converted into carbon-rich solid fuel at temperature around 180–280°C under water saturation pressure. The process occurred above HTC temperature and below critical temperature (374°C) is known as hydrothermal liquefaction (HTL), where biocrude is the desired product. Finally, supercritical water gasification (SCWG) of biomass takes place in supercritical region of water to produce methane, synthesis gas, or hydrogen gas, depending on SCWG temperature and applied catalysts. Unlike the HTC, HTL, SCWG, where the reaction is kept under inert atmosphere to prevent oxidation, both wet air oxidation (WAO) and supercritical water oxidation (SCWO) apply excess oxygen pressure to combust feedstocks and produce heat. Both WAO and SCWO are also applied for destruction of toxic, hazardous, and organic pollutants. This chapter covers the fundamentals of HTC, HTL, SCWG, WAO, and SCWO processes based on the current knowledges. Reaction mechanism, chemistry, and kinetics are compared for these hydrothermal processes. The economic and environmental impacts of hydrothermal processes based on the current state-of-the-art knowledge are discussed in the later part of the chapter.

7.1   INTRODUCTION

Over the years, fossil fuels have been the cheapest energy source as well as the feedstock for millions of petroleum-based products. As a result, the world oil demand in 2014 was 93 million barrels per day, which has been increased more than 20% in the last decade [14]. Carbon dioxide (CO_2) emission from the petroleum usage alone was 11,830 Million Metric Tons in 2013. Alarming greenhouse gas (GHG), especially CO_2 accumulation caused the earth's temperature more than 0.85°C in the last century [15].

The global warming causes various disturbances of the world's environment as well as threats submerging several countries. As the world is accustomed with its energy consumption, the energy generation needs to be consistent. However, to save the world from the disastrous global warming and GHG accumulation, alternative energy sources are the only hope. Alternative energy, preferably renewable and sustainable energy sources e.g., solar, wind, tide, and biomass have enough potentials to mitigate the world's energy demand without causing any additional GHG emission [16]. However, the current cost for energy harvesting and transportation from alternative energy sources are much higher than fossil-based energy sources. In fact, the world's energy infrastructure is based for fossil fuels and it is reasonable to understand why alternative energy production cost is much higher compared to fossil fuel. However, the scientists over the world are developing cutting-edge alternative energy research. As a result, alternative energy is making its way into competitive energy market and the progress is very promising.

Biofuel is one of the major alternative energy sources, which is making great advance over the last decade especially in the form of ethanol. Currently, we can get a synthetic blend of 10% ethanol in every gas station in the US. The feedstock behind ethanol is biomass. Biomass is considered as renewable and sustainable energy source, as biomass has a close-carbon cycle. Biomass converts atmospheric CO_2 to O_2 while alive, and produce CO_2 when produce energy from it. One can argue the slow growth of biomass over time, however, biofuel derived from biomass especially short rotation coppices and energy crops are proved as net negative GHG emission source. Moreover, more than a billion ton of biomass is available in the US for biofuel production [16]. Effective use of biomass can potentially replace a big part fossil fuel. However, inefficient biofuel conversion technology is still incompatible with fossil fuel price. As a result, biofuel has been upgrading into third generation. Food versus fuel was another major concern that drives first generation corn ethanol fuels to third generation algae-derived biofuel.

Environmental and social issues are the other triggers for biomass utilization, which can boost clean environment and social well-being of less developed areas. Certain advantages in using biomass as an alternative energy include: (i) CO_2-free substitute of fossil fuel, (ii) SO_X and NO_X trimmer, and (iii) biodiversity and social prospects. Plants consume carbon dioxide during photosynthesis, which helps to reduce greenhouse gasses (GHG CO_2 emissions on g/KWh electricity generation bases are the lowest in case of biomass

(17–27) compared to coal (955), oil (818) and gas (446) [17]. With improved biomass utilization technology in future, biomass is expected to emit only 15–18 g/KWh of CO_2 supporting its CO_2 neutral nature [17]. However, by maintaining a balance between biomass production and its utilization, it is possible to achieve almost zero GHG emissions [16].

Biomass is an organic substance mainly composed of carbon, hydrogen, nitrogen, oxygen, and trace metals. Chemically, biomass consists of hemi-celluloses, cellulose, lignin, extractives (e.g., starch, lipids, and proteins), and ash. Examples of biomass include trees, algae, corn, wheat, rye straw, grass, vegetable wastes, plant-based waste, urban waste and agro-industrial waste. Due to moderate carbon content (~30–50% dry basis), biomass has a high utilization potential among renewable energy resources. Biomass has always been a major source of energy for mankind; it still accounts for 10–14% of worldwide energy demand [14]. There are two routes of energy production from biomass, namely dry and wet routes. In the dry route for energy production from biomass, direct combustion in order to obtain heat or power is the most common and primitive yet the most inefficient way. Direct combustion also produces harmful chemicals like particulates (e.g., PM 2.5), polycyclic aromatic hydrocarbons (PAHs), and dioxins, which can contribute to air pollution significantly [18–19]. Biomass can also be gasified (CO and H_2) to generate liquid fuel via Fisher-Tropsch process or to combust in an internal combustion engine (ICE) for power production. Gasification is somewhat better than combustion in terms of energy efficiency and PAH emissions, however, additional reaction unit makes this a more capital cost intensive process. For instance, the liquid fuel produced from biomass via Fisher-Tropsch is several times more expensive than fossil-based liquid fuel (gasoline). Biomass can also be pyrolyzed under inert atmosphere (He, N_2, or Ar) to produce solid fuel, often called biochar, which is also considered for soil amendment and carbon sequestration [20, 21]. Fast pyrolysis also produces liquid biocrude, which can be upgraded to liquid fuel [22, 23]. Now, all the dry route conversion technologies require relatively dry (max. 15% moisture) or bone-dry feedstock. Unfortunately, biomass usually found in "wet" form, where moisture content may vary from 50–95%. Drying biomass feedstock prior to thermochemical processing is energy intensive, therefore, it often limits the application of wet biomass to energy production.

In contrary to dry route, biomass can be converted to biofuel without drying in wet route. Wet route consists of biochemical and hydrother-mal processing. Biochemical processing includes anaerobic digestion to produce biogas (CH_4-rich) and enzymatic hydrolysis to produce ethanol. Transesterification of microalgae-derived lipids to produce biodiesel is also considered as wet route [24]. Hydrothermal treatments of biomass are similar to dry thermochemical treatment except water in this case used as reaction medium [25]. Based on the oxygen content in the reaction medium, hydrothermal processes can be divided into carbonization and oxidation. Carbonization processes include hydrothermal carbonization (HTC), hydrothermal liquefaction (HTL), and supercritical water gasification (SCWG), where reactions are maintained in inert atmosphere. Meanwhile, oxidation processes include wet air oxidation (WAO) and supercritical water oxidation (SCWO), where excess oxygen or air is added during the processes [26]. The main advantage of hydrothermal treatments over the other biofuel production technologies is the usage of wet biomass as feedstock. The processes do not require preprocessing and many of the processes can take heterogeneous biomass feedstock and produce homogeneous fuel intermediates or fuel. The only downside of the hydrothermal treatments is the presence of high pressure. The reactor pressure should be maintained at least equal to the vapor pressure to ensure the water in its liquid form. As a result, the reaction pressure increases significantly with reaction temperature. Continuous process design, therefore, becomes complicated and the capital cost of the hydrothermal processes is often higher than dry route processes.

For water, the critical point is at 374°C and 22.1 MPa. Subcritical water is classified below the critical point at a 100–374°C temperature range and under sufficient pressure to remain liquid-phase. Supercritical water occurs when the temperature is above 374°C and the pressure is above 22.1 MPa. Subcritical and supercritical water have several advantages because of their unique thermodynamic properties. Solvent properties of water can be changed as a function of temperature and pressure. Near the critical point, the ionic product of water is much higher than that of room temperature. Therefore, water can be an effective medium for acid–base-catalyzed organic reactions under subcritical conditions. Meanwhile, viscosity of water decreases significantly with the increase of temperature and has a value close to the viscosity of water vapor near the critical point. A low viscosity provides a high diffusion coefficient, leading to high reaction rates. In addition, water at high temperatures can also behave as a reactant in the hydrothermal reaction medium. Under hydrothermal conditions, water molecules may participate in hydrolysis reactions and can act as a hydrogen source.

Hydrothermal processes between 100–374°C at their saturation pressure or above are known as subcritical hydrothermal processes. Meanwhile, hydrothermal processes above 374°C at or above the saturation pressures are known as supercritical hydrothermal processes. SCWG and SCWO are considered as supercritical hydrothermal processes. As shown in Figure 7.1, reaction temperature plays significant role for specific biofuel product. For example, with no supply of oxygen, biomass undergoes for HTC around 180–280°C, where volatile organic fraction is released and solid product is carbonized with time. In most cases, solid HTC product, also known as hydrochar, has similar fuel properties as lignite to bituminous coal. The fuel properties depend preliminary on HTC temperature, pressure, reaction time, and feedstock. At higher hydrothermal temperature than HTC, formation of carbon-rich mostly hydrophobic biocrude occurs during HTL. Like HTC, HTL depends on reaction time, temperature, and feedstock as well as catalyst

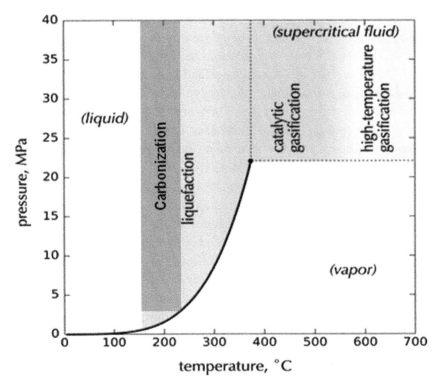

FIGURE 7.1 Overview of different hydrothermal biomass conversion processes and the vapor pressure curve of water. Reprinted with the permission from Ref. [1].

and extracting solvents. Supercritical water behaves like gas but has density similar to liquid. As a result, the reactivity of supercritical water increases significantly. Supercritical water can convert biomass components into gaseous product like CH_4, H_2, CO, and/or CH_4 depending of catalyst, reaction condition, and feedstock properties. Therefore, the main product of SCWG is gaseous fuel either CH_4 or H_2-rich gas. One of the major advantages SCWG is product separation compare to HTC and HTL. The application of hydrothermal gasification to biomass with a moisture content of at least 30% under supercritical conditions requires less energy than that required for pre-drying the same biomass [27]. Therefore, it is an appropriate process for utilization of biomass wastes with high moisture content that are generated by the agriculture and food industries. The disadvantage is the need for extremely high pressure as well as the corrosiveness of water. Often SCWG reaction vessel are made of corrosion resistant alloys like Hastalloy-C or Inconel, in which case the reactor material cost increases significantly than reactor made of carbon steel.

Other hydrothermal technologies, where oxygen is fed into the reactor during the reaction stage are mainly for hydrothermal degradation of organics or production of heat directly from the reactor. WAO as well as SCWO are similar to incineration except the reaction medium is compressed hot sub-or supercritical water. Supplying oxygen or air in the hydrothermal reactor is the main challenge. Also, mass transfer effect plays a significant role as well. Therefore, applications for these oxidation processes are limited to hazardous waste disposal rather than focusing on heat optimization.

Figure 7.2 is another way to interpret the hydrothermal processes especially HTC, HTL, and SCGW. Above the boiling point, biomass experiences hydrolysis predominantly under subcritical water. This results the cleavage of hydrogen bonds among starch, hemicellulose, and even cellulose. The degraded products then undergo for dehydration followed by hydrogenation. If the hydrothermal temperature is high enough, dehydrated biomass-derived components contribute to aqueous-phase reforming, where biocrude starts to form. Bio-crude is a hydrophobic organic liquid with a reduced oxygen content and a high-energy density [28]. It may contain hundreds of compounds depending on the nature of the raw material and experimental conditions. This bio-crude can replace heavy petroleum oil and can directly be used as fuel for co-firing with coal or converted into high-quality distillate fuels, such as diesel and gasoline. Hydrocarbons with high oxygen contents have lower energy contents, higher melting points, higher boiling points, and

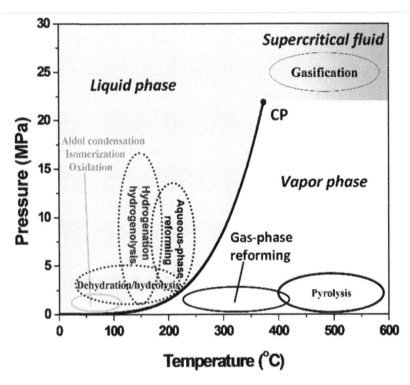

FIGURE 7.2 Phase diagram for water indicating the temperature and pressure regimes for reactions of interest in the conversion of biomass derived molecules. *Note*: CP is critical point. Reprinted with the permission from Ref. [10].

greater viscosities than other hydrocarbons with the same molecular weight. Therefore, the oxygen content of bio-oils is reduced by decarboxylation and hydrodeoxygenation reactions to improve the quality of the fuel [29]. It is also feasible to obtain valuable chemicals from bio-oils by various purification and separation methods. Aqueous phase reforming continues until critical point. Beyond that biomass components as well as intermediate products experience gasification, depending on the type of catalyst use.

7.2 PROPERTIES OF WATER

Water, the universal solvent, is a polar solvent at ambient condition, which is capable to dissolve salts, sugar, acids, and bases. Water at ambient temperature and pressure is a very weak solvent for the non-polar solutes like oil, grease, and hydrocarbons [30]. However, liquid water at higher temperatures than boiling point, i.e., subcritical and supercritical water has completely different properties than water at room temperature. Sub- and supercritical water are more reactive as they behave like mild acid and base at the same time [30]. The solvent properties of sub and supercritical water shifts from polar to nonpolar solvent. As a result, hot pressurized liquid water is capable of dissolving oils, grease, and hydrocarbons (see Figure 7.3). The main benefit for using water medium is with the release of pressure or decrease of temperature shifts the properties of water into benign (polar) again, which first, enhances the separation, second, eases of regeneration of water, third, collects and stores water, and fourth, is harmless for the environment at ambient condition. That's why water is considered as green solvent and processes using water as solvent or reaction medium are green processes.

$$2H_2O(l) \leftrightarrow H_3O^+(aq) + OH^-(aq) \tag{1}$$

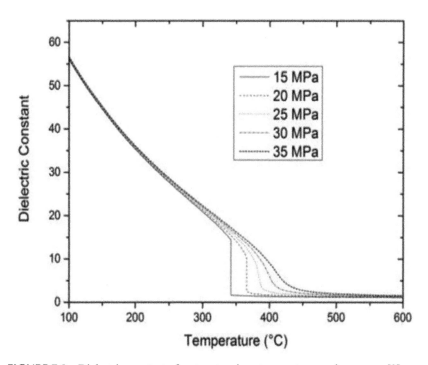

FIGURE 7.3   Dielectric constant of water at various temperatures and pressures [9]

$$K_w = \left[H_3O^+\right]\left[OH^-\right] \qquad (2)$$

$$pK_w = pH + pOH \qquad (3)$$

When water is heated up under pressure, density decreases with temperature as shown in Figures 7.4 and 7.6. Because of the increase of thermal movement of water molecules, interference between water molecules becomes weaker. This leads to weaker hydrogen bonds, although clusters by hydrogen bonds still exist at high temperature. Notably, density decrease is severe just below critical point [31]. The decrease of density affects other thermodynamics properties of water like dielectric constant. Dielectric constant is the indicator of nonpolarity of a solvent. The lower the dielectric constant, the stronger nonpolar solvent it becomes. Dielectric constant often influences solubility and chemical reactions. In this case, an intermediate

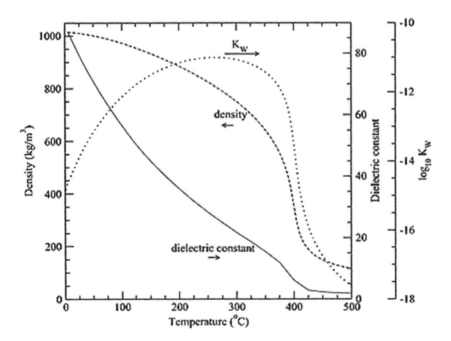

FIGURE 7.4 Properties (density, ionic product and relative static dielectric constant) of water as function of temperature at 25 MPa. Adapted from Ref. [1].

state of chemical species during a certain reaction has higher polarity. The macroscopic dielectric constant or a local dielectic constant created by the solvent effects is different at elevated temperature and pressure. As shown in the Figure 7.3, Solvent shells around organic compounds influence organic reactions in supercritical water. Concerning the influence on chemical reactions, it is experimentally very difficult to distinguish which property of water is relevant, because they all change with densities and temperatures [4, 32, 33]. Overall, water is very reactive at elevated temperature and pressure. This influences solubility and the stability of ions makes the environmentally benign water at room temperature into a nonpolar solvent.

Besides density and dielectric constant, subcritical water also behaves as a weak acid and base simultaneously. Therefore, the ionic product (as shown in Eqs. 1–3) is higher at subcritical conditions as shown in the Figure 7.5. In contrary, the low density of water at supercritical condition leads to breakdown of the solvent shell and the ionic product decreases drastically at low densities. At supercritical conditions at, e.g., 550°C and 20 MPa, water behaves as a nonpolar organic solvent like pentane with good solubility for organic components and gases and low solubility for salts [2,

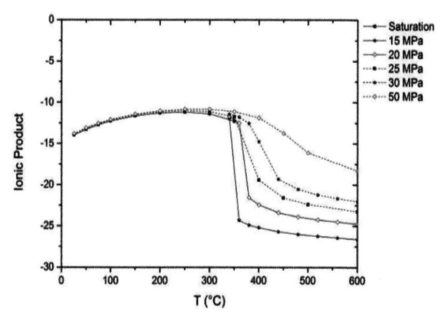

FIGURE 7.5 Ionic product of water at various temperatures and pressures [19].

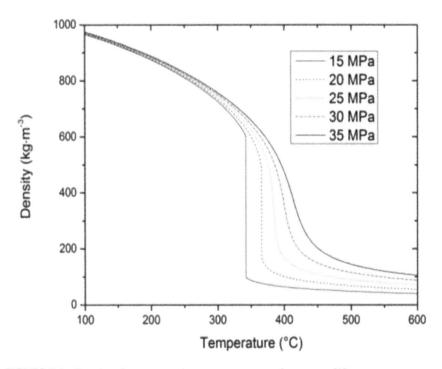

FIGURE 7.6   Density of water at various temperatures and pressures [9].

11]. However, the single water molecules are still polar. In the presence of a polar compounds or ions, water molecules in its nearer environment are attracted (Figure 7.7). The attraction is stronger for higher multivalent cations and the strong interaction to the oxygen atom leads to an elimination of H^+ and a strong acidic behavior. In contrary, the hydrogen atom comes closer to the monovalent anion than the oxygen of the water molecule in the solvent shell to a cation. This leads to the observation that salts, which are usually neutral like NaCl become basic by formation of HCl. Solubilities of various salts in sub-and supercritical water are shown in Figure 7.8 Self-dissociation of water molecule as well as the formation of H^+ and OH^- is influenced by the strong clustering effect [34]. This leads to a high "local concentration" of H^+ and OH^- ions accelerating, e.g., the Beckmann and Pincol-Pinacolone rearrangement, and monoterpene alcohol synthesis as well as the Cannizzaro and Heck reaction, especially slightly above or very close to the critical point of water [2, 35]. Here, the H^+ and OH^- ions can move very fast inside one cluster leading to a high reactivity slightly above

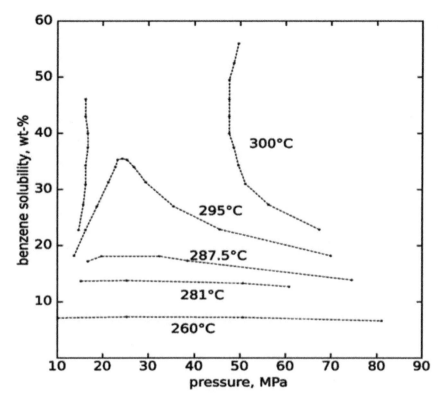

FIGURE 7.7 Benzene solubility in high-pressure water. Reprinted with permission from Ref. [1]. Note that at 300°C and above, the phases become completely miscible between 17 and 47 MPa. Reprinted with the permission from Ref. [1]

the critical temperature, although the total concentration is lower than in subcritical water.

7.3 HYDROTHERMAL PROCESSES

7.3.1 HYDROTHERMAL CARBONIZATION

Biomass naturally transforms into coal or peat underground but the process takes from hundreds (peat) to millions (anthracite) of years. Presumably, wet biomass treated under geothermal conditions of high pressure and temperature converts to coal. HTC, also known as hydrothermal pretreatment or wet torrefaction, is a thermo-chemical conversion technique that uses

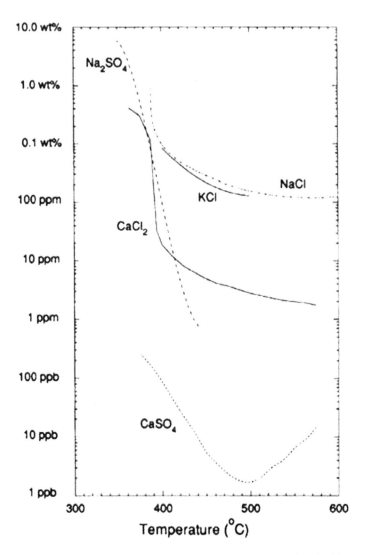

FIGURE 7.8 The solubility of limits of various salts at 25 MPa. Reprinted with permission from Ref. [1].

subcritical liquid water as a reaction medium for conversion of wet biomass and waste streams into a valuable carbon-rich solid product [36, 37]. It is usually performed at temperatures ranging from 180–260°C, at pressures slightly higher than water saturation pressure to ensure water is in a liquid state, and under an inert atmosphere. Reaction time has been reported to be

1 min to several hours, although most of the reaction seems to occur within the first 20 min [3, 38, 39]. Higher heating value (HHV) of solid hydrochar is reported as high as 27–30 MJ kg^{-1}, whereas the HHV of raw feedstock is around 15–19 MJ kg^{-1} [3, 36, 40–43]. Additives, such as acids or bases, can affect the products formed [44]. Wet biomass and water may be used in this process.

During hydrothermal pretreatment, hemicelluloses and cellulose are hydrolyzed to oligomers and monomers [45], while lignin is mostly unaffected. The solid product, hydrochar, also known as HTC biochar, has reduced equilibrium moisture content, so it is less likely to deteriorate in storage [46]. The pretreated solid is quite friable and can be made into pellets that could be fed to a gasifier or coal power plant. The other uses of HTC products are for the production of liquid fuel or bio-oil; carbon sequestration; carbon material that could be either activated to work as a low cost adsorbent or permeable reactive barrier for uranium(VI); copper and cadmium contaminated waters; nanostructured carbon catalyst, which could be used in the production of fine chemicals; and lastly, a carbon material that could increase a fuel cell's efficiency [3, 47–56]. The liquid products can also be further fractionated by means of extraction with polar organic solvent(s), or anaerobic digestion [57–59]. Another recent development of the HTC process is the use of hydrochar for soil amendment [37]. When it is added to soil, the carbon content of the soil can be significantly increased and it remains in the soil for a prolonged time period. Hydrochar has very high meso- and micro porous surface area and the nano-sized spherical carbon structure promotes water encapsulation [26, 54–55, 60–64]. The water-holding capacity of hydrochar is thus much higher than that of regular soil [60], so that the fertility of sandy soils might be improved with the introduction of hydrochar [65]. Moreover, its porous structures along with its sorption capacity promote microbial colony growth in the hydrochar, which becomes a nutrient storage space.

Hydrolysis is the first step of the HTC reaction, where water reacts with extractives, hemicellulose, or cellulose and breaks ester and ether bonds (mainly β-(1-4) glycosidic bonds), resulting in a wide range of products including soluble oligomers like (oligo-) saccharides from cellulose, and hemicellulose as shown in Figure 7.9 [3]. Hemicellulose starts hydrolyzing at HTC temperatures above 200°C, but cellulose hydrolysis starts above 220°C [66–71]. Cellulose can degrade into oligomers, a portion of which hydrolyzes into glucose and fructose. Other components like extractives,

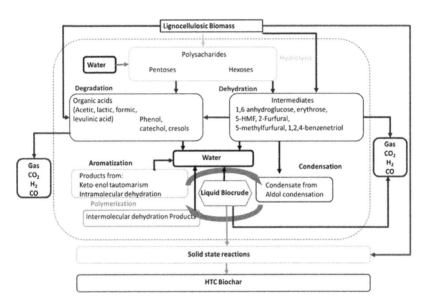

FIGURE 7.9   HTC reaction pathways for lignocellulosic biomass. Note: Liquid biocrude is a complex liquid solution of condensation, aromatization [3].

which are monomeric sugars (mainly glucose and fructose) along with various alditols, aliphatic acids, oligomeric sugars, and phenolic glycosides, are very reactive in hydrothermal media [72, 73]. A very small portion of lignin reacts at higher HTC temperature (260°C) and releases phenol and phenolic derivatives. Inorganic components are very stable and probably remain unchanged by HTC at 200–260°C, however, the degradation of polymeric components might release inorganics from the solid structure to liquid [72, 73]. Dehydration and decarboxylation of hydrolyzed products likely take place immediately after hydrolysis [39, 45]. Reduction of carboxyl groups, mainly from extractives, hemicellulose, and cellulose could be the main reason for the significant decrease in oxygen content. Dehydration and decarboxylation happen simultaneously. Under hydrothermal conditions, hydrolyzed products degrade into furfurals like 5-HMF, erythrose, and aldehydes, of which furfural and corresponding derivatives are further dehydrated and decarboxylated into H_2O and CO_2, respectively [29, 32]. For instance, each mole of 5-HMF production from glucose yields two moles of water. Moreover, the polymerization of hydrolyzed intermediates can yield water, too. For example, the retro-condensation of 5-HMF into aldol condensation or keto-enol condensation of n monomers yields n moles of water. Most of the intermediate compounds (5-HMF, anhydroglucose, furfural, erythrose, 5-methyl furfural) produced from dehydration and decarboxylation reactions of monomers undergo condensation, polymerization, and aromatization. The products of these simultaneous condensation, polymerization, and aromatization are called bio-crude. The liquid biocrude, after successive polymerization and aromatization, converts into solid product with or without auto-nucleation, as shown in Figure 7.10.

Hydrochar, is the desired product from HTC. Hydrochar can be produced from a liquid-liquid (liquid biocrude), a liquid-solid (resulting from a liquid biocrude and solid lignin residue), or even a solid-solid reaction. Hydrochar is a cross-linked polymer, and has similar acid digestion properties as lignin,

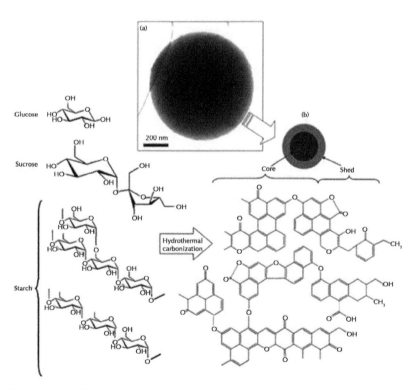

FIGURE 7.10 (a) TEM image of a starch-based hydrochar microsphere, and (b) schematic illustration of the hydrophobic/hydrophilic core–shell chemical structure of the hydrochar microspheres resulting from the hydrothermal carbonization of saccharides [13].

so that the hydrochar is almost impossible to distinguish from unreacted lignin fraction. Thus, a linear polymer like cellulose can convert into a cross-linked polymer similar to lignin. HTC reactions in the liquid state make it unique among thermochemical conversion processes of biomass. The reaction chemistry of liquid state HTC reactions will determine the usage of HTC process streams. Reza et al. (2013) reported that the mass yield of hydrochar becomes steady after only 1 min at 260°C [44]. Other researchers use HTC reaction times of more than 6 h under otherwise similar reaction conditions [37, 60, 63, 65, 69, 74–75]. Possibly, lignin degradation and hydrochar formation rates are similar after 1 min for HTC at 260°C, so that the mass yield is constant. Condensation reactions of monosaccharides are slower, since cross-linked polymerization competes with recondensation to oligosaccharides. Condensation polymerization is most likely governed by step-growth polymerization, which is enhanced by higher temperatures and reaction times. Moreover, condensing fragments within the biomass matrix are able to 'block' remaining biomacromolecules, preventing water access and subsequent hydrolysis, a phenomenon that makes the remaining hydrochar hydrophobic [63]. Condensation precursors are reported to be toxic substances for soil usage, requiring an extended reaction time to ensure degradation of these reactive intermediates. Thus, optimum HTC reaction conditions must be based on the end use of HTC products.

Reaction temperature and time are undoubtedly the main process parameters for HTC. However, the type of biomass can also affect HTC products. These products vary depending on feedstock even when the reaction time and temperature are similar. However, agricultural residues perform more similarly to grassy biomass than woody biomass when undergoing HTC. Their sensitivity to small reaction temperature changes is noteworthy. Mass yields for these biomass tend to be lower, particularly at higher reaction temperatures. Agricultural biomass are also similar to grassy biomass in that both have higher ash (inorganic) content than woody biomass. Overall, softwoods give results for HTC similar to hardwoods, except that softwood lignin is more resistant to hydrolysis. HTC hydrolyzes the hemicellulose out of both types of woody biomass at temperatures near 180°C and hydrolyzes cellulose at higher temperatures. To remove substantial amounts of lignin requires even higher temperatures.

HTC has been performed in large pilot scale in Switzerland, Germany, France, and Japan. Several start-up companies like AVA-CO$_2$, TerraNova, SmartCarbon etc. as well as large companies like Mitsubishi Heavy Industries performed HTC. Most of the cases, the HTC temperature was maintained below 220°C and waste biomass (e.g., sewage sludge, manure, and municipal solid wastes) are preferable for large scale HTC. Up until now, almost all HTC has been performed aiming to produce solid fuel, although a very few researchers attempted to produce energy either direct combustion or via gasification [76–83]. Main hurdles for HTC as solid fuel production include low and stable price of coal, lack of HTC process development, high pressure and high temperature process, and use or disposal of HTC process liquid. As a result, HTC research is remaining in the laboratory, where scientists are now focusing on value-added applications of hydrochar such as energy storage, solid adsorbent, nutrient recovery, and soil amendment.

7.3.2 HYDROTHERMAL LIQUEFACTION

HTL is very similar to HTC in terms of reaction medium and reactions, except HTL takes place at higher temperature (>260°C) than HTC. HTL temperature can be as high as the critical point of the water. During HTL of biomass, a nonpolar oil phase, often called biooil or biocrude, a polar aqueous based organic, and a gaseous phase with predominantly CO_2 are formed. Biooil is the desirable product of HTL, which can be further upgraded to drop-in liquid fuel (jet fuel or biodiesel). Usually, biooil yield is around 10–25% of the total dry biomass, while rest of it becomes gas (5–20%), polar organic substances (10–30%), and solid char (20–50%). Presence of catalyst often higher yields, although regeneration of catalysts is often challenging. Biooil contains nitrogen and sulfur depending on the biomass feedstock. Heating value of biooil is in the range of 30–37 MJ/kg. The heating value is not as high as gasoline (30–42 MJ/kg). One of the main reasons is the presence of oxygen (10–20%). High oxygen content is not only reducing the heating value bit also contributes towards corrosive properties and thermal instability. Therefore, the quality of biooil is usually improved by hydrodeoxygenation and thermal catalysis.

Overall HTL reaction chemistry is complex as discussed in the HTC. As the severity increases with the higher reaction temperature, the reaction does not yield the solid macromolecules, instead transformation into crude oil-like products. Although biomass contains lignin, cellulose, hemicellulose, carbohydrates, proteins, and fats, which are reported HTL reactions individually, the overall HTL reaction kinetics and mechanism are different for biomass feedstocks. In general, the decomposition of biomass compo-nents in subcritical water conditions yield different products, but degrada-tion mechanisms comprise the following steps [84–86]: (i) Hydrolysis or depolymerization of the biomass; (ii) degradation of hydrolyzed products via cleavage, dehydration, and decarboxylation; and (iii) condensation, polymerization, isomerization, and recombination of fragmented com-ponents. Macromolecules in the structure of biomass first dissociate into water-soluble oligomers and monomers by hydrolysis. The monomers and oligomers may also undergo further degradation, repolymerization or have their functional groups reduced [17, 87–89]. As shown in Figure 7.11, water at subcritical conditions breaks down the β-1-4 glycosidic hydrogen bonded structure and causes the formation of glucose monomers. As a result of the decomposition of cellulose, glucose and other oligomers of cellulose may form. Some of these oligomers may be further hydrolyzed and converted into glucose. The hydrolysis of glucose takes place very quickly (within sec-onds) in hydrothermal media, and depending on the conditions, a wide range

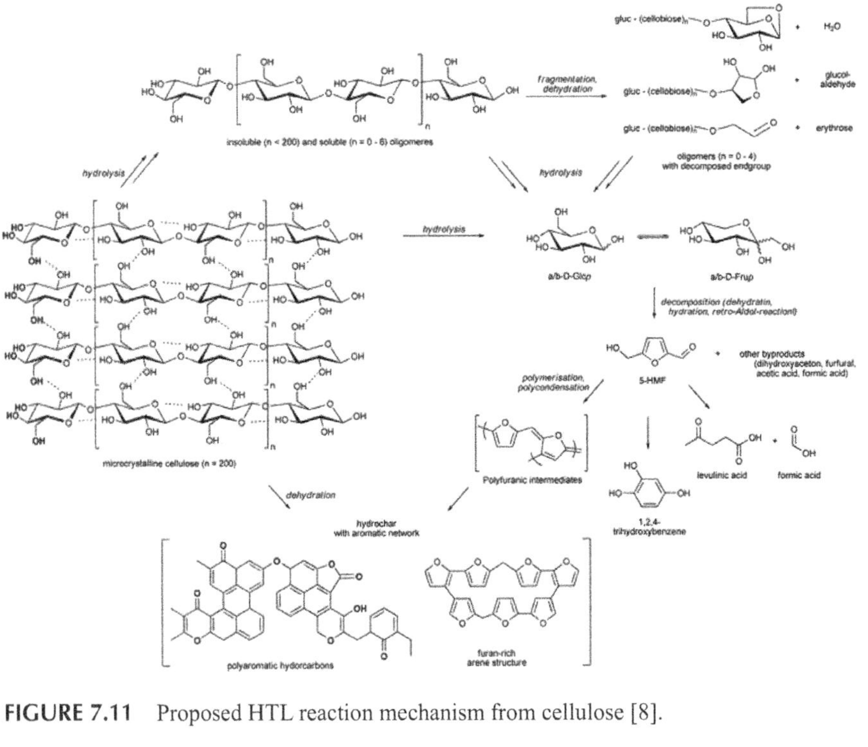

FIGURE 7.11   Proposed HTL reaction mechanism from cellulose [8].

of products, including acetic acid, acetaldehyde, glyceraldehyde, glycolaldehyde, and furfural derivatives, can be formed [8].

Hemicellulose consists of a wide range of sugar monomers, such as xylose, mannose, glucose, and galactose, and may also have side chains. Due to its complex nature, hemicellulose does not have the same crystal structure and resistance as cellulose. It is therefore more conducive to hydrolysis, and can readily dissolve in water at 180°C and higher temperatures [44]. Xylose from hemicellulose is found in water as a pyranose ring, a furanose ring or an open chain structure [1]. Furfural may form from the pyranose ring state of xylose, whereas compounds such as glyceraldehyde, pyruvaldehyde, formic acid, lactic acid and acetol may form from its open chain structure [3]. Lignin, which is another component contained in the structure of the lignocellulosic materials, has a much more irregular structure and higher molecular weight than hemicellulose.

HTL reaction pathway for lignin as feedstock is shown in Figure 7.12. As the density of water decreases and ionic product increases in a hydrothermal environment, hydrolysis of lignin increases, causing an increase in decomposition of lignin to its low molecular weight components [6]. Usually phenolic compounds form as a result of the hydrothermal degradation of lignin [90]. However, degradation of lignin only occurs at temperature more than 260°C when water molecules become involved in chemical reactions [91,

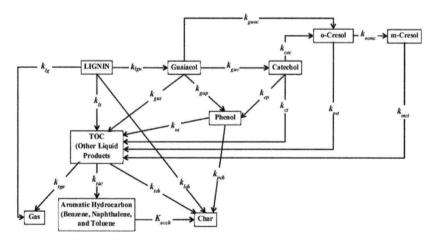

FIGURE 7.12 Lignin conversion and guaiacol reaction mechanism in supercritical water at temperatures between 390 and 450°C as proposed by Yong and Matsumura [35].

92]. Though most of the compounds within lignin, including benzyl aryl ethers, benzonitriles, pyridine carbonitriles, benzamides, and cyclohexyl phenyl compounds remain in the crosslinked structure of lignin below 260°C, the cleavage occurs after that the compounds react at the subrcritical medium. Often, they react with the cellulose, hemicellulose, and carbohydrate derived intermediates to form condensation and polymerization products, which eventually forms a bio-oil. Degradation of lignin is the main key factor that separates HTL from HTC and SCWG. In fact, a major portion of bio-oil contains phenolic compounds, which is derived from lignin.

Besides temperature, various other factors, such as pressure, reaction time, biomass type, size of biomass particles, use of catalyst, and reaction medium, influence the yield and composition of resulting bio-oils [93]. In general, there is an increase in bio-oil yield up to approximately 300–350°C; the gaseous product yield increases at higher temperatures (i.e., >350°C) [94–97]. Although bio-oils from HTL have lower oxygen contents, they cannot be used directly as a fuel for transportation [98]. For a fuel to be used in transportation, it needs to have additional physical characteristics, includes high-energy content, high boiling point and auto-ignition point, low freezing point, a good combustibility, and the ability to conveniently store in an effective manner [28, 99–101]. The oxygen content of biomass is 40–60%, which reduced to 5–10% in the bio-oil, however, still oxygen content is still quite high compare to high-quality liquid fuel (<1%) [100]. A significant amount of biomass oxygen is removed by dehydration or decarboxylation reactions [6]. Though there is excess water in the reaction medium, dehydration reactions usually occur in hydrothermal media at high temperatures and pressures. Decarboxylation reactions also remove biomass oxygen as CO_2, which is an exothermic reaction. Therefore, some heat is added towards the overall HTL reaction energy balance. A higher CO_2 production may produce enough heat to make the HTL autothermal, however, the higher CO_2 also reduce the carbon content from the bio-oil, which is more favorable in HTL [24, 102–103]. Therefore, HTL usually considered as slightly endothermic reaction and the reaction temperature is kept under 350°C so that less gaseous product formed. Bio-oils obtained as a result of a hydrothermal process can be improved and used instead of gasoline or diesel. Improvement procedures for obtaining high-quality liquid fuels from bio-oils can be conducted by physical (i.e., separation, extraction or solvent addition), chemical or catalytic means [28, 84, 104–107]. Hydrodeoxygenation is the major bio-oil improvement method and is conducted at 300–600°C under high pressure

H_2 in the presence of a heterogeneous catalyst [108]. During hydrodeoxygenation, oxygen in the bio-oil reacts with H_2 to form water and saturated C–C bonds. In this manner, the energy content and the stability of the fuel is significantly increased [109].

In recent years, microalgae have received increasing attention and HTL might be a promising process for conversion to a liquid energy carrier. In general, algae are relatively rich in protein and/or lipids. In contrary to transesterification using NaOH or KOH base to recover lipids from algae, HTL offers more bio-oil yield as both proteins and lipids as well as carbohydrates contribute to HTL reaction. The maximum bio-oil yield is reported around 25–35% of the whole dry algae, which depends heavily on the choice of solvent and bio-oil extraction procedure [110–113]. Both Na_2CO_3 and K_2CO_3 were proved to be effective catalysts for HTL of microalgae due to the carbonic acid concentration of HTL, which shifts the HTL reaction towards more bio-oil routes than charring. The produced oil from all microalgae was found to have high heating values (HHVs) of approximately 22.8–36.9 MJ/kg. The elementary composition depended on catalyst and algae type, but a typical composition was C: 70–75%, H: 5–11%, N: 3–7%, O: 8–19% and S: 0–1%. Elliott et al. at the Pacific North-west National Laboratory (PNNL) performed a detailed technoeconomic analysis of HTL of microalgae and subsequent bio-oil upgrading [28, 99–101]. However, the current HTL technology is still facing challenge to reduce the U.S. Department of Energy (US DoE) target biofuel cost of $3/gallon gasoline equivalent [28]. The current price of the gasoline price as well as the availability of shale natural gas and no carbon credit may hinder the development of HTL technology even more in the upcoming years.

7.3.3 SUPERCRITICAL WATER GASIFICATION

Supercritical water gasification (SCWG) process is similar to HTC and HTL, except the treatment temperature is above critical temperature of water (>374°C). Whereas, HTC and HTL produce main products as solid or liquid fuels, SCWG disintegrates biomass into gaseous fuels, predominantly as synthesis gas (CO + H_2) or methane (CH_4) depending on catalyst type and process conditions. Unlike thermal gasification with limited oxygen supply into a dry biomass bed, SCWG uses supercritical water as reaction medium for gasification. The main advantage of SCWG is the application of wet feedstock without any drying. Therefore, SCWG is fairly common for gasification of wet wastes including biomass, municipal waste, digestate, and wastewater sludge [11, 114, 115]. SCWG process, introduced late 1970s, SCWG sees very little processing and reactor modeling and design [116–118]. Unlike thermal gasification options, SCWG can be designed as an exothermal process, which positively addresses high-moisture wet biomass [11, 119]. Because of unique thermodynamic properties of supercritical water as described in earlier section, supercritical water disintegrates wet biomass and organic aqueous wastes rapidly and produces H_2 and Cl_2 rich gases. Application of acid catalyst shifts the production of gas towards CH_4. Likewise, application of basic or novel catalyst shifts the reaction towards synthesis gas ($CO+H_2$) or hydrogen at higher SCWG temperature (>550°C). The assumed expected reaction kinetics using glucose as a model compound are represented by the equations (9.4 and 9.5) listed below [120, 121]:

Theoretically:

$$C_6H_{12}O_6 + 6H_2O \leftrightarrow 6CO_2 + 6H_2 \quad \Delta H = 158 \; kj \; mol^{-1} \quad\quad (4)$$

Experimentally:

$$2C_6H_{12}O_6 + 10H_2O \leftrightarrow 11CO_2 + CH_4 + 20H_2 \quad \Delta H = 152 \; kj \; mol^{-1} \quad (5)$$

Theoretically, if glucose is fully converted into CO_2 and H_2, 158 kJ mol^{-1} energy will be produced, however during SCWG, partial carboxylation occurs with 152 158 kJ mol^{-1} along with H_2 and CH_4. Gaseous fuel composition under both catalytic and noncatalytic conditions approximate values of H_2: 40%–60%, CO_2: 30%–70%, CH_4: 15%–25%, and CO: 5%–30%, with noncatalytic conditions favoring CO production over CH_4[115]. Synthesis gas (H_2 and CO), the same desired product as of thermal gasification, can be converted to drop in liquid hydrocarbons via Fischer-Tropsch or catalytic reforming. Therefore, the unwanted moist wastes like sewage sludge can be used for producing liquid biofuels via SCWG [122–124].

Like HTC and HTL, supercritical water simultaneously fulfills multiple roles in SCWG process. SCWG of model compound glucose reaction pathway is shown in Figure 7.13. Initially, water serves as the solvent for hydrolysis reactions, which quickly polymerizes the major biomass components

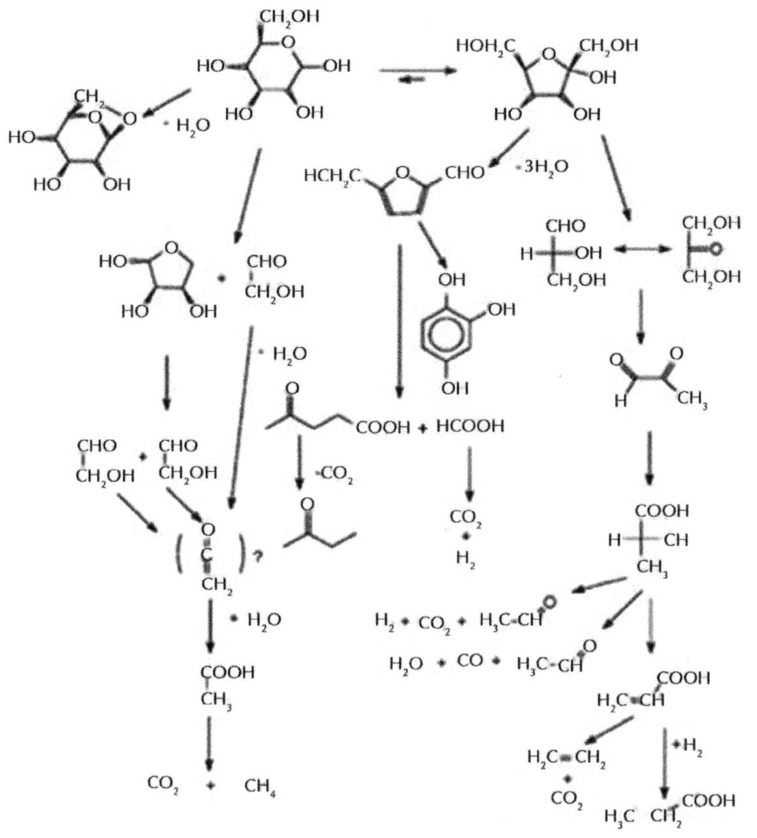

FIGURE 7.13 Proposed reaction pathways of hydrothermal biomass gasification with primary intermediates [11].

(e.g., hemicellulose, cellulose, polysaccharides and fatty acids) into simple monomers like fructose, glucose, and short-chain organic acids [125]. Gasification occurs after hydrolysis, wherein supercritical water quickly pyrolyzes simple sugars and organic products to produce H_2-rich fuel gas and carbon oxides [126]. Water acts as H_2 donor during water-gas shift reactions due to the weaker H_2 bonds of supercritical water. Therefore, overall concentration of H_2 and O_2 availability increases rapidly during SCWG and so as corresponding H_2 yield [11]. The increase in O_2 availability also facilitates slightly exothermic reactions, which improve SCWG energy efficiency [27, 127]. However, the excess O_2 shifts the reaction toward the complete combustion and produce CO_2. The process would then be defined supercritical wet air oxidation (SCWO), which is discussed in later section.

Under supercritical conditions, water's hydrolysis solvation characteristics quickly give way to a secondary role as a reactant as well as a H_2 source [2, 11]. The severity of supercritical water is much higher than subcritical water as H_2 production can be increased as much as 80% for only 30°C increase from subcritical conditions to 380°C supercritical conditions [11, 125]. Understanding water molecule interaction at supercritical conditions can help us predicting surface-bound, intermediate species, and reaction mechanism. Superior solvation and dilution properties prevent polymerization of double-bond intermediates, mainly by spatial distancing and reduced collisions between reactant molecules [11]. As a result, supercritical water suppresses tar and coke formation, which is a large concern for thermal gasification, pyrolysis, or even HTL.

SCWG reaction pathways for a biomass are depicted in Figure 7.14. In supercritical water gasification, water-gas shift reaction is the key reaction as well [11]. The presence of alkali salts is necessary to attain the low CO and high hydrogen yields calculated by thermodynamic studies [128]. Alkali salts catalyze the water-gas shift reaction so as other heterogeneous catalysts like Nickel [128]. The catalytic effect was connected with the basic character of salts although such argumentation causes problems if the changes in acidity/basicity in near- and supercritical water are considered. Although,

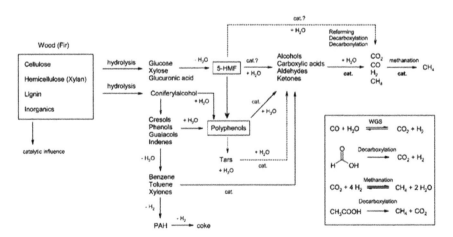

FIGURE 7.14 The influence of catalyst on the reaction pathway of wood gasification under supercritical conditions [5].

it is not fully clear how the alkali salts catalyze the water-gas shift reaction, the result is obvious. Only in the presence of salts the thermodynamic predicted gas composition is reached (below 650°C). In addition, the hydrogen formed via this reaction is very reactive and influences further reactions. The hydrogen, formed via the water-gas shift reaction, hydrogenates organic compounds were shown be the reaction of deuterated glucose in normal water. Here, H_2 was added to double bonds formed via the degradation of glucose, and it could only be formed via the water-gas shift reaction of water. Surplus H_2 availability also positions supercritical water as the natural upgrading medium for lipid containing sludge, coal pitch, and petroleum coke. Prevailing dogma, however, asserts that H_2-production costs via SCWG of wet biomass (e.g., sludge) are several times higher than the costs of H_2 production via steam CH_4 or natural gas reforming [129–131]. The H_2-production argument is based solely on fuel (e.g., H_2) as the cost reference point. When nested within the revenue framework of waste disposal as the primary objective, secondary H_2 fuel conversion costs via SCWG is actually estimated to be a full two magnitudes less than that of natural gas reforming [129]. The conversion costs are constant, regardless of the feedstock origin. However, the bottom-line product production costs are also largely driven by feedstock production and extraction costs, which in the case of natural gas have dropped significantly as a result of shale-based, strata fracturing (fracking), albeit fraught with controversy [27, 130].

7.3.4 WET AIR OXIDATION

Hydrothermal processes discussed above (HTC, HTL, and SCWG) are occurred at inert atmosphere to prevent the carboxylation of the biomass. However, biomass can be carboxylated with excess oxygen under hydrothermal condition. Carboxylation yields heat, which can be used directly in Rankine or Bryton cycle. The process is called wet air oxidation (WAO). Process condition of WAO is very similar to HTC and HTL, except oxygen or air in excess amount (1.2–1.5 times more than stoichiometry of feed carbon content) is introduced to the system. The idea of the WAO process is to incinerate waste carbon molecules in water medium. The concept is to enhance contact between molecular oxygen and the organic matter to be oxidized and then to eliminate organic compounds by oxidizing them to carbon dioxide and water with oxygen in the liquid phase [132–135]. WAO reactions also produce low molecular weight organic compounds including carboxylic acids, acetaldehydes and alcohols [136]. In WAO process, either pure oxygen gas or air is used as an oxidant, therefore, the latter case is also called WAO. The WAO process includes two steps, which are the physical and the chemical step. In the physical step oxygen is transferred from the gas phase to the liquid phase. According to Debellefontaine et al. [137], the only significant transfer resistance will occur at the gas-liquid interface. There are few limiting cases for mass transfer [137, 138]. For example, oxygen can react already within the film, it can react within the bulk liquid or the oxygen concentration within the bulk liquid can be equal to the interface concentration. The second step, the chemical step, there are many factors influence WAO rate and product distribution. The most important factors are temperature, oxygen partial pressure, pH of the solution, reactor type, and in some extent composition of the reactors walls. The general agreement is that the reactions in WAO proceed through free-radical chemical reactions. Free-radical chemical reactions have three main types: initiation, propagation and termination [139]. In Figure 7.15, a simplified reaction pathway for toluene degradation by WAO is shown.

In wet air oxidation it is also possible to use catalysts. The use of a catalyst can reduce the capital-intensive process conditions (e.g., high pressure) but still reaching almost complete oxidation. In addition, the use of catalyst can reduce material costs. The catalyst can be either heterogeneous or homogeneous. The phase of heterogeneous catalyst differs from the other

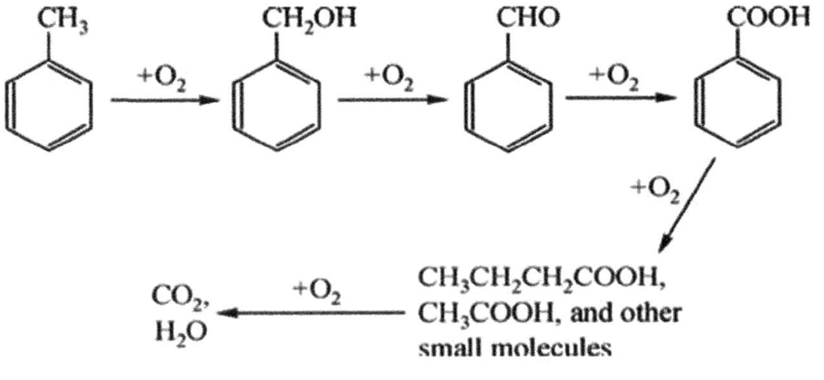

FIGURE 7.15   Proposed mechanism for toluene degradation under wet air oxidation [12].

reactants and homogeneous catalyst is in same phase as the reactants. Copper ion is an effective homogeneous catalyst. Copper ion can be used for the practical treatment of wastewater discharged from petrochemical industries [57]. Nowadays, most of WAO plants are treating waste streams from petro-chemical, chemical and pharmaceutical industries and residual sludge from wastewater treatment [137, 140–147]. Plants can operate either for complete oxidative decomposition or for partial oxidation of pollutants. In partial oxi-dation the feed is oxidized to low-molecular weight compounds and after that they are treated by biological processes.

A typical WAO plant is composed primarily of a high-pressure pump, an air or oxygen compressor, a heat-exchanger and also a reactor with a relief valve and a downstream separator [141, 145–146]. Even though WAO pro-cess has a wide range of advantages, there is still one big disadvantage. The process needs very high temperature and pressure to work properly, so that the organic compounds will obtain a high degree of oxidation in a reason-able amount of time. These conditions will require large amounts of capital and the operating costs are also high. However, without the necessary tem-perature and pressure, there will be only partial oxidation. To improve WAO process more efficient oxidizers should be used. This can be accomplished by using homogeneous catalysts (for example, transition metal salts) or to use hydrogen peroxide as the oxidizer instead of oxygen.

7.3.5 SUPERCRITICAL WATER OXIDATION

Supercritical water oxidation (SCWO) is similar to SCWG in terms of reaction parameters (temperature and pressure) but also similar to WAO in terms of oxygen loading. The goal of SCWO is to destroy hazardous wastes like nitrocellulose based propellants, nuclear wastes, and organic pathogens and antibiotic compounds. Although, SCWO first introduced in 50's, the main push was in early 80's when NASA was conducting studies on feasibility of human living on moon [148–151]. Even the early studies of SCWO show an unexpected high reaction rate of the water-gas shift reaction. Kinetics of the gas phase water-gas shift reaction, the main reaction of SCWO is faster as supercritical water enhances the thermodynamics (La Chatelier's phenomenon) in favor of water-gas shift reaction. The reactions of small free radicals at increased pressures are faster because of higher collision numbers leading to better energy inflation [152, 153]. To consider this, the reaction rate coefficient can be set to the so-called high-pressure limit. By doing so, the reaction rate of the measured water-gas shift reaction was still very high. Early studies assumed lower activation energies by water some shell forms around the activated complex [154, 155]. Later this was specified by assuming formic acid as intermediate and a lowering of activation energy for the formation of CO_2 and H_2 by solvation of the activated complex [156]. In the second case water as solvent changes selectivity, because the lowering of activation energy is different for the two possible reaction pathways of formic acid in both directions of the water-gas shift reaction. Here formic acid is forced to form CO_2 and H_2 instead of CO and H_2O, because the activated complex formed with water has a lower energy in the first case [156].

When organic compounds and oxygen are dissolved in water above the critical point they are immediately brought into intimate molecular contact in a single homogeneous phase, with no interface transport limitations and, for sufficiently high temperatures, the kinetics is fast and the oxidation reaction proceeds rapidly to completion. Figure 7.16 shows the degradation mechanism of model compound phenol. The kinetics of SCWO of organics is frequently considered as a first-order or pseudo first-order kinetics

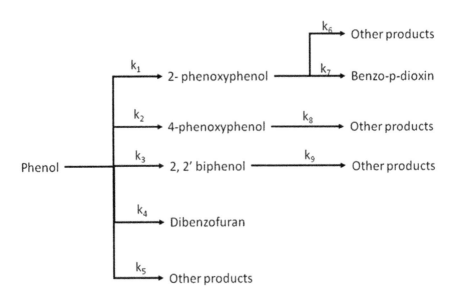

FIGURE 7.16 Proposed mechanism for phenol degradation under supercritical water oxidation [1].

with respect to the concentration of the organic compounds [7]. The oxidation rate is frequently considered independent or weakly dependent on the oxidant concentration. SCWO kinetics is controlled by the formation and destruction of rate controlling intermediates: some organics compounds are directly destroyed into the final oxidation products, whereas others are transformed into stable intermediates [150, 151]. By-product analyzes have indicated that short-chain carboxylic acids, ketones, aldehydes, and alcohols are the main oxidation intermediates, of which the most frequent are acetic acid and ammonia for nitrogen-containing reagents. These intermediates are more stable and their oxidation rate is slower.

The SCWO process is suitable for treating wide range of wastewaters and organic hazardous and toxic compounds. If destruction of waste is the main goal not heat generation, excess oxygen and additional heating are provided to ensure the maximum destruction with very low partial oxidation products from targeted wastes. At the appropriate pressures, temperatures, and residence times a great variety of organic compounds have been oxidized to CO_2, water, and N_2, without detectable formation of partial oxidation products. Until now, SCWO technology has been applied to organic compounds such as ammonia, cyanides, trinitrotoluene, nitrocellulose, insecticides, pesticides, antibiotics, hormones, etc. [157–161]. SCWO has been studied as an alternative for the destruction of military wastes. Both the U.S. Department of Defense (US DoD) and the U.S. Department of Energy (US DoE) have contributed the most to the development of the SCWO process [162]. National Aeronautics and Space Administration (NASA) has investigated the SCWO process applied to the destruction of the biomass produced in spatial trips. The study has been extended to other materials such as ion-exchange resin decomposition, biomass, and industrial and urban sludges, with an important energy recovery in the waste destruction [163]. At the industrial scale, the AquaCat® process of Chematur recovers oxidized metals from the SCWO of catalyst in Johnson Matthey, Brimsdown, UK.

Two main challenges that SCWO encounter are pumping oxygen or air at very high temperature and pressure, and corrosion of the reactor and pipelines. Plugging problems also occur in almost every existing SCWO industrial plants and the plant needed to stop and cleaned-up after a few months of operation. The extreme operational conditions along with the corrosive environment make necessary an extensive study of the materials behavior on duty. A challenge in SCWO is the application of new construction materials that are able to withstand the harsh operational conditions in the main equipment, valves, and fittings. From the perspective of energetics, SCWO can be performed in an energetically profitable way but the capital cost to install a SCWO is still very high compare to thermal incineration. Development of cheaper corrosion resistant materials may improve the SCWO process significantly.

7.4 SUMMARY

Hydrothermal technologies, where water is used as solvent, medium, and/or catalyst, are green processes to produce renewable energy, biomaterials, heat, or destruction of hazardous and unwanted organic wastes. Thermodynamic properties of water change substantially from ambient conditions to sub- and supercritical conditions. Polar water becomes nonpolar with increased ionic constants and less density until critical point. Therefore, subcritical water acts as mild acid, mild base, and nonpolar solvent. The alteration of thermodynamic properties influence water to react with biomass and degraded products. With the absence of oxygen, biomass releases oxygen-rich volatile components to produce solid hydrochar at around 180–260°C and process is known as hydrothermal carbonization (HTC). Hydrochar has the properties similar to lignite or bituminous coal. Although HTC process is exothermic but the product is competing directly with coal, therefore HTC economics is questionable. Also, HTC is lacking scale-up results, as the process parameters are often debatable. Also, coal, the direct compatible product of hydrochar, application for energy is reducing in the USA. With the increase of temperature, lignin starts to degrade and reacts with the other hydrolyzed products to produce a viscous carbon-rich mostly nonpolar biocrude. The process is now called hydrothermal liquefaction (HTL), as liquid is the feasible product. The biocrude itself is not a final product but it can be hydrodeoxygenated to produce drop-in gasoline-range products. The technology is well developed for microalgae and scaled-up tests are performed. However, the cheap crude oil price is hampering the prosperity of the HTL. Once water crosses critical point, a single phase appears with more reactive nature. Biomass in this condition, degraded into gaseous products, therefore, the process is called supercritical water gasification (SCWG). At lower temperature (374–450°C) with noble metal catalyst biomass converts into methane rich gas. To produce hydrogen, the SCWG temperature needs to be higher than 600°C. SCWG is a very quick process to produce methane or hydrogen from wet waste biomass. However, corrosion turns out to be a huge issue for designing the reaction. Designing a SCWG process with corrosion resistive material involves tremendous amount of capital investment. Now, the other hydrothermal processes where oxygen or air is fed to the reactor are called wet air oxidation (WAO) operated at subcritical conditions and supercritical air oxidation (SCWO) operated at supercritical conditions. Both processes are promising for producing direct heat or destroying hazardous, toxic, and organic compounds. However, mass transfer limitations and corrosions are the drawbacks for WAO and SCWO processes, respectively. Overall, the hydrothermal processes are promising green technologies to produce biofuel and biopower. More research and governmental support and initiative (e.g., carbon tax) will be necessary to advance the development of water-based environment friendly biofuel production.

KEYWORDS

- **biomass (wood, grass, municipal solid waste, sewage sludge)**
- **higher heating value**
- **hydrothermal carbonization**
- **hydrothermal liquefaction**
- **methane (CH_4)**
- **supercritical water gasification**
- **supercritical water oxidation**
- **synthesis gas ($CO + H_2$)**
- **wet air oxidation**

REFERENCES

1. Peterson, A. A., Vogel, F., Lachance, R. P., Froling, M., Antal, M. J., & Tester, J. W. (2008). Thermochemical biofuel production in hydrothermal media: A review of sub and supercritical water technologies. *Energ Environ Sci, 1* (1), 32–65.
2. Kruse, A., & Dahmen, N. (2015). Water - A magic solvent for biomass conversion. *J Supercrit Fluid, 96*, 36–45.

3. Reza, M. T., Andert, J., Wirth, B., Busch, D., Pielert, J., Lynam, J. G., & Mumme, J. (2014). Hydrothermal carbonization of biomass for energy and crop production. *Applied Bioenergy*, 1(1).

4. Yakaboylu, O., Harinck, J., Smit, K. G., & De Jong, W. (2013). Supercritical Water Gasification of Biomass: A thermodynamic equilibrium modeling approach. *Biomass Bioenergy*, 59, 253–263.

5. Waldner, M. H., & Vogel, F. (2005). Renewable production of methane from woody biomass by catalytic hydrothermal gasification. *Ind Eng Chem Res.*, *44* (13), 4543–4551.

6. Yong, T. L. K., & Matsumura, Y. (2012). Reaction Kinetics of the Lignin Conversion in Supercritical Water. *Ind Eng Chem Res.*, *51*(37), 11975–11988.

7. Ghoreishi, S. M., Mortazavi, S. M. S., & Hedayati, A. (2015). Modeling of Non-catalytic Supercritical Water Oxidation of Phenol. *Chem Prod Process Mo.*, *10*(4), 243–251.

8. Moller, M., Harnisch, F., & Schroder, U. (2013). Hydrothermal liquefaction of cellulose in subcritical water-the role of crystallinity on the cellulose reactivity. *Rsc Adv.*, *3*(27), 11035–11044.

9. Yakaboylu, O., Harinck, J., Smit, K. G., & de Jong, W. (2014). Supercritical Water Gasification of Manure: A Thermodynamic Model for the Prediction of Product Compounds at Equilibrium State. *Energ Fuel*, *28*(4), 2506–2522.

10. Xiong, H. F., Pham, H. N., & Datye, A. K. (2014). Hydrothermally stable heterogeneous catalysts for conversion of biorenewables. *Green Chem .*, *16* (11), 4627–4643.

11. Kruse, A. (2008). Supercritical water gasification. *Biofuel Bioprod Bior.*, *2*(5), 415–437.

12. Bo, L. L., Liao, J. B., Zhang, Y. C., Wang, X. H., & Yang, Q. (2013). CuO/zeolite catalyzed oxidation of gaseous toluene under microwave heating. *Front Env Sci Eng.*, *7*(3), 395–402.

13. Sevilla, M., & Fuertes, A. B. (2009). Chemical and Structural Properties of Carbonaceous Products Obtained by Hydrothermal Carbonization of Saccharides. *Chem-Eur J.*, *15*(16), 4195–4203.

14. EIA, Independent statistics and analysis, US Energy Information Administration. EIA: 2016.

15. IPCC *Climate Change (2014): Impacts, Adaptation, and Vulnerability: Part A: Global and Sectoral Aspects. Contribution of Working Group II to the Fifth Assessment Report of the Intergovernmental Panel on Climate Change*, pp. 1132.

16. Energy, U. D. O. (2016). *Billion Ton Update: Biomass Supply for a Bioenergy and Bioproducts Industry*, Oak Ridge National Laboratory,

17. Akhtar, J., & Amin, N. A. S. (2011). A review on process conditions for optimum bio-oil yield in hydrothermal liquefaction of biomass. *Renew Sust Energ Rev.*, *15*(3), 1615–1624.

18. Acelas, N. Y., Lopez, D. P., Brilman, D. W. F., Kersten, S. R. A., & Kootstra, A. M. J. (2014). Supercritical water gasification of sewage sludge: Gas production and phosphorus recovery. *Bioresource Technol.*, *174*, 167–175.

19. Yakaboylu, O., Harinck, J., Smit, K. G., & de Jong, W. (2015). Supercritical Water Gasification of Biomass: A Literature and Technology Overview. *Energies*, *8*(2), 859–894.

20. Anjum, R., Krakat, N., Reza, M. T., & Klocke, M. (2014). Assessment of mutagenic potential of pyrolysis biochars by Ames Salmonella/mammalian-microsomal mutagenicity test. *Ecotox Environ Safe*, *107*, 306–312.

21. Hognon, C., Delrue, F., & Boissonnet, G. (2015). Energetic and economic evaluation of Chlamydomonas reinhardtii hydrothermal liquefaction and pyrolysis through thermochemical models. *Energy*, *93*, 31–40.

22. Reza, M. T. (2011). Hydrothermal carbonization of lignocellulosic biomass. Univeristy of Nevada Reno.

23. Reza, M. T. (2013). Upgrading biomass by hydrothermal and chemical conditioning. University of Nevada Reno, Reno,

24. Barreiro, D. L., Beck, M., Hornung, U., Ronsse, F., Kruse, A., & Prins, W. (2015). Suitability of hydrothermal liquefaction as a conversion route to produce biofuels from macroalgae. *Algal Res.*, *11*, 234–241.

25. Coronella, C. J., Lynam, J. G., Reza, M. T., & Uddin, M. H. (2014). Hydrothermal Carbonization of Lignocellulosic Biomass. In *Application of Hydrothermal Reactions to Biomass Conversion, Jin., F., Ed.,* Springer Berlin Heidelberg.

26. Kruse, A., Funke, A., & Titirici, M. M. (2013). Hydrothermal conversion of biomass to fuels and energetic materials. *Curr Opin Chem Biol.*, *17*(3), 515–521.

27. Gasafi, E., Reinecke, M. Y., Kruse, A., & Schebek, L. (2008). Economic analysis of sewage sludge gasification in supercritical water for hydrogen production. *Biomass Bioenerg.*, *32*(12), 1085–1096.

28. Elliott, D. C., Biller, P., Ross, A. B., Schmidt, A. J., & Jones, S. B. (2015). Hydrothermal liquefaction of biomass: Developments from batch to continuous process. *Bioresource Technol.*, *178*, 147–156.

29. Wang, Z. H., Adhikari, S., Valdez, P., Shakya, R., & Laird, C. (2016). Upgrading of hydrothermal liquefaction biocrude from algae grown in municipal wastewater. *Fuel Process Technol.*, *142*, 147–156.

30. Matubayasi, N., Wakai, C., & Nakahara, M. (1999). Structural study of supercritical water. II. Computer simulations. *The Journal of Chemical Physics*, *100*, 8000.

31. Bandura, A. V., & Lvov, S. N. (2006). The ionization constant of water over wide ranges of temperature and density. *J Phys Chem Ref Data*, *35*(1), 15–30.

32. Franck, E. U., Rosenzweig, S., & Christoforakos, M. (1990). Calculation of the Dielectric-Constant of Water to 1000-Degrees-C and Very High-Pressures. *Ber Bunsen Phys Chem.*, *94*(2), 199–203.

33. Wu, G., Heilig, M., Lentz, H., & Franck, E. U. (1990). High-Pressure Phase-Equilibria of the Water-Argon System. *Ber Bunsen Phys Chem.*, *94*(1), 24–27.

34. Wernet, P., Testemale, D., Hazemann, J. L., Argoud, R., Glatzel, P., Pettersson, L. G. M., Nilsson, A., & Bergmann, U. (2005). Spectroscopic characterization of microscopic hydrogen-bonding disparities in supercritical water. *J Chem Phys.*, *123*(15).

35. Tsujino, Y., Wakai, C., Matubayashi, N., & Nakahara, M. (1999). Noncatalytic Cannizzaro-type reaction of formaldehyde in hot water. *Chem. Lett.*, (4), 287–288.

36. Lynam, J., Reza, M. T., Yan, W., Vásquez, V., & Coronella, C. (2014). Hydrothermal carbonization of various lignocellulosic biomass. *Biomass Conversion and Biorefinery*, 1–9.

37. Mumme, J., Titirici, M. M., Pfeiffer, A., Luder, U., Reza, M. T., & Masek, O. (2015). Hydrothermal Carbonization of Digestate in the Presence of Zeolite: Process Efficiency and Composite Properties. *Acs Sustain Chem Eng.*, *3*(11), 2967–2974.

38. Reza, M. T., Rottler, E., Herklotz, L., & Wirth, B. (2015). Hydrothermal carbonization (HTC) of wheat straw: Influence of feedwater pH prepared by acetic acid and potassium hydroxide. *Bioresource Technol.*, *182*, 336–344.

39. Reza, M. T., Wirth, B., Luder, U., & Werner, M. (2014). Behavior of selected hydrolyzed and dehydrated products during hydrothermal carbonization of biomass. *Bioresource Technol.*, *169*, 352–361.

40. Reza, M. T., Uddin, M. H., Lynam, J. G., & Coronella, C. J. (2014). Engineered pellets from dry torrefied and HTC biochar blends. *Biomass Bioenerg.*, *63*, 229–238.

41. Reza, M. T., Yang, X., Coronella, C. J., Lin, H., Hathwaik, U., Shintani, D., Neupane, B. P., & Miller, G. C. (2015). Hydrothermal Carbonization (HTC) and Pelletization of Two Arid Land Plants Bagasse for Energy Densification. *ACS Sustainable Chemistry and Engineering.*

42. Alvarez-Murillo, A., Ledesma, B., Roman, S., Sabio, E., & Ganan, J. (2015). Biomass pyrolysis toward hydrocarbonization. Influence on subsequent steam gasification processes. *J. Anal. Appl. Pyrol., 113*, 380–389.

43. Alvarez-Murillo, A., Roman, S., Ledesma, B., & Sabio, E. (2015). Study of variables in energy densification of olive stone by hydrothermal carbonization. *J Anal Appl Pyrol., 113*, 307–314.

44. Reza, M. T., Yan, W., Uddin, M. H., Lynam, J. G., Hoekman, S. K., Coronella, C. J., & Vasquez, V. R. (2013).Reaction kinetics of hydrothermal carbonization of loblolly pine. *Bioresource Technol., 139*, 161–169.

45. Reza, M. T., Uddin, M. H., Lynam, J., Hoekman, S. K., & Coronella, C. (2014). Hydrothermal carbonization of loblolly pine: reaction chemistry and water balance. *Biomass Conversion and Biorefinery., 4*(4), 311–321.

46. Reza, M. T., Lynam, J. G., Vasquez, V. R., & Coronella, C. J. (2012). Pelletization of Biochar from Hydrothermally Carbonized Wood. *Environmental Progress & Sustainable Energy., 31*(2), 225–234.

47. Fuertes, A. B., Arbestain, M. C., Sevilla, M., Macia-Agullo, J. A., Fiol, S., Lopez, R., Smernik, R. J., Aitkenhead, W. P., Arce, F., & Macias, F. (2010). Chemical and structural properties of carbonaceous products obtained by pyrolysis and hydrothermal carbonisation of corn stover. *Aust J Soil Res., 48*(6–7), 618–626.

48. Fuertes, A. B., Ferrero, G. A., & Sevilla, M. (2014). One-pot synthesis of microporous carbons highly enriched in nitrogen and their electrochemical performance. *J. Mater Chem. A., 2*(35), 14439–14448.

49. Andert, J., & Mumme, J., (2015). Impact of pyrolysis and hydrothermal biochar on gas-emitting activity of soil microorganisms and bacterial and archaeal community composition. *Appl. Soil Ecol., 96*, 225–239.

50. Dicke, C., Lanza, G., Mumme, J., Ellerbrock, R., & Kern, J. (2014).Effect of Hydrothermally Carbonized Char Application on Trace Gas Emissions from Two Sandy Soil Horizons. *J. Environ. Qual., 43*(5), 1790–1798.

51. Dicke, C., Luhr, C., Ellerbrock, R., Mumme, J., & Kern, J. (2015). Effect of Hydrothermally Carbonized Hemp Dust on the Soil Emissions of CO2 and N2O. *Bioresources, 10*(2), 3210–3223.

52. Hu, B., Wang, K., Wu, L. H., Yu, S. H., Antonietti, M., & Titirici, M. M. (2010). Engineering Carbon Materials from the Hydrothermal Carbonization Process of Biomass. *Adv Mater., 22*(7), 813–828.

53. Regmi, P., Moscoso, J. L. G., Kumar, S., Cao, X. Y., Mao, J. D., & Schafran, G. (2012). Removal of copper and cadmium from aqueous solution using switchgrass biochar produced via hydrothermal carbonization process. *J. Environ. Manage, 109*, 61–69.

54. Titirici, M. M., White, R. J., Brun, N., Budarin, V. L., Su, D. S., del Monte, F., Clark, J. H., & MacLachlan, M. J. (2015). Sustainable carbon materials. *Chem. Soc. Rev., 44*(1), 250–290.

55. White, R. J., Brun, N., Budarin, V. L., Clark, J. H., & Titirici, M. M. (2014). Always Look on the "Light" Side of Life: Sustainable Carbon Aerogels. *Chemsuschem 7* (3), 670–689.

56. White, R. J., Yoshizawa, N., Antonietti, M., & Titirici, M. M. (2011). A sustainable synthesis of nitrogen-doped carbon aerogels. *Green Chem., 13*(9), 2428–2434.

57. Reza, M. T., Freitas, A., Yang, X., & Coronella, C. J. (2016). Wet Air Oxidation of Hydrothermal Carbonization (HTC) Process Liquid. *Acs Sustain Chem Eng.,* In press.

58. Uddin, M. H., Reza, M. T., Lynam, J. G., & Coronella, C. J. (2014). Effects of water recycling in hydrothermal carbonization of loblolly pine. *Environmental Progress & Sustainable Energy, 33*(4), 1309–1315.

59. Wirth, B., & Reza, M. T., (2016). Continuous anaerobic degradation of liquid condensate from steam-derived hydrothermal carbonization of sewage sludge. *ACS Sustainable Chemistry and Engineering.*

60. Erdogan, E., Atila, B., Mumme, J., Reza, M. T., Toptas, A., Elibol, M., & Yanik, J. (2015). Characterization of products from hydrothermal carbonization of orange pomace including anaerobic digestibility of process liquor. *Bioresource Technol., 196,* 35–42.

61. Reza, M. T., Borrego, A. G., & Wirth, B. (2014). Optical texture of hydrochar from maize silage and maize silage digestate. *Int. J. Coal Geol., 134,* 74–79.

62. Reza, M. T., Mumme, J., & Ebert, A. (2015). Characterization of hydrochar obtained from hydrothermal carbonization of wheat straw digestate. *Biomass Conversion and Biorefinery.*

63. Reza, M. T., Rottler, E., Tolle, R., Werner, M., Ramm, P., & Mumme, J. (2015). Production characterization, and biogas application of magnetic hydrochar from cellulose. *Bioresource Technol., 186,* 34–43.

64. Ferrero, G. A., Preuss, K., Fuertes, A. B., Sevilla, M., & Titirici, M. M. (2016). The influence of pore size distribution on the oxygen reduction reaction performance in nitrogen doped carbon microspheres. *J. Mater Chem. A., 4*(7), 2581–2589.

65. Laube, H., & Reza, M. T. (2016). Application of biosorbents for ion removal from sodium lactate fermentation broth. *Journal of Environmental Chemical Engineering, 4*(1), 10–19.

66. Negandar, L., Delidovich, I., & Palkovits, R. (2016). Aqueous-phase hydrolysis of cellulose and hemicelluloses over molecular acidic catalysts: Insights into the kinetics and reaction mechanism. *Appl. Catal. B-Environ., 184,* 285–298.

67. Grenman, H., Eranen, K., Krogell, J., Willfor, S., Salmi, T., & Murzin, D. Y. (2011). Kinetics of Aqueous Extraction of Hemicelluloses from Spruce in an Intensified Reactor System. *Ind Eng Chem Res., 50*(7), 3818–3828.

68. Rissanen, J. V., Grenman, H., Willfor, S., Murzin, D. Y., & Salmi, T. (2014). Spruce Hemicellulose for Chemicals Using Aqueous Extraction: Kinetics, Mass Transfer, and Modeling. *Ind Eng Chem Res., 53*(15), 6341–6350.

69. Lynam, J. G., Coronella, C. J., Yan, W., Reza, M. T., & Vasquez, V. R. (2011). Acetic acid and lithium chloride effects on hydrothermal carbonization of lignocellulosic biomass. *Bioresource Technol., 102*(10), 6192–6199.

70. Reza, M. T., & Becker, W. (2014). Sachsenheimer, K., Mumme, J., Hydrothermal carbonization (HTC): Near infrared spectroscopy and partial least-squares regression for determination of selective components in HTC solid and liquid products derived from maize silage. *Bioresource Technol., 161,* 91–101.

71. Diakite, M., Paul, A., Jager, C., Pielert, J., & Mumme, J. (2013). Chemical and morphological changes in hydrochars derived from microcrystalline cellulose and investigated by chromatographic, spectroscopic and adsorption techniques. *Bioresource Technol., 150,* 98–105.

72. Reza, M. T., Freitas, A., Yang, X., Hiibel, S., Lin, H., & Coronella, C. J., (2016). Hydrothermal Carbonization (HTC) of Cow Manure: Carbon and Nitrogen Distributions in HTC products. *Environmental Progress & Sustainable Energy.*, In-press.
73. Reza, M. T., Lynam, J. G., Uddin, M. H., & Coronella, C. J., (2013). Hydrothermal carbonization: Fate of inorganics. *Biomass Bioenerg.*, *49*, 86–94.
74. Lynam, J. G., Reza, M. T., Vasquez, V. R., & Coronella, C. J., (2012). Effect of salt addition on hydrothermal carbonization of lignocellulosic biomass. *Fuel*, *99*, 271–273.
75. Reza, M. T., Werner, M., Pohl, M., & Mumme, J., (2014). Evaluation of Integrated Anaerobic Digestion and Hydrothermal Carbonization for Bioenergy Production. *Jove-J Vis Exp* (88).
76. Areeprasert, C., Coppola, A., Urciuolo, M., Chirone, R., Yoshikawa, K., & Scala, F., (2015). The effect of hydrothermal treatment on attrition during the fluidized bed combustion of paper sludge. *Fuel Process Technol.*, *140*, 57–66.
77. Areeprasert, C., Scala, F., Coppola, A., Urciuolo, M., Chirone, R., Chanyavanich, P., & Yoshikawa, K., (2016). Fluidized bed cocombustion of hydrothermally treated paper sludge with two coals of different rank. *Fuel Process Technol.*, *144*, 230–238.
78. Areeprasert, C., Zhao, P. T., Ma, D. C., Shen, Y. F., & Yoshikawa, K., (2014). Alternative Solid Fuel Production from Paper Sludge Employing Hydrothermal Treatment. *Energ Fuel*, *28*(2), 1198–1206.
79. Makela, M., & Yoshikawa, K., (2016). Simulating hydrothermal treatment of sludge within a pulp and paper mill. *Appl Energ.*, *173*, 177–183.
80. Zhao, P. T., Shen, Y. F., Ge, S. F., & Yoshikawa, K., (2014). Energy recycling from sewage sludge by producing solid biofuel with hydrothermal carbonization. *Energ Convers Manage.*, *78*, 815–821.
81. Tremel, A., Stemann, J., Herrmann, M., Erlach, B., & Spliethoff, H., (2012). Entrained flow gasification of biocoal from hydrothermal carbonization. *Fuel.*, *102*, 396–403.
82. Erlach, B., Harder, B., & Tsatsaronis, G., (2012). Combined hydrothermal carbonization and gasification of biomass with carbon capture. *Energy.*, *45* (1), 329–338.
83. Steurer, E., & Ardissone, G., (2015). Hydrothermal Carbonization and Gasification Technology for Electricity Production using Biomass, *2015 International Conference on Alternative Energy in Developing Countries and Emerging Economies 79*, 47–54.
84. Cao, L. C., Luo, G., Zhang, S. C., & Chen, J. M. (2016). Bio-oil production from eight selected green landscaping wastes through hydrothermal liquefaction. *Rsc Adv.*, *6*(18), 15260–15270.
85. Li, Z. X., Hong, Y. M., Cao, J. F., Huang, Z. T., Huang, K., Gong, H., Huang, L. Y., Shi, S., Kawashita, M., & Li, Y. (2015). Effects of Mild Alkali Pretreatment and Hydrogen-Donating Solvent on Hydrothermal Liquefaction of Eucalyptus Woodchips. *Energ Fuel*, *29*(11), 7335–7342.
86. Tian, C. Y., Liu, Z. D., Zhang, Y. H., Li, B. M., Cao, W., Lu, H. F., Duan, N., Zhang, L., & Zhang, T. T. (2015). Hydrothermal liquefaction of harvested high-ash low-lipid algal biomass from Dianchi Lake: Effects of operational parameters and relations of products. *Bioresource Technol.*, *184*, 336–343.
87. Albrecht, K. O., Zhu, Y. H., Schmidt, A. J., Billing, J. M., Hart, T. R., Jones, S. B., Maupin, G., Hallen, R., Ahrens, T., & Anderson, D. (2016). Impact of heterotrophically stressed algae for biofuel production via hydrothermal liquefaction and catalytic hydrotreating in continuous-flow reactors. *Algal Res.*, *14*, 17–27.
88. Li, F., Liu, L., An, Y., He, W. Z., Themelis, N. J., & Li, G. M. (2016). Hydrothermal liquefaction of three kinds of starches into reducing sugars. *J Clean Prod.*, *112*, 1049–1054.

89. Li, R. D., Xie, Y. H., Yang, T. H., Li, B. S., Wang, W. D., & Kai, X. P. (2015). Effects of Chemical-Biological pretreatment of corn stalks on the bio-oils produced by hydrothermal liquefaction. *Energ Convers Manage., 93*, 23–30.

90. Su, Y., Zhu, W., Gong, M., Zhou, H. Y., Fan, Y. J., & Amuzu-Sefordzi, B. (2015). Interaction between sewage sludge components lignin (phenol) and proteins (alanine) in supercritical water gasification. *Int J Hydrogen Energ., 40* (30), 9125–9136.

91. Zhang, B., Huang, H. J., & Ramaswamy, S. (2012). A Kinetics Study on Hydrothermal Liquefaction of High-diversity Grassland Perennials. *Energ Source Part A., 34*(18), 1676–1687.

92. Zhang, B., von Keitz, M., & Valentas, K. (2008). Thermal effects on hydrothermal biomass liquefaction. *Appl Biochem Biotech., 147* (1–3), 143–150.

93. Yang, X., Lyu, H., Chen, K. F., Zhu, X. D., Zhang, S. C., & Chen, J. M. (2014). Selective Extraction of Bio-oil from Hydrothermal Liquefaction of Salix psammophila by Organic Solvents with Different Polarities through Multistep Extraction Separation. *Bioresources., 9*(3), 5219–5233.

94. Chen, K. F., Lyu, H., Hao, S. L., Luo, G., Zhang, S. C., & Chen, J. M. (2015). Separation of phenolic compounds with modified adsorption resin from aqueous phase products of hydrothermal liquefaction of rice straw. *Bioresource Technol., 182*, 160–168.

95. Chen, W. T., Zhang, Y. H., Zhang, J. X., Yu, G., Schideman, L. C., Zhang, P., & Minarick, M. (2014). Hydrothermal liquefaction of mixed-culture algal biomass from wastewater treatment system into bio-crude oil. *Bioresource Technol., 152*, 130–139.

96. Chen, W. T., Zhang, Y. H., Zhang, J. X., & Zhang, P. (2013). Hydrothermal liquefaction of waste water algae mixtures into biocrude oil. *Abstr. Pap. Am. Chem. S., 246.*

97. Li, C. J., Yang, X., Zhang, Z., Zhou, D., Zhang, L., Zhang, S. C., & Chen, J. M. (2013). Hydrothermal Liquefaction of Desert Shrub Salix psammophila to High Value-added Chemicals and Hydrochar with Recycled Processing Water. *Bioresources, 8*(2), 2981–2997.

98. Biller, P., Sharma, B. K., Kunwar, B., & Ross, A. B. (2015). Hydroprocessing of biocrude from continuous hydrothermal liquefaction of microalgae. *Fuel, 159*, 197–205.

99. Elliott, D. C., Hart, T. R., Schmidt, A. J., Neuenschwander, G. G., Rotness, L. J., Olarte, M. V., Zacher, A. H., Albrecht, K. O., Hallen, R. T., & Holladay, J. E. (2013). Process development for hydrothermal liquefaction of algae feedstocks in a continuous-flow reactor. *Algal Res., 2*(4), 445–454.

100. Zhu, Y. H., Albrecht, K. O., Elliott, D. C., Hallen, R. T., & Jones, S. B. (2013). Development of hydrothermal liquefaction and upgrading technologies for lipid-extracted algae conversion to liquid fuels. *Algal Res., 2*(4), 455–464.

101. Zhu, Y. H., Biddy, M. J., Jones, S. B., Elliott, D. C., & Schmidt, A. J. (2014). Techno-economic analysis of liquid fuel production from woody biomass via hydrothermal liquefaction (HTL) and upgrading. *Appl Energ., 129*, 384–394.

102. Anastasakis, K., & Ross, A. B., (2011). Hydrothermal liquefaction of the brown macroalga Laminaria Saccharina: Effect of reaction conditions on product distribution and composition. *Bioresource Technol., 102*(7), 4876–4883.

103. Audo, M., Paraschiv, M., Queffelec, C., Louvet, I., Hemez, J., Fayon, F., Lepine, O., Legrand, J., Tazerout, M., Chailleux, E., & Bujoli, B., (2015). Subcritical Hydrothermal Liquefaction of Microalgae Residues as a Green Route to Alternative Road Binders. *Acs Sustain Chem Eng., 3*(4), 583–590.

104. Cheng, X., Ooms, M. D., & Sinton, D., (2016). Biomass-to-biocrude on a chip via hydrothermal liquefaction of algae. *Lab Chip., 16*(2), 256–260.

105. Christensen, P. R., Morup, A. J., Mamakhel, A., Glasius, M., Becker, J., & Iversen, B. B., (2014). Effects of heterogeneous catalyst in hydrothermal liquefaction of dried distillers grains with solubles. *Fuel, 123*, 158–166.

106. Costanzo, W., Hilten, R., Jena, U., Das, K. C., & Kastner, J. R., (2016). Effect of low temperature hydrothermal liquefaction on catalytic hydrodenitrogenation of algae bio-crude and model macromolecules. *Algal Res., 13*, 53–68.

107. Duan, P. G., & Savage, P. E., (2011). Hydrothermal Liquefaction of a Microalga with Heterogeneous Catalysts. *Ind. Eng. Chem. Res., 50* (1), 52–61.

108. Li, H. Y., Hu, J., Zhang, Z. J., Wang, H., Ping, F., Zheng, C. F., Zhang, H. L., & He, Q., (2014). Insight into the effect of hydrogenation on efficiency of hydrothermal liquefaction and physicochemical properties of biocrude oil. *Bioresource Technol., 163*, 143–151.

109. Sato, T., (2014). Upgrading of Heavy Oil by Hydrogenation through Partial Oxidation and Water-gas Shift Reaction in Supercritical Water. *J Jpn Petrol Inst 57.*, (1), 1–10.

110. Lavanya, M., Meenakshisundaram, A., Renganathan, S., Chinnasamy, S., Lewis, D. M., Nallasivam, J., & Bhaskar, S., (2016). Hydrothermal liquefaction of freshwater and marine algal biomass: A novel approach to produce distilate fuel fractions through blending and coprocessing of biocrude with petrocrude. *Bioresource Technol., 203*, 228–235.

111. Leow, S., Bradley, I., Vardon, D. R., Sharma, B. K., Guest, J. S., & Strathmann, T. J., (2013). Hydrothermal liquefaction of Chlamydomonas reinhardtii: Influence of varying cell composition on liquid fuel yield and quality. *Abstr Pap Am Chem S., 246*.

112. Leow, S., Witter, J. R., Vardon, D. R., Sharma, B. K., Guest, J. S., & Strathmann, T. J., (2015). Prediction of microalgae hydrothermal liquefaction products from feedstock biochemical composition. *Green Chem., 17*(6), 3584–3599.

113. Li, H., Liu, Z. D., Zhang, Y. H., Li, B. M., Lu, H. F., Duan, N., Liu, M. S., Zhu, Z. B., & Si, B. C., (2014). Conversion efficiency and oil quality of low-lipid high-protein and high-lipid low-protein microalgae via hydrothermal liquefaction. *Bioresource Technol., 154*, 322–329.

114. Kruse, A., Krupka, A., Schwarzkopf, V., Gamard, C., & Henningsen, T., (2005). Influence of proteins on the hydrothermal gasification and liquefaction of biomass. 1. Comparison of different feedstocks. *Ind Eng Chem Res., 44*(9), 3013–3020.

115. Kruse, A., Maniam, P., & Spieler, F., (2007). Influence of proteins on the hydrothermal gasification and liquefaction of biomass. 2. Model compounds. *Ind Eng Chem Res., 46*(1), 87–96.

116. Castello, D., Kruse, A., & Fiori, L., (2015). Low temperature supercritical water gasification of biomass constituents: Glucose/phenol mixtures. *Biomass Bioenerg., 73*, 84–94.

117. Castello, D., Kruse, A., & Fiori, L., (2014). Supercritical water gasification of hydrochar. *Chem Eng Res Des., 92*(10), 1864–1875.

118. Dinjus, E., Dahmen, N., & Kruse, A., (2009). Refining biomass into chemical energy. *Przem Chem., 88*(8), 856–860.

119. Kruse, A., Bernolle, P., Dahmen, N., Dinjus, E., Maniam, P., (2010). Hydrothermal gasification of biomass: consecutive reactions to long-living intermediates. *Energ. Environ. Sci., 3*(1), 136–143.

120. Gasafi, E., Meyer, L., & Schebek, L., (2007). Exergetic efficiency and options for improving sewage sludge gasification in supercritical water. *Int J. Energ. Res., 31*(4), 346–363.

121. Schmieder, H., Abeln, J., Boukis, N., Dinjus, E., Kruse, A., Kluth, M., Petrich, G., Sadri, E., & Schacht, M., (2000).Hydrothermal gasification of biomass and organic wastes. *J. Supercrit Fluid, 17*(2), 145–153.

122. Demirbas, A., (2010). Hydrogen Production from Biomass via Supercritical Water Gasification. *Energ Source Part A., 32*(14), 1342–1354.

123. Demirbas, A., (2005). Hydrogen production from biomass via supercritical water extraction. *Energ Source., 27*(15), 1409–1417.

124. Demirbas, A., (2004). Hydrogen-rich gas from fruit shells via supercritical water extraction. *Int J Hydrogen Energ., 29*(12), 1237–1243.

125. Demirbas, A., (2010). Sub- and Super-critical Water Depolymerization of Biomass. *Energ Source Part A., 32*(12), 1100–1110.

126. Castello, D., Kruse, A., & Fiori, L., (2014). Supercritical Water Gasification of Glucose/Phenol Mixtures as Model Compounds for Ligno-Cellulosic Biomass. *Iconbm: International Conference on Biomass, Pts 1 and 2., 37*, 193–198.

127. Yanik, J., Ebale, S., Kruse, A., Saglam, M., & Yuksel, M., (2008). Biomass gasification in supercritical water: II. Effect of catalyst. *Int J Hydrogen Energ., 33*(17), 4520–4526.

128. Sheikhdavoodi, M. J., Almassi, M., Ebrahimi-Nik, M., Kruse, A., & Bahrami, H., (2015). Gasification of sugarcane bagasse in supercritical water, evaluation of alkali catalysts for maximum hydrogen production. *J. Energy Inst., 88*(4), 450–458.

129. Demirbas, A., (2009). Biorefineries: Current activities and future developments. *Energ Convers Manage, 50*(11), 2782–2801.

130. Demirbas, A., (2008). Biohydrogen generation from organic waste. *Energ Source Part A., 30*(5), 475–482.

131. Demirbas, A., (2007). Progress and recent trends in biofuels. *Prog Energ Combust., 33*(1), 1–18.

132. Wang, J. B., Fu, W. T., He, X. W., Yang, S. X., & Zhu, W. P., (2014).Catalytic wet air oxidation of phenol with functionalized carbon materials as catalysts: Reaction mechanism and pathway. *J Environ Sci-China., 26*(8), 1741–1749.

133. Wang, S. Z., Yang, Q., Bai, Z. Y., Wang, S. D., Chen, H., & Cao, Y., (2015). Catalytic Wet Air Oxidation of Wastewater of the Herbicide Fomesafen Production with CeO2-TiO2 Catalysts. *Environ. Eng. Sci., 32*(5), 389–396.

134. Yang, J., Wang, J. B., Yang, S. X., Wang, Y. H., & He, X. W., (2015). Catalytic Wet Air Oxidation of Phenol Over the Graphene Oxide as Catalysts. *International Conference on Energy and Environment Engineering (Iceee 2015)., 334–340.

135. Zhang, Z., Yang, R. Y., Umar, A., Gao, Y. S., Wang, J. Y., Lu, P., Guo, Z. H., Huang, L., Zhou, T. T., & Wang, Q., (2014). Synthesis of ZnMoO4/Na2Mo4O13/alpha-MoO3 Hybrid Catalyst for the Catalytic Wet Air Oxidation of Dye Under Room Condition. *Sci Adv Mater 6* (10), 2159–2164.

136. Luck, F., (1996). A review of industrial catalytic wet air oxidation processes. *Catal Today., 27* (1–2), 195–202.

137. Debellefontaine, H., Chakchouk, M., Foussard, J. N., Tissot, D., & Striolo, P., (1996). Treatment of organic aqueous wastes: Wet air oxidation and wet peroxide oxidation(R). *Environ Pollut., 92*(2), 155–164.

138. Fajerwerg, K., & Debellefontaine, H., (1996). Wet oxidation of phenol by hydrogen peroxide using heterogeneous catalysis Fe-ZSM-5: A promising catalyst. *Appl Catal B-Environ., 10*(4), L229-L235.

139. Bhargava, S. K., Tardio, J., Prasad, J., Foger, K., Akolekar, D. B., & Grocott, S. C., (2006). Wet oxidation and catalytic wet oxidation. *Ind Eng Chem Res., 45*(4), 1221–1258.

140. Arena, F., Di Chio, R., Gumina, B., Spadaro, L., & Trunfio, G., (2015). Recent advances on wet air oxidation catalysts for treatment of industrial wastewaters. *Inorg. Chim. Acta., 431*, 101–109.

141. Hii, K., Baroutian, S., Parthasarathy, R., Gapes, D. J., & Eshtiaghi, N., (2014). A review of wet air oxidation and Thermal Hydrolysis technologies in sludge treatment. *Bioresource Technol., 155*, 289–299.

142. Li, X. Y., Xu, Y., & Sun, D. Z., (2014). Study on coupling with catalytic wet air oxidation and membrane separation in the treatment of cationic red GTL. *Desalin Water Treat., 52*(4–6), 816–823.

143. Malik, S. N., Saratchandra, T., Tembhekar, P. D., Padoley, K. V., Mudliar, S. L., & Mudliar, S. N., (2014). Wet air oxidation induced enhanced biodegradability of distillery effluent. *J. Environ Manage, 136*, 132–138.

144. Sriprom, P., Neramittagapong, S., Lin, C., Wantala, K., Neramittagapong, A., & Grisdanurak, N., (2015). Optimizing chemical oxygen demand removal from synthesized wastewater containing lignin by catalytic wet-air oxidation over CuO/Al2O3 catalysts. *J. Air Waste Manage, 65*(7), 828–836.

145. Weber, B., Chavez, A., Morales-Mejia, J., Eichenauer, S., Stadlbauer, E. A., & Almanza, R., (2015). Wet air oxidation of resorcinol as a model treatment for refractory organics in wastewaters from the wood processing industry. *J. Environ Manage, 161*, 137–143.

146. Zhong, S. J., & Dong, G. W., (2014). Research on wet air oxidation sludge treatment system using nongrid-connected wind power. *Chin. Cont .Decis. Conf.,* 4801–4804.

147. Ledesma, B., Roman, S., Sabio, E., & Alvarez-Murillo, A., (2015). Improvement of spent activated carbon regeneration by wet oxidation processes. *J. Supercrit Fluid, 104*, 94–103.

148. Chen, Z., Wang, G. W., Yin, F. J., Chen, H. Z., & Xu, Y. J., (2015). A new system design for supercritical water oxidation. *Chem. Eng. J., 269*, 343–351.

149. Feng, C. T., & Wang, J., (2015). Treatment of Oily Wastewater Via Supercritical Water Gasification (Scwg). *Oxid Commun 38* (3), 1384–1390.

150. Qian, L. L., Wang, S. Z., & Li, Y. H., (2014). Review of Supercritical Water Oxidation in Hydrothermal Flames. *Materials Science, Environment Protection and Applied Research, 908*, 239–242.

151. Qian, L. L., Wang, S. Z., Xu, D. H., Guo, Y., Tang, X. Y., & Wang, L. F., (2015). Treatment of sewage sludge in supercritical water and evaluation of the combined process of supercritical water gasification and oxidation. *Bioresource Technol., 176*, 218–224.

152. Zhang, J. L., Gu, J. T., Han, Y., Li, W., Gan, Z. X., & Gu, J. J., (2015). Supercritical Water Oxidation vs Supercritical Water Gasification: Which Process Is Better for Explosive Wastewater Treatment? *Ind. Eng. Chem. Res., 54*(4), 1251–1260.

153. Zhang, Y. R., Zhang, L. J., & Zhao, T. T., (2015). Supercritical Water Gasification of Oily Wastewater. *Oxid Commun 38* (2), 803–807.

154. Chen, S. Y., Qu, X., Zhang, R., & Bi, J. C., (2015). Destruction of representative submarine food waste using supercritical water oxidation. *Environ. Sci. Pollut. R., 22*(6), 4527–4533.

155. Dong, X. Q., Wang, Y. Q., Li, X. Q., Yu, Y. Z., & Zhang, M. H., (2014). Process Simulation of Laboratory Wastewater Treatment via Supercritical Water Oxidation. *Ind. Eng. Chem. Res. 53*(18), 7723–7729.

156. Zhang, J. L., Gu, J. T., Han, Y., Li, W., Gan, Z. X., & Gu, J. J., (2015). Analysis of degradation mechanism of disperse orange 25 in supercritical water oxidation using molecular dynamic simulations based on the reactive force field. *J. Mol. Model, 21*(3).

157. Bermejo, M. D., & Cocero, M. J., (2006).Supercritical water oxidation: A technical review. *Aiche., J., 52* (11), 3933–3951.
158. Cabeza, P., Al-Duri, B., Bermejo, M. D., & Cocero, M. J., (2014). Co-oxidation of ammonia and isopropanol in supercritical water in a tubular reactor. *Chem. Eng. Res. Des., 92*(11), 2568–2574.
159. Cabeza, P., Queiroz, J. P. S., Criado, M., Jimenez, C., Bermejo, M. D., Mato, F., & Cocero, M. J., (2015). Supercritical water oxidation for energy production by hydrothermal flame as internal heat source. Experimental results and energetic study. *Energy. 90,* 1584–1594.
160. Garcia-Rodriguez, Y., Mato, F. A., Martin, A., Bermejo, M. D., & Cocero, M. J., (2015). Energy recovery from effluents of supercritical water oxidation reactors. *J. Supercrit. Fluid, 104,* 1–9.
161. Queiroz, J. P. S., Bermejo, M. D., Mato, F., & Cocero, M. J., (2015). Supercritical water oxidation with hydrothermal flame as internal heat source: Efficient and clean energy production from waste. *J., Supercrit. Fluid. 96,* 103–113.
162. Shaw, R. W., & Dahmen, N., (2000). Destruction of toxic organic materials using supercritical water oxidation: Current state of the technology. *Nato., Adv., Sci., I E-App., 366,* 425–437.
163. Akai, Y., Yamada, K., & Sako, T., (2001). Ion-exchange resin decomposition in supercritical water. *High Pressure Res., 20*(1–6), 515–524.

CHAPTER 8

SUSTAINABLE BIOFUELS AND CHEMICALS PRODUCTION USING IONIC LIQUIDS

P. N. AMANIAMPONG,[1] R. BEHLING,[1] N. ARAJI,[1] S. VALANGE,[1] K. DE OLIVEIRA VIGIER,[1] and G. CHATEL[2]

[1]IC2MP UMR CNRS 7285, Université de Poitiers, ENSIP, B1, 1 rue Marcel Doré TSA 41105, 86073 Poitiers Cedex 9, France

[2]Univ. of Savoie Mont Blanc, LCME, F-73000 Chambéry, France

CONTENTS

ABSTRACT

In the last two decades, the use of ionic liquids (ILs) in different areas of chemistry has increased considerably, especially for biomass conversion into fuels and chemicals. This chapter describes the investigations in strategies and innovations based on ILs in terms of dissolution and pretreatment methods and their uses as reaction solvents, catalysts and extraction solvents in biorefinery. Relevant literature examples related to the design of ILs for the valorization of cellulose, lignin and vegetable oil are reported, with emphasis on their impact on the reactivity and reaction pathways to further improve chemical yields. Additionally, several parameters involved in these processes such as the choice of the anion or/and cation of ILs are thoroughly discussed. Significant improvements have been made in recyclability of ILs for a wide range of reactions. This chapter also discusses the renewability and sustainability aspects related to biorefinery processes, where ILs are involved.

8.1   INTRODUCTION ON IONIC LIQUIDS

In the recent years, the use of ionic liquids (ILs), salts with low or no melting point (typically less than 100°C at atmospheric pressure), attracted a lot of interest in different areas of chemistry, especially from the Green Chemistry community [1]. ILs have indeed been identified as a new class of solvents offering opportunities to transfer the traditional chemical processes to new, clean and ecofriendly technologies [2]. They exhibit specific properties that could be used judiciously for the replacement of volatile organic solvents such as low vapor pressure, air and moisture stabilities, high polarity, chemical and electrochemical stabilities, etc. [3, 4].

The application of ILs as reaction media is currently a very active field of research. New strategies involving ILs have been proposed for many applications in organic and pharmaceutical chemistry [5], preparation of materials [6], analytical chemistry [7], energy chemistry [8], electrochemistry [9], microextraction [10], and biomass valorization [11]. Such aspects will be subsequently discussed in the next sections.

Interestingly, Holbrey and Seddon made the estimation of nearly 1 million simple ILs that can be easily prepared in the laboratory, leading to 10^{18} possible ILs, and even more if multiionic systems are considered [12]. In addition, double-salt ionic liquids (DSILs), defined as unique ionic liquid as a function of the composition of each ions (several ions), let imagine many applications or uses as a function of their physicochemical, thermal and solvent properties [13]. This represents a great advantage in terms of tunability for these solvents, but also a limiting drawback in terms of the lack of theoretical and fundamental data about their properties to guide their use.

The most used ILs are generally composed of a bulky organic cation (ammonium, phosphonium and sulfonium) with an alkyl chain associated to an organic or inorganic anion (several cations and anions in the case of DSILs). The synthesis of ILs is generally performed through the first alkylation of an amine, phosphine or sulfide through a quaternization reaction leading to an intermediate salt, followed by anion exchange with a Lewis acid, a metal salt, a Brønsted acid or *via* an ion exchange resin (Figure 8.1) [2–4]. The purification of ILs during and after their synthesis is a challenging step since impurities can have important effects, even at trace levels, for example when biomass is involved in ILs-based processes [14].

The most commonly used cations are 1-alkyl-3-methylimidazolium, 1-alkyl-pyridinium, 1-alkyl-1-methylpyrrolidinium, tetraalkylammonium, tetraalkylphosphonium, and trialkylsulfonium and the common anions are chlorides,

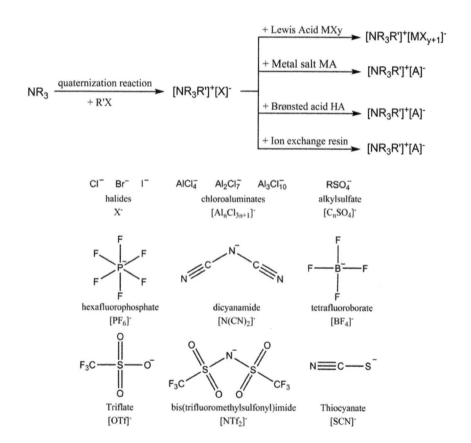

FIGURE 8.1   Principle of the synthesis of ammonium based ILs.

chloroaluminates, hexafluorophosphate, tetrafluoroborate, triflate (or trifluo-romethanesulfonate), thiocyanate, dicyanamide, bis(trifluoromethylsulfonyl) imide, etc. (Figure 8.2). The alphanumeric nomenclature allows naming an IL as a function of the cation and its alkyl chain and the nature of the anion [4]. For example, the 1-butyl-3-methylimidazolium chloride is noted [C_4C_1im]Cl and *N*-octylpyrrolidinium hexafluorophosphate is noted [C_8pyrr][PF_6].

Many recent studies have been exploring the feasibility of using ILs to dissolve, separate, and recover cellulose, hemicellulose, and lignin from lig-nocellulosic biomass [15–22] or also for biofuel production from vegetable oils [23–25].

8.2 DECONSTRUCTION OF LIGNOCELLULOSIC BIOMASS WITH IONIC LIQUIDS (DISSOLUTION AND PRETREATMENT)

Majority of our current energy, liquid fuels and chemicals production are emanating from nonrenewable fossil sources. However, it is anticipated that the nonrenewable resources will eventually run out and cannot be considered as sustainable resources. Nonetheless, lignocellulosic biomass are promising alternatives to the dwindling fossil fuel resources, and been extensively discussed as one of the alternative feedstocks for the energy and chemicals production because of its high energy content, sustainability and

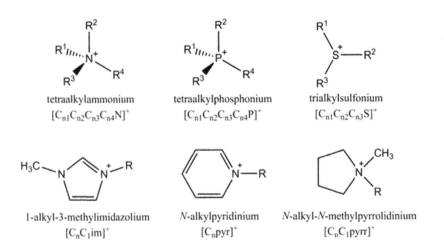

FIGURE 8.2 Names and structures of the most common anions and cations used in the literature.

biodegradability. Lignocellulose consists largely of polymeric carbohydrates (cellulose, accounting for about 40-50% by composition, and hemicellulose) and the aromatic polymer lignin (Figure 8.3) [26]. The exact composition of lignocellulose depends on the species, the plant tissue and the growth conditions.

Traditionally, lignocellulose treatment was focused on the production of a cellulose-enriched pulp for the manufacture of paper and fiber board. Therefore, the current industrially most developed lignocellulose treatment processes are in the area of paper production [27]. Several biomass deconstruction techniques have been developed, such as mechanical, thermal, chemical, and biological methods [18]. For example, in Kraft pulping, the lignocellulosic biomass is subjected to high temperature heating (130–180°C) in an aqueous mixture of sodium hydroxide and sodium hydrogen sulfide for several hours to dissolve most of the lignin and part of the hemicellulose. The main aim for biomass deconstruction processes is to alter the structure of cellulosic biomass to make cellulose more accessible to enzymatic and catalytic actions that convert the carbohydrate polymers into fermentable sugars as shown in Figure 8.4 [28].

The full potential for plant biomass, more specifically lignocellulose, has not been yet fully explored due to the availability of cheap petroleum based polymers, the lack of environmentally friendly techniques

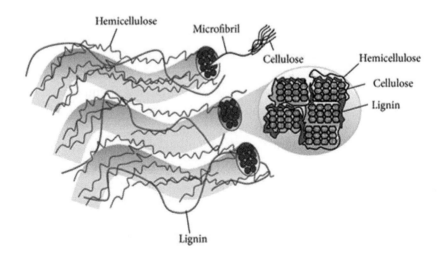

FIGURE 8.3   Plant cell wall structure and microfibril cross-section, with strands of cellulose molecules embedded in a matrix of hemicellulose and lignin [175].

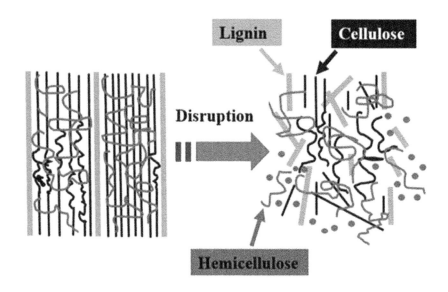

FIGURE 8.4   Disruption of cellulosic biomass by pretreatment.

of extracting cellulose from plant biomass, the challenges in modifying cellulose and the lack of suitable solvent capable of dissolving lignocelluloses [29]. This is a significant drawback that needs to be overcome in order to reach a widespread utilization of lignocelluloses. To render lignocellulose more susceptible to further reactions and processes, pretreatment and or dissolution steps are often required [30, 31]. The primarily goal for these processes is to distort or break the lignin seal and disrupt the crystalline structure of cellulose to make it more reactive to further reactions. To achieve this, the structural and chemical obstacles that hamper the release of carbohydrates must be overcome. A key challenge, however remains; namely, achieving the efficient and selective removal of near native lignin coupled with the enhanced biodegradability of cellulose and hemicellulose. This has been the main concern for recent investigation into finding suitable solvents capable of dissolving cellulose.

It is often suggested that the ability of a solvent to dissolve cellulose is related to its facility to cleave the intermolecular hydrogen bonds present in cellulose polymers [26, 32]. Hydrophobic interactions between cellulose and the dissolving solvent have also been reported to be a key factor for effective dissolution of cellulose [33]. Cellulose has been shown to consist of both hydrophilic and hydrophobic parts [34], and it is also in fact considered to be amphiphilic [34]. This suggests that cosolvents have the ability to weaken the hydrophobic interactions in cellulose or amphiphilic solvents, like ILs should preferably be used to increase the degree of cellulose dissolution [34]. Therefore, understanding the interactions is thus important for the processing of lignocellulosic biomass in ionic liquids.

Developments on the use of ILs for cellulose dissolution in industrial processes, has become an established approach only in the last few years. However, the dissolution of cellulose using ILs is not a novel concept. ILs like ammonium nitrate, $[C_2H_3N][NO_3]$, were mentioned in the early 1900's [35] and the ability of ILs to dissolve cellulose was recognized in 1934 by Graenacher [36]. The importance of the research made by Graenacher was not fully recognized at that time due to the high melting point of the used benzylpyridinium chloride. It was later revealed that ILs with lower melting temperatures may also be used as nonderivatizing solvents for cellulose [37, 38]. Many ILs possess the ability to dissolve cellulose and it has been confirmed both by means of NMR [39, 40], molecular dynamic studies [41] and simulation studies [42] that anions interact with hydroxyl groups of cellulose by forming strong hydrogen bonds between them. This effectively cleaves the intermolecular glycosidic bonds that exist between the individual cellulose molecules. This phenomenon is believed to be the major contributing factor that enables cellulose dissolution in ILs [43] and has also been reported to occur between cellulose and the cation ends of ILs as well [23, 42].

The intermolecular hydrogen bonds cleavage ability is corroborated to its basicity. A strong basicity will result in strong hydrogen bond interaction with the hydrogen on the hydroxyl groups of cellulose and this basicity is primarily influenced by the anion [44]. The importance of the anion's hydrogen-bond basicity is demonstrated in Figure 8.5. Here, cellulose solubilities derived from a plethora of publications are plotted against the Kamlet-Taft β parameters of these liquids, where only dialkylimidazolium cations were considered. One of the anions with the highest basicity is $[CH_3COO]^-$ with a Kammel-Taft β value of 1.2, this anion combined with the cation $[C_2C_1im]^+$ renders the IL $[C_2C_1im][CH_3COO]$ that is known to be one of the best ILs noted for dissolving cellulose [45].

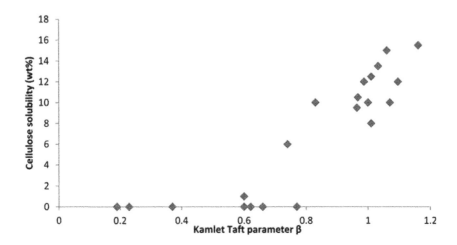

FIGURE 8.5   The Kammel-Taft beta value of dialkylimidazolium-based ILs (a measurement of the ILs basicity) correlated to the cellulose solubility of different ILs. (Reprinted with permission from Brandt, A., Gräsvik, J., Hallett, J. P., & Welton, T. (2013). *Green Chem.*, 15, 550–583. © 2012 Royal Chemistry Society.)

Rogers and co-workers also examined a range of 1-alkyl-3-methylimid-azolium cations and inorganic anions for their abilities to dissolve cellulose. $[C_4C_1im]Cl$ was found to be the most effective room temperature IL capable of dissolving up to 25 % (w/w) cellulose [39]. However, replacing the Cl^- with Br^- or $[SCN]^-$ resulted in substantial lower cellulose dissolution while $[BF_4]^-$ and $[PF_6]^-$ were unable to dissolve cellulose. High-throughput systems have also been developed to identify effective room temperature ILs that solubilize lignocellulose components, based on transmitted light and light scattering measurements. A recent work by Zavrel et al. [31] revealed that, despite the fact that chloride-based ILs were known to be effective solvents for cellulose, $[C_2C_1im][OAc]$ was found to be a good solvent for cellulose for up to 4 % (w/w) at 80°C (Figure 8.6). They also observed and reported that although $[C_2C_1im][BF_4]$ was not an ideal IL solvent for dissolving cel-lulose, $[C_2C_1im]Cl$, $[C_4C_1im]Cl$ and $[(C_1=C_2)C_1im]Cl$ exhibited appreciable dissolution degrees of cellulose. The intrinsic ability of $[C_2C_1im][OAc]$, as well as those of chloride-containing ILs to dissolve cellulose revealed the unique interactions *via* hydrogen bonds and subsequently disruption of the robust crystalline structure of the polysaccharide [31].

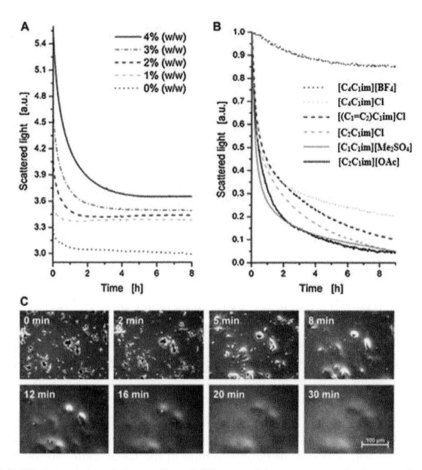

FIGURE 8.6 (a) Dissolution profiles of different weight percentages of microcrystalline cellulose in [C₂C₁im][OAc] at 60°C; (b) Comparison of ionic liquids ability to dissolve 4% (w/w) microcrystalline cellulose at 80°C; (c) *In situ* microscopy pictures of [C₂C₁im][OAc] with 1% (w/w) microcrystalline cellulose. (Reprinted with permission from Zavrel, M., Bross, D., Funke, M., Büchs, J., & Spiess, A. C. (2009). *Biores. Technol., 100*, 2580–2587. © 2008 Elsevier.)

8.3   USE OF IONIC LIQUIDS IN BIOREFINERY

A biorefinery is a facility where different low-value renewable biomass materials are the feedstock to the processes where they are transformed, in multiple steps including fractionation, separation and conversion, to several higher-value bio-based products. In biorefining, one can find similarities to oil refining, with the exception that in the latter case, the raw materials come from fossil resources. The lignocellulosic biorefinery uses naturally dry biomass such as cellulose biomass and agriculture waste to produce biofuels and other bioproducts. Here, the raw material is first cleaned, pretreated to improve accessibility of sugars for subsequent processing and then broken down into its primary constituents (cellulose, hemicellulose and lignin) through biochemical or chemical routes.

The unique and especially easily tuneable properties of ILs make them ideal candidates for reactions media for bio- and chemo-conversion as well as solvents for downstream processing. ILs are used to pretreat biomass through a recalcitrance reduction process to enhance downstream biofuel and chemical production. This pretreatment process typically allows for much higher hydrolysis rates and yields, based on the saccharide content of the feedstock. Furthermore, by applying an ILs treatment to lignocellulosic feedstock the crystallinity of cellulose can be significantly reduced or converted into the more digestible cellulose.

8.3.1 IONIC LIQUIDS AS REACTION SOLVENTS

The usefulness and scope of ILs as reaction solvents in organic reactions, carbohydrate chemistry and catalysis has been extensively reviewed [3, 46]. Lignocellulosic biomass dissolution involving ionic liquids, especially those containing Cl⁻ anion has also been extensively reported in literature [32, 48]. Heinze et al. reported that without using any catalyst, cellulose derivatives with high degree of substitution could be prepared in IL solutions [49]. Also, cellulose with a degree of polymerization in the range from 290 to 1200 could be dissolved in $[C_4C_1im]Cl$ to relatively high concentration (up to ~ 20%) without degradation [50]. The wide range of availability of ILs (cation-anion combinations) offers an attractive option to improve the reactants solubility in the catalyst phase when ILs are used as reaction solvents. It is also often possible to find biphasic IL/organic system for which the catalyst is dissolved and immobilized in the IL (Figure 8.7) [51]. The ideal situation is often seen when IL displays partial miscibility with the substrates and when the products have negligible miscibility with the IL.

The isomerization of 3,4-epoxybut-1-ene to 2,5-dihydrofuran has been described in literature as a reaction step involved in the production of tetrahydrofuran, a valuable chemical compound useful as a chemical process solvent. This reaction process requires simultaneous activation by Lewis base and acid. Phosphonium iodide ionic liquid has hence been employed as

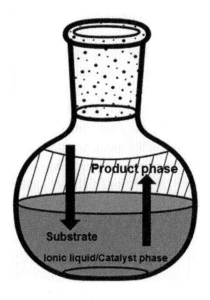

FIGURE 8.7   IL-Liquid/liquid-biphasic concept.

reaction solvents for this isomerization process due it its high thermal stability and as well as its high hydrophobic character, with respect to ammonium analogs [52]. The use of IL as reaction solvents also affords milder reaction conditions, simplified product separation and the ability to remove and replenish the catalyst system.

8.3.2   IONIC LIQUIDS AS CATALYSTS

The potentially most efficient way in which an IL can be used in catalysis is as a combination of solvent and catalyst. Whenever changing solvents leads to a faster reaction, the new solvent can be viewed as a catalyst. ILs has recently been used as reaction catalysts for transesterification of vegetable oils. Typically, Li and co-workers [53] reported a biodiesel yield of 95%, when $[C_6C_1im][HSO_4]$ or $[HSO_3-C_5C_1im][HSO_4]$ ILs were used as catalysts. Ranu et al. [54] employed 1-butyl-3-methylimidazolium hydroxide $[C_4C_1im][OH]$ as an efficient catalyst for the Knoevenagel condensation without the requirement of any organic solvent. The $[C_4C_1im][OH]$ catalyst was recycled for five runs without any loss of efficiency. Their results confirmed the versatility of using ILs as solvents and catalyst at the same time in a one-pot reaction.

8.3.3   IONIC LIQUIDS AS EXTRACTION SOLVENTS

As a favorable separation technique for engineers and chemists, extraction is an energy-efficient technology using two immiscible phases (conventionally an organic phase and an aqueous phase). However, many organic solvents involved in this processes are toxic and flammable volatile organic compounds (VOCs). Therefore, to improve the safety and environmental friendliness of this conventional separation technique, ILs can be used as ideal substitutes because of their stability, nonvolatility and adjustable miscibility and polarity. The ILs based on $[PF_6]^-$ and $[NTf_2]^-$ (bis [(trifluoromethyl)sulfony]amide) are water immiscible, therefore, they are solvents of choice for forming biphasic systems in most IL extraction applications [55]. Typically, the hydrophobic character of ILs allows them to extract hydrophobic compounds in biphasic separations. The use of ILs as extraction solvents has been reported for metal ion extractions that have particular industrial significance [56, 57]. The high degree of solubility of charged organic molecules in ILs has also stimulated the development of organic product recovery by ILs. Furthermore, IL biphasic systems are widely used to separate many biologically important molecules such as carbohydrates (Figure 8.7), [58, 59] organic acids including lactic acid, [58] butyl alcohol [58] and polyketide antibiotic erythromycin-A [62].

8.4   DESIGN OF IONIC LIQUIDS FOR BIOMASS VALORIZATION

The current section is not attempted to be exhaustive on the complete review of existing literature, but rather to focus on precise and relevant examples to show how ILs can be a solvent/catalyst of choice for the chemical valorization of cellulose, lignin or vegetable oils.

8.4.1   CELLULOSE VALORIZATION

The adventure started with the discovery of Rogers et al. at the beginning of the 2000s, reporting the use of ILs as an efficient nonderivatizing solvent for cellulose [39]. They particularly showed that ILs incorporating anions which are hydrogen bond acceptors were most effective, especially in combination with microwave heating. $[C_4C_1im]Cl$, $[C_6C_1im]Cl$, $[C_8C_1im]Cl$ appeared to be the most effective solvents compared to $[BF_4]^-$, $[PF_6]^-$ or $[SCN]^-$ based ILs, presumably solubilizing cellulose through hydrogen-bonding from hydroxyl functions to the chloride of the solvent [39]. From this work, several research groups investigated the role of different ILs on cellulose dissolution, chemical modification or even for the preparation of new cellulosic materials [63]. The valorization of cellulose through the use of ILs was recently widely reviewed [26, 30, 64] as a result, only recent and innovative examples from literature are reported here in this current chapter. H-bonding seems to play a paramount role: several computational studies on cellulose dissolution/regeneration in ILs reported that the dissolution in ILs is initiated by the disruption of H-bonds in cellulose, driven by the formation of H-bonds between cellulose and anions, as well as the hydrophobic interactions with cations [65]. This strong role of H-bonding was also shown in different studies investigating the addition of other organic solvents in ILs media [66, 67].

Indeed, the ability of ILs to dissolve cellulose with no derivatization under mild conditions, and the easy regeneration of the same molecular weight cellulose with any given shape, rheology or function, provide a platform for a wide variety of new advanced materials [65]. In addition, several chemical modifications of cellulose dissolved in ILs have been investigated to obtained functions such as ester, ether, amine, sulfate, hemicacetal, silylether, carbanilate, etc. [68–70]. To resume, ILs represents an innovative platform for the conversion of cellulose into valuable chemicals, either as a pretreatment method (see Section 8.2) or as a conversion solvent, essentially for its hydrolysis and fermentation to ethanol or biofuels.

Some catalytic hydrolyses of cellulose were reported in the literature. For example, Zhang et al. showed the use of a magnetic core–shell $Fe_3O_4@SiO_2$–SO_3H acid catalyst to hydrolyse Avicel PH-101 (DP 220) in $[C_4C_1im]$ Cl at 130°C during 8 h with a 73% yield of reduced sugars of (51% of glucose, 11% of cellobiose, 7% of cellotriose, 4% of cellotetraose and traces of cellopentaose and cellohexose). HMF and levulinic acid were also produced with 8% and 5%, yields, respectively [71].

Petrich et al. performed the enzymatic hydrolysis of cellulose using a pure cellulase (endo-1,4-glucanase) in the tris-(2-hydroxyethyl)-methylammonium methylsulfate IL [72]. Interestingly, they showed the increase of heat tolerance of the enzyme in the selected IL by fluorescence studies (the transition temperature shifted from 55°C in buffer solution to 75°C in the IL). Viscosity, pH, and polarity had also been studied.

Itoh et al. reported the use of halogen-free ILs, consisting of a nontoxic ammonium cation and a natural amino acid [73]. Thus, the biodegradation of cellulose regenerated from a N,N-diethyl-N-(2-methoxyethyl)-N-methylammonium alanine [N$_{221ME}$][Ala] solution to glucose using cellulose (Accellerase DUET) proceeded very quickly. The conversion reached 88% after 10 h reaction at 50°C at pH 5.0 when regenerated cellulose was subjected to the hydrolysis, while the conversion was less than 40% when original cellulose was used as substrate. Interestingly, the cellulose regenerated from the IL was only of the Type II form, indicating that the transformation of cellulose from Type I to Type II occurred after the dissolution and regeneration in [N$_{221ME}$][Ala], facilitating the hydrolysis reaction.

The hydrolysis of cellulose was also directly performed in homogeneous conditions by the addition of a catalytic amount of HCl in the dissolve cellulose in [C$_4$C$_1$im]Cl. After stirring for 180 min at 378 K, the cellulose was fully converted, leading to a total selectivity to glucose + cellobiose of about 99% [74]. In this study, the IL exhibited a unique role as reaction solvent in dissolving cellulose under stirring for 60 min at 378 K and favored the homogeneous catalytic acidic hydrolysis of cellulose. Interestingly, Xia et al. proposed the use of SO$_3$H-functionalized acidic ILs as acid catalyst to promote the hydrolysis of microcrystalline cellulose (MCC) in [C$_4$C$_1$im] Cl [75]. Triethyl-(3-sulfo-propyl)-ammonium hydrogen sulfate (Figure 8.8) was the optimum ionic liquid for the study of cellulose hydrolysis, with a maximum of total reducing sugars yield up to 99% at 100°C. In this case, the relatively cheap [C$_4$C$_1$im]Cl is use for dissolution process, and the miscible SO$_3$H-functionalized IL plays the role of acidic catalyst. Authors also highlighted that the water content in [C$_4$C$_1$im]Cl can have negative effect on cellulose hydrolysis, that is why a strict purification procedure for the synthesis and recycling of ILs is required for this kind of processes [76].

The patent on homogeneous synthesis of cellulose ethers reported the functionalization in different ILs, especially [C$_2$C$_1$im][OAc], [C$_2$C$_1$C$_1$im] [OAc] and [C$_2$C$_1$C$_1$im]Cl under mild conditions (Table 8.1, Entry 1) [76]. Due to the absence of organic and inorganic bases, only minor degradation of chain length of the cellulose ether was observed. In addition, it is possible to control the degree of substitution by varying the molar ratio of etherification reagent per anhydroglucose unit, reaction time and temperature.

The acylation of cellulose was also investigated with the fatty acid chloride lauroyl chloride leading to cellulose laurates with a degree of substitution from 0.34 to 1.54 (Table 8.1, Entry 2) [77]. The reaction starts homogeneously and continues heterogeneously. The synthesis of cellulose carbanilates succeeds in the ionic liquid [C$_4$C$_1$im]Cl without any catalyst. This homogeneous path gives pure cellulose carbanilates. All reactions are carried out under mild

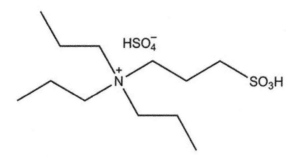

FIGURE 8.8   Structure of the triethyl-(3-sulfo-propyl)-ammonium hydrogen sulfate IL.

conditions, low excess of reagent and a short reaction time (< 2 h). The reaction media applied can be easily recycled and reused. The dilution of ILs with DMSO led to the carboymethylation of cellulose (Table 8.1, Entry 4) in presence of solid NaOH and sodium monochloroacetate [78].

The homogeneous acetylation of cellulose was also efficiently performed in 1-allyl-3-methylimidazolium chloride presenting interesting advantages such as catalyst-free, rapid, degree of substitution value-controllable, and solvent recyclable (Table 8.1, Entry 3) [79]. Other cellulose esters, such as propionates, butyrates, inorganic acid esters, and/or mixed cellulose esters, also can be obtained through homogeneous esterification of cellulose by using corresponding acylating agents.

An example of glutarylation of sugarcane bagasse cellulose in 1-butyl-3-methylimidazolium chloride in the absence of catalyst was reported under low frequency ultrasound irradiation (Table 8.1, Entry 5) [80]. The degree of substitution ranging from 0.22 to 1.20 was obtained in one-step homogeneous modification, which increased with ultrasound irradiation time, temperature and the molar ratio of glutaric anhydride/anhydroglucose unit in cellulose. Even if the mechanisms were not really investigated, a synergetic effect of the ultrasound/IL combination was noted. The physical effects of the cavitation seem to be responsible of these improvements in the reactivity [81].

Interestingly, ILs was investigated for the conversion of cellulose into 5-hydroxymethylfurfural (HMF), which is considered to a valuable and versatile intermediate in the synthesis of plastics, pharmaceuticals, and fine chemicals (Figure 8.9) [82, 83]. As HMF is the dehydration product of glucose, it is preferable to covert cellulose directly into HMF without the separation of glucose.

TABLE 8.1 Recent Functionalization of Dissolved Cellulose in ILs

Entry	Reaction	Used ILs	Conditions	Observations	Ref.
1	Etherification	$[C_2C_1im][OAc]$, $[C_2C_1im][OAc]$, $[C_2C_1im]C_1$	20 to 130°C, 7 to 20 h, etherification reagent (ex: propylene oxide)	The obtained cellulose ethers show a novel substitution pattern which gives rise to alternative interesting properties of the cellulose ethers.	[77]
2	Acetylation and carbanilation	$[C_2C_1im]Cl$, $[C_4C_1im]C_1$, $[C_4C_1im]C_1$, $[(C_1=C_2)C_1C_1]Br$	80°C, 2 h, acetyl chloride or phenyl isocyanate	Cellulose acetates with different degrees of substitution can be obtained by varying the molar ratio and the reaction time.	[78]
3	Acetylation	$[(C_1=C_2)C_1]C_1$	80 to 100°C, 15 min to 23 h, under N_2 atmosphere, acetylating reagent (acetic anhydride)	The degree of substitution of the products increases as reaction time prolongs. The reaction can be accelerated through raising the temperature. Increasing the molar ratio of acetic anhydride/D-anhydroglucopyranose units generally increases the degree of substitution of the product.	[80]
4	Carboxymethylation	$[C_4C_1im]C_1$, $[C_4C_1pyr]C_1$, $[BzC_{14}C_1C_1N]C_1$	80°C, 2 h, DMSO, NaOH, ClCH2COONa	The clear solution of cellulose in $[C_4C_1im]$ Cl/DMSO showed optical anisotropic phases between crossed polarizing filters.	[79]
5	Glutarylation	$[C_4C_1im]C_1$	70 to 90°C, 20 to 120 min, glutaric anhydride	Synergetic effects of the ultrasound and IL combination.	[81]

For example, K. C.-W Wu et al. used mesoporous titania nanoparticles for the conversion of cellulose into glucose and HMF in $[C_2C_1im]Cl$ during 3 h at 120°C, leading to maximum yields of glucose and HMF of 13% and 18%, respectively [84]. Enhanced HMF yield (29%) was reached in the presence of mesoporous zirconia nanoparticles at 450°C, due to a strong acidity of the catalyst.

Y. Wu et al. investigated the use of metal chlorides ($CrCl_3$, $CuCl_2$, $SnCl_4$, WCl_6) in $[C_4C_1im]Cl$ for the conversion of microcrystalline cellulose [85]. $CrCl_3$ exhibited the best performance with more than 63% yield of HMF obtained at 120°C after 4 h at atmospheric pressure. However, when filter paper or cotton was used as the raw material, a low yield of HMF (40% for filter paper and 12% for cotton) was obtained. Authors also demonstrated that low content of water in reaction mixture is beneficial for the production of HMF. In addition, the system has been reused nine times in this study.

Zhao et al. combined the use of $ZrCl_4$ as catalyst and $[C_4C_1im]$ Cl as ionic liquid, with the microwave irradiations, showing a clear synergetic effect [86]. Under optimal conditions, a high HMF yield up to 51.4% was obtained from cellulose in only 3.5 min under microwave irradiations (400 W) while 18.2% was obtained under classical conditions (without microwave irradiations), showing the importance of the thermal effect of microwave in the reaction.

Y. Wu et al. also proposed the innovative approach to catalyze the conversion of cellulose to HMF using bifunctional ionic liquids, preparing by mixing 1-(3-sulfonic acid) propane-3-methylimidazole hydrosulfate IL ($[C_3\text{-}SO_3HC_1im][HSO_4]$) with $CrCl_3$ or $CrCl_3$-$CuCl_2$ [87]. Interestingly, a solvent-catalyst $Cr([C_3\text{-}SO_3HC_1im][HSO_4])_3$ led to a maximum yield of HMF of 53% with 95% conversion of cellulose after 5 h at 120°C. This catalytic system has been reused several times. However, a detailed reaction mechanism of this system is needed and the reusability of the IL has to be deeply studied to improve the economical route of the process.

In summary, the use of ILs in cellulose processing has become a topic of burgeoning interest. The scientific discovery of the dissolution of cellulose in ILs is being translated into new processing technologies, cellulose functionalization methods and new cellulose materials including blends, composites, fibers and ion gels [64]. The functionalization of cellulose using ILs generally allows the reduction of reaction time, the reduction or absence of catalyst amount, the possibility to control the yield of cellulose derivatives and the degree of substitution. In addition, due to the use of IL, the separation and purification step are improved, with in many cases, the possibility of

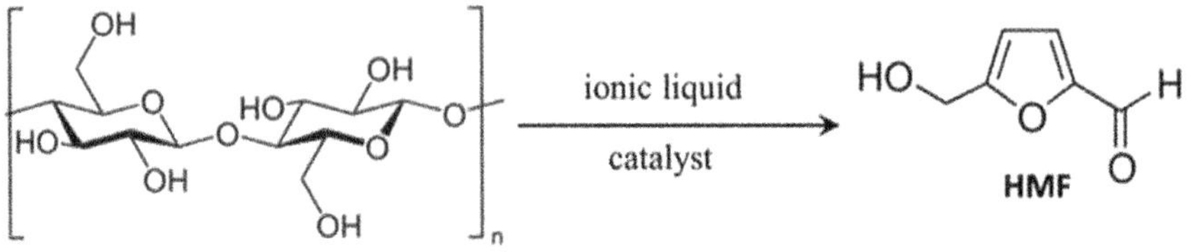

FIGURE 8.9   Investigation of the use of ILs for the conversion of cellulose into HMF.

recycle the solvent for several runs [49]. Additionally, the presence of water (an important contaminant of biomass) is known to have a negative effect on the dissolution of cellulose in ILs. As a consequence, most of the ILs require to be dried prior to dissolving cellulose, which dramatically raises their price to an unacceptable level for use on a large scale. By changing the nature of anions and cations, the water tolerance properties of ILs can be designed. For example, Boissou et al. recently reported various technical grade alkyl ammonium-derived ILs based on levulinate anion showing a great tolerance to the presence of water (up to 18 wt%) [88].

8.4.2   LIGNIN VALORIZATION

Lignin is an aromatic cross-linked biopolymer with a complex amorphous heterogeneous structure comprising phenylpropane type units. It accounts for 20 up to 30% of the organic carbon in the Earth's biosphere. Lignin represents an integral part of the secondary cell walls of lignocellulosic biomass such as wood, annual plants and some algae, with variable content depending on the species. The most common linkage between the lignin building units is the β-O-4 ether bond, representing from 50% (softwood lignin) to 65% (hardwood lignin) of all intersubunit bonds of this type. Lignin is of great value because it is the only renewable source for the production of key and high-volume aromatic compounds in the chemical industry. However, essentially due to its complex recalcitrant polyphenolic structure, this naturally occurring macromolecule is traditionally employed for heat and power purposes through combustion in the pulp and paper industry. Today, the valorization of lignin into the production of chemical feedstocks represents a real challenge both in terms of sustainability and environmental protection [89]. Novel strategies and techniques to chemically valorize lignin are continuously being reported in the literature, among which ILs are being given a lot of attention to. Mainly used to extract lignin from lignocellulosic biomass, ILs have also recently emerged as a reaction media strategy to valorize lignin into value-added chemicals. Task-specific ILs are not only able to extract and dissolve lignin at low temperatures and pressures, but they can also be used as a catalyst for lignin surface modifications or conversion of lignin into functional materials.

In 2013, Yinghuai et al. reviewed the applications of ILs in lignin chemistry [90]. Regarding lignin extraction from plants with ionic liquids, they reported that the ideal IL should possess the following properties: (1) high dissolution capacity for lignin; (2) low melting point; (3) good thermal stability; (4) nonvolatile; (5) nontoxic; (6) chemically stable; (7) not conducive to lignin decomposition; (8) easy lignin regeneration and (9) low cost and simple process. The extracted lignin can then be chemically modified to generate value-added aromatic compounds through oxidation, dehydration or esterification. When small aromatics are desired, a depolymerization process should take place. However, still a major point that needs to be further explored is the recover and regeneration of ILs. Due to the π-π interaction between ILs and lignin, removal of lignin from ILs is indeed a complex process that requires multiple steps [91]. A particular attention should therefore be paid to the recycling of ILs in order to improve the greenness of the dissolution–separation process.

In another recent review, the use of ILs was reported as an innovative strategy to form renewable chemicals from the oxidation of lignin and lignin model compounds [92]. It has been shown that most of the ILs-based oxidation experiments on lignin samples were carried out with organosolv or soda lignins (Table 8.2, entries 1–6, [93–98]). The reason is that such technical lignins have compositions and structures close to natural lignin, while having a high chemical purity. Among the ILs used, ILs mainly based on phosphate and sulfonate anions proved to be stable against oxidation while able to dissolve lignin. More importantly, some ILs were shown to induce selectivity in lignin oxidation processes. The access to new compounds was also reported in the presence of such ILs. The possible control of this selectivity to a specific reactivity by changing the experimental conditions (IL nature, reaction temperature, catalyst loading, extracting solvent, etc.) needs to be investigated more in depth to provide new insight into IL-promoted lignin oxidation to value-added chemicals.

The beneficial roles of ILs for lignin depolymerization processes have been recently compiled in an extensive overview by Luque and co-workers [99]. Regarding the design of ILs for lignin depolymerization strategies, it has been demonstrated that anions mostly affect the structural integrity of lignin while cations only have spectator roles. Alkylsulfonate anions are the most effective in terms of reducing the polydispersity of the biopolymer. The anion nucleophilicity seems to be the prominent property for lignin depolymerization, since the anion can possibly attack highly electron deficient protonated C–O bonds.

In addition to these comprehensive reviews, here we wish to highlight the most recent use of ILs as solvent or catalyst that have afforded opportunities to efficiently convert raw lignin into platform aromatic chemicals. Zhang and co-workers reported on the conversion of a series of lignin β–O–4 model compounds and organosolv lignin to aromatic chemicals over methyltrioxorhenium (MTO) in ILs without any oxidant and reducing agent under mild conditions [100]. Various ILs were studied for the β–O–4 model compounds ($[C_4C_1im]Cl$, $[C_4C_1im][BF_4]$, $[C_4C_1im][PF_6]$, $[C_4C_1C_1im]$ Cl, $[C_4C_1im][NTf_2]$), but the reaction with organosolv lignin was performed only with $[C_4C_1im][NTf_2]$. The reaction mixture was subjected to microwave irradiation of 240 W at 180°C (Table 8.3, entry 1). The lignin model compounds were converted to their corresponding phenols as the primary products with yields as high as 69%. Depolymerization of a birch wood derived organosolv lignin under microwaves produced a wide range of aromatic compounds, with 34.2% yield of the main phenolic syringyl and guaiacyl monomers only within 2 min. Besides being able to dissolve lignin, $[C_4C_1im][NTf_2]$ exhibited excellent dielectric properties for transformation of microwave energy into heat. Microwave irradiation was shown to accelerate the cleavage of aryl ether bonds, thereby shortening the reaction time to 2 min.

With the aim of circumventing difficulties in product separation and catalyst recycling, a novel and efficient water/oil (W/O) emulsion reactor for organosolv lignin depolymerization was recently reported using $[C_4\text{-}SO_3C_4im][HSO_4]$ as ionic liquid catalyst [101]. Several types of lignin (tapioca, rice straw, bagasse, corn stalk and corncob) were studied (Table 8.3, entry 2). During the reaction process, lignin could stabilize the emulsion and be degraded simultaneously at the W/O interface. The main depolymerization products identified were phenol, 4-ethylphenol, 4-ethyl-2-methoxyphenol and 2,6-dimethoxyphenol. Such emulsion reactor demonstrated a

TABLE 8.2 Lignin Valorization Using Ionic Liquids—Works Covering Years 2010–2013.

Entry	Type of lignin	Catalyst	Reaction	Conditions	IL	Role of IL	Recycling	Products	Ref
1	Alcell Organosolv Soda	Co(salen) CoCl$_2$.6H$_2$O	Homogeneous Oxidation	80°C, 3h O$_2$ (0.5 MPa) NaOH	[C$_2$C$_1$im] [Et$_2$PO$_4$]	Easy dissolution of catalyst and lignin samples	Not investigated	Oxidated lignin	[94]
2	Organosolv	Mn, Fe and Cu salts	Homogeneous Oxidation	100°C, 24h air (8 MPa)	[C$_2$C$_1$im] [CF$_3$SO$_3$] [C$_2$C$_1$im] [MeSO$_3$] [C$_2$C$_1$im] [EtSO$_4$] [C$_1$C$_1$im] [MeSO$_4$]	Solvent of the reaction	Attempted IL recycling	Syringol Vanillin DMBQ Syringaldehyde Coniferyl-fragment Sinapinic acid Vanillic acid	[95]
3	Alkali Lignin	Use of an active Ru/V/ Ti mixed oxide as electrodes	Electro-catalytic oxidative cleavage	1.0, 1.3, 1.5 and 1.7V oxidation potentials investigated	[C3HN] [MeSO3]	Easy dissolution of lignin sample, solvent of the reaction	IL easily regenerated	3-Methylfuran 3-Methylfuraldehyde Benzaldehyde Acetovanillone m-Tolualdehyde 2,6-Di-tert-butyl -4-methyl-phenol 2-Methoxy-4-vinylphenol Diphenylether Vanillic acid Syringaldehyd	[96]

TABLE 8.2 (Continued)

Entry	Type of lignin	Catalyst	Reaction	Conditions	IL	Role of IL	Recycling	Products	Ref.
								Vanillin	
								4-Methoxy-biphenyl	
								Guaiacol	
								Syringol	
4	Organosolv	Nanopalladium pyridinium salt of iron bis(dicarbollide)	Oxidation	120°C, 18h O2 (0.4 MPa)	[C4C1im][PF6]/ [C4C1im][MeSO4] (2:1, v/v)	Stabilization of NPs, solubilization of lignin samples	Catalyst reused five times	Syringaldehyde Vanillin p-Hydroxy-benzaldehyde 2,6-Dimethoxy-1,4-benzoquinone	[97]
5	Rubber wood	-	Oxidation	O2 (9.4 L.min−1)	[C1C1im][MeSO4]	Solvent of the reaction	Not investigated	Vanillin	[98]
6	Organosolv	CuSO4	Homogeneous Oxidation	175°C, 1.5h O2 (2.5 MPa)	[C1C1im][Me2PO4] [C1pyr][Me2PO4] [C1C2C2C2N][Me2PO4] [C1morph][Me2PO4]	Solvent Easy separation	IL phase used six times	Vanillin Syringaldehyde p-Hydroxy-benzaldehyde	[99]

more significant process intensification effect on lignin depolymerization, with 3.3 times more desired phenolic compounds than for a reactor without emulsification. Another advantage of this water/oil emulsion reactor is that both the organic solvent (n-butanol) and the IL catalyst can be recycled easily. The enriched ionic liquid water phase can be reused directly.

Yan et al. [102] investigated the treatment of enzymatically hydrolyzed lignin (EHL) in dialkylimidazolium-based ionic liquid (IL)–water mixtures (50–100 wt% IL content) at 150°C for 3 h (Table 8.3, entry 3). Besides the reaction pH, IL anion (chloride, acetate and methylsulfonate) and IL content were found to greatly influence the degradation and chemical transformation of the lignin structure. 1-Butyl-3-methylimidazolium methylsulfonate–water mixtures with low pH promoted lignin depolymerization, but destroyed the regenerated lignin substructure. Structural variations of lignin were thoroughly characterized by 2D ^{1}H-^{13}C heteronuclear single quantum coherence (2D-HSQS) NMR, GPC and elemental analysis. Regenerated lignin with low molecular weight and narrow polydispersity index (2.2–7.7) was obtained using a 1-butyl-3-methylimidazolium acetate-based system. Water addition was shown to inhibit lignin depolymerization at IL content of 50–100 wt%, except for 70% 1-butyl-3-methylimidazolium chloride-water mixture. Compared with sole IL treatment, the beneficial role of IL–water mixture in the breakdown of interunit linkages and ratio of syringyl to guaiacyl units in regenerated lignin was demonstrated.

In a very recent work reported by Prado et al., two ILs, namely butylimidazolium hydrogensulfate $[C_4C_1im][HSO_4]$ and triethylammonium hydrogensulfate $[C_2C_2C_2HN][HSO_4]$ were used for the delignification of *Miscanthus Giganteus* and subsequent lignin depolymerization by oxidation with H_2O_2 directly applied to the black liquors [103]. Due to imidazolium-derived ILs toxicity, they compared the obtained results with the ammonium derived IL in order to get a greener process (Table 8.3, entry 4). It was observed that lignins derived from butylimidazolium hydrogen sulfate were more susceptible to degradation. The $[C_2C_2C_2HN][HSO_4]$ IL was less reactive thereby leading to lower lignin yields in the pretreatment, but generated no contaminated phenolics. The highest phenolic yield was obtained for 5% H_2O_2 with guaiacol as the main product.

In addition to ILs recycling, more attention must be also paid to the development of energy-efficient lignin processing (Table 8.3, entry 5). In this respect, Croft and co-workers evaluated very recently, through electrochemical oxidation, the mediator 2,2'-azinobis (3-ethylbenthiazoline-6-sulfonic

TABLE 8.3 Most Recent Examples of Lignin Valorization (Oxidative and Reductive Depolymerization) Using ILs (On 2014–2016 Period)

Entry	Type of lignin	Catalyst	Reaction	Conditions	IL	Role of IL	Recycling	Products	Ref
1	Organosolv	Methyltrioxorhenium (MTO)	Oxidative cleveage	180°C MW (240W), 2 min	[C4C1im][NTf2]	Solvent of the reaction	Not investigated	Vanillin Vanillin; 2,6-Dimethoxy-phenol; 2,6-Dimethoxy-4-methyl-benzaldehyde; 2,6-Di-*tert*-butyl-4-methylphenol; 2,6-Dimethoxy-4-butyl-phenol; 3,5-Dimethoxy-4-hydroxy-benzaldehyde; 3,5-Dimethoxy-4-hydroxyaceto-phenone	[101]
2	Organosolv	Ionic liquid	Emulsion Reactor Process	250°C, 30min Water-n-heptane-n-hexane	[C4SO3-C4im][HSO4]	Catalyst of the reaction	IL easily recycled	Phenol, 4-Ethyl-phenol; 4-Ethyl-2-methoxy-phenol; 2,6-Dimethoxyl-phenol	[102]

3	Enzymatically hydrolyzed lignin (EHL)	Ionic liquid	150°C 3h IL–water mixtures (50–100 wt% IL content)	[C4C1im]Cl [C4C1im][OAc] [C4C1im][MeSO3]	Dissolution of lign-in/Reaction catalyst	Not investigated	Lignin with low molecular weight and narrow polydispersity index (2.2–7.7)	[103]
4	Organosolv	-	Oxidation 120°C, 1h, 0–10% H2O2	[C4Him][HSO4] [C2C2-C2HN][HSO4]	Solvent of the reaction	[C4Him][HSO4] (oxidized) [C2C2C-2HN][HSO4] (recycled)	Phenol o-Cresol Guaiacol Catechol Methoxycatechol Syringol Vanillin Acetovanillone 4-Hydroxy-3-methoxyphenyl acetone Vanillic acid Syringaldehyde 3,5-Dimethoxy-4-hydroxy acetophenone	[104]

TABLE 8.3 (Continued)

Entry	Type of lignin	Catalyst	Reaction	Conditions	IL	Role of IL	Recycling	Products	Ref
5	Organosolv Kraft Lignosulfonate	2,2'-azinobis (3-ethylbenthiazoline-6-sulfonic acid) diammonium salt (ABTS)	Electro-oxidation	10–50 mV.s−1 5–20% (V/V) buffer + IL + ABTS	[C_2C_1im] [EtSO$_4$]	-	Not investigated	Not specified	[105]
6	Dealkalized Lignin and Organosolv	NPs: Pd, Pt, Rh, Ru	Reduction Reductive cleaveage	130°C 10h H2 (5 MPa) H3PO4	[C_4C_1im] [PF$_6$]	Solvent of the reaction	Yes (but with model compound)	Cyclohexane	[106]

acid) diammonium salt (ABTS), commonly used with enzyme degradation systems, for enhancing the oxidation of three types of lignin (organosolv, Kraft and lignosulfonate) in the ionic liquid 1-ethyl-3-methylimidazolium ethyl sulfate, ($[C_2C_1im][EtSO_4]$) [104]. It appeared that electrochemical techniques can be quickly and easily applied to study ionic liquid/lignin/ mediator systems for prediction and selection of an appropriate ionic liquid and mediator combination for the lignin degradation process.

Regarding C–O selective reductive cleavage and hydrodeoxygenation lignin reactions, ILs were also reported to stabilize noble metal (Pd, Pt, Rh, Ru) nanoparticles, acting as a pseudohomogeneous catalyst system [105]. Using the best combination of Pt and $[C_4C_1im][PF_6]$ for dealkalized lignin and organosolv lignin reactions, the liquid products yield is only 5% and 3%, respectively. The selectivity to the main product cyclohexane is accounting for 68% and 49%. No loss of activity was observed for this pseudohomogeneous catalyst for at least 3 runs, thereby confirming its recyclability (Table 8.3, entry 6).

ILs and their unique property sets make them interesting candidates to develop new methods to extract, oxidize and isolate chemicals stemming from the oxidation of lignin. However, challenges still remain to be addressed for developing attractive processes at the industrial scale, with respect to the recyclability, costs and investment points of view.

8.4.3 VEGETABLE OIL VALORIZATION

Vegetable oils, composed of triglycerides, can be converted to fatty acids or fatty acid esters. The most known reaction in oleochemistry is the transesterification of vegetable oils with alcohol to produce biodiesel. However some others fatty acid esters like carbohydrates fatty acid esters can be obtained by esterification reaction. Numerous reactions can be then afforded from fatty acids or fatty acid esters such as epoxidation, Diels-Alder, metathesis, etc. All these reactions can be performed in the presence of ionic liquids. Some examples of ILs used in the conversion of vegetable oils are reported below.

8.4.3.1 Synthesis of Biodiesel

Fatty acid methyl esters (FAME) are commonly used as additive to biodiesel (Figure 8.10). The commonly route to obtained FAME from vegetable oils is the used of homogeneous catalysts such as alkali hydroxides, methoxides or strong mineral acids [106]. The drawbacks of this synthesis are the use of corrosive media, generation of water or soap [107]. Hence a high interest has been devoted to the use of ILs to catalyze the synthesis of biodiesel. The first used of ILs was reported in 2004, using a suspension of sodium methoxide in 1-butyl-3-methylimidazolium tetrafluoroborate $[C_4C_1im][BF_4]$ to afford the synthesis of biodiesel [108]. Later Seddon et al. have studied several ILs and they have shown that ILs containing choline derived cations were active in the synthesis of biodiesel [109]. ILs can be used as a catalyst or as a solvent (enzymatic catalysis) in this reaction.

8.4.3.1.1 Ionic Liquids as Catalysts

Brønsted acid ILs were investigated in the synthesis of biodiesel (Figure 8.11). Hence, transesterification of cottonseed oil with methanol to biodiesel was investigated in various Brønsted acidic ILs with an alkane sulfonic acid group. Among all the ILs investigated, 1-(4-sulfonic acid) butylpyridinium hydrogen sulfate exhibited a high yield of fatty acid methyl esters of 92% at 170°C after 5 h of reaction which was ascribed to its strong Brønsted acidity. The separation of the biodiesel was performed by simple decantation [110]. In 2010, a recyclable 1-methyl-3-(3-sulfopropyl)-imidazolium hydrogen sulfate ionic liquid ($[C_3\text{-}SO_3HC_1im][HSO_4]$) was used in the synthesis of biodiesel [111]. The synthesis of biodiesel from soybean oil was carried out in the presence of $[C_3\text{-}SO_3HC_1im][HSO_4]$ ionic liquid achieving 94% yield of biodiesel at 120°C after 8.5 h reaction [112]. This IL was highly stable and could be reused six times without noticeable drop in activity. A novel strong Brønsted acidic IL with four $-SO_3H$ groups was synthesized from hexamethylenetetramine and 1,4-butane sulfonate leading to a yield of 98% of biodiesel from rapeseed oil [113]. The authors have studied the recyclability of the IL catalyst by simple centrifugation and up to 10 cycles were performed without significant loss in the yield of the reaction. Li et al. have used butylsulfonic pyridinium ILs for the production of biodiesel from Jatropha oil leading to a 92% yield of biodiesel at 100°C [114].

One can note that the hydrolysis of vegetable oils was studied in similar ILs family and the trend was as follows: 1-(4-sulfonic group)butylcap-rolactamium hydrogen sulfate ($[HSO_3\text{-}C_4CPL][HSO_4]$) > 1-(4-sulfonic

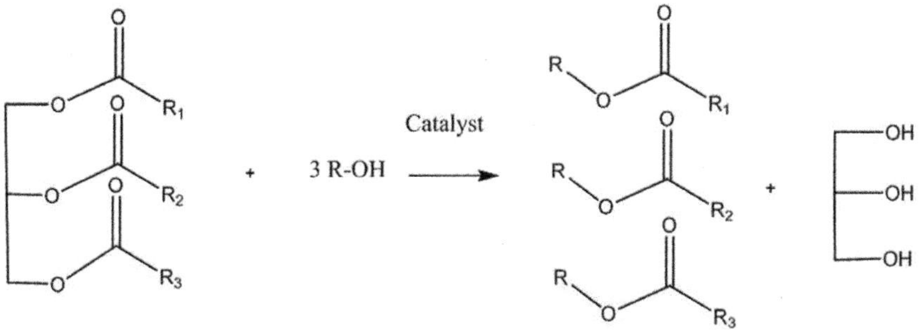

FIGURE 8.10   Synthesis of biodiesel from vegetable oils.

group)butylpyridinium hydrogen sulfate ($[HSO_3$-$C_4pyr][HSO_4]$) > 1-(4-sul-fonic group)butyl-3-methylimidazolium hydrogen sulfate ($[HSO_3$-$C_4C_1im]$ $[HSO_4]$) > 1-(4-sulfonic group)butyltriethylaminium hydrogen sulfate ($[HSO_3$-$C_4C_2C_2C_2N][HSO_4]$) [115]. In optimized conditions (180°C, water/ oil molar ratio of 10:1, 6 h of reaction), the yield of fatty acids was greater than 95 wt% in the presence of 8 wt% $[HSO_3$-$C_4CPL][HSO_4]$. The yield to fatty acids was similar even after six times of IL recycling.

Highly Brønsted acidic ILs based on 1-benzyl-1H-benzimidazole were also studied for the transesterification of canola oil with methanol [24]. The authors have shown that in the presence of 5% (based on the num-ber of mmol of oil) of 3,3'-(hexane-1,6-diyl)bis(6-sulfo-1-(4-sulfobenzyl)-1H-benzimidazolium) hydrogen sulfate catalyst, 95% of canola oil was converted at 60°C in a MeOH/oil molar ratio of 9, after 5 h of reaction. This IL was recyclable and can be used in the transesterification of palm, soybean, sunflower oils with a conversion range between 84 and 95% in the presence of methanol, ethanol or butanol. Recently, an imidazole-type solid acidic ionic liquid polymer (PIL) has been synthesized and investigated in the biodiesel synthesis (94%) from vegetable oil at 70°C for 4 h with the solvent–oil ratio of 1:1 [25]. The PIL could be reused for four times dem-onstrating its stability.

Waste oils transesterification was also studied using an acid IL catalyst (Figure 8.12). Generally, alkaline-based catalysts are used to catalyze the transesterification reaction, but for waste cooking oil where it contains high free fatty acids, direct usage is not possible due to separation of layers and saponification problems. Hence, a Brønsted acidic IL with an alkane sulfonic

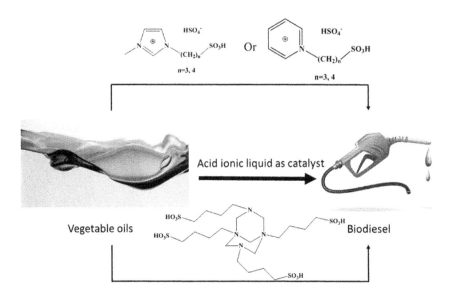

FIGURE 8.11   Synthesis of biodiesel from vegetable oils in the presence of acid ionic liquid catalysts.

acid group (N-methyl-2-oxopyrrolidonium methyl sulfonate ([C_1oxopyrro] [MeSO$_3$])) was used as a catalyst for the preparation of biodiesel from waste oils (cottonseed, Swill, Sewer, acidic and soybean sediment oils) [116]. They have shown that at 170°C, the yield of fatty acid methyl esters can reach 93% in a methanol:oils:ionic liquid molar ratio of 12:1:0.06 after 4 h of reaction. After distillation, the ionic liquid was reused and the yield of FAME decreased slightly after nine runs.

In a similar manner, the production of biodiesel from waste palm cooking oil using butyl-methyl imidazolium hydrogen sulfate [C_4C_1im][HSO$_4$] acidic ionic liquid as a catalyst was investigated [117]. In this study, a two-step process i.e., esterification and transesterification, was performed. The highest biodiesel yield was obtained with 5 wt% [C_4C_1im][HSO$_4$], methanol:oil of 15:1, 60 min reaction time, at 160°C, and agitation speed of 600 rpm. The second step of transesterification catalyzed by KOH at 60°C, 1.0 wt% and 60 min of reaction time. The final yield was 96 wt%. This study demonstrates that acid ILs are also suitable for the transesterification reaction of waste oils containing free fatty acids. This reaction can be also performed in a two-step reaction where the free fatty acids are converted to ester in the presence of methanol or ethanol and then the transesterification reaction can occur. The first step can be carried out in the presence of Brønsted acidic ionic liquid with sulfonic acids groups [118–120]. An interesting study has shown that using dicationic Brønsted ionic liquids, bearing dialkylsulfonic acid groups in acyclic diamine cations the esterification of free long chain fatty acids or their mixtures with low molecular weight alcohol was carried out leading to 93–96% yield at 70°C for 6 h of reaction [121]. The recycling of these dicationic Brønsted ILs was investigated and after simple decantation the catalysts were reused after removal of water for the next reaction. Up to 6 cycles were performed without significant loss of yield. An amphiphilic ionic liquid containing acid sulfonic groups and oxyethylene was used in the synthesis of biodiesel from fatty acids and methanol achieving a yield of 90% at a temperature above 150°C [122]. In another study, two ILs1-methyl-3-propane sulfonic-imidazolium and 1-methyl-3-propane sulfonic-imidazolium hydrogen sulfate were mixed with heteropolyacid $Cs_{2.5}H_{0.5}PW_{12}O_{40}$ at the mass ratio of 1:1 and was used as catalysts for esterification of cooking oil for preparation of 97% of biodiesel at 70°C after 3.5 h of reaction [123].

From all these studies, it is clear that acid ionic liquid catalysts containing sulfonic acid group are effective for the synthesis of biodiesel. Some studies have also used microwaves or ultrasound irradiations for the synthesis of biodiesel in presence of acidic ionic liquids. Guo et al. have shown that ultrasound irradiations of soybean in methanol and Brønsted acid ILs afforded a yield of 93% to biodiesel [124]. In the presence of acidic

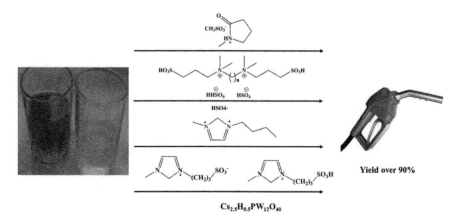

FIGURE 8.12   Synthesis of biodiesel from waste oils in the presence of acid ionic liquid catalysts

symmetrical acidic ionic liquid, $[C_1C_1benzoim][HSO_4]$, the transesterification of oils having high free fatty acid content to biodiesel was studied (Figure 8.13) [125]. A comparison was made between conventional, microwave and ultrasonic conditions. Microwave conditions afforded the highest yield to biodiesel (97%) in 10 min.

The use of basic ionic liquid catalysts is not so largely reported in the literature. However some studies reported the use of a basic IL catalyst for such reaction. Most of the used ILs contained a hydroxyl group such as $[C_xC_1im][OH]$ and led to 95% yield of biodiesel [126, 127]. Moreover, an ionic liquid containing an imidazole anion was effective in the synthesis of biodiesel, a yield of 99 % was obtained at 60°C after 2.5 h of reaction [128]. Although this ionic liquid was effective in the synthesis of biodiesel, it is sensitive to the presence of water and of free fatty acids leading to a decrease in the yield of biodiesel.

8.4.3.1.2   Ionic Liquids as Solvents

The use of ILs as solvents in the biodiesel synthesis in the presence of conventional catalysts was explored to a few extend. For example, Sn complex was used, dissolved in $[C_4C_1im][PF_6]$ [129] or in $[C_4C_1im][InCl_4]$ [130]. The yield of biodiesel obtained was over 80% but the recycling was hampered by the loss of active Sn complex. In $[C_4C_1im][NTf_2]$, using K_2CO_3 or H_2SO_4 as a catalyst the yield to biodiesel was over 90% [131, 132].

If the use of ILs in the presence of conventional catalysts is scarcely reported, a lot of examples of their use in enzymatic catalysis can be found in the literature (Figure 8.14) [133, 135]. Hence the use of ILs as solvents reduces the deactivation of enzymes [136].

The most commonly used enzyme was *Candida antarctica* lipases commercially available as Novozyme 435. Short chain alkyl imidazolium ILs such as $[C_2C_1im]X$ or $[C_4C_1im]X$ with strong hydrophobic fluoride anions such as $[BF_4]^-$, $[PF_6]^-$, $[OTf]^-$ and $[NTf_2]^-$ were used in the enzymatic synthesis of biodiesel leading to a yield over 80% [137]. Some studies have shown that in the presence of $[BF_4]^-$ as an anion, the selectivity to biodiesel was higher than in the presence of $[PF_6]^-$ [138–140]. One can note that the use of water was required to recover the catalyst at the end of the reaction [141, 142]. Some studies were devoted to the use of long alkyl chain ILs leading to an increase of the lipophilicity of the ILs increasing the solubility of ILs in glycerides.

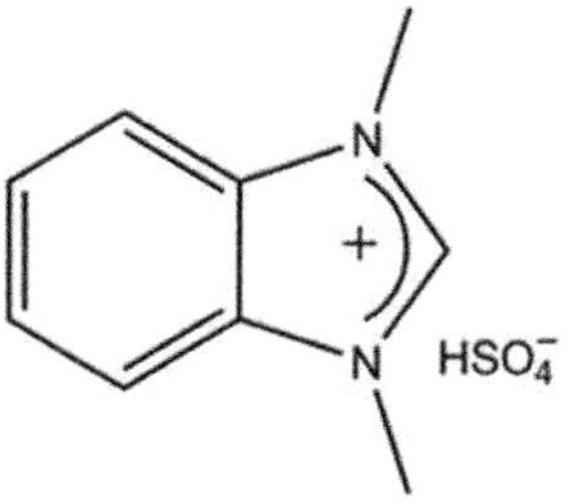

[C₁C₁benzoim][HSO₄]   [C₁C₁im][HSO₄]

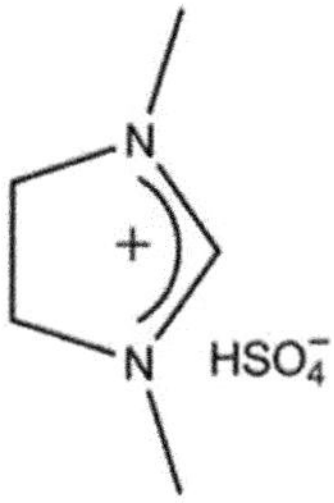

FIGURE 8.13   Acidic symmetrical ionic liquids [126].

Quantitative yield of methyl esters were obtained in a single phase-system. At the end of the reaction, the presence of three phases allows the catalyst and the reaction products to be easily recovered [143]. Another study has shown that amphiphilic ILs had a positive effect on the transesterification reaction of glycerides in the presence of methanol leading to 98% yield of biodiesel [144]. The viscosity of the ILs is also of prime importance and De Diego et al. [144] have shown that the synthesis of biodiesel in the presence of an enzyme was favored by ILs containing [NTf₂]⁻ and [OTf]⁻ as anions, owing to their lower viscosity. The use of microwave irradiations in the synthesis of biodiesel in the presence of Novozyme 435 and [C₂C₁im][BF₄] led to 98% yield of biodiesel while without microwave activation the yield did not exceed 70% [145].

8.4.3.2   Synthesis of Fatty Acid Esters Derivatives in the Presence of ILs

Fatty acid esters can be synthesized from esterification of fatty acids with alcohols in the presence of acid ILs as reported below in the synthesis of biodiesel when free fatty acids were present in the reaction media. For example, the esterification of fatty acids with methanol was carried out in the presence of sulfonic acid [146] and arylsulfonic acid ILs [147] leading to high conversion of fatty acids (lauric acid, stearic acid…) at 70°C. The esterification of lauric acid with methanol was studied in the presence

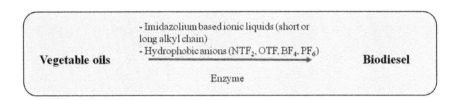

FIGURE 8.14   ILs as solvents in the enzymatic catalytic transesterification of vegetable oils to produce biodiesel.

of [C₄C₁im][NTf₂] along with H₂SO₄ and gave high activity (>85%) and selectivity (100%) after 2 h reaction at 70°C [148].

The synthesis of carbohydrates fatty acid esters is also carried out in ILs in the presence of enzymes [149–151]. Hence, the use of enzymes allows the utilization of water. In this synthesis, neutral ILs are preferred and the most studied anions are [BF₄]⁻, [PF₆]⁻, [TfO]⁻ and [NTf₂]⁻. In the presence of [C₄C₁im][OTf], a yield of 33% to glucose palmitate was obtained using a lipase B as a catalyst [152]. If [C₄C₁im][BF₄] was used, in the presence of Novozyme 435, glucose esters were obtained with a yield of 60% at 60°C [153]. At 55°C, for an enzyme concentration of 20 mg/mL, a mole ratio of glucose/11-dodecenoic ethyl ester of 1:2, the water content of the system being 2%. Lipase Novozym-435 can use repeatedly seven times. In the presence of [C₄C₁im][OTf] ionic liquid and lipase Novozym-435 as a catalyst, 75% yield of lauryl ester of glucose was observed [154]. It was shown that the addition of a small amount of water in the system Lipase/[C₄C₁im][OTf] increased the solubility of glucose leading to a conversion of glucose of 90% [155]. Glucose fatty acid ester synthesis with poly(ethylene glycol)-modified *Candida antarctica* lipase B (CAL-B) was also studied in pure [C₄C₁im][BF₄] (30% conversion) as well as in pure [C₄C₁im][PF₆] (35% conversion). In a biphasic system of [C₄C₁im][PF₆] in the presence of 40% *t*-BuOH, conversions up to 90% and isolated yields up to 89% were achieved using fatty acid vinyl esters as acyl donors and commercial *Candida antarctica* CAL-B [156]. The same authors have shown that 64% of carbohydrate fatty acid esters were obtained in the presence of Chirazyme L-2 [157]. Esterification of starch with palmitic acid was also studied in the presence of *Candida rugose* lipase in a mixture of [C₄C₁im][OAc] and [C₄C₁im][BF₄] [158]. A series of starch palmitate was obtained with a degree of substitution (DS) from 0.034 and 0.153. Flavanoids (Rutin, esculin...) were also investigated in the esterification of fatty acids in the presence of novozyme 435 Lipase in the presence of hydrophobic ILs $[C_4C_1im][BF_4]$, $[C_4C_1im]$ $[PF_6]$, $[C_4C_1im]$ [OTf], or $[C_4C_1im]$ $[NTf_2]$ [159]. The conversion of flavonoids was over 85%.

8.4.3.3   Use of Ionic Liquids in Other Oleochemical Processes

ILs were used in several reactions (isomerization, epoxidation, Diels-Alder reaction, and metathesis) in oleochemistry (Figure 8.15). The reactivity of the double bond of fatty acid chains was studied in the presence of ILs. For example, the isomerization of unsaturated fatty acids was carried out in the presence of chloroaluminate ILs $[C_4C_1im][Al_nCl_{3n+1}]$ [160]. A recent study has shown that in the presence of 5% Ru on $MgAl_4$-LDH (layered double hydroxide) and 1-butyl-3-methyl imidazolium chloride using toluene as solvent for 12 h at 90°C, a 42% conversion of ethyl linoleate was observed with 29% yield of isomerized products [161].

Diels-Alder reaction was investigated from ethyl linoleate and methylvinylketone in the presence of $[C_4C_1im][BF_4]$ and $[C_4C_1im][PF_6]$ and scandium triflate as a catalyst [162]. Without any cosolvent, the best yield was obtained (49%) in the presence of $[C_4C_1im][PF_6]$ at 40°C after 24 h of reaction for 72% of ethyl linoleate conversion. In the presence of a mixture of dichloromethane and ILs, above 80% of ethyl linoleate was converted with 50% yield to cycloadduct. The authors have also showed that in the presence of $[C_4C_1im]$ $[AlCl_4]$, 98% of conversion was observed but the selectivity was only 36%.

Epoxidation of unsaturated fatty acids and their derivatives was also studied in the presence of ILs. This reaction was carried out in the presence of H_2O_2 using ILs as a solvent. Cai et al. have shown that the epoxidation of a technical mixture of methyl oleate and methyl linoleate with H_2O_2, catalyzed by $MoO(O_2)2 \cdot 2QOH$ (QOH = 8-quinilinol) and $NaHCO_3$ as a cocatalyst in a hydroxyl functionalized ionic liquid $[C_2\text{-}OHC_1im][BF_4]$ led to high conversion of methyl oleate (95%) and methyl linoleate (89%), as well as ta 95% total selectivity of their respective oxidation products [163]. IL phases containing the Mo(VI) catalyst was recycled and the Mo(VI) catalyst can be reused at least five times. Later the same authors have studied the epoxidation of oleic acid methyl ester in the presence of SO$_3$H-functional Brønsted acidic ionic liquid as a catalyst in the presence of a mixture of H$_2$O$_2$ and acetic acid [164]. They have obtained a selectivity and conversion higher than 90%. The epoxidation of methyl oleate was also performed in the presence of an enzymatic catalyst in the presence of hydrophobic and hydrophilic ILs and hydrogen peroxide [165]. They have shown that in the presence of hydrophobic ILs such as [C$_4$C$_1$im][NTf$_2$], [C$_4$C$_1$im][PF$_6$], the epoxide product was obtained with high yields and within a few hours and, in many cases, in just one hour of reaction in the presence of various enzymes. However, the highest yield (89%) was obtained using the enzyme from *Aspergillus niger* in this medium. In the presence of the hydrophilic [C$_4$C$_1$im][BF$_4$] IL, it has been shown that the diol formation competes directly with the epoxide formation. The reaction takes place in just one hour. Moreover, the diol yield can be increased in hydrophilic ILs.

Another extensive reaction studied in oleochemistry is the metathesis reaction leading to the production of important intermediates such as polymers and lubricants. For example, the ethenolysis of methyl oleate carried out under mild conditions with ruthenium-alkylidene catalysts in toluene and C2-methylated imidazolium cation 1-butyl-2,3-dimethylimidazolium [C$_4$C$_1$C$_1$im][NTf$_2$] led to 89% conversion of methyl oleate with 100% selectivity to 1-decene and methyl-9-decenoate [166]. The catalyst was recyclable at least for three runs.

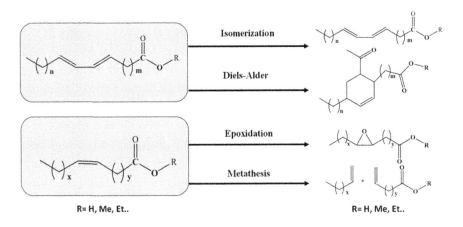

FIGURE 8.15 Reactions from fatty acids and fatty acid esters in ILs.

ILs were also used as extractants in oleochemistry. For example, extraction of crude oils from microalgae biomass was carried out in the presence of mixtures of ILs and methanol [167, 168]. $[C_4C_1im][MeSO_4]$ or $[C_4C_1im]$ [OTf] ILs allow the extraction of C16:0, C16:1, C18:2, and C18:3 fatty acids. This study has shown that dipolarity/polarizability and hydrogen bond acidity of ILs are more important than their hydrogen bond basicity for effectively extracting lipids from algal biomass. Several studies were devoted to the extraction of polyunsaturated fatty acids or their methyl esters in the presence of ILs. A mixture of Ag salts ILs($[C_8C_1im][PF_6]$) was selective to the extraction of polyunsatured fatty acid methyl esters [169, 170]. Another study has shown that using AMMOENG100 (Cocos alkyl pentaethoximethylammonium methylsulfate) and $[C_4C_1im][N(CN)_2]$ (1-butyl-3-methylimidazolium dicyanamide), linoleic acid was extracted from soybean oil [171]. These solvents exhibit a complete miscibility with free fatty (linoleic) acid and a very low solubility in soybean oil.

8.5 CONCLUSION

To resume, the use of ILs for sustainable biofuels and chemicals production was increasingly investigated during the last decade, essentially due to the ability of several ILs to dissolve and pretreat biomass. Interestingly, ionic liquids-based dissolution processes compared to other pretreatment options allow one to recrystallize the cellulose portion of lignocellulosic biomass and simultaneously disrupt the lignin and hemicellulose network. The low volatility of ILs can favor the pretreatment of biomass at atmospheric pressure even at temperatures surpassing the boiling point of water. As an environmental point of view, ILs allow one to perform nonodorous treatment without production of vapors, compared to organic solvents.

However, deconstruction with ILs is not viable yet because of some current drawbacks to solve, as for example their costs (production and energy costs) in comparison with the value of the substrate processed by them. A recent techno-economic analysis modeling of ILs deconstruction has determined that among the investigated variables the order of importance/sensitivity is IL price > biomass loading > recycling rate [172]. In addition, the ability to sell the lignin and/or its products will heavily impact on the process costs.

Further investigations are required to develop the actual ILs-based processes at a larger scale, in particular on:

1. The reduction of the ILs cost (ideally less than $2.50 kg^{-1});
2. The increase of biomass loading;
3. The decrease of pretreatment times in order to save energy;
4. The increase of yield and selectivity to compete with classical processes;
5. The possibility to apply IL-technologies to a wider range of feedstocks depending on the type of biomass, geographical location, season, etc;
6. The increase of moisture tolerance;
7. The reduction of IL losses and optimization of its recycling;
8. The deep investigation of the end of life of residual ionic liquids, as well as the collection of data on their impact in terms of toxicity and risks for health and environment. Indeed, it is very difficult to determine accurately the toxicity of ILs towards cells and the environment with the current available data. Moreover, the millions of possible cation/anion combinations also contribute to a complex evaluation of their toxicity [173, 174].

Several recycling processes were reported in this chapter, but the development of much more efficient and energy-saving methods is required. Indeed, the current methods to recycle ILs in biomass processing are mainly centered on evaporation of the antisolvents, which can consume a lot of energy, especially in the case of IL/water solutions.

At a fundamental level, a better understanding of the mechanisms of dissolution is needed (roles of the cation and anion in the treatment of biomass, etc) to design more efficient ILs. The collection of a more comprehensive database on the physicochemical properties of the ILs will be also an important step in the future applications of ILs in industrial scale processes.

Nonetheless, the design of ILs and their unique property sets give us an opportunity to develop truly new methods to produce fuels and added-value chemicals from biomass (cellulose, lignin, vegetable oils, etc.) facilitating extraction and separation steps. We believe that ionic liquids-based processes should offer a much greater valorization of biomass in the future.

ACKNOWLEDGMENTS

The authors gratefully acknowledge the CAPES Foundation (Brazilian Ministry of Education) for the awarding of the PhD scholarship (13342-13-4) to Ronan Behling through the Science without Borders program, and the French Ministry of Higher Education and Research for the awarding of the PhD scholarship to Nahla Araji through the France-Canada Research Fund program. The authors also acknowledge the International Consortium on Ecoconception and renewable resources (INCREASE FR CNRS 3707) for the funding of the postdoctoral fellowship of Prince N. Amaniampong.

KEYWORDS

- biofuels
- chemicals
- dissolution
- ionic liquids
- pretreatments

REFERENCES

1. Rogers, R. D., & Seddon, K. R. (2003). *Science*, 302, 792–793.
2. Rogers, R. D., & Seddon, K. (2003). *Ionic Liquids as Green Solvents: Progress and Prospects*, American Chemical Society, Washington, D.C.
3. Wasserscheid, P., & Welton, T. (2011). *Ionic Liquids in Synthesis*, Wiley-VCH, Weinheim, 2008.
4. Hallett, J. P., & Welton, T. (2011) *Chem. Rev.,* 111, 3508–3576.
5. Cojocaru, O. A., Bica, K., Gurau, G., Narita, A., McCrary, P. D., Shamshina, J. L., Barber, P. S., & Rogers, R. D., (2013). *Med. Chem. Comm, 4,* 559–563.
6. Zhang, P., Wu, T., & Han, B. (2014). *Adv. Mater., 26,* 6810–6827.
7. T. D. Ho, C. Zhang, L. W. Hantao, J. L., & Anderson, (2014). *Anal. Chem., 86,* 262–285.
8. MacFarlane, D. R., Tachikawa, N., Forsyth, M., Pringle, J. M., Howlett, P. C., Elliot, G. D., Davis Jr., J. H., Watanabe, M.: Simon, P., & Austen Angell, C., (2014). *Energy Environ. Sci., 7,* 232–250.
9. Torriero, A. A. J. (2015). *Electrochemistry in Ionic Liquids*, Springer International Publishing: 738 p.

10. Stanisz, E., Werner, J., & Zgoła-Grześkowiak, A. (2014). *TrAC, Trends Anal. Chem., 61*, 64–66.

11. Tadesse, H., & Luque R. (2011). *Energy Environ. Sci., 4*, 3913–3929.

12. Holbrey, J. D., & Seddon, K. R. (1999). *Clean Products and Processes* (Ed. T. Matsunaga), Vol. *1*, Springer-Verlag, New York, p. 223.

13. Chatel, G., Pereira, J. F. B., Debbeti, V., Wang H., & Rogers, R. (2014). *Green Chem., 16*, 2051–2083.

14. Stark, A., Behrend, P., Braun, O., Müller, A., Ranke, J., Ondruschka, B., & Jastorff, B. (2008). *Green Chem., 10*, 1152–1161.

15. Fort, D. A., Remsing, R. C., Swatloski, R. P., Moyna, P., Moyna, G., & Rogers, R. D. (2007). *Green Chem., 9*, 63–69.

16. Sun, N., Rahman, M., Qin, Y., Maxim, M. L., Rodríguez, H., & Rogers, R. D. (2009). *Green Chem., 11*, 646–655.

17. Kilpeläinen, I., Xie, H., King, A., Granstrom, M., Heikkinen, S., & Argyropoulos, D. S. J. (2007). *Agric. Food Chem., 55*, 9142–9148.

18. Lee, S. H., Doherty, T. V., Linhardt, R. J., & Dordick, J. S. (2009). *Biotechnol. Bioeng., 102*, 1368–1376.

19. Doherty, T. V., Mora-Pale, M., Foley, S. E., Linhardt, R. J., & Dordick, J. S. (2010). *Green Chem., 12*, 1967–1975.

20. George, A., Brandt, A., Tran, K., Nizan S. Zahari, S. M. S., Klein-Marcuschamer, D., Sun, N., Sathitsuksanoh, N., Shi, J., Stavila, V., Parthasarathi, R., Singh, S., Holmes, B. M., Welton, T., Simmons, B. A., & Hallett, J. P. (2015). *Green Chem., 17*, 1728–1734.

21. Da Costa Lopes, A. M., & Bogel-Łukasik, R. (2015). *Chem. Sus. Chem., 8*, 947–965.

22. Cheng, F., Wang, H., Chatel, G., Gurau, G., & Rogers, R. D. (2014). *Biores. Technol., 164*, 394–401.

23. Liu, C.-Z., Wang, F., Stiles, A. R., & Guo, C. (2012). *Appl. Energy, 92*, 406–414.

24. Ghiaci, M., Aghabarari, B., Habibollahi, S., & Gil, A. (2011). *Biores. Technol., 102*, 1200–1204.

25. Wu, H., Gao, Y., Zhang, W., Tang, A., Tan, Y., & Men, Y. (2015). *Chem. Eng. Process. Process Intensif., 93*, 61–65.

26. Brandt, A., Gräsvik, J., Hallett, J. P., & Welton, T. (2013). *Green Chem., 15*, 550–583.

27. Ragauskas, A. J., Nagy, M., Kim, D. H., Eckert, C. A., Hallett, J. P., & Liotta, C. L. (2006). *Ind. Biotechnol., 2*, 55–65.

28. Mosier, N., Wyman, C., Dale, B., Elander, R., Lee, Y., Holtzapple, M., & Ladisch, M. (2005). *Biores. Technol., 96*, 673–686.

29. Zhu, S., Wu, Y., Chen, Q., Yu, Z., Wang, C., Jin, S., Ding, Y., & Wu, G., (2006). *Green Chem., 8*, 325–327.

30. Mora-Pale, M., Meli, L., Doherty, T. V., Linhardt, R. J., & Dordick, J. S. (2011). *Biotechnol. Bioengin., 108*, 1229–1245.

31. Zavrel, M., Bross, D., Funke, M., Büchs, J., & Spiess, A. C. (2009). *Biores. Technol., 100*, 2580–2587.

32. Zhang, L., Ruan, D., & Gao, S. J. (2002). *Polym. Sci., Part B: Polym. Phys., 40*, 1521–1529.

33. Lindman, B., Karlström, G., & Stigsson, L. J. (2010). *Mol. Liq., 156*, 76–81.

34. Yamane, C., Aoyagi, T., Ago, M., Sato, K., Okajima, K., & Takahashi, T. (2006). *Polym. J., 38*, 819–826.

35. Walden, P. (1914). *Bull. Acad. Imper. Sci.(St. Petersburg), 8*, 405-422.

36. Graenacher, C., (1934). Cellulose solution. Google Patents.

37. Swatloski, R., Rogers, R., & Holbrey, J., (2003). University of Alabama. *USA, WO Patent, 3*, 029329.

38. Swatloski, R. P., Spear, S. K., Holbrey, J. D., & Rogers, R. D. (2002). . *Amer. Chem. Soc., 124*, 4974–4975.

39. Vancov, T., Alston, A.-S., Brown, T., & McIntosh, S. (2012). *Renewable Energy, 45*, 1–6.

40. Remsing, R. C., Swatloski, R. P., Rogers, R. D., & Moyna, G., (2006). *Chem. Commun.,* 1271–1273.

41. Liu, H., Sale, K. L., Holmes, B. M., Simmons, B. A., & Singh, S. (2010). *J. Phys. Chem. B., 114*, 4293–4301.

42. Youngs, T., Hardacre, C., & Holbrey, J. (2007). *J. Phys.Chem. B., 111*, 13765-13774.

43. Zhang, J., Zhang, H., Wu, J., Zhang, J., He, J., & Xiang, J. (2010). *Phys. Chem. Chem. Phys., 12*, 1941–1947.

44. Ab Rani, M., Brant, A., Crowhurst, L., Dolan, A., Lui, M., Hassan, N., Hallett, J., Hunt, P., Niedermeyer, H., & Perez-Arlandis, J. (2011). *Phys. Chem. Chem. Phys., 13*, 16831–16840.

45. Brandt, A., Hallett, J. P., Leak, D. J., Murphy, R. J., & Welton, T. (2010). *Green Chem., 12*, 672–679.

46. Murugesan, S., & Linhardt, R. J. (2005). *Curr. Org. Synth., 2*, 437–451.

47. El Seoud, O. A., Koschella, A., Fidale, L. C., Dorn, S., & Heinze, T. (2007). *Biomacromol., 8*, 2629–2647.

48. Feng, L., & Chen, Z.-l. (2008). *J. Mol. Liq., 142*, 1–5.

49. Heinze, T., Schwikal, K., & Barthel, S., (2005). *Macromol. Biosci., 5*, 520–525.

50. Barthel, S., & Heinze, T. (2006). *Green Chem., 8*, 301–306.

51. Olivier-Bourbigou, H., Magna, L., & Morvan, D., (2010). *Appl. Catal., A 373*, 1–56.

52. Falling, S. N., Godleski, S. A., & McGarry, L. W. (1993). Google Patents.

53. Li, H., Wang, Q., Lan, X., Wang, X., & Song, H., (2008). *China oils and fats, 4*, 021.

54. Ranu, B. C., & Jana, R. (2006). *Eur. J. Org. Chem.,* 3767–3770.

55. Zhao, H., Xia, S., & Ma, P. (2005). *J. Chem. Technol. Biotechnol., 80*, 1089–1096.

56. Dai, S., Ju, Y., & Barnes, C. (1999). *J. Chem. Soc., Dalton Trans., 8*, 1201–1202.

57. Visser, A. E., Swatloski, R. P., Reichert, W. M., Griffin, S. T., & Rogers, R. D. (2000). *Ind. Eng. Chem. Res., 39*, 3596–3604.

58. Spear, S., Visser, A., & Rogers, R. (2002). In: *Ionic liquids: green solvents for carbohydrate studies, Advances in the chemistry and processing of beet and cane sugar,* Proceedings of the Sugar Processing Research Conference, New Orleans, Louisiana, USA, 10–13 March (2002)., Sugar Processing Research, Institute, Inc., pp. 336–340.

59. Liu, Q., Janssen, M. H., van Rantwijk, F., & Sheldon, R. A. (2005). *Green Chem., 7*, 39–42.

60. Matsumoto, M., Mochiduki, K., Fukunishi, K., & Kondo, K., (2004). *Sep. Purif. Technol., 40*, 97–101.

61. Fadeev, A. G., & Meagher, M. M. (2001). *Chemical Commun., 3*, 295–296.

62. Cull, S., Holbrey, J., Vargas-Mora, V., Seddon, K., & Lye, G., (2000). *Biotechnol. Bioeng., 69*, 227–233.

63. Isik, M., Sardon, H., & Mecerreyes, D. (2014). *Int. J. Mol. Sci., 15*, 11922–11940.

64. Wang, H., Gurau, G., & Rogers, R. D. (2012). *Chem. Soc. Rev., 41*, 1519–1537.

65. Gupta, K. M., & Jiang, J. (2015). *Chem. Engin. Sci., 121*, 180–189. .

66. Medronho, B., & Lindman, B. (2014). *Curr. Opin. Colloid Interface Sci., 19*, 32–40.

67. Andanson, J.-M., Bordes, E., Devémy, J., Leroux, F., Pádua, A. A. H., & Costa Gomes M. F. (2014). *Green Chem., 16*, 2528–2538.
68. Kohler, S., & Heinze, T. (2007). *Cellulose,* 14, 489–495.
69. Bose, S., Armstrong D. W., & Petrich J. W. J. (2010). *Phys. Chem., B 114*, 8221–8227.
70. Gericke, M., & Fardim, P., Heinze, T. (2012). *Molecules,* 17, 7458 –7502.
71. Xiong, Y., Zhang, Z., Wang, X., Liu, B., & Lin, J. (2014). *Chem. Eng. J., 235,* 349 –355.
.
72. Bose, S., Barnes, C. A., & Petrich, J. W. (2012). *Biotechnol. Bioeng., 109,* 434–443. .
73. Ohira, K., Abe, Y., Kawatsura, M., Suzuki, K., Mizuno, M., Amano, Y., & Itoh, T. (2012). *Chem. Sus. Chem., 5,* 388–391.
74. Morales-delaRosa, S., Campos-Martin, J. M., & Fierro, J. L. G. (2012). *Chem. Eng. J., 181–182,* 538–541. .
75. Liu, Y., Xiao, W., Xia, S., & Ma, P. (2013). *Carbohydr. Polym., 92,* 218–222.
76. Moellmann, E., Heinze, T., Liebert, T., & Koehler, S. (2013). Patent US 8541571 B2. *Homogeneous synthesis of cellulose ethers in ionic liquids,*
77. Barthel, S., & Heinze, T. (2006). *Green Chem., 8,* 301–306. .
78. Heinze, T., Schwikal, K., & Barthel, S. (2005). *Macromol. Biosci., 5,* 520–525.
79. Wu, J., Zhang, J., Zhang, H., He, J., Ren, Q., & Guo, M. (2004). *Biomacromol., 5,* 266–268.
80. Ma, S., Xue, X.-L., Yu, S.-J., & Wang, Z.-H. (2012). *Ind. Crops Prod., 35,* 135–139.
81. Chatel, G., & MacFarlane, D. R. (2014). *Chem. Soc. Rev., 43,* 8132–8149.
82. Rosatella, A. A., Simeonov, S. P., Frade R. F. M., & Afonso, C. A. M. (2011). *Green Chem., 13,* 754–793.
83. Kazi, F. K., Patel, A. D., Serrano-Ruiz, J. C., Dumesic, J. A., & Anex, R. P. (2012). *Chem. Eng. J., 169,* 329–338.
84. Kuo, I.-J., Suzuki, N., Yamauchi, Y., & W. K. C.-W. (2013). *RSC Adv., 3,* 2028–2034.
85. Zhou, L., He, Y., Ma, Z., Liang, R., Wu, T., & Wu, Y. (2015). *Carbohydr. Polym., 117,* 694–700.
86. Liu, B., Zhang, Z., & Zhao, Z. K. (2013). *Chem. Eng. J., 215–216,* 517–521.
87. Zhou, L., Liang, R., Ma, Z., Wu, T., & Wu, Y. (2013). *Bioresour. Technol., 129,* 450–455.
88. Boussou, F., Mühlbauer, A., De Oliveira Vigier, K., Leclercq, L., Kunz, W., Marinkovic, S., Estrine, B., Nardello-Rataj, V., & Jérôme, F. (2014). *Green Chem., 16,* 2463–2471. .
89. Behling, R., Valange, S., & Chatel, G. (2016). *Green Chem., 18,* 1839–1854.
90. Yinghuai, Z., Yuanting, K. T., & Hosmane, N. S. (2013). *Ionic liquids – New aspects for the future, In: Applications of ionic liquids in lignin chemistry,* InTech, Chap., 13, p. 315–346.
91. Zakzeski, J., Bruijnincx, P. C., Jongerius, A. L., & Weckhuysen, B. M. (2010). *Chem. Rev., 110,* 3552–3599.
92. Chatel, G., & Rogers, R. D. (2014). *ACS Sustainable Chem. Eng., 2,* 322–339.
93. Zakzeski, J., Jongerius, A. L., & Weckhuysen, B. M. (2010). *Green Chem., 12,* 1225–1236.
94. Stärk, K., Taccardi, N., Bösmann, A., & Wasserscheid, P. (2010). *Chem. Sus. Chem., 3,* 719–723.
95. Reichert, E., Wintringer, R., Volmer, D. A., & Hempelmann, R. (2012). *Phys. Chem. Chem. Phys., 14,* 5214–5221.
96. Zhu, Y., Chuanzhao, L., Sudarmadji, M., Min, N. H., Biying, A. O., Maguire, J. A., & Hosmane, N. S. (2012). *Chemistry Open. 1,* 67–70.

97. Shamsuri, A. A., & Abdullah, D. K. (2012). *Oxidation Comm., 35*, 767–775.

98. Liu, S., Shi, Z., Li, L., Yu, S., Xie, C., & Song, Z. (2013). *RSC Adv., 3*, 5789–5793.

99. Xu, C., Arancon, R. A. D., Labidi, J., & Luque R. (2014). *Chem. Soc. Rev., 43*, 7485–7500.

100. Zhang, B., Li, C., Dai, T., Huber, G. W., Wang, A., & Zhang, T. (2015). *RSC Adv., 5*, 84967–84973.

101. Cai, Z., Li, Y., He, H., Zeng, Q., Long, J., Wang, L., & Li, X. (2015). *Ind. Eng. Chem. Res., 54*, 11501–11510.

102. Yan, B., Li, K., Wei, L., Ma, Y., Shao, G., Zhao, D., Wan, W., & Song, L. (2015). *Bioresource Technol., 196*, 509–517.

103. Prado, R., Brandt, A., Erdocia, X., Hallet, T., Welton, T., & Labidi, J. (2016). *Green Chem., 18*, 834–841.

104. Eshtaya, M., Ejigu, A., Stephens, G., Walsh, D. A., Chen, G. Z., & Croft, A. K. (2016). *Faraday Discuss. Advance Article*, DOI: 10.1039/C5FD00226E.

105. Chen, L., Xin, J., Ni, L., Dong, H., Yan, D., Lu, X., & Zhang, S. (2016). *Green Chem., 18*, 2341–2352.

106. Schuchardt, U., Sercheli, R., & Vargas, R. M. J. (1998). *Braz. Chem. Soc., 9*, 199-210.

107. Muhammad, N., Elsheikh, Y. A., Mutalib, M. I. A., Bazmi, A. A., Khan, R. A., Khan, H., Rafiq, S., Man, Z., & Khan, I. J. (2015). *Ind. Eng. Chem., 21*, 1–10.

108. Verkade, J. G. (2004). International *Conference on Phosphorous Chemistry (ICPC)*, Birmingham England, OP 074.

109. Earle, M. J., Plechkova, V. N., & Seddon, K. R. (2006). *WO 2006095134. Production of bio-diesel.*

110. Wu, Q., Chen, H., Han, M., Wang, D., & Wang, J. (2007). *Ind. Eng. Chem. Res., 46*, 7955–7960. .

111. Zhou, J., Lu, Y., Huang, B., Huo, Y., & Zhang, K. (2011). *Adv. Mater. Res., 314-316*, 1459–1462.

112. Du, H., Fang, M., Song, L., Tan, Z., He, Y., & Han, X. (2010). *Asian J. Chem., 2014, 26*, 7575–7580.

113. Liang, X., Yang, Z. *Green Chem., 12*, 201–204.

114. Li, K., Chen, L., Yan, Z., & Wang, H. (2010). *Catal. Lett., 139*, 151–156.

115. Luo, H., Xue, K., Fan, W., Li, C., Nan, G., & Li, Z. (2014). *Ind. Eng. Chem. Res., 53*, 11653–11658.

116. Han, M., Yi, W., Wu, Q., Liu, Y., & Wang, D. (2009). *Bioresour. Technol., 100*, 2308–2310.

117. Ullah, Z., Bustam, M. A., & Man, Z. (2015). *Renewable Energy. 77*, 521–526.

118. Zhang, L., Xian, M., He, Y., Li, L., Yang, J., Yu, S., & Xu, X. (2009). *Bioresour. Technol., 100*, 4368–4373. .

119. Elsheikh, Y. A., Man, Z., Bustam, M. A., Yusup, S., & Wilfred, C. D. (2011). *Energy Convers. Manage, 52*, 804–809. .

120. Man, Z., Elsheikh, Y. A., Bustam, A. M., Yusup, S., Mutalib, M. I. A., & Muhammad, N. A. (2013). *Ind. Crops Prod., 41*, 144–149.

121. Fang, D., Yang, J., & Jiao, C. (2011). *ACS Catal., 1*, 42–47.

122. Wu, Q., Wan, H., Li, H., Song, H., & Chu, T. (2013). *Catal. Today. 200*, 74–79.

123. Wu, J., Gao, Y., Zhang, W., Tan, Y., Tang, A., Men, Y., & Tang, B. (2014). *Appl. Petrochem. Res., 4*, 305–312.

124. Guo, W., Li, H., Ji, G., & Zhang, G. (2012). *Bioresour. Technol., 125*, 332–334.

125. Soni, S. S., Kotadia, D. A., Patel, V. K., & Bhatt, H. (2014). *Biomass Convers. Bioref., 4*, 301–309. .
126. Zhou, S., Liu, L., Wang, B., Xu, F., & Sun, R. C. (2012). *Chin. Chem. Lett., 23*, 379–382. .
127. Liang, J., Rem., V., Wang, J., Jinag, M., & Li, Z. J. (2010). *Fuel. Chem. Technol., 38*, 275–280.
128. Fan, M., Yang, J., Jiang, P., Zhang, P., & Li, S. (2013). *RSC Adv., 3*, 752–756.
129. Abreu, F. R., Alves, M. B., Macedo, C. C. S., Zara, L. F., & Suarez, A. Z. J. (2005). *Mol. Cat. A: Chem., 227*, 263–267.
130. Neto, B. A. D., Alves, M. B., Lapis, A. A. M., Nachtigall, F. M., Eberlin, M. N., Dupont, J., & Suarez, P. A. Z. J. (2007). *Catal., 249*, 154–161.
131. Lapis, A. A. M., De Oliveira, L. F., Neto, B. A. D., & Dupont, J. (2008). *Chem. Sus. Chem., 1*, 759–762. .
132. Fang, D., Jiang, C., & Yang, J. (2013). *Energy Technol., 1*, 135–138.
133. Bajaj, A., Lohan, P., Jha, P. N., & Mehrotra, R. J. (2010). *Mol. Catal. B: Enzym., 62*, 9–14. .
134. Bisen, P. S., Sanodiya, B. S., Thakur, G. S., Baghel, R. K., & Prasad, G. B. K. S. (2010). *Biotechnol. Lett., 32*, 1019–1030.
135. Gog, A., Roman, M., Tos, M., Paizs, C., & Irmie, F. D. (2012). *Renewable Energy, 39*, 1019–1030.
136. De Diego, T., Manjon, A., Lozano, P., & Iborra, J. L. (2011). *Bioresour. Technol., 102*, 6336–6339.
137. Ha, S. H., Lan, M. N., Lee, S. H., Hwang, S. M., & Koo, Y. M. (2007). *Enzyme Microbiol. Technol., 41*, 480–483.
138. Sunitha, S., Kanjilal, S., Reddy, P. S., & Prasad, R. B. N. (2007). *Biotechnol. Lett., 29*, 1881–1885.
139. Gamba, M., Lapis, A. A. A. M., & Dupont, J. (2008). *Adv. Synth. Catal., 350*, 160–164.
140. Arai, S., Nakashima, K., Tanino, T., Ogino, C., Kondo, A., & Fukuda, H. (2010). *Enzyme Microbiol. Technol., 46*, 51–55.
141. Yang, Z., Zhang, K., Huang, Y., & Wang, Z. J. (2010). *Mol. Cat. B: Enzym., 63*, 23–30.
142. Zhang, K., Lai, J. Huang, Z., & Yang, Z. (2011). *Bioresour. Technol., 102*, 2767–2772.
143. De Diego, T., Manjon, A., Lozano, P., Vaultier, M., & Iborra, J. R. (2011). *Green Chem., 13*, 444–451.
144. Devi, B. L. A. P., Guo, Z., & Xu, X. (2011). *AIChEJ 57*, 1628–1637.
145. Yu, D., Wang, C., Yin, Y., Zhang, A., Gao, G., & Fang, X. (2011). *Green Chem., 13*, 1869–1875. .
146. Zhao, Y., Long, J., Deng, F., Liu, X., Li, Z., Xia, C., & Peng, J. (2009). *Catal. Commun., 10*, 732–736.
147. Li, X., & Eli, W. J. (2008). *Mol. Catal. A: Chem., 279*, 159–164.
148. Yaacob, Z., Nordin, N. A. M., & Yarmo, M. A. (2011). *Malaysian J. Anal. Sci., 15*, 46–53.
149. Kennedy, J. F., Kumar, H., Panesar, V., Marwaha, S. S., Goyal, S. S., Parma, A., & Kaur, S. J. (2006). *Chem. Technol. Biotechnol., 81*, 866–876.
150. Galonde, N., Nott, K., Debuigne, A., Deleu, M., Jerome, C., Paquot, M., & Wathelet, J. P. J. (2012). *Chem. Technol. Biotechnol., 87*, 451–471.
151. Yang, Z., & Huang, Z. (2012). *Cat. Sci. Technol., 2*, 1767–1775.
152. Liang, J., Zeng, P., Yao, P., & Wei, Y. (2012). *Adv. Biol. Chem., 2*, 226–232.
153. Yao, P., Huang, G., Yan, W., Zhang, X., Li, Q., & Wei, Y. (2012). *Adv. Chem. Eng. Sci., 2*, 204–211.

154. Ye, R., Pyo, S., & Hayes, D. G. (2010). *J. Am. Chem. Oil Soc., 87*, 291–293.

155. Lee, S. H., Dang, D. T., Ha, S. H., Chang, W., & Koo, Y. (2008). *Biotechnol. Bioeng., 99*, 1–8.

156. Ganske, F., & Bornscheuer, U. T. (2005). *Org. Lett., 7*, 3097–3098.

157. Ganske, F., & Bornscheuer, U. T. (2005). *J. Mol. Catal. B-Enzym., 36*, 40–42. .

158. Lu, X., Luo, Z. Yu, S., & Fu, X. (2012). *J. Agr. Food Chem., 60*, 273–9279.

159. Lue, B. M., Guo, Z., & Xu, X. (2010). *Process. Biochem., 45*, 1375–1382.

160. Adams, C. A., Earle, M. E., Hamill, J., Lok, C. M., Roberts, G., & Seddon, K. R. (1998). *WO Patent 1998007679 A1*.

161. Sankaranarayanan, S., Selvama, G., & Srinivasan, K. (2015). *RSC Adv., 5*, 36075–36082.

162. Behr, A., Naendrup, F., & Nave, S. (2003). *Eng. Life Sci., 3*, 325–327.

163. Cai, S.-F., Wang, L.-S., & Fan, C.-L. (2009). *Molecules, 14*, 2935–2946.

164. Cai, S.-F., & Wang, L.-S. (2011). *Chin. J. Chem. Eng., 19*, 54–63.

165. Wendylene, S. D., Silva, W. S. D., Lapis, A. A. M., Suarez, P. A. Z., & Neto, B. A. D. (2011). *J. Mol. Catal. B-Enzym., 68*, 98–103.

166. Thurier, C., Fischmeister, C., bruneau, C., Olivier-Bourbigou, H., & Dixneuf, P. H. (2008). *Chem. Sus. Chem., 1*, 118–122.

167. Young, G., Nippgen, F., Titterbrandt, S., & Cooney, M. (2010). *J. Sep. Purif. Technol., 72*, 118–121.

168. Kim, Y. H., Choi, Y. K., Park, J., Lee, S., Yang, Y. H., Kim, H. J., Park, T. J., Kim, Y. H., & Lee, S. H. (2012). *Bioresource Technol., 109*, 312–315.

169. Li, M., & Li, T. (2008). *Sep. Sci. Technol., 43*, 2072–2089.

170. Li, M., Pittman, Jr., C. U., & Li, T. (2012). *Talanta., 78*, 1364–1370.

171. Manic, M. S., Nadjanovic-Visak, V., Da Ponte, V. N., & Visak, Z. P. (2012). *AIChEJ 57*, 1344–1355. .

172. Klein-Marcuschamer, D., Simmons, B. A., & Blanch, H. W. (2011). *Biofuels, Bioprod. Bioref., 5*, 562–569.

173. Jastorff, B., Störmann, R., Ranke, J., Mölter, M., Stock, F., Oberheitmann, B., Hoffman, W., Hoffmann, J., Nüchter, M., Ondruschka, B., & Filser, J. (2003). *Green Chem., 5*, 136–142.

174. Bubalo, M. C., Radosevic, K., Redovnikovic, I. R., Halambek, J., & Srcek, V. G. (2014). *Ecotoxicol. Environ., Saf. 99*, 1–12.

175. Lee, H. V., Hamid, S. B. A., & Zain, S. K., (2014). "Conversion of Lignocellulosic Biomass to Nanocellulose: Structure and Chemical Process," *The Scientific World Journal*, vol. Article ID 631013, 20 pages, 2014. doi:10.1155/2014/631013.

PART III

BIOFUELS FROM MICROALGAE AND OTHER WASTE SOURCES AND BIOREFINERY CONCEPTS

CHAPTER 9

ALGAE AS A SUSTAINABLE FEEDSTOCK FOR BIOFUEL PRODUCTION

MARTIN GROSS, ASHIK SATHISH, and ZHIYOU WEN

Department of Food Science and Human Nutrition – AGLS, Iowa State University, Ames, IA 50011, USA

CONTENTS

ABSTRACT

Microalgae have been investigated as a potential feedstock for a variety of biofuels among, which biodiesel production has been most commonly researched. In general, the production chain for algal biofuels includes strain development, mass cultivation of algal cells, harvesting and dewatering of algal biomass, extraction of desired components from the biomass, and conversion of the target components into fuel products. In recent years, the use of thermochemical-based methods particularly the hydrothermal liquefaction to treat the whole biomass has also gained interest in recent years. This chapter will provide an overview of the algal biofuel production chain and discuss the current hurdles to commercialization and possible solutions.

9.1 INTRODUCTION AND SCOPE

Microalgae are photosynthetic microorganisms capable of growing in a variety of environments including fresh and salt water. Although microalgae primarily use water, CO_2, and sunlight for phototrophic growth, some species are capable of heterotrophic growth. Compared with terrestrial plants, microalgae have a high growth rate. Algal cells generally contain 5–20% oil (dry basis), but can contain as high as 86% lipid depending on algal species and growth conditions [1, 2]. Mass cultivation of microalgae can be performed in a diverse range of environments including unexploited lands using saline water in arid regions, thus avoiding competition for limited arable land. This can address the commonly discussed "food versus fuel" argument that many traditional oil or energy crops face [3]. Due to these merits, microalgae have long been considered a promising alternative and renewable feedstock for biofuels production.

It is believed that over 200,000 species of algae exist but only about 50,000 have been described [4], and each of these species have their own unique growth and compositional profiles. The diversity of microalgae leads to a range of possibilities in terms of biofuel production pathways. Depending on the biomass composition, microalgae can be processed into biodiesel, alcohol, biogas, and/or bio-crude. However, current algal biofuel production is not economical due to several major challenges associated with the development of optimal strain traits and engineering challenges faced in mass cultivation of microalgae. This chapter provides an overview of the algal biofuels production pathway including strain development, mass cultivation, harvesting and dewatering, and the conversion processes to make biofuels. The various types of biofuels that can be produced from algae are also discussed.

9.2 ALGAL PHYSIOLOGY AND COMPOSITION

9.2.1 ALGAL PHYSIOLOGY

Microalgae are commonly grown phototrophically by using CO_2 and sunlight as carbon and energy source, and require nutrients, primarily nitrogen, phosphorus, mineral salts, and silicon (for diatoms). The algal cells in phototrophic culture system is often implemented in open raceway ponds or photobioreactors and is often limited by the light due to the mutual shading of algal cells. Heterotrophic microalgae use organic carbon as carbon source, and are commonly grown in fermenters. Due to the elimination of the light limited problem, heterotrophic algal culture can reach much higher cell densities than phototrophic algal cultures [5]. Microalgae have also been grown mixotrophically, a method that combines both phototrophic and heterotrophic growth, allowing for higher cell densities than pure phototrophic systems [6].

Compared to terrestrial plants microalgae have a much faster growth rate with a higher lipid content. For example, it has been reported that certain algal species can accumulate lipid contents up to 77% (dry basis) [3, 7]. Compared to some terrestrial energy crops such as corn, soybean, or canola, the algal oil yield can reach to 136,900 L/ha (with 70% lipid in the algal biomass) or 58,000 L/ha (with 30% lipid in biomass) [3], these oil yield was around 10–90 folds higher than the oil yield in those terrestrial oil plants [3].

In addition to the high oil content, microalgae can grow in areas with nonarable lands using saline water, and use waste CO_2 generated from power plants and nutrients from wastewater [8]. On the contrary, terrestrial plants require fertile soil and ample freshwater to grow, Due to these advantages, algae has long been considered an ideal vehicle for the conversion of solar energy into biofuels.

9.2.2 ALGAL COMPOSITION AND UTILIZATION

Three major components of microalgae are lipids (10–20%), proteins (30–60%), and carbohydrates (20–40%) [7]. Under certain conditions, some algae can accumulate high levels of lipid (>70%) [3, 7] or protein (>70%) [9] or carbohydrates (>75%) [10]. In addition to the main components microalgae also contain smaller amounts (1–5%) of nucleic acids and pigments [7]. The biomass compositional profile usually varies with algal species and growth conditions. For example, under nitrogen limiting conditions, algae tend to accumulate more lipids with less protein and carbohydrates [3].

Algal lipids are an attractive feedstock for biofuel production due to the high-energy density of algal oil (~29 KJ/Kg) [11]. Lipids can be characterized into two groups, polar (primarily glycolipids and phospholipids) and neutral (primarily triacylglycerol (TAG), monoacylglycerol, diacylglyc-erol photosynthetic pigments and sterols). Algal cells produce polar lipids to incorporate into their cellular structure. Under stressful conditions, the cells alter their metabolism and produce neutral lipids particularly TAG as energy storage. TAGs are preferred in the production of biodiesel due to the higher ratio of fatty acids than other types of lipids such as glycolipids or phospholipids [12]. The fatty acids that make up TAGs can be converted into biodiesel via transesterification. The fatty acid profile of microalgae var-ies widely in terms of chain length and saturation [1, 2], which can affect the melting and boiling point, cetane number, and viscosity of the biodiesel generated from the algal lipid [13]. Algal fatty acid chain length commonly ranges from 16 to 18 carbons and the major fatty acids are C16:0, C18:1, and C18:2 or C18:3 in green algae, C16:0 and C16:1 in diatoms, and C16:0, C16:1, C18:1, C18:2 in cyanobacteria. Some species are capable of produc-ing fatty acids with longer chains (>C18). The two most widely studied long chain unsaturated fatty acids are eicosapentaenoic acid (EAP, C20:5, n3) and docosahexaenoic acid (DHA,C22:6, n3), which have beneficial effects on human health [14].

Algal carbohydrates are another potential feedstock for biofuel produc-tion. The carbohydrates found in microalgae are quite diverse. In general, green algae have plant-like carbohydrate composed of mostly starch and cellulose, whereas diatomic algae accumulate laminaran, fucoidin and man-nitol [14]. Algal carbohydrate composition can be altered by manipulating medium compositions and culture conditions. For example, algae can accu-mulate up to 75% of their cell mass (dry weight) as carbohydrate (60% as starch) by manipulating macronutrient levels (sulfur, phosphorus, and nitro-gen) and/or adding cyclohexamide to block protein generation [10]. These carbohydrates, primarily starch and cellulose, can be fermented to produce ethanol via yeast fermentation [10].

Algal proteins as another major component have not been largely explored as a feedstock for biofuels but can be a potentially viable animal or aquaculture feed [15]. As a matter of fact, algae biomass is often processed to extract lipids and/or carbohydrates as biofuel feedstock with the remaining protein rich fraction (algae meal) being used as a feed supplement [16, 17]. In recent years, use algal protein for fuel production has also been attempted. For example, the nitrogen flux of microalgae was engineered to deaminate hydrolyzed proteins and convert them into C4 and C5 alcohols [18].

9.3   ALGAL PRODUCTION PIPELINE

A complete algal production pipeline needs to be developed prior to the economic conversion of algal biomass into fuel products. This pipeline includes strain selection, mass cultivation of algae cells, harvesting, dewatering and drying of algal biomass, and biofuel conversion processes.

9.3.1   ALGAL STRAIN SELECTION

The first step in the algal production pipeline is the selection of an algal strain with desirable characteristics. Each strain has innate characteristics dictating its growth rate, cell size, robustness, nutrient requirements, and cellular composition. When selecting algal strain for biofuel production purpose, lipid content, and the biomass productivity are important parameters to evaluate the strain's biofuel production potential. A comprehensive list of the algal strains investigated for the biofuel production is summarized in a review literature [19]. In general, biomass productivity is represented as volumetric productivity (unit: g/L/day) and areal productivity (unit: g/m^2/day). Most algal strains have volumetric biomass productivity ranging from 0.02–1.5 g/L/day and areal biomass productivity ranging 3–25 g/m^2/day, although some strains were reported with a super higher productivities than this range [19].

Algal strain can be naturally occurring or genetically modified. Cell collections such as The Culture Collection of Algae at the University of Texas at Austin (UTEX) and the Bigelow Laboratory for Ocean Sciences maintain a large bank of natural strains. However, some of the strains in these culture collections have been maintained for decades and it is likely that they have lost their original properties resulting in a decrease in robustness [4]. An alternative approach to attaining a natural algae strain is to isolate from natural habitats. For specific applications, such as wastewater treatment, a polyculture of native algae is usually preferred.

Genetic modification of naturally occurring algal species is a tool to enhance desirable traits. Common applications of genetic engineering include (1) increasing cellular lipid concentrations by promoting the fatty acid synthesis pathway [20], and (2) enhancing photosynthetic efficiency and growth rate of the algal cells [21]. Other applications of the genetic engineering include the improvement of the robustness of the culture by enhancement of the algal strain to be resistant to certain algaecides or fungicides in order to maintain contaminate free monocultures [21]. In addition to the above strategy, genetic modification was also applied to enable cyanobacteria to secrete ethanol in the culture medium [22]. This would help with the economics of the algae to biofuels production process by negating the need for cell rupture [23].

9.3.2 ALGAL MASS CULTIVATIONS

Microalgae can be grown in suspended growth systems (open raceway ponds or closed photobioreactors) or attached growth systems (biofilm based reactors). Both saltwater and freshwater strains of algae are commercially grown. Currently the most common algal cultivation systems are open raceway ponds and closed photobioreactors. However, in recent years biofilm based technologies have received heightened interest. Each of these cultivation methods has its relative advantages and disadvantages.

9.3.2.1 Open Raceway Ponds

Open raceway ponds are the oldest and simplest suspension based cultivation systems and are configured in an oval shape with the culture liquid circulating in a continuous loop using a paddlewheel. The liquid level is commonly shallow, typically 30 cm deep. The foundation of the ponds are made of a water impermeable material such as concrete, or are simply dug into the earth and lined with a plastic liner. Baffles can be used to provide additional turbulence to improve distribution of light and allow mass transfer of gases into and out of the liquid medium. The size of these systems can vary from a few meters to thousands of meters in length [25].

Temperature, evaporation, and light intensity in open raceway ponds are difficult to control due to their large size and open nature. Algal cells in open raceway ponds are also very susceptible to contamination by native strains and/or predators. Light is usually the growth-limiting factor in these systems because the penetration of the light is limited by vertical mixing and mutual cell shading. As a result, the cell densities in open raceway pond cultures are generally low ($0.1–1.5$ g L^{-1}), which increases the cost to harvest the algal biomass [26].

9.3.2.2 Closed Photobioreactors

Closed photobioreactors (PBRs) are closed vessels made of transparent glass or plastic with the most common designs being tubular or flat panel based. PBRs were established to overcome major issues associated with open raceway pond systems such as low cell densities, water evaporation, contamination, and large land requirements [27]. Regarding the issue of cell density, PBR systems can achieve cell densities that are 13 times greater than that in open raceway ponds [3]. PBRs usually have a high surface to volume ratio that increases the light illumination area and reduces light attenuation. In addition, PBRs are usually very versatile in design configuration and can be placed indoors with artificial light or outdoors with natural sunlight [28].

Although PBRs have multiple benefits, this type of culture system usually requires higher capital investments and is costly expensive to scale up. In addition, a separate degassing system is often needed to remove O_2 produced during photosynthesis and light limitation is again an issue as the culture density increases [29].

9.3.2.3 Biofilm-Based Systems

Biofilm-based systems are an alternative to suspended algal growth systems in which algae cells are attached on the surface of a supporting material and harvested by scraping. Biomass harvested from a biofilm-based system can have water content between 80–90%, similar to centrifuged algal biomass [30–32]. Research has demonstrated that a biofilm-based system could outperform an open raceway pond by 694% in a pilot-scale yearlong side-by-side study [33].

Various biofilm systems have been reported in recent years [33]. In general, biofilm systems can be classified as either a stationery biofilm, in which liquid flows over a stationary biofilm, or a moving biofilm, in which biofilm is moved through the culture liquid. An example of a stationery biofilm system would be algae turf scrubbers, which are similar to a spillway with a very mild slope [34]. A typical example of a moving biofilm system is the revolving algal biofilm (RAB) system, which essentially contains a vertical conveyor belt on which a biofilm forms and rotates in and out of a culture broth reservoir [35, 36].

Compared to suspended culture systems, algal biofilm systems exhibit several advantages such as high biomass productivity, cost effective harvesting, low water requirements, enhanced light utilization efficiency, and enhanced mass transfer of CO_2 and O_2 [33, 37]. However, biofilm systems can be mechanically complex, which incurs additional cost and the potential for mechanical failures. In general, algal biofilm systems still require additional research prior to commercial deployment.

9.3.3 ALGAE DOWNSTREAM PROCESSING

Algae grown in mass cultivation systems will be subject to multiple processes before they can be processed into biofuels. These downstream processes include harvesting, dewatering, drying, and lysis of algal cells. In some processes such as anaerobic digestion or hydrothermal liquefaction, drying and lysis may not be required.

9.3.3.1 Algae Harvesting

Selecting an appropriate harvesting technology is largely based on the cultivation system and the strain of algae. In suspension culture systems, algal cells are harvested from the culture liquid (0.05–0.5% solids) as an algal slurry (2–7% solids) through a sedimentation, flocculation, or floatation process [26, 29]. Sedimentation is usually the first step in the harvesting process. The size and physicochemical characteristics of algal cells play an important role in sedimentation efficiency. A clarifier commonly used in wastewater treatment can be used for sedimentation for strains that have naturally high sedimentation rates. In the case of algae with low sedimentation rates, flocculants can be used to promote aggregation of cells into larger clumps that can be more rapidly settled [38].

Flocculation can be achieved through auto/bio-flocculation, chemical flocculants, or electroflocculation. Autofloculation (i.e., natural aggregation of the cells) can be induced by limiting the CO_2 supply or allowing the pH to rise in the culture [28, 39]. Chemical flocculants can be used to force the algal cells to aggregate by acting on the algal cell's physiochemical properties. In general, algal cells carry a negative charge that prevents aggregation in suspension. The surface charge can be neutralized or reduced by adding flocculants such as multivalent cations or cationic polymers (polyelectrolytes).

Aluminum or iron (III) ions are commonly used in algal cells flocculation. However, using chemical flocculants may lead to the accumulation of undesirable metal-containing biomass. Electro-flocculation is another method for algal cell flocculation by adding an electric current to the culture to neutralize cell charge and force cells to aggregate [38, 40].

Dissolved air floatation (DAF) is another technology used for algae harvesting. DAF is achieved by dissolving air into the liquid under high pressure. This supersaturated liquid containing dissolved air is then pumped into the vessel holding the algal culture. When the liquid reaches atmospheric pressure the dissolved air is forced out of solution in the form of small bubbles that are capable of lifting the algal flocs to the surface of the water. Once on the surface the floating algal particles can be skimmed off the top and collected [38].

It should be noted that in certain cultures the harvesting step based on sedimentation, flocculation, or flotation operations can be skipped if the cell density is high enough. In these situations, the dense algae culture can be directly dewatered in a centrifuge or filtration device.

9.3.3.2   Algae Dewatering and Drying

Once the algae are concentrated into a slurry, it needs to be further dewatered to approximately 20% solid content prior to thermal drying. This process is usually accomplished by centrifugation or filtration. Depending on the size of the algal cells, centrifugation is able to achieve >90% separation efficiency and 20% solids [41]. However, centrifugation is very expensive and is associated with high capital, operational, and energy costs [42]. Filtration is another method for dewatering algae where separation efficiency is based on the size of the filtration membrane pores (size exclusion principle). Various types of filtration systems can be used to separate algae cells including dead end, tangential flow, pressure filtration, and microfiltration [43]. In general filtration has a lower cost and energy requirement than centrifugation. However, this separation method can have problems with filter fouling and clogging [38, 41].

Following the dewatering step the biomass may need to be further dried to at least a 90% solid content prior to processing the biomass to produce biofuels. A variety of thermal processes are available to accomplish this goal, but the most popular drying methods are drum and oven drying. Air drying can also be used in low-humidity climates, but requires extra time and space and can lead to lipid degradation. In general, thermal drying is very energy intensive; therefore, biofuel conversion processes that do not require excessive drying are preferred [42, 44].

It should be noted that in algal biofilm systems the biomass can be harvested through a simple and inexpensive mechanical scrape harvester system. This negates the need for complicated harvesting and dewatering processes previously described, and the harvested biomass resembles centrifuged algal biomass in terms of solids content. This is a significant advantage of the algal biofilm systems when considering that up to 30% of the total capital and operational costs related to algal biomass production are associated with dewatering of the algal biomass [45].

9.3.3.3   Algal Cell Lysing

Lysis of the algal cells provides the means to access intracellular components, such as lipids and carbohydrates, which can be converted to biofuels. Various methods are available to disrupt the cell membrane and lyse the cells, including mechanical-based homogenization, milling, and ultra-sonication. Non-mechanical methods such as freezing, use of organic solvents, osmotic shock, enzymatic degradation, and acid and/or base treatments can also be used [19]. A recent study was conducted to evaluate lipid extraction efficiency using bead beating, sonication, autoclaving, osmotic shock, or microwaves and it was found that microwave disruption results in the best cell lysing and lipid extraction efficiency [46].

9.4   CONVERSION PATHWAYS FOR ALGAL BIOFUELS

Algal biomass can be converted into biofuels through various pathways. In general, these biofuel production pathways can be classified into three categories: (1) conversion of cellular substances such as lipids and carbohydrates, (2) conversion of whole (or defatted) algae biomass, and (3) production of extracellular metabolites as fuel products during algal cultivation. It is also possible that different pathways can be combined to create a more economical or sustainable pathway.

9.4.1 BIODIESEL PRODUCTION FROM ALGAL LIPIDS

The algal biodiesel production process is composed of a lipid extraction step followed by conversion of the extracted transesterifiable lipids to fatty acid methyl esters (FAMEs). Several processes associated with the extraction and conversion of algal lipids to biodiesel have been proposed [2, 19, 47–49]. Typically dried algal biomass (~90 wt% solids) is treated with an organic solvent such as hexane, chloroform, or other solvent mixture to solubilize the transesterifiable lipids. The solvent phase can be separated from the defatted algae residue and the dissolved lipid material can then be isolated by evaporating the organic solvent.

The extracted lipid is reacted with an alcohol (commonly methanol) to form biodiesel via transesterification. In this reaction triacylglycerols (TAG) react with methanol to form FAMEs with glycerol as a byproduct [2]. A strong acid catalyst, such as sulfuric acid, is required in the reaction. Alkali catalysts are not typically used for transesterification due to the high free fatty acid content of algal oils, which leads to soap formation [50–52]. Biodiesel formed by transesterification can be separated and collected as an organic phase, washed with water to remove aqueous impurities, and finally purified [53]. The biodiesel must meet ASTM D6751 in the United States and EN 14214 standards in the European Union for use as a fuel [54].

Unlike traditional oil crops, algal biomass is harvested with high moisture content. This results in an energetic hurdle due to the need to dry the biomass prior to lipid extraction [42, 55]. Supercritical carbon dioxide extraction is capable of extracting lipids from wet algal biomass with up to 70 wt% moisture [47, 56–58]. Other methods have also been developed to extract lipids from wet biomass such as the use of switchable polarity solvents [59, 60] and hydrolysis based lipid extraction [61].

Direct transesterification with simultaneous extraction and conversion of algal lipids to biodiesel can simplify the biodiesel production process, reducing the amount of solvent used, with higher conversion efficiencies [62–65]. For example, dried algal biomass was mixed with a strong catalyst and alcohol to produce biodiesel [62, 65, 66]. Several variations of this method have also been presented [11, 63, 64]. This method can accommodate certain level of moisture content in the algal biomass, although moisture content greater than 20% can inhibit the reaction [17, 18, 67, 68].

9.4.2   ALCOHOL PRODUCTION FROM ALGAL CARBOHYDRATES

Certain species of microalgae are capable of accumulating high levels of carbohydrates, such as starch, which can be used as an ideal substrate for fermentation into fuel products such as ethanol. Corn, sugar cane, and sugar beets are common feedstocks of fermentable sugars for fuel ethanol production. However, the use of food-based crops for fuel production is controversial. The use of algae derived starch avoids this concern because algae are not considered a food crop [69].

In addition to starch, algae also contain cellulose, which is another feedstock for ethanol production. Lignocellulosic materials such as switchgrass and corn stover are being used as fuel ethanol feedstocks, but a major challenge regarding these feedstocks is the presence of hemicellulose and lignin, which requires additional pretreatment and disposal costs. Algae does not contain lignin, which reduces the recalcitrance of the algal cellulosic materials to microbial degradation [70]. In addition to being used as a fuel ethanol feedstock, microalgae can also be used as a biocatalyst in the conversion of sugars by directly secreting ethanol into growth medium. This pathway of producing ethanol will be discussed in Section 9.4.6.

9.4.3   ANAEROBIC DIGESTION OF ALGAL BIOMASS FOR BIOGAS PRODUCTION

Anaerobic digestion (AD) converts carbon-based feedstocks into biogas, a mix of CH_4 and CO_2 with small amounts of N_2, H_2, H_2S and ammonia. AD is a straightforward process that does not require complex processing or significant energy input. The biogas produced from AD usually has an energy density of 25 MJ/kg [71], which is approximately 40% as energy dense as natural gas. Similar to natural gas, biogas can be used to produce heat and electricity and it can also be compressed and used as transportation fuels.

Whole algal biomass or lipid extracted algae meal can be used as an AD feedstock. It can also be blended with other feedstocks to improve the C:N ratio of the feedstock, which is an important factor affecting ammonia inhibition and methane production in the AD process [72]. A major advantage of algae-based AD is that the algae biomass does not need to be dried prior to anaerobic digestion. Depending on rigidity of the algal cell wall, a cell-lysing step may be needed to enhance the algae digestibility [73].

Using AD to produce biogas has several synergies with algae cultivation. For example, the effluent from the digester can be used as a nitrogen- and phosphorus-rich nutrient source for algal growth [71]. Algae can also be used to consume or scrub out the CO_2 in the biogas stream and thus increase the CH_4 content and energy density of the biogas [74].

AD of algal biomass also has several challenges. Algal biomass generally contains a high protein content leading to high levels of NH_3 production, which will be eventually inhibit the anaerobic bacteria [72]. The high salinity in marine algae can also lead to inhibition. Lastly, AD can be slowed due to strong algal cell walls.

9.4.4 BIO-CRUDE PRODUCTION VIA HYDROTHERMAL LIQUEFACTION OF ALGAL BIOMASS

Thermochemical processing of algal biomass is another approach to convert algal biomass into fuel products. Hydrothermal liquefaction (HTL) is one of the most popular methods for production of biofuels from microalgae. HTL is the process in which high moisture biomass is subjected to elevated temperatures (250–350°C) and pressures (10–20 MPa) for 20–60 minutes to decompose biomass into bio-crude in an oxygen-limited environment. Essentially the HTL process converts macromolecules such as protein, lipids and carbohydrates into bio-crude, which contains smaller chemicals such as phenols, hydrocarbons, sugars, and amino acids [75, 76]. The process mimics the natural geological process, which produced current fossil fuel reserves from ancient organic material.

HTL is an ideal process for algae-based fuel production as this process does not need to dry algal biomass prior to processing and HTL has been used to convert both whole cell and defatted algal cells. The reactor temperature, heating rate, pressure, and residence time all affect bio-crude quality and yield as well as the feedstock composition [76]. Catalysts such as salts and transition metals (Ni, Pd, and Pt) have been used to increase bio-crude yields [77]. Following the conversion process, the residual water, or aqueous phase, separates from the bio-crude phase. Bio-crude generally has an energy density of 30–40 MJ/kg, which is similar to petroleum crude (44 MJ/kg) and can be burned in boilers or further upgraded to drop in fuels [75].

Water is not only allowable in the HTL process, but also critical in the depolymerization of the biomass. In HTL conditions water becomes a highly reactive medium, which promotes the depolymerization of macromolecules into monomers and the subsequent conversion of these chemicals into bio-crude [75, 78]. It is also desirable to separate oxygen, nitrogen, and phosphorus from the bio-crude in order to produce a high-energy density bio-crude rich in hydrogen and carbon. The aqueous phase, which is rich in nitrogen and phosphorus can possibly be used as a nutrient source for algal growth [79, 80].

Several improvements are still needed for HTL processing to be commercially viable. For example the process requires a pressurized vessel and pumps capable of handling high pressures. The protein contained in algae cells results in nitrogen in the bio-crude, which decreases stability and quality of the bio-crude [75]. The nutrient rich aqueous phase contains various compounds that are inhibitory to microbial cells when used as a nutrient source [79, 80].

9.4.5   ALGAL BIO-OIL VIA FAST PYROLYSIS AND SYNGAS VIA GASIFICATION

Pyrolysis and gasification are two other thermochemical processes that can be used for converting algae into fuel products. Pyrolysis of algae is the thermochemical decomposition of algal biomass at (400–600°C) at atmospheric pressure with the absence of oxygen [75]. The major product from algal biomass pyrolysis is crude liquor (bio-oil) with small amount of incondensable gases (syngas) and carbonaceous charcoal (biochar). Similar to bio-crude, bio-oil can be either used in boilers or refined into liquid transportation fuels, but it has a much lower energy density (~21.1 MJ/kg) [81].

Gasification of algal biomass is the thermochemical decomposition of biomass at temperatures >700°C with limited amounts of oxygen. The major product from the gasification process is a mixture of gases (syngas) composed of carbon monoxide (30–60%) and hydrogen (25–30%), with lesser amounts of methane (0–5%) and CO_2 (5–15%). Syngas has an energy density of ~27 KJ/kg and can be used similarly to natural gas for heating and electricity generation. It can also be upgraded into liquid fuels using either the Fischer-Tropsch process [82] or through the fermentation of syngas to fuel products such as ethanol [83].

A major limitation with pyrolysis and gasification of algal biomass in comparison to HTL is that the biomass must be dried prior to processing, which consumes significant amounts of energy. To address this concern, researchers are evaluating the ability to capture process heat released from these processes to dry the algae, which may provide a cost effective pyrolysis or gasification process for conversion of algae to biofuel [84].

9.4.6 DIRECT PRODUCTION OF RECOVERABLE FUEL MOLECULES

In addition to being a feedstock for biofuel production, algal cells can also serve as a biocatalyst to produce and secrete molecules directly into the growth medium, which can be separated from the broth and purified into fuels such as alcohols, alkanes, and hydrogen. A major advantage in using this approach is it does not require expensive biomass harvesting and dewatering steps. An example is the use of genetically modified phototrophic cyanobacteria to produce and secrete ethanol directly into the culture broth [85]. This technology has been estimated to yield 4,000–6,000 gallons of ethanol per acre and it is projected that one ton of CO_2 is converted into 60–70 gallons of ethanol [26].

The production of hydrogen is another example. Hydrogen is an energy rich gas (120 MJ/kg) that can be directly used as a biofuel or used in hydrogenation processes to upgrade biofuels [26, 86–88]. Algal biohydrogen production, however, has several challenges as outlined in the DOE National Algal Biofuels Technology Roadmap, including the "accumulation of a proton gradient, competitive inhibition by CO_2, requirement for bicarbonate binding at photosystem II (PSII), and competitive drainage of electrons by oxygen" [26]. Alkanes are another fuel product secreted by microalgae [21]. The algae derived alkanes are similar to light petroleum and can be heterotrophically produced, secreted, and recovered from the culture broth. However, heterotrophic algal growth requires an organic carbon source and does not directly mitigate CO_2 emissions.

9.5 PERSPECTIVES

Producing biofuels from microalgae has several advantages such as high biomass productivity and ability to grow on salt water with marginal land. However, currently algal biofuel production is still not economically feasible due to several limitations associated with algal strain characteristics and engineering challenges such as high costs of harvesting biomass. For example, it was estimated that a 100-ha open raceway pond system in Netherlands produces algal biomass at a cost of \$6.86/kg (€4.95/kg) [89], while harvest cost estimated accounting for 21% of the total biomass production cost [90]. The conversion technologies from biomass to fuel products are also immature. Therefore, a variety of opportunities exist that can improve the economics of algal production.

One approach to decrease the cost of algal biofuels is to lower the production cost of the biomass feedstock. One method to accomplish this is to increase the biomass productivity, which can be accomplished by using genetically modified algal species or by optimizing culture conditions such as lighting and CO_2 supply. Algal production costs can also be reduced by decreasing the capital and operating costs associated with cultivation, harvesting, dewatering, and conversion processes.

Another approach to improve the economics of algal fuel production is to explore high value coproducts. In fact, in some cases the primary value driver for creating algal biofuel is not the actual biofuel, but rather a high value coproduct. The concept of value added coproducts is critical in processes such as corn grain ethanol production, where the ethanol, DDGS, and corn oil are all required to achieve profit. It is expected that a similar biorefinery approach will be required to achieve profitable algal biofuel production.

Coupling algal production with wastewater treatment or CO_2 mitigation can also increase the economic viability of the algal production processes. Effective production of algal biomass needs a concentrated CO_2 source to maximize biomass productivity and industrial facilities, such as power generation and ethanol fermentation plants, produce large quantities of CO_2. If algal cultivation can be coupled with such industries, additional value could be derived for CO_2 removal. Algae also needs nitrogen and phosphorus to grow and currently municipal and industrial wastewater treatment facilities are paying to remove these nutrients. If algae can effectively remove these nutrients from wastewater, it is expected that these entities would pay for such a service, helping to improve the economics of algal biomass production.

9.6 CONCLUSION

Algae biomass is among the most promising feedstocks for biofuel production. The biofuels that can be produced from algae range from gaseous fuels such as biogas and syngas to liquid fuels such as ethanol and biodiesel. Many methods have been developed to grow and convert algae into biofuels. However, the current processes available for producing algae-based biofuels are still not economically viable. Significant improvements in strain development and in engineering issues related with mass culture and harvesting are needed to lower the cost of algal biofuel production. Deriving coproducts and/or coupling algae cultivation with pollution treatment could serve as an intermediate step for developing long-term economical algal biofuels.

KEYWORDS

- **bio-crude**
- **biofuels**
- **dewatering**
- **hydrothermal liquefaction**
- **microalgae**
- **photobioreactors**

REFERENCES

1. Mandal, S., & Mallick, N. (2009). Microalga Scenedesmus Obliquus as a Potential Source for Biodiesel Production. *Appl. Microbiol. Biotechnol., 84* (2), 281–291.
2. Huang, G., Chen, F., Wei, D., Zhang, X., & Chen, G. (2010). Biodiesel Production by Microalgal Biotechnology. *Appl. Energy, 87* (1), 38–46.
3. Chisti, Y. (2007). Biodiesel from Microalgae. *Biotechnol. Adv., 25* (3), 294–306.
4. Guiry, M. D. (2012). How Many Species of Algae Are There? *J. Phycol., 48* (5), 1057–1063.
5. Xu, H., Miao, X., & Wu, Q. (2006). High Quality Biodiesel Production from a Micro-alga Chlorella Protothecoides by Heterotrophic Growth in Fermenters. *J. Biotechnol., 126*(4), 499–507.
6. Garc'ia, M. C., Camacho, G. F., Mirón, S. A., Sevilla, J. F., Chisti, Y., & Grima, M. E. (2006). Mixotrophic Production of Marine Microalga Phaeodactylum Tricornutum on Various Carbon Sources. *J. Microbiol. Biotechnol., 16*(5), 689.
7. Singh, A., Nigam, P. S., & Murphy, J. D. (2011). Mechanism and Challenges in Com-mercialization of Algal Biofuels. *Bioresour. Technol., 102*(1), 26–34.
8. Kesaano, M., & Sims, R. C. (2014). Algal Biofilm Based Technology for Wastewater Treatment. *Algal Res., 5*, 231–240.

9. Becker, E. W. (2007). Micro-Algae as a Source of Protein. *Biotechnol. Adv., 25*(2), 207–210.

10. Branyikova, I., Marsalkova, B., Doucha, J., Branyik, T., Bisova, K., Zachleder, V., & Vtova, M. (2011). Microalgae-Novel Highly Efficient Starch Producers. *Biotechnol. Bioeng., 108*(4), 766–776.

11. Ahmad, A. L., Yasin, N. H. M., Derek, C. J. C., & Lim, J. K. (2011). Microalgae as a Sustainable Energy Source for Biodiesel Production: A Review. *Renew. Sustain. Energy Rev., 15*(1), 584–593.

12. MacDougall, K. M., McNichol, J., McGinn, P. J., O'Leary, S. J. B., & Melanson, J. E. (2011). Triacylglycerol Profiling of Microalgae Strains for Biofuel Feedstock by Liquid Chromatography-High-Resolution Mass Spectrometry. *Anal. Bioanal. Chem., 401*(8), 2609–2616.

13. Knothe, G. (2005). Dependence of Biodiesel Fuel Properties on the Structure of Fatty Acid Alkyl Esters. *Fuel Process. Technol., 86*(10), 1059–1070.

14. Wen, Z., Liu, J., & Chen, F. (2011). 3.12 - Biofuel from Microalgae A2 - Moo-Young, Murray. In *Comprehensive Biotechnology (Second Edition)*, Academic Press: Burlington, pp. 127–133.

15. Kang, J., & Wen, Z. (2015). Use of Microalgae for Mitigating Ammonia and CO2 Emissions from Animal Production Operations — Evaluation of Gas Removal Efficiency and Algal Biomass Composition. *Algal Res., 11*, 204–210.

16. Lum, K. K., Kim, J., & Lei, X. G. (2013). others. Dual Potential of Microalgae as a Sustainable Biofuel Feedstock and Animal Feed. *J Anim Sci Biotechnol., 4*(1), 53.

17. Lodge-Ivey, S. L., Tracey, L. N., & Salazar, A. (2014). RUMINANT NUTRITION SYMPOSIUM: The Utility of Lipid Extracted Algae as a Protein Source in Forage or Starch-Based Ruminant Diets. *J. Anim. Sci., 92*(4), 1331–1342.

18. Huo, Y.-X., Cho, K. M., Rivera, J. G. L., Monte, E., Shen, C. R., Yan, Y., & Liao, J. C. (2011). Conversion of Proteins into Biofuels by Engineering Nitrogen Flux. *Nat. Biotechnol., 29*(4), 346–351.

19. Mata, T. M., Martins, A. A., & Caetano, N. S. (2010). Microalgae for Biodiesel Production and Other Applications: A Review. *Renew. Sustain. Energy Rev., 14*(1), 217–232.

20. Radakovits, R., Eduafo, P. M., & Posewitz, M. C. (2011). Genetic Engineering of Fatty Acid Chain Length in Phaeodactylum Tricornutum. *Metab. Eng., 13*(1), 89–95.

21. Radakovits, R., Jinkerson, R. E., Darzins, A., & Posewitz, M. C. (2010). Genetic Engineering of Algae for Enhanced Biofuel Production. *Eukaryot. Cell, 9*(4), 486–501.

22. Deng, M.-D., & Coleman, J. R. (1999). Ethanol Synthesis by Genetic Engineering in Cyanobacteria. *Appl. Environ. Microbiol., 65*(2), 523–528.

23. Samarasinghe, N., Fernando, S., Lacey, R., & Faulkner, W. B. (2012). Algal Cell Rupture Using High Pressure Homogenization as a Prelude to Oil Extraction. *Renew. Energy, 48*, 300–308.

24. Jorquera, O., Kiperstok, A., Sales, E. A., Embiruçu, M., & Ghirardi, M. L. (2010). Comparative Energy Life-Cycle Analyses of Microalgal Biomass Production in Open Ponds and Photobioreactors. *Bioresour. Technol., 101*(4), 1406–1413.

25. Rogers, J. N., Rosenberg, J. N., Guzman, B. J., Oh, V. H., Mimbela, L. E., Ghassemi, A., Betenbaugh, M. J., Oyler, G. A., & Donohue, M. D. (2014). A Critical Analysis of Paddlewheel-Driven Raceway Ponds for Algal Biofuel Production at Commercial Scales. *Algal Res., 4*, 76–88.

26. U.S. Department of Energy, Office of Energy Efficiency and Renewable Energy. National Algal Biofuels Technology Roadmap. (2010).

27. Molina Grima, E., Fernández, F. G. A., García Camacho, F., & Chisti, Y. (1999). Photobioreactors: Light Regime, Mass Transfer, and Scaleup. *J. Biotechnol., 70*(1–3), 231–247.

28. Chen, C.-Y., Yeh, K.-L., Aisyah, R., Lee, D.-J., & Chang, J. S. (2011). Cultivation, Photobioreactor Design and Harvesting of Microalgae for Biodiesel Production: A Critical Review. *Bioresour. Technol., 102*(1), 71–81.

29. Rawat, I., Ranjith Kumar, R., Mutanda, T., & Bux, F. (2013). Biodiesel from Microalgae: A Critical Evaluation from Laboratory to Large Scale Production. *Appl. Energy, 103*, 444–467.

30. Gross, M., Henry, W., Michael, C., & Wen, Z. (2013). Development of a Rotating Algal Biofilm Growth System for Attached Microalgae Growth with in Situ Biomass Harvest. *Bioresour. Technol., 150*, 195–201.

31. Johnson, M. B., & Wen, Z. (2010). Development of an Attached Microalgal Growth System for Biofuel Production. *Appl. Microbiol. Biotechnol., 85*(3), 525–534.

32. Christenson, L. B., & Sims, R. C. (2012). Rotating Algal Biofilm Reactor and Spool Harvester for Wastewater Treatment with Biofuels by-Products. *Biotechnol. Bioeng., 109*(7), 1674–1684.

33. Gross, M., Jarboe, D., & Wen, Z. (2015). Biofilm-Based Algal Cultivation Systems. *Appl. Microbiol. Biotechnol., 99*(14), 5781–5789.

34. Mulbry, W., Kondrad, S., & Buyer, J. (2008). Treatment of Dairy and Swine Manure Effluents Using Freshwater Algae: Fatty Acid Content and Composition of Algal Biomass at Different Manure Loading Rates. *J. Appl. Phycol., 20*(6), 1079–1085.

35. Gross, M., Mascarenhas, V., & Wen, Z. (2015). Evaluating Algal Growth Performance and Water Use Efficiency of Pilot-Scale Revolving Algal Biofilm (RAB) Culture Systems. *Biotechnol. Bioeng., 112*(10), 2040–2050.

36. Gross, M., & Wen, Z. (2014). Yearlong Evaluation of Performance and Durability of a Pilot-Scale Revolving Algal Biofilm (RAB) Cultivation System. *Bioresour. Technol., 171*, 50–58.

37. Genin, S. N., Stewart Aitchison, J., & Grant Allen, D. (2014). Design of Algal Film Photobioreactors: Material Surface Energy Effects on Algal Film Productivity, Colonization and Lipid Content. *Bioresour. Technol., 155*, 136–143.

38. Uduman, N., Qi, Y., Danquah, M. K., Forde, G. M., & Hoadley, A. (2010). Dewatering of Microalgal Cultures: A Major Bottleneck to Algae-Based Fuels. *J. Renew. Sustain. Energy, 2*(1), 012701.

39. Sukenik, A., & Shelef, G. (1984). Algal Autoflocculation-Verification and Proposed Mechanism. *Biotechnol. Bioeng., 26*(2), 142–147.

40. Anthony, R. J., & Sims, R. C. (2013). Optimization of Cationic Amino Starch Synthesis Using Biogenic Amines. *Carbohydr. Polym., 98*(2), 1409–1415.

41. Christenson, L., & Sims, R. (2011). Production and Harvesting of Microalgae for Wastewater Treatment, Biofuels, and Bioproducts. *Biotechnol. Adv., 29*(6), 686–702.

42. Sander, K., & Murthy, G. S. (2010). Life Cycle Analysis of Algae Biodiesel. *Int. J. Life Cycle Assess., 15*(7), 704–714.

43. Harun, R., Singh, M., Forde, G. M., & Danquah, M. K. (2010). Bioprocess Engineering of Microalgae to Produce a Variety of Consumer Products. *Renew. Sustain. Energy Rev., 14*(3), 1037–1047.

44. Xu, L., (Wim) Brilman, D. W. F., Withag, J. A. M., Brem, G., & Kersten, S. (2011). Assessment of a Dry and a Wet Route for the Production of Biofuels from Microalgae: Energy Balance Analysis. *Bioresour. Technol., 102*(8), 5113–5122.

45. Molina Grima, E., Belarbi, E.-H., Acién Fernández, F. G., Robles Medina, A., & Chisti, Y. (2003). Recovery of Microalgal Biomass and Metabolites: Process Options and Economics. *Biotechnol. Adv., 20*(7), 491–515.

46. Lee, J.-Y., Yoo, C., Jun, S.-Y., Ahn, C.-Y., & Oh, H.-M. (2010). Comparison of Several Methods for Effective Lipid Extraction from Microalgae. *Bioresour. Technol., 101*(1), S75–S77.

47. Gong, Y., & Jiang, M. (2011). Biodiesel Production with Microalgae as Feedstock: From Strains to Biodiesel. *Biotechnol. Lett., 33*(7), 1269–1284.

48. Vyas, A. P., Verma, J. L., & Subrahmanyam, N. (2010). A Review on FAME Production Processes. *Fuel, 89*(1), 1–9.

49. Marchetti, J. M., Miguel, V. U., & Errazu, A. F. (2007). Possible Methods for Biodiesel Production. *Renew. Sustain. Energy Rev., 11*(6), 1300–1311.

50. Lotero, E., Liu, Y., Lopez, D. E., Suwannakarn, K., Bruce, D. A., & Goodwin, J. G. (2005). Synthesis of Biodiesel via Acid Catalysis. *Ind. Eng. Chem. Res., 44*(14), 5353–5363.

51. Miao, X., & Wu, Q. (2006). Biodiesel Production from Heterotrophic Microalgal Oil. *Bioresour. Technol., 97*(6), 841–846.

52. Ataya, F., Dubé, M. A., & Ternan, M. (2007). Acid-Catalyzed Transesterification of Canola Oil to Biodiesel under Single- and Two-Phase Reaction Conditions. *Energy Fuels, 21*(4), 2450–2459.

53. Ma, F., & Hanna, M. A. (1999). Biodiesel Production: A Review. *Bioresour. Technol., 70*(1), 1–15.

54. Moser, B. R. (2009). Biodiesel Production, Properties, and Feedstocks. *Vitro Cell. Dev. Biol. Plant, 45*(3), 229–266.

55. Lardon, L., Helias, A., Sialve, B., & Steyer, J.-P., (2009). Bernard, O. Life-Cycle Assessment of Biodiesel Production from Microalgae. *Environ. Sci. Technol., 43*(17), 6475–6481.

56. Halim, R., Danquah, M. K., & Webley, P. A. (2012). Extraction of Oil from Microalgae for Biodiesel Production: A Review. *Biotechnol. Adv., 30*(3), 709–732.

57. Herrero, M., Cifuentes, A., & Ibanez, E. (2006). Sub- and Supercritical Fluid Extraction of Functional Ingredients from Different Natural Sources: Plants, Food-by-Products, Algae and microalgaeA Review. *Food Chem., 98*(1), 136–148.

58. Halim, R., Gladman, B., Danquah, M. K., & Webley, P. A. (2011). Oil Extraction from Microalgae for Biodiesel Production. *Bioresour. Technol., 102* (1), 178–185.

59. Kusdiana, D., & Saka, S. (2004). Effects of Water on Biodiesel Fuel Production by Supercritical Methanol Treatment. *Bioresour. Technol., 91*(3), 289–295.

60. Reddy, H. K., Muppaneni, T., Patil, P. D., Ponnusamy, S., Cooke, P., Schaub, T., & Deng, S. (2014). Direct Conversion of Wet Algae to Crude Biodiesel under Supercritical Ethanol Conditions. *Fuel, 115*, 720–726.

61. Sathish, A., Marlar, T., & Sims, R. C. (2015). Optimization of a Wet Microalgal Lipid Extraction Procedure for Improved Lipid Recovery for Biofuel and Bioproduct Production. *Bioresour. Technol., 193*, 15–24.

62. Haas, M. J., & Wagner, K. (2011). Simplifying Biodiesel Production: The Direct or in Situ Transesterification of Algal Biomass. *Eur. J. Lipid Sci. Technol., 113*(10), 1219–1229.

63. Griffiths, M. J., van Hille, R. P., & Harrison, S. T. L. (2010). Selection of Direct Transesterification as the Preferred Method for Assay of Fatty Acid Content of Microalgae. *Lipids, 45*(11), 1053–1060.

64. Wahlen, B. D., Willis, R. M., & Seefeldt, L. C. (2011). Biodiesel Production by Simultaneous Extraction and Conversion of Total Lipids from Microalgae, Cyanobacteria, and Wild Mixed-Cultures. *Bioresour. Technol., 102*(3), 2724–2730.

65. Ehimen, E. A., Sun, Z. F., & Carrington, C. G. (2010). Variables Affecting the in Situ Transesterification of Microalgae Lipids. *Fuel 89* (3), 677–684.

66. Johnson, M. B., & Wen, Z. (2009). Production of Biodiesel Fuel from the Microalga *Schizochytrium Limacinum* by Direct Transesterification of Algal Biomass. *Energy Fuels, 23*(10), 5179–5183.

67. Sathish, A., Smith, B. R., & Sims, R. C. (2014). Effect of Moisture on *in Situ* Transesterification of Microalgae for Biodiesel Production: Effect of Moisture on Biodiesel Production from Microalgae. *J. Chem. Technol. Biotechnol., 89*(1), 137–142.

68. Liu, Y., Lotero, E., & Goodwin, J. G. (2006). Effect of Water on Sulfuric Acid Catalyzed Esterification. *J. Mol. Catal. Chem., 245*(1–2), 132–140.

69. Schenk, P. M., Thomas-Hall, S. R., Stephens, E., Marx, U. C., Mussgnug, J. H., Posten, C., Kruse, O., & Hankamer, B. (2008). Second Generation Biofuels: High-Efficiency Microalgae for Biodiesel Production. *BioEnergy Res., 1*(1), 20–43.

70. John, R. P., Anisha, G. S., Nampoothiri, K. M., & Pandey, A. (2011). Micro and Macroalgal Biomass: A Renewable Source for Bioethanol. *Bioresour. Technol., 102*(1), 186–193.

71. Collet, P., Hélias, A., Lardon, L., Ras, M., Goy, R.-A., & Steyer, J.-P. (2011). Life-Cycle Assessment of Microalgae Culture Coupled to Biogas Production. *Bioresour. Technol., 102*(1), 207–214.

72. Chen, Y., Cheng, J. J., & Creamer, K. S. (2008). Inhibition of Anaerobic Digestion Process: A Review. *Bioresour. Technol. 99* (10), 4044–4064.

73. Samson, R., & Leduy, A. (1983). Influence of Mechanical and Thermochemical Pretreatments on Anaerobic Digestion ofSpirulina Maxima Algal Biomass. *Biotechnol. Lett., 5*(10), 671–676.

74. Xia, A., Herrmann, C., & Murphy, J. D. (2015). How Do We Optimize Third-Generation Algal Biofuels? *Biofuels Bioprod. Biorefining, 9*(4), 358–367.

75. López Barreiro, D., Prins, W., Ronsse, F., & Brilman, W. (2013). Hydrothermal Liquefaction (HTL) of Microalgae for Biofuel Production: State of the Art Review and Future Prospects. *Biomass Bioenergy, 53*, 113–127.

76. Biller, P., & Ross, A. B. (2011). Potential Yields and Properties of Oil from the Hydrothermal Liquefaction of Microalgae with Different Biochemical Content. *Bioresour. Technol., 102*(1), 215–225.

77. Duan, P., & Savage, P. E. (2011). Hydrothermal Liquefaction of a Microalga with Heterogeneous Catalysts. *Ind. Eng. Chem. Res., 50*(1), 52–61.

78. Tian, C., Li, B., Liu, Z., Zhang, Y., & Lu, H. (2014). Hydrothermal Liquefaction for Algal Biorefinery: A Critical Review. *Renew. Sustain. Energy Rev., 38*, 933–950.

79. Biller, P., Ross, A. B., Skill, S. C., Lea-Langton, A., Balasundaram, B., Hall, C., Riley, R., & Llewellyn, C. A. (2012). Nutrient Recycling of Aqueous Phase for Microalgae Cultivation from the Hydrothermal Liquefaction Process. *Algal Res., 1*(1), 70–76.

80. Jena, U., Vaidyanathan, N., Chinnasamy, S., & Das, K. C. (2011). Evaluation of Microalgae Cultivation Using Recovered Aqueous Co-Product from Thermochemical Liquefaction of Algal Biomass. *Bioresour. Technol., 102*(3), 3380–3387.

81. Kim, S. W., Koo, B. S., & Lee, D. H. (2014). A Comparative Study of Bio-Oils from Pyrolysis of Microalgae and Oil Seed Waste in a Fluidized Bed. *Bioresour. Technol., 162*, 96–102.

82. Okabe, K., Murata, K., Nakanishi, M., Ogi, T., Nurunnabi, M., & Liu, Y. (2008). Fischer–Tropsch Synthesis over Ru Catalysts by Using Syngas Derived from Woody Biomass. *Catal. Lett., 128*(1–2), 171–176.

83. Shen, Y., Brown, R., & Wen, Z. (2014). Syngas Fermentation of Clostridium Carboxidivoran P7 in a Hollow Fiber Membrane Biofilm Reactor: Evaluating the Mass Transfer Coefficient and Ethanol Production Performance. *Biochem. Eng. J., 85*, 21–29.

84. Scott, D. S., Majerski, P., Piskorz, J., & Radlein, D. (1999). A Second Look at Fast Pyrolysis of Biomass—the RTI Process. *J. Anal. Appl. Pyrolysis., 51*(1–2), 23–37.

85. Luo, D., Hu, Z., Choi, D. G., Thomas, V. M., Realff, M. J., & Chance, R. R. (2010). Life Cycle Energy and Greenhouse Gas Emissions for an Ethanol Production Process Based on Blue-Green Algae. *Environ. Sci. Technol., 44*(22), 8670–8677.

86. Zhao, Y.-F., Rousseau, R., Li, J., & Mei, D. (2012). Theoretical Study of Syngas Hydrogenation to Methanol on the Polar Zn-Terminated ZnO(0001) Surface. *J. Phys. Chem. C., 116*(30), 15952–15961.

87. Das, S. K., Majhi, S., Mohanty, P., & Pant, K. K. (2014). CO-Hydrogenation of Syngas to Fuel Using Silica Supported Fe–Cu–K Catalysts: Effects of Active Components. *Fuel Process. Technol., 118*, 82–89.

88. Serrano-Ruiz, J. C., & Dumesic, J. A. (2009). Catalytic Upgrading of Lactic Acid to Fuels and Chemicals by Dehydration/hydrogenation and C–C Coupling Reactions. *Green Chem., 11*(8), 1101–1104.

89. Norsker, N., Barbosa, M., Vermue, M., & Wijffels, R. (2011). Microalgal production- A close look at the economics. *Biotechnol. Adv., 29*, 24–27.

90. Davis, R., Aden, A., & Pienkos, P. (2011). Techno-economic analysis of autotrophic microalgae for fuel production. *Appl. Energy, 88*, 3524–3531.

CHAPTER 10

BIOENERGY FROM ACTIVATED SLUDGE AND WASTEWATER

ANDRO MONDALA,[1] RAFAEL HERNANDEZ,[2] TODD FRENCH,[3] EMMANUEL REVELLAME,[4] DHAN LORD FORTELA,[2] and MARTA AMIRSADEGHI[5]

[1]*Department of Chemical and Paper Engineering, Western Michigan University, Kalamazoo, MI 49008, USA*

[2]*Department of Chemical Engineering, University of Louisiana at Lafayette, Lafayette, LA, 70504, USA*

[3]*Dave C. Swalm School of Chemical Engineering, Mississippi State University, Mississippi State, MS, 39759, USA*

[4]*Department of Industrial Technology, University of Louisiana at Lafayette, Lafayette, LA, 70504, USA*

[5]*Department of Chemical and Materials Engineering, California State Polytechnic University Ponoma, Ponoma, CA, 91768, USA*

CONTENTS

ABSTRACT

Wastewater treatment operations present significant opportunities for integration of sustainable bioenergy production technologies. This chapter outlines and discusses research efforts on the utilization of activated sludge, municipal and industrial wastewaters, and treatment facilities for the production of lipidic biofuels (i.e., biodiesel and renewable diesel) and nonfood-based lipid feedstock. Lipidic fractions of sewage sludges have been extracted, characterized, and subjected to transesterification and catalytic cracking for production of biodiesel and renewable diesel, respectively. Wastewaters from municipal and industrial sources have been used as carbon and nutrient source and cultivation media for the cultivation of oleaginous yeasts, which produce substantial quantities of microbial oils for extraction and conversion to biofuels. The same approach has been applied for enhancing the oil contents of activated sludge microbial biomass for increased lipid feedstock and biodiesel or renewable diesel yield via cultivation in wastewater media with increased carbon content through the addition of sugars derived from renewable lignocellulosic biomass wastes. Short chain fatty acids have been evaluated as carbon sources to oil-accumulating activated sludge cultures.

10.1   INTRODUCTION

Interest and application of biofuels continue to increase due to concerns about the volatility of oil supplies and costs as well as increased air pollution and greenhouse gas emissions associated with their use. Current biofuels production research endeavors heavily involve the search for resources that are low-cost, renewable, and does not compete with the food industry. Recent studies focused on the use of agricultural, industrial, and domestic solid residues and wastewaters as raw materials for chemical or biological conversion biofuels in order to reduce production costs.

The use of bio-based petroleum diesel alternatives such as biodiesel and renewable diesel continue to be popular as the total annual U.S. consumption reached a record high of 2.1 billion gallons in 2015 [145]. However, a continuing major challenge to the commercialization of biodiesel is its relatively higher production cost compared with petroleum-based diesel [223], around 70–85% of which could be attributed to the cost of the feedstock [81]. The major biodiesel feedstocks used are crop seed oils such as soybean oil and animal fats. Crop oil supplies are also limited by planting and harvesting seasons. Recycled used cooking oils and trap grease are also increasingly being used but these will require substantial cleanup and refining prior to conversion to biodiesel. To overcome these limitations and to help make biodiesel more cost-competitive with petroleum diesel, recent studies have been exploring low-cost and abundant nonfood-based lipid feedstocks that are readily available all-year round.

The focus of this chapter is the utilization of municipal wastewater treatment systems as a resource base and biorefinery platform for the sustainable production of biodiesel and renewable diesel and their lipidic substrates. Municipal or domestic wastewater treatment plants (WWTPs) process significant quantities of organic-rich wastewaters, producing large quantities of sludges as an unwanted by-product. The organic content of these sludges can be harnessed for the production of biofuels such as biodiesel via chemical or biological processes. The activated sludge process requires large amounts of energy for aeration while sewage biosolids continue to pose disposal and reuse issues. Current research efforts and studies in the past decade are aimed to address these sustainability challenges through the development of a WWTP biorefinery platform in which influent wastewaters and generated sewage sludges during the treatment processes are used as resources for biofuels production. This chapter discusses the envisioned WWTP biorefinery platform, findings of recent research activities related to platform development, and future perspectives.

10.2   CHEMISTRY AND SUSTAINABILITY ASPECTS

10.2.1   WASTEWATER TREATMENT USING THE ACTIVATED SLUDGE PROCESS

According to the U.S. Environmental Protection Agency, there are currently 14,748 municipal WWTPs in the U.S. treating a combined flow of 28.3 billion gallons of wastewater per day [206]. Majority of these publicly owned treatment plants employ the activated sludge process. The activated sludge process was first described over a hundred years ago by Ardern and Lockett [11] as a means of bioremediation of domestic sewage and industrial wastewaters based on the principle of using aerobic heterotrophic microbial biomass for oxidizing dissolved organic matter in the influent wastewater. At present, modified activated sludge-based wastewater treatment processes are also being used for specific wastewater nutrient removal applications such as enhanced biological phosphorus removal, nitrification-denitrification, and anaerobic oxidation of ammonium [190].

The activated sludge process works in this manner: wastewater influents are first screened and primary sludges composed of floating grease, fecal matter, fibers, and other bulk solids not removed by the screening process are separated. The screened and bulk solids-free wastewater influent is then sent into an aeration basin or bio-oxidation ditch in which air is bubbled through the wastewater to allow heterotrophic microbes to grow, proliferate, and consume the organic contaminants in the wastewater. The process results in the production of a treated effluent with reduced biochemical oxygen demand (BOD), primary sludges, and the suspended microbial biomass generated during the aerobic bio-oxidation process, which is called activated sludge or secondary sludge. The activated sludges are separated from the treated effluent by sedimentation or gravity filtration. Majority of the separated activated sludge are recycled back into the aerobic bio-oxidation process in order to maintain a sufficient level of active microbial biomass required for a specific treatment level. The excess activated sludge is typically combined with primary sludges for further treatment and stabilization most commonly by anaerobic digestion, generating sewage biosolids in the process [178, 199]. Throughout this chapter, the term "primary sludge" pertains to semisolids captured from primary clarifier, while "activated sludge" and "secondary sludge" are used interchangeably to refer to semisolid materials produced from the secondary or biological processes of wastewater treatment operations (see Figure 10.1). Furthermore, the term "sewage sludge" refers to both primary and secondary sludges.

Although currently established and widely used, the activated sludge technology faces two major sustainability challenges. First, activated sludge-based biological wastewater treatment processes consume considerable amounts of electrical energy for supplying air/oxygen to the bio-oxidation process via aeration. The goal for addressing this challenge involves increasing energy efficiency and sustainability of aeration processes through the use of renewable alternative energy sources or minimization of air requirements

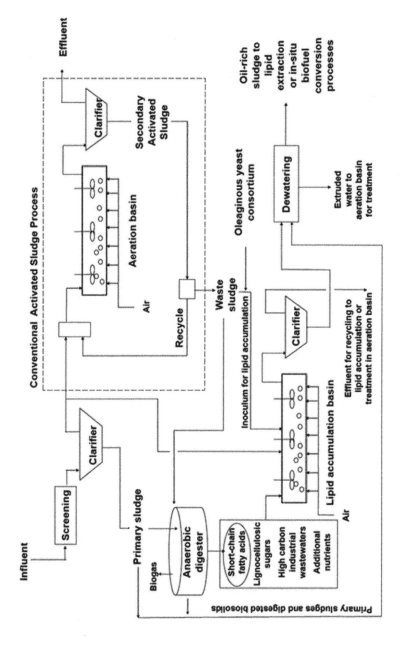

FIGURE 10.1 Activated sludge wastewater treatment plant biorefinery platform for lipidic biofuels production from wastewater and sludges.

for bio-oxidation process. The second challenge is the generation of large amounts of sewage biosolids, which present severe challenges for disposal. The most recent available data according to the U.S. EPA estimates an 8.2 million-ton production of sewage sludge biosolids in 2010 [205]. This amount is expected to increase in the coming years due to increasing urbanization and industrialization resulting into population growth in urban areas. Sewage biosolids are typically used or disposed through incineration, landfilling, and composting. Together, these issues present high operating costs and environmental issues related to increased greenhouse gas emissions and the potential for accumulation of heavy metals and other toxic organic compounds in the soil, air, and groundwater [205]. In order to address these major challenges and improve sustainability of activated sludge wastewater treatment operations, research and development efforts in the last decade have sought to harness wastewater and biosolids generated during wastewater treatment as sources of value-added biofuel substrates and compounds, including biodiesel and renewable diesel.

10.2.2 BIODIESEL AND RENEWABLE DIESEL

Biodiesel is a petroleum diesel substitute produced via the transesterification or esterification of lipidic materials such as triacylglycerides (TAGs) and/ or free fatty acids (FFAs) with short chain alcohols to yield fatty acid alkyl esters, which are essentially the diesel fuel compounds, and glycerol [207]. When methanol is used as the alcoholic reactant, the resulting compounds are called fatty acid methyl esters or FAMEs. Biodiesel has been extensively studied and produced commercially as a petroleum diesel fuel substitute due to its environmental benefits (i.e., biodegradability and reduced emissions of CO_2, unburned hydrocarbons, carbon monoxide, and particulates), enhanced safety properties (i.e., lower flashpoint than petroleum diesel), the use of renewable domestic feedstocks, and good performance characteristics (i.e., comparable energy content with petrodiesel and improved lubricity) [144]. Biodiesel is defined under the American Society for Testing and Materials (ASTM) Standard D6751 as "a fuel comprised of mono-alkyl esters of long chain fatty acids derived from vegetable oils or animal fats."

On the other hand, renewable diesel or green diesel is different from biodiesel in that the former is more chemically similar to petroleum diesel and does not contain ester groups that are characteristic of biodiesel compounds.

Renewable diesel or green diesel can be produced by hydrotreating or hydroprocessing, thermal depolymerization, or the biomass-to-liquid (BTL) with Fischer-Tropsch process [222]. In the hydrotreating process, the lipid feedstock is reacted with hydrogen in the presence of a catalyst to convert TAGs into paraffinic hydrocarbons with similar properties to petrodiesel. Thermal depolymerization processes involves subjecting carbon-containing substrates to high-temperature and –pressure conditions to convert them into "bio-oil," which is then refined into petrodiesel-like fuel. The BTL process involves high temperature gasification of biomass substrates into syngas, which is then condensed into liquid fuels via the Fischer-Tropsch process.

As mentioned earlier, one of the major sustainability challenges in the use of these bio-based petrodiesel compounds is the cost and source of the feedstock. Current trends for achieving sustainability indicate the diversion from crop oils or animal fats that are also used in food production towards nonfood or waste derived sources of lipidic raw materials. The use of sewage sludge and biosolids and microbial oils generated by oleaginous microbes grown in wastewater as an oil feedstock source for biodiesel or renewable diesel production offers advantages of having low to zero costs, year-round availability, and renewability of sources.

10.2.3   WASTEWATER TREATMENT PLANT BIOREFINERY PLATFORM FOR BIO-BASED DIESEL FUEL PRODUCTION

The envisioned biorefinery platform (see Figure 10.1) integrates biofuels production technologies into a conventional activated sludge process-based wastewater treatment process with anaerobic digestion for biosolids handling. This biorefinery concept was designed with concepts of resource recovery and waste minimization as the primary motivating factors in order to use influent wastewater and sludge streams for bioenergy recovery through conversion to biofuel compounds and/or precursors. The key features of this WWTP biorefinery include the following: (1) Extraction of adsorbed oils and lipidic materials from sewage sludges or biosolids using conventional solvent based extraction processes and subsequently converted to biodiesel or renewable diesel. Alternatively, sewage sludges or biosolids can be subjected to *in situ* chemical conversion processes (e.g., transesterification, hydrotreating, gasification, etc.) for direct production of biodiesel and/or renewable diesel compounds without prior oil extraction and recovery. (2) Influent wastewater can be supplemented with additional renewable carbon and nutrient sources and used as growth media for oleaginous microorganisms capable of synthesizing high amounts of lipid storage compounds, which can then be extracted and converted to biodiesel or renewable diesel. The oleaginous microbes can be sourced from a specialized oleaginous consortium or generated from within the activated sludge microbial community under certain cultivation conditions. This process produces sludge biomass with increased oil content, which can be subjected to sequential extraction and conversion or *in situ* conversion to biodiesel or renewable diesel. The fundamental aspects and specific features of the WWTP biorefinery concepts and the related research and development efforts conducted on this area are discussed in the next sections of this chapter.

10.2.4   SUSTAINABILITY OF APPROACH

This WWTP biorefinery approach applies sustainability principles of maximizing resource recovery from waste streams, producing value added products from waste streams, leveraging existing process equipment and facilities, and integrating wastewater treatment and resource recovery. These approaches are viable alternatives to conventional sludge disposal and low-value use practices and could potentially offset the energy use due to aeration by the production of energy-rich molecules such as microbial storage lipids and conversion to fuel compounds such as biodiesel and renewable diesel. It should be noted that the approaches presented in this chapter are not intended to replace existing wastewater operations (see Figure 10.1). Rather, the intent is to integrate these approaches into existing WWTPs without jeopardizing the quality of the effluents from these facilities.

10.3   EXTRACTION AND FRACTIONATION OF LIPIDIC MATERIALS FROM ACTIVATED SLUDGE

10.3.1   INTRODUCTION

Extraction of materials (i.e., lipids) from activated sludge for renewable fuel applications is commonly accomplished by solvent extraction. Similar to extraction of any materials, the solubility of the compound of interest is the main criterion in solvent selection. For biodiesel application, TAGs are the most attractive lipid feedstock due to their amenability to base-catalyzed transesterification [175]. TAGs are nonpolar in nature and thus, can be extracted with common nonpolar solvents such as hexane or slightly polar solvents such as chloroform. Although TAGs are present in significant quantity, they comprise only a small portion of the extractable materials from activated sludge. The remainder includes compounds with varying polarity including hydrocarbons, wax esters (WEs), polyhydroxyalkanoates (PHAs), phospholipids (PLs), diacylglycerides (DAGs), monoacylglycerides (MAGs), FFAs, sterols and fatty alcohols [173, 174]. Maximizing the yield of biodiesel from this feedstock is synonymous to maximizing the recovery of all these compound classes. Thus, it is critical to have an extraction protocol that can efficiently recover both polar and nonpolar compounds. This is commonly accomplished by using a mixture of solvents with different polarities or by sequential extraction using solvents with varying polarities [55, 173]. In addition, pretreatment strategies are equally important in maximizing extraction yields from activated sludges. This section describes different extraction techniques as well as pretreatment strategies to maximize the yield of extractables from activated sludge (see Figure 10.2).

10.3.2 PRE-TREATMENTS AND EXTRACTION TECHNIQUES

Prior to extraction, activated sludges are usually subjected to various pretreatments including drying, size reduction, homogenization, sonication, acidification and subcritical-water treatment (see Table 10.1). The choice of pretreatment strategy (except drying) does not depend on the targeted extraction technique, which for activated sludge includes Soxhlet extraction, accelerated solvent extraction (ASE®), Bligh and Dyer (BD), solvent extraction and supercritical fluid extraction (SFE). Among these extraction techniques, only BD does not require sludge drying since water (in addition to methanol and chloroform) is one of the extraction solvents (Bligh and

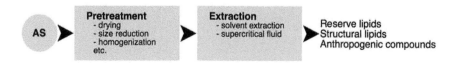

FIGURE 10.2 Generalized schematic for the extraction of lipidic materials from activated sludge (AS).

TABLE 10.1 Lipid Content of Raw Activated Sludge Using Different Extraction Techniques[a]

Extraction Technique	Extraction Solvent	Sludge Dewatering and Pre-Treatment	Moisture Content (wt.%)	Extraction Yield (wt.% of dry sludge)	Esterifiable Lipids (wt.% of dry sludge)	Reference
Soxhlet	Chloroform	Drying	1.5–2.0	11.96	—	[25]
Soxhlet	Toluene	Drying	1.5–2.0	11.78	—	[25]
Soxhlet	Hexane	Drying with $MgSO_4 \cdot H_2O$	—	9 ± 1	—	[150]
Soxhlet	Hexane	Acidification to pH 2 (HCl), drying with $MgSO_4 \cdot H_2O$	—	7 ± 1	—	[150]
Soxhlet	Hexane	Sonication, drying with $MgSO_4 \cdot H_2O$	—	10 ± 1	—	[150]
Soxhlet	Hexane	Sonication, acidification using HCl, drying with $MgSO_4 \cdot H_2O$	—	9.3 ± 1.3	2.9 ± 0.5	[151]
Soxhlet	Hexane	Sonication, acidification to pH 2 (HCl), drying with $MgSO_4 \cdot H_2O$	—	8 ± 1	—	[150]
Soxhlet	Hexane	Homogenization, drying with $MgSO_4 \cdot H_2O$	—	9 ± 1	—	[150]

Soxhlet	Hexane	Homogenization, acidification to pH 2 (HCl), drying with MgSO$_4$;H$_2$O	—	8 ± 1	—	[150]
Soxhlet	Hexane	Oven drying	—	3.70	0.70	[27]
Soxhlet followed by dewaxing and degumming	Hexane	Sun drying, milling, oven drying	2.60	2.10	1.41 ± 0.03	[93]
Soxhlet followed by dewaxing and degumming	Hexane	Sun drying, milling, oven drying, subcritical-water treatment	2.60	7.87	5.15 ± 0.15	[93]
ASE®	Hexane	Gravity-settling, centrifugation, pressure filtration	12–14	1.94	0.38	[55]
ASE®	Methanol	Gravity-settling, centrifugation, pressure filtration	12–14	19.39 ± 3.20	2.76 ± 0.39	[55]
ASE®	60/20/20 vol. Hexane/Methanol/Acetone	Gravity-settling, centrifugation, pressure filtration	12–14	27.43 ± 0.98	4.41 ± 0.63	[55]
ASE®	65/35 Dichloromethane/Methanol	Freeze drying, sieving	—	5.25–14.23[b]	3.21–16.21[c]	[97]
—					2.16–19.62[d]	
					6.00–10.28[e]	

TABLE 10.1 (Continued)

Extraction Technique	Extraction Solvent	Sludge Dewatering and Pre-Treatment	Moisture Content (wt.%)	Extraction Yield (wt.% of dry sludge)	Esterifiable Lipids (wt.% of dry sludge)	Reference
Sequential ASE	Methanol followed by Hexane	Gravity-settling, centrifugation, pressure filtration	12–14	21.96 ± 2.28	3.07 ± 0.33	[55]
Bligh and Dyer	Methanol, Chloroform and Water	Gravity-settling, centrifugation, freeze drying	5	11.0 ± 1.7	2.84 ± 0.45	[141]
Bligh and Dyer	Methanol, Chloroform and Water	Gravity-settling, centrifugation, freeze drying	5	—	2–3	[139]
Bligh and Dyer	Methanol, Chloroform and Water	Gravity-settling, centrifugation, freeze drying	5	—	1–2	[138]
Bligh and Dyer	Methanol, Chloroform and Water	Heating	10	5.3 ± 0.2	4.2	[184]
Bligh and Dyer	Methanol, Chloroform and Water	Gravity-settling, centrifugation	84–92	3.80–13.14	—	[161]
Modified Bligh and Dyer	Methanol, Chloroform and Phosphate buffer	Freeze drying	—	—	0.20	[83]
Bligh and Dyer followed by Solid Phase Extraction	Methanol, Chloroform and Water	Gravity-settling, centrifugation, freeze drying	—	5.1–10.4	1.4–2.3	[175]

Method	Solvent	Pretreatment				Reference
Bligh and Dyer followed by Solid Phase Extraction	Methanol, Chloroform and Water	Gravity-settling, centrifugation/ vacuum filtration, (freeze drying)	84–92 (4.6)	5.45–17.58	1.13–3.79	[174]
Solvent extraction	Hexane	Settling, centrifugation, vacuum drying	6	3.04	0.82	[193]
Solvent extraction	Methanol	Settling, centrifugation, vacuum drying	6	10.04	3.04	[193]
Solvent extraction	Hexane	—	—	18–20	—	[113]
Solvent Extraction	Methanol	Settling, centrifugation, oven-drying	—	2.1	1.74	[132]
Boiling Solvent Extraction	Chloroform	Drying	1.5–2.0	17.80	—	[25]
Boiling Solvent Extraction	Toluene	Drying	1.5–2.0	17.23	12.47	[25]
Liquid-liquid extraction	Hexane	Acidification to pH 2 (HCl), drying with $MgSO4 \cdot H2O$	—	7.7 ± 0.1	—	[149]
Supercritical Fluid Extraction	CO_2	Fluid-bed drying	5	3.55	0.28	[55]
Supercritical Fluid Extraction	CO_2 with 10 vol.% Methanol	Freeze drying	—	—	0.19	[83]
Supercritical Fluid Extraction	CO_2 with 1.96 wt.% Methanol	Fluid-bed drying	5	4.19	1.12	[55]

TABLE 10.1 (Continued)

Extraction Technique	Extraction Solvent	Sludge Dewatering and Pre-Treatment	Moisture Content (wt.%)	Extraction Yield (wt.% of dry sludge)	Esterifiable Lipids (wt.% of dry sludge)	Reference
Supercritical Fluid Extraction	CO_2 with 13.04 wt.% Methanol	Fluid-bed drying	5	13.56	2.31	[55]
In situ transesterification	Methanol containing 1% H_2SO_4	Fluid-bed drying	5	—	6.23 ± 0.11	[55]
In situ transesterification	Methanol containing 4 vol.% H_2SO_4	Gravity-settling, centrifugation, freeze drying	5	—	4.79 ± 0.02	[170]
In situ transesterification	Methanol containing 4 vol.% H_2SO_4	Sun drying, sieving, heating	4.88	45.42^e	35	[203]
In situ transesterification	Methanol containing 4 vol.% H_2SO_4	Drying	—	66.64 ± 1.2^e	58.99 ± 1.34	[94]
In situ transesterification	Methanol (+water) containing 10 vol.% H_2SO_4	Gravity-settling, centrifugation, freeze drying	5–84.5	—	3.93 ± 0.15	[171]
In situ transesterification	Methanol containing 1 and 5 vol.% H_2SO_4 with Hexane as cosolvent	Gravity-settling, centrifugation, Freeze drying	5	—	2.5	[140]

In situ transesterification	Methanol containing 5% H_2SO_4 with Hexane as cosolvent	Furnace drying, sieving	< 5	—	9.68 ± 0.39	[38]
In situ transesterification	Methanol with 0.25 vol.% H_2SO_4	Centrifugation, freeze drying	—	4	1.9	[158]
In situ transesterification	Methanol with Zr-SBA-15 catalyst	Settling, centrifugation, oven drying	—	—	10	[132]
Subcritical in situ transesterification	Methanol with 15% acetic acid as catalyst	Sun drying, sieving, heating	4.88	45.42ᵉ	30.11	[203]
Subcritical in situ transesterification	Methanol and water	Drying	—	66.64 ± 1.2ᵉ	45.58 ± 3.52	[94]
Supercritical in situ transesterification	Methanol	Filtration/ Centrifugation, freeze drying	5	—	7.78 ± 4.15	[41]

[a] Sludges were obtained from wastewater treatment plant treating residential wastewater unless specified.

[b] Rural sludges.

[c] Small urban sludges.

[d] Urban sludges.

[e] Sludge from food processing wastewater treatment plant.

Dyer, 1959). The other techniques require relatively dry activated sludge (typically $\leq$ 15 wt.% moisture content) to reduce the required solvent for the extraction. Waste activated sludge from wastewater treatment facilities typically contains 1–2 wt.% solid and removal of the huge amount of water is not economically attractive [55].

Among the extraction techniques that have been used for activated sludge, only solvent extraction and SFE can possibly be applied in large-scale operations. Soxhlet and ASE® extraction techniques are common laboratory protocols for the extraction of materials from a variety of sources. Soxhlet is a long exhaustive solvent extraction technique that could last for a period of 6–48 hours while ASE® is a solvent extraction at elevated temperature (ambient – 200°C) and pressure (500–3000 psi) [129, 177, 190]. Because of these disadvantages, Soxhlet and ASE® might not be an economical option for larger scale operation. Correspondingly, BD extraction is a commonly used technique for extraction of lipids from biological sources. However, since sludge drying is not required, BD could be a reasonable option for commercial extraction. A discussion on BD extraction of activated sludge, which can be adapted for large-scale operation, is detailed elsewhere by Revellame [173]. The main disadvantage of the BD extraction is the hazardous nature of chloroform and toxicity of methanol. However, a study conducted by Hara and Radin [84] indicated that chloroform and methanol could be replaced by hexane and isopropanol, respectively. The substitutions resulted to less toxic solvents, easier phase separation and cheaper solvents.

To maximize biodiesel yield from activated sludge, researchers have also explored supercritical and subcritical reactive extraction technique specifically termed "*in situ* transesterification." This process combines lipid extraction and biodiesel conversion steps into one step that could result into reduced process costs [81]. Sludge drying is often required prior to this reactive extraction process. However, based on the study conducted by Revellame and colleagues [171], the *in situ* transesterification process can tolerate up to 84.5 wt.% moisture suggesting that this process might be the most suitable one for biodiesel from activated sludge. In fact, to date, this is the only process with an almost complete economic analysis for biodiesel produced from this feedstock [55, 140, 171]. Studies involving the use of *in situ* transesterification process for direct biodiesel production from sewage sludge will be discussed in more detail in Section 10.4.

There is no direct correlation between pretreatment and yield of extracted materials as shown in Table 10.2. This is also true for extraction technique and extraction yields. This might be due to the inherent variability of extractable materials from activated sludge. On a study conducted by Revellame and co-workers [174], they found that within a municipal WWTP, the profile of extractable materials from activated sludge stays similar throughout the year. However, the amount that can be extracted varies, which is possibly due to dissimilar wastewater characteristics at different times of the year. For example, rainy season and seasonal diet could affect the BOD loading of wastewater, consequently affecting the amount of extractable materials from activated sludge. This suggests that extraction yield is dependent on the type of wastewater being treated. As shown in Table 10.2, activated sludges obtained from treatment facilities for domestic or residential wastewater can have as much as ~30 wt.% (dry sludge) extraction yield while those obtained from food processing wastewater treatment facilities could have extraction yields twice as high. With respect to esterifiable lipid yield, the highest recorded was ~10 wt.% (dry sludge) for domestic sludges while as high as 60 wt.% (dry sludge) was obtained for food processing sludges.

10.3.3 COMPOSITION OF ACTIVATED SLUDGE EXTRACT

Activated sludge is composed of a wide variety of microorganisms including bacteria, fungi, protozoa, rotifers and nematodes. Among these groups, bacteria (*Eubacteria* and *Archaebacteria*) are the ones responsible for biological wastewater treatment and thus, they comprise a dominant portion in activated sludge [173]. As general classification, compounds present in activated sludge extract can be divide into four classes: (i) lipid storage compounds such as

TABLE 10.2 Compound Classes Present in Raw Activated Sludge Extract [174, 175]

Compound Class	Concentration (wt.% of extract)	
	Conventional	**Oxidation Ditch**
Hydrocarbons	0.8–7.9 ppm	1.1–6.2 ppm
PHAs	1.1–4.1	1.5–5.7
TAGs	1.0–2.9	1.0–2.2
Fatty Alcohols (from WEs)	0.3–5.9	0.8–3.3
Sterols (from SEs)	0.1–3.0	0.1–0.4
Free Sterols	0.4–18.7	0.9–1.8
FAMEs[a]	16.6–19.0	23.8–26.8

[a]Total FAMEs from FFAs, DAGs, MAGs, WEs, SEs and PLs.

TAGs, WEs and PHAs; (ii) compounds associated with cellular structure (i.e., PLs, sterols); (iii) intermediate compounds from metabolic pathways (i.e., DAGs, MAGs and FFAs); and (iv) other compounds which are present in wastewaters due to anthropogenic contributions such as hydrocarbons, sterols, steryl esters (SEs) and fatty alcohols [173, 174]. Lipid storage compounds serve as energy and carbon reserves and are known to accumulate as inclusion bodies when bacteria are subjected to stressful conditions (i.e., N-limited environment) [174]. The functions of the other compound classes in living bacterial cells are self-explanatory, but a comprehensive discussion on functions as well as associated bacterial species is detailed elsewhere [174].

10.3.3.1   Raw Activated Sludge

Activated sludge extract is composed of a wide variety of compounds, which are often dictated by the influent wastewater being treated. As an example, Jardé and colleagues (2005) found out that among 48 sewage sludges they tested, linear alkyl benzenes are only present in domestic sludges while sterols are present in both food-processing and domestic sludges. In terms of lipidic compounds, bacteria are characterized by fatty acids in the C_{12}–C_{20} chain length, which could be saturated and monounsaturated. These fatty acids however, are usually associated (moiety) with other compounds (i.e., TAGs, WEs, PLs, etc.) [80, 173].

A comprehensive compilation of organic chemicals found in sewage sludges showed a list that includes 516 compounds such as aliphatic, chlorinated, and aromatic hydrocarbons, nitrosamines, phenolics, pesticides, sterols, surfactants and compounds from personal care products [85]. The compounds included in the list were detected in sludges from different WWTs and most of them are present in trace quantities and thus, will not be included here. To have an idea of the relative concentration of compounds in activated sludge extract that are useful for biofuel applications, a summary of datasets obtained from two domestic wastewater treatment facilities is presented in Table 10.2. These two facilities use different configurations of the activated sludge process: one operates using the conventional activated process (CAS) while the other uses the oxidation ditch process (ODP). The data in Table 10.2 is far from a complete characterization of activated sludge extract. However, this is considerably the most wide-ranging data available in the literature with respect to compound classes present in sludge extract of the same origin.

The almost similar profile of compounds detected in the two raw sludges considered in Table 10. 2 is advantageous for the downstream processing of the extracts prior to their use as commodity chemicals or as precursors to other products. This indicates that similar downstream/separation processes could be applied to both of these extracts to separate them into various fractions for different applications, i.e., hydrocarbons and FAMEs as fuel, PHAs as commodity bioplastics, TAGs and fatty alcohols as oleochemical feedstocks, and sterols as bioactive compounds [174]. To have a variety of products obtainable from the extracts makes activated sludge similar to crude petroleum and thus a very attractive potential replacement for it.

10.3.3.2 Lipid-Enhanced Activated Sludge

The common pathway for the utilization of activated sludge extract as fuel is through alcoholysis or esterification to produce biodiesel or FAMEs. Utilization of activated sludges produced in the United States as biodiesel feedstock requires two main conditions: (i) similar biodiesel properties, and (ii) economic competitiveness. Biodiesel properties such as cold flow and cetane number are highly dictated by the feedstock's fatty acid profile [175]. Thus, all the activated sludges must have similar profiles so they can be blended without affecting the properties of the resulting mixture. Figure 10.3a shows a scatter plot to compare the fatty acid profiles of the extract from the two plants (CAS and ODP) in Table 10.2. A diagonal line ($y = x$) was added to visually compare the two profiles. Similarity in these profiles would mean that the points representing fatty acids lining up along the diagonal line. The figure clearly shows otherwise, suggesting that the two feedstocks cannot be blended together without jeopardizing the properties of the resulting biodiesel. Studies also indicated that a biodiesel (FAMEs) yield of more than 10 wt.% (dry sludge) is necessary for this feedstock to be competitive with petroleum diesel [171]. The yield of biodiesel from the two plants (CAS and ODP) in Table 10.2 ranges from 1.4 to 2.3 wt.% (dry sludge) indicating economic unattractiveness of this feedstock. It should be noted however, that the presence of other useful compounds (i.e., PHAs, sterols and fatty alcohols) were not considered in the economic analysis of this feedstock.

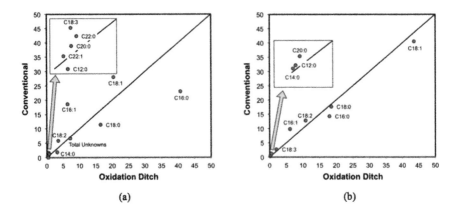

FIGURE 10.3 Illustration of fatty acid homogenization of sludges from conventional and oxidation ditch activated sludge processes (wt.% of total fatty acids as FAMEs). (a) Raw sludges, (b) Enhanced sludges. Data were obtained from Revellame et al. [175]. (Note: Homogeneous samples are characterized by fatty acid distribution points along the $y = x$ line).

To increase the biodiesel yield from this feedstock, researchers proposed subjecting the activated sludge microorganisms to a N-limited environment. This strategy required addition of carbon source to stimulate lipid accumulation and have resulted to an "enhanced sludge" with increased biodiesel yield of 8–20 wt.% (dry sludge) [139]. A more detailed discussion on the production of enhanced sludges is provided in Section 10.7. The resulting biodiesel from enhanced sludges from the two plants also showed very similar fatty acid profiles as shown in Figure 10.3b. Furthermore, the resulting extracts showed a cleaner profile of products as shown in Table 10.3 signifying the suitability of the proposed strategy for countrywide utilization of activated sludge as biofuel feedstock.

TABLE 10.3 Compound Classes Present in Lipid-Enhanced Activated Sludge Extract [175]

Compound Class	Concentration (wt.% of extract)	
	Conventional	Oxidation Ditch
PHAs	0.5–2.1	0.5–4.5
TAGs	10.4–18.4	19.1–24.6
FAMEs[a]	5.7–13.6	8.3–16.8

[a]Total FAMEs from FFAs, DAGs, MAGs, WEs, SEs and PLs.

10.4 BIODIESEL PRODUCTION FROM SLUDGES

10.4.1 INTRODUCTION

As discussed in the previous section, municipal sewage sludge contains substantial amounts of lipidic materials such as TAGs, DAGs, DAGs, PLs, and FFAs that can be used as feedstock for biodiesel production [25, 97, 169, 178]. These lipidic materials were either directly adsorbed into the sludge, particularly in primary sludge, or originated from heterotrophic microbial biomass as in the case of activated sludge. Exploiting sewage sludges and biosolids as biodiesel feedstock yields a previously untapped source of cheap oil feedstock and can help solve both energy and environmental sustainability issues. It provides a viable nonfood source of biofuel feedstock but also a sustainable sludge and biosolids disposal and beneficial reuse method that could replace land application [101]. It was estimated that integrating lipid extraction and transesterification processes for recovering sludge lipids and converting them to biodiesel in 50% of WWTP facilities in the US could produce around 1.8 billion gallons of biodiesel and replace roughly 0.5% of annual petroleum diesel demand [55]. In this section, recent efforts in producing biodiesel from lipids derived from sewage sludges as feedstock are discussed. The two main approaches that have been used are presented in Figure 10.4. The first approach involves extracting the lipids out of the sludge matrix and then subjecting these lipids to transesterification reactions to convert them to biodiesel compounds or FAMEs. The second approach that has been mostly studied is the use of an *in situ* transesterification process, in which the lipids are converted to FAMEs within the sludge matrix without prior separation or extraction.

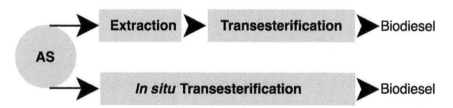

FIGURE 10.4 Generalized schematic for the production of biodiesel from activated sludge (AS).

10.4.2 SEQUENTIAL EXTRACTION AND TRANSESTERIFICATION

Dufreche and colleagues [55] first studied sequential extraction and transesterification of sewage sludge lipids for the production of biodiesel. They used different types and combinations of extraction solvents including hexane, methanol, acetone, and supercritical carbon dioxide (SC-CO$_2$). The results indicated that using a cosolvent system of (in vol.) 60% hexane, 20% methanol, and 20% acetone gave the highest total oil extraction yield of 27.4 wt.% (dry sludge) compared with individual solvent systems and combinations with SC-CO$_2$. This good extraction yield could be attributed to the balance of polar and nonpolar solvents in the cosolvent system that led to the extraction of both polar and nonpolar lipid fractions of the sewage sludges. The extracted sludge oil using this extraction system also showed the highest biodiesel conversion yield of 4.41 wt.% (dry sludge) in terms of the dry weight of the sludge after transesterification of the extracted sludge oil. Gas chromatography with flame ionization detection (GC-FID) analysis of the extracted sludge oil and methyl esters produced showed the dominance of C16:0 (palmitate) and C18:1 (oleate) methyl esters (45 and 35 wt.% based on total FAMEs, respectively). This composition profile indicates that sludge-derived oils have similar composition with most crop oils and are thus suitable for biodiesel production. A more recent study by Zhu and co-workers [232] compared acid hydrolysis, Soxhlet extraction, and water bath shaking for extracting lipids from sewage sludge for subsequent conversion to biodiesel and found that Soxhlet extraction led to a the highest overall biodiesel yield of 6.35 wt.% (dry sludge). Extracting the oils from the sludge prior to conversion to biodiesel can provide the opportunity to refine the oil feedstock before conversion to methyl esters and thus, can result into better biodiesel quality. However, this can add additional processing steps and may increase the biodiesel production cost.

10.4.3 IN SITU TRANSESTERIFICATION

In situ transesterification can circumvent the need for separating lipids from the sludge matrix before transesterification. This process combines the lipid extraction and transesterification reaction in a single step and can thus reduce overall biodiesel production costs. The *in situ* transesterification process involves the direct conversion of lipids within the sludge matrix by adding the alcohol reactant and catalyst directly into the sludge followed by reacting the mixture under a specified temperature, reaction time, and alcohol and catalyst-to-sludge ratio. A cosolvent such as hexane is typically added to the reaction mixture to immediately separate the generated FAMEs from the alcohol phase. After the reaction has been completed, the cosolvent and alcohol/glycerol phases are allowed to separate and the FAMEs are recovered from the cosolvent phase.

Dufreche and co-workers [55] conducted the first known attempt for producing FAMEs via *in situ* transesterification of waste activated sludge and obtained an overall biodiesel yield of 6.23 wt.% (dry sludge) under the following conditions: 5:1 volume-to-mass ratio of methanol-to-dried sludge, 1 vol.% H_2SO_4 catalyst in methanol, and 50°C reaction temperature with no cosolvent added. The investigators showed that the overall biodiesel yield from the sewage sludge using the *in situ* transesterification process were significantly higher than when using conventional sequential lipid extraction and conversion process. In addition to activated sludge, Mondala and colleagues [140] tested the *in situ* transesterification process under different conditions of reaction temperature, catalyst concentration, and methanol levels for biodiesel generation from primary sludges. The latter were expected to have higher amounts of adsorbed oils for higher conversion yields to FAMEs. This study showed maximum biodiesel yields of 14.5% and 2.5% by dry weight from dried primary and activated sludges, respectively obtained under the following acid-catalyzed transesterification reaction conditions: 75°C reaction temperature, 5 vol.% H_2SO_4 catalyst in methanol, and 12:1 volume-to-mass ratio of methanol to dried sludge. Hexane was also added as a cosolvent at a 5:1 volume-to-sludge dry mass ratio. The authors also investigated the kinetics of the *in situ* transesterification process for biodiesel production from sewage sludge and found that only the acid catalyst level had a significant effect on the specific rate of the pseudo second-order *in situ* transesterification reaction. However, the temperature tested at 75°C is higher than the boiling points of methanol and hexane (64.7 and 68°C, respectively). Although the vaporized solvents were refluxed into the reaction mixture using a condenser apparatus, there were concerns about loss of methanol in the liquid reaction phase, which could have reduced the biodiesel yield from the reaction mixture.

Revellame and colleagues [170] conducted response surface designed experiments to optimize the *in situ* transesterification process for dried activated sludge conversion to biodiesel. Their study found a maximum of 4.8 wt.% (dry sludge) FAMEs yield under the optimum reaction conditions of 55°C, 25:1 methanol volume-to-dry sludge mass ratio, and 4 vol.% H_2SO_4

catalyst level in methanol. The resulting biodiesel yield from activated sludge in this study was higher than what was obtained by Mondala et al. [140], but lower than that obtained by Dufreche et al. [55]. Although the sludges they used originated from the same wastewater treatment facility, variations in treatment plant operating conditions during the different experimental time frames of these studies could have caused a fluctuation in the lipidic contents of the activated sludge microbial biomass. Another possible factor could be differences in laboratory sludge dewatering and drying process conditions used by these investigators for preparing the activated sludge samples prior to the *in situ* transesterification process.

10.4.3.1   Wet vs. Dried Sludge

Sludge dewatering and drying processes are considered major contributors to the sewage sludge biodiesel production costs. Typically, activated sludges collected from the municipal WWTP to be used in the biodiesel production studies contain ∼ 98 wt.% water and thus have a liquid consistency. In the laboratory, the sludges were dewatered by centrifugation and then oven-dried or lyophilized to achieve up to 95 wt.% dry solids concentration. Reducing the dewatering and drying requirements could reduce energy and processing costs and potentially the overall sewage biodiesel price per gallon to enhance its economic competitiveness with crop oil- and animal fat-based biodiesel or petroleum diesel. The study by Revellame and co-workers [171] tested *in situ* transesterification of wet activated sludge with up to 84.5 wt.% moisture and found a maximum biodiesel yield of 3.93 wt.% (dry sludge) under conditions of 75°C reaction temperature, 30 mL/g methanol volume-to-sludge mass ratio, and 10 vol.% acid catalyst concentration. Compared with earlier studies using dried sewage sludge, conditions for processing wet sludge for biodiesel production required higher energy and reagent (i.e., methanol, catalyst, and cosolvent) expenditures due to higher total mass of the wet sludge.

Choi and colleagues [38] used xylene in place of hexane as a cosolvent in the *in situ* transesterification of wet activated sludge. With xylene as cosolvent, they obtained a FAMEs yield of 8.12 wt.% (dry sludge), which was 2.5 times higher than when hexane was used as cosolvent. This yield was comparable to the maximum biodiesel yield from *in situ* transesterification of dried sludge (9.68 wt.% dry sludge) used in their study. The higher boiling point of xylene allowed higher reaction temperature (105°C), which resulted to vaporization of water during the reaction and consequently enhancing biodiesel yield. In addition, the use of xylene as cosolvent resulted to reduced reaction time and methanol consumption when compared to hexane for achieving a similar biodiesel yield.

10.4.3.2   Acid vs. Enzymatic Catalysis

In situ transesterification processes for biodiesel production from sewage sludge typically employ acids instead of bases as catalyst to prevent soap formation due to the expected high FFA content of sewage sludges. However, the use of acid catalysts can be disadvantageous in commercial applications due to issues such as equipment corrosion, high methanol consumption, and biodiesel washing [114]. Sangaletti-Gerhard and co-workers [184] used a commercially available lipase Novozyme 435 from the *Candida antartica* B yeast as an alternative catalyst for biodiesel production from sewage sludge via *in situ* transesterification. Although biodiesel yields using this biocatalyst were comparable with the acid-catalyzed processes, the enzymatic process was deemed uneconomical due to the high cost of lipase enzymes.

10.4.4   SLUDGE BIODIESEL CHARACTERISTICS

The fatty acid methyl ester profiles of sewage sludge-derived biodiesel have been characterized via gas chromatography methods. Previous studies showed biodiesel produced by either sequential extraction-transesterification or *in situ* transesterification of sewage sludges were dominated by 16- and 18-carbon chain length fatty acid methyl esters. Biodiesel from primary sludge contained up to (based on total FAMEs) 40 wt.% palmitate (C16:0) methyl esters and up to 25 wt.% oleate (C18:1) methyl esters followed by up to 10 wt.% of both stearate (C18:0) and linoleate (C18:2) methyl esters [140]. Activated sludge biodiesel have typically the same FAME profile with varying proportions of the C_{16} and C_{18} FAMEs, particularly with palmitate and oleate and higher C16:1 (palmitoleate) methyl esters than primary sludge biodiesel [55, 140, 170]. This composition was found to be the same for both dried and wet sludges [171] or when using acid or lipase enzyme as *in situ* transesterification catalysts [184]. On the other hand, the study by Choi et al. [38] showed a substantial difference in the FAME profile when using xylene as the *in situ* transesterification cosolvent.

Greater quantities of saturated fatty acid methyl esters C14:0 (myristate), C15:0 (pentadecyclate), and C18:0 (stearate) were obtained compared to when hexane was the cosolvent. It was speculated that the higher reaction temperature made possible through the use of the high boiling solvent xylene caused the generation of more saturated and less unsaturated fatty acid methyl esters.

Biodiesel properties such as ignition quality (cetane number), cold flow properties and oxidative stability are highly dictated by its fatty acid profile. Thus, producing a biodiesel with the right balance of saturated and unsaturated FAMEs is important for achieving a fuel with desirable properties [29]. As discussed in Section 10.3.3.2, the FAMEs profile of biodiesel that can be obtained from raw activated sludge varies significantly with respect to WWTPs biological treatment configuration. However, enhancement of the activated sludge produces a biodiesel with uniform FAMEs profile regardless of the source of the raw activated sludge (see also Figure 10.3). The enhancement strategies that can be used to accomplish this are presented in Sections 10.6–10.8. Having uniform FAMEs implies that the biodiesel produced from the enhanced sludges can be blended without affecting the properties of the resulting biodiesel mix. On the average, the biodiesel produced from the enhanced sludges discussed in Section 10.3.3.2 contains (as wt.% of total FAMEs) 16.1% C16:0, 18.1% C18:0, 8.0% C16:1, 42.0% C18:1, 11.8% C18:2, 2.4% C18:3 and minute quantities of C12:0, C14:0 and C20:0. This profile is very similar to that of biodiesel obtained from lard which at 20% blend (B20) has slightly higher viscosity, better oxidation stability, and higher cold filter plugging and cloud point compared to canola biodiesel B20 blend. However, at B10 blend, the properties of the resulting fuel are similar to those of soy biodiesel at the same blend [106]. From the FAMEs profile, the cetane number of the biodiesel is around 57 as estimated by the empirical equation developed by Bamgboye and Hansen [13]. This is higher than the required cetane number specification of 47 (minimum) required by ASTM D6751.

10.4.5   ECONOMIC CHALLENGES

In general, the major challenge for making activated sludge-derived biodiesel more cost-competitive with conventional crop oils and animal fats and petroleum diesel is to reduce the cost below the $3.00 per gallon benchmark set by previous studies in the last decade. However, price per gallon estimates provided by previous studies showed that current processes for producing biodiesel from sewage sludges are still not competitive with petroleum diesel. The benchmark is even lower with petrodiesel costs dropping to around $2 per gallon in early 2016 [59]. Dufreche et al. [55] and Mondala et al. [140] previously estimated the sewage biodiesel cost (in 2008 USD) at $3.11 and $3.23 per gallon, respectively. At the time of publication of these findings, this cost estimate was lower than petrodiesel ($4.80 per gallon) and soybean oil biodiesel ($4 – $4.50 per gallon). However, the cost estimates were calculated based on a 10 wt.% (dry sludge) yield of FAMEs, which is yet to be achieved for activated sludges obtained directly from existing WWTPs.

Although the production cost attributed to the oil feedstock has been off-set due to the waste nature and wide availability of sewage sludge, calculations by Dufreche et al. [55] and Mondala et al. [140] showed that 53–74% of the production costs can be attributed to sludge dewatering and drying. This consumes significant amounts of energy due to the high water content of sewage sludges as obtained directly from the WWTP. Thus, using sludge with minimal dewatering and no drying could be a viable option to reduce production costs. Despite this, the study of Revellame and colleagues [171] showed that (with up to 84.5 wt.% moisture) despite using less energy for dewatering and drying, the biodiesel produced from wet sludge could cost up to $14 per gallon (in 2010 U.S. dollars) due to higher reactant (methanol) and catalyst (acid) needed to compensate for the increased sludge volume. A minimum biodiesel cost of $7 per gallon could be achieved if the wet sludge water content was lowered to 50 wt.%. On the other hand, Choi and co-workers [38] showed that the cost of biodiesel produced via *in situ* transesterification of wet sludge could be reduced by 50 wt.% through the use of xylene as a cosolvent ($3.52 per gallon) instead of hexane ($7.12 per gallon). However, these calculations did not include capital costs, which is important since the *in situ* transesterification process using xylene as cosolvent would require a specialized reactor that can separate the vaporized water from the reaction mixture.

Cost sensitivity analysis of the *in situ* transesterification process for biodiesel production from sludge conducted by Revellame et al. [171] showed that overall, the sludge biodiesel per gallon price can be reduced to $3 per gallon if the expected biodiesel yield from sludge was increased to 10 wt.% (dry sludge). The target biodiesel yield is expected to be higher nowadays if the current price of petrodiesel ($2 per gallon) was to be used as the benchmark for economic competitiveness. Controlling the sludge characteristics to increase its lipid content is a formidable challenge, especially in the context of maintaining normal WWTP operating conditions. The lipid content of primary sludge is mainly a result of external factors that are beyond the plant operator's control (i.e., the amounts of oils, fats, and grease dumped into the sewers). Further improvements and optimization of extraction and transesterification conditions could help improve primary sludge biodiesel yield and reduce production costs. On the other hand, the amount of lipids in activated sludge can be influenced by the characteristics of the influent wastewater (i.e., carbon and nutrient loading) or the sludge residence time in the aerobic bio-oxidation basin. Controlling these conditions could in theory influence the amount of stored lipids that can be extracted from the activated sludge microbial biomass while targeting a specific wastewater organic pollution removal level.

10.5 CATALYTIC CRACKING OF ACTIVATED SLUDGE LIPIDS

10.5.1 INTRODUCTION

A significant fraction of activated sludge extracts are compounds that cannot be converted to FAMEs or biodiesel. In fact, this nonesterifiable portion could account for as high as 86 wt.% of the extract (see Table 10.1), and contains hydrocarbons, fatty alcohols, sterols, and glycerol (from TAGs, DAGs, MAGs and PLs) (see Table 10.2). Even the extract from the lipid-enhanced activated sludge could have significant quantity of glycerol that is usually wasted during biodiesel production. Conversion of these nonesterifiables to fuel-compatible compounds could have a tremendous impact on the economics of this feedstock. Biodiesel is an excellent solvent and cannot be used in existing diesel engines without blending with petroleum diesel. Additionally, biodiesel requires a separate distribution pipeline to avoid problems with the existing ones that are used for petroleum. Alternatively, the esterifiable lipidic compounds can be subjected to catalytic cracking to produce green gasoline and green diesel, which are chemically similar to petroleum fuels [21].

Catalytic cracking is the most extensively used process in petroleum refinery to produce valuable products like gasoline and other lighter products. Catalytic cracking reactions are normally carried out at 290–400°C and 1200–2000 psig [72]. Cracking of lipidic compounds is commonly accomplished using zeolites as catalyst, particularly H$^+$ZSM5 [32, 95, 146, 182]. ZSM5 is a shape selective catalyst that produces higher proportion of liquid relative to gaseous products and is selective towards octane-boosters (aromatic hydrocarbons) [19, 198]. Most catalytic cracking studies involving lipidic materials are limited to fatty acids (including their esters) and vegetable oils (e.g., canola, rapeseed), which are mainly TAGs.

These studies indicated that fatty acids and vegetable oils can be converted to gasoline range organics and diesel range organics [1, 21, 102, 103]. The same range of products was obtained by Benson and colleagues [20] on the catalytic cracking of DAG and MAG using H⁺ZSM5. However, the feedstocks used in these studies are ideal/pure ones. Dealing with activated sludge extract for catalytic cracking is completely different due to its complexity. On the other hand, it can be concluded that the esterifiable portion of activated sludge extract can be converted to green fuels through catalytic cracking.

10.5.2 CATALYTIC CRACKING OF NON-ESTERIFIABLE COMPOUNDS IN ACTIVATED SLUDGE

In the utilization of activated sludge extract for green fuel production, it would be advantageous if all the materials can be catalytically cracked. This would eliminate possible downstream fractionation processes to separate the esterifiable and nonesterifiable compounds.

10.5.2.1 Glycerol

Several catalysts have been tested on the catalytic cracking of glycerol. This includes fluid catalytic cracking catalyst, a mesoporous Al_2O_3, an USY zeolite, ZSM5, ZSM22, SiC and modernite [42, 43, 86, 99, 221]. Among these catalysts, ZSM5 cracking produced the highest level of olefins and aromatics and lowest level of coke formation [43]. Acrolein (propenal) was the major ZSM5 cracking product, which resulted from dehydration of glycerol. Longer contact times and higher reaction temperatures and pressures increased production of gasoline range aromatics up to a yield of 60% [42, [86].

10.5.2.2 Sterols

Dehydration was identified to be the primary thermal degradation reaction of sterols (i.e., cholesterol, stigmasterols and sitosterol) [73]. Above 275°C, hydrous pyrolysis of cholesterol showed further degradation as indicated by formation of aromatic compounds [180]. Catalytic cracking of cholesterol over HY and ZSM5 produced less coke than rapeseed oil. Consequently, cracking of cholesterol – rapeseed oil mixture over the two zeolite catalysts resulted in the decrease in both coke deposition and gaseous products formation. Cracking of the mixture over Pd/C catalyst produced a liquid product similar to ultra-low sulfur diesel with high levels of alkanes and increased alkane to aromatic ratio [209].

10.5.2.3 Fatty Alcohols

Similar to sterols, thermal degradation of fatty alcohols starts with dehydration reaction. Dehydration was also believed to be the primary steps in catalytic cracking of 1-octadecanol over H^+ZSM5. The reaction produced octadecene, which then undergoes further cracking forming products similar to catalytic cracking of alkenes. The products include significant proportion of olefins, paraffins and aromatic hydrocarbons [173].

10.5.2.4 Phospholipids

PLs are phosphorus-containing lipids that can be esterified to produce esters and glycerol, both of which can be catalytically cracked. It is however important to consider cracking of PL molecule as a whole due to the inherent characteristic of phosphorus as catalyst poison [56]. Cracking of phosphatidylglycerol and phosphatidic acid over H^+ZSM5 resulted to cleavage of their fatty acid moieties and significant formation of aromatic compounds. No phosphorus-containing compounds were detected in the products, suggesting that the phosphorus was deposited in the catalyst [176]. Phosphorus poisoning was considered to be irreversible due to its reaction to the catalyst framework (Al_2O_3, SiO_2) producing phosphates [9].

10.5.2.5 Activated Sludge Extracts

Catalytic cracking of actual activated sludge extract at 450°C over activated alumina produced low viscosity liquid, noncondensable gases, semisolids and water. The liquid product contained mainly alkanes in the C_6–C_{20} range while the gaseous product included CO, CO_2, and C_1–C_5 compounds. However, the extract was recovered using toluene as solvent and most probably contains mainly esterifiable lipids with traces of PHAs, PLs and sterols [109]. Nevertheless, this is indicative of the amenability of activated sludge extract to catalytic cracking.

10.5.3   FLUIDIZED BED CATALYSIS OF ACTIVATED SLUDGE

In WWTPs, activated sludge disposal entails water removal, which could be accomplished through mechanical means (e.g., centrifuge, filter press) followed by fluidized bed drying. This process operates between 300 and 900°C using air or steam in the presence of fluidization medium such as quartz sand as heat carriers and dispersion enhancer. This is an avenue that can be exploited to integrate the production of green fuels. By using catalyst as fluidization medium, existing infrastructures for sludge drying could be transformed into a fluidized bed catalytic cracking unit that will benefit waste treatment facilities: (i) by producing fuel that can be used within the plant; and (ii) by minimizing solid management issues [176]. A general schematic for this process, which can be applied on both raw and enhanced activated sludges is presented in Figure 10.5.

Fluidized bed catalysis of raw activated sludge with helium as fluid-izing gas over H^+ZSM5 at 500°C can tolerate up to 15 wt.% moisture. However, a higher yield was obtained at a lower moisture content of 5 wt.% (see Table 10.4). Sludge conversion was in the 34–48% range with tremendous production of fuel compatible compounds during the process. Utilization of the raw activated sludge for biodiesel production will typi-cally yield 3–6 wt.% (dry sludge) of biodiesel [175], whereas 10–15 wt.% (dry sludge) of fuel compatible components is produced through fluidized bed catalysis [176].

Fluidized bed catalytic cracking of enhanced activated sludge at similar con-ditions boosted reaction conversion to 60–75% and fuel yield to 40–55 wt.% (dry sludge). This is possibly due to higher amount of extractables in enhanced sludge that can be converted to fuel. Table 10.4 summarizes the distribution of the compounds produced from catalytic cracking of both activated sludges.

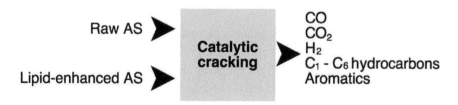

FIGURE 10.5   Generalized schematic for the production of biofuels from activated sludge (AS) through catalytic cracking.

TABLE 10.4 Gaseous Product Yields from Fluidized Bed Catalytic Cracking of Activated Sludges with 5 wt.% Moisture Over H$^+$ZSM5 at 500°C

Product	Yield (mg/g dry sludge)	
	Raw Sludge[a]	Enhanced Sludge[b]
CO_2	141.0 ± 1.8	184.1 ± 12.1
CO	73.7 ± 5.5	89.9 ± 20.0
Hydrogen	2.6 ± 1.5	0.6
Methane	3.3 ± 0.8	8.9 ± 0.3
Ethylene	2.4 ± 0.2	5.4 ± 0.1
Ethane	10.1 ± 1.6	7.5 ± 0.7
Olefins		
C3	3.0 ± 0.5	10.0 ± 1.2
C4	3.9 ± 0.3	9.6 ± 1.2
C5	3.3 ± 0.8	3.7 ± 0.4
C6	1.8 ± 0.9	5.7 ± 1.9
Paraffins		
C3	10.4 ± 3.7	33.4 ± 4.4
C4	5.5 ± 3.3	18.6 ± 5.4
C5	1.4 ± 0.4	6.5 ± 1.1
C6	-	0.1
Acetonitrile	14.7 ± 3.6	5.3 ± 1.9
Benzene	22.6 ± 2.8	119.7 ± 22.4
Toluene	51.6 ± 8.3	169.6 ± 21.2
Xylenes	32.0 ± 4.6	108.2 ± 16.4
Linear Alkyl Benzene	-	0.1
FAMEs	0.2 ± 0.1	-
PAH	0.1	0.3

[a]Data obtained from Revellame et al. [176].

[b]Data obtained from Revellame et al. [172].

Among the fuel compatible compounds produced from raw sludge, 9 wt.% accounts for olefins, 20 wt.% for paraffins, and 69 wt.% for aromatics on a dry sludge basis. On the other, cracking of enhanced sludge is more selective towards aromatic hydrocarbons with distributions of (base on dry sludge) 7 wt.% olefins, 15 wt.% paraffins and 78 wt.% aromatics. The enhanced sludge is cleaner than the raw sludge, which could contain unwanted species that could deactivate the catalyst (i.e., heavy metals in raw sludge). With shape-selective H$^+$ZSM5 as catalyst, low molecular weight hydrocarbons act as precursors to formation of aromatics. The eventual catalyst deactivation results to higher proportion of olefins and paraffins and lower aromatics fraction. Catalyst deactivation is probably present in the enhanced sludge as well, but is not as severe as in the raw sludge. Decarboxylation and decarbonylation are the two deoxygenation reactions observed for the process as indicated by high amount of CO_2 and CO formation for both sludges. Cracking of both sludges also resulted to formation of acetonitrile. Acetonitrile is an important solvent in chemical syntheses that could contribute to the economics of this process [172, 176].

10.6 CULTIVATION OF OLEAGINOUS YEASTS IN WASTEWATER

10.6.1 INTRODUCTION

Operational WWTPs maintain ideal carbon and nutrients (e.g., N, P) levels in the aerobic biological treatment units to promote microbial biomass growth and multiplication; hence, treatment of wastewaters. In municipal wastewaters, however, the levels of carbon and nutrients (particularly N) do not trigger the accumulation of storage lipids in activated sludge microflora due to low molar carbon-to-nitrogen ratio (C/N). Research studies have proven that high C/N ratio induces lipid accumulation in oleaginous microbes such as those in activated sludge, bacteria and yeasts. The high C/N ratio required for microbial lipid production could be attained by using high carbon-containing industrial wastewater streams. As shown in Figure 10.6, oleaginous yeasts can be cultivated in these high C/N wastewaters to accumulate high amounts of storage lipids (i.e., TAGs) through feeding on carbon and nitrogen in the wastewater. This approach addresses two important research objectives: (i) low-cost carbon

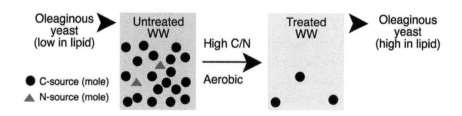

FIGURE 10.6 Generalized schematic for the utilization of different waste streams to produce microbial lipids using oleaginous yeasts.

sources for lipid enhancement, and (ii) treatment of wastewaters. This section focuses on the strategy of using high C-containing wastewaters as a growth medium for an oleaginous microbial consortium to supplement activated sludge microflora for generating sludge biomass with higher amounts of lipids that can be used as feedstock for biodiesel and renewable diesel production.

10.6.2 LIPID PRODUCTION BY OLEAGINOUS MICROORGANISMS

10.6.2.1 Oleaginous Species and Types of Lipid Compounds

Lipids from microorganisms, or "single-cell oils" have been studied for over 100 years, primarily for the purpose of supplementing edible oils and fats for human consumption. Oleaginous microorganisms are those that are capable of accumulating 20–80 wt.% of their dry biomass as lipids under stress exerted by the limitation of a key nutrient (usually nitrogen) relative to an excess supply of the carbon source [164]. Table 10.5 shows a list of representative strains from different microbial groups that have been known to accumulate large amounts of storage lipids, which could then be extracted and potentially used for biodiesel production. The types of storage lipids produced also vary between prokaryotes and eukaryotes. Eukaryotes such as yeasts, fungi, and algae typically synthesize TAGs, which contain polyunsaturated fatty acids similar to vegetable oils that can be used for biodiesel or renewable diesel production [127, 166, 211]. In oleaginous fungi such as *Mucor circinelloides* however, FFAs and PLs comprise 32 and 21 wt.% of the total lipids, respectively as opposed to TAG, which comprised around 14 wt.% [208]. Many algal species have also been shown to accumulate substantial amounts of neutral lipids (20–50 wt.%), majority of which is TAG [90]. On the other hand, most prokaryotic bacteria tend to manufacture specialized lipids such as PHAs, glycolipids, lipoproteins, and WEs [7, 147, 188, 210], although TAG accumulation has been reported in a few bacterial strains belonging to the actinomycetes group such as *Mycobacterium, Streptomyces, Rhodococcus,* and *Nocardia* [4, 28, 192]. WEs as energy storage compounds were speculated to be widespread in bacteria belonging to the genus *Acinetobacter* while TAG biosynthesis has been detected only in aerobic heterotrophic bacteria and cyanobacteria, specifically the actinomycetes group including the

TABLE 10.5 Lipid Accumulation by Different Oleaginous Microorganisms

Species	Oil yield (wt.% of dry biomass)	Reference
Microalgae		
C. vulgaris	56.6	[125]
C. vulgaris	40	[96]
C. emersonii	63	[96]
C. minutissima	57	[96]
C. sorokiniana	22	[96]
B. braunii	21	[230]
Yeast		
L. starkeyi	52.6	[110]
C. curvatus	34.6	[227]
Y. lipolytica	58.5	[204]
R. glutinis	72	[133]
R. glutinis	40	[154]
R. toruloides	67.5	[118]
C. echinula	37.6	[54]
C. albidus	65	[133]
C. protothecoides	55.3	[216]
Fungi		
M. isabellina	51.7	[156]
M. isabellina	65	[61]
C. enchinulata	57.7	[61]
M. vinacea	66	[196]
M. circinelloides	25	[214]
M. alpina	40	[214]
Bacteria		
R. opacus	87	[4]
R. opacus	24–25	[196]
R. rhodochrous	50	[6]
B. alcalophilus	18–24	[196]
A. calcoaceticus	27–38	[133]
P. aeruginosa	38	[47]

genera *Streptomyces, Nocardia, Rhodococcus, Mycobacterium, Dietzia*, or *Gordionia*. To date, *Rhodococcus opacus* is the only bacteria in its native form that is shown to be able to accumulate more than 20 wt.% of its dry biomass as lipids, producing as high as 87 wt.% (dry biomass) lipids containing TAG [4]. On a similar study, Kurosawa et al. [112] conducted a high- cell-density batch cultivation of *R. opacus* PD630 on glucose (240 g/L) which resulted to 77.6 g/L of biomass concentration containing 38 wt.% (dry biomass) TAGs. This suggests the great potential of *R. opacus* for production of biodiesel from cellulosic feedstock containing primarily glucose.

In addition to food and feed applications, microbial oils have been used as feedstocks for biodiesel production [44, 57, 77, 90, 116, 123, 133, 208]. Microbial oils are considered more advantageous over vegetable oils and animal fats because of their short life cycle; less labor requirements for production; minimal influence by location, season, and climate; and ease of process scale-up [117]. Furthermore, as shown in Table 10.6, the fatty acid profiles of these microbial oils are similar with representative animal- and plant-based biodiesel feedstocks tallow and soybean oil in terms of the dominance of oleic (C18:1) and palmitic (C16:0) acids, which is ideal in attaining improved biodiesel characteristics such as cold flow, oxidative stability, ignition quality (cetane number), and reduced emissions of nitrogen oxides (NOx) [29].

10.6.2.2   Metabolic Regulation of Lipid Accumulation in Oleaginous Microorganisms

The basic requirement for lipid accumulation to occur in oleaginous microorganisms is an excess of carbon over a limiting nutrient, usually nitrogen (high C/N). In batch cultures, there is an initial phase of balanced cell proliferation and lipid biosynthesis in the presence of sufficient nitrogen. Following the exhaustion of the limiting nutrient, cell proliferation ceases and the excess carbon supply is continually assimilated by the cells and converted into storage lipids, mostly TAGs. The stored TAG can be extracted from the cells and converted to biodiesel. Other lipid classes (i.e., PLs, glycolipids, etc.) are also produced and can be used to produce biodiesel. The limitation of nitrogen in the culture initiates a cascade of biochemical events that lead to the accumulation of lipids. This phenomenon

TABLE 10.6 Relative Fatty Acid Composition of Oils from Different Sources (wt.% of Total Fatty Acids)

Source	Reference	Fatty acids							
		C16:0	C16:1	C18:0	C18:1	C18:2	C18:3	Others
Yeasts								
L. starkeyi	[116]	33	4.8	4.7	55.1	1.6	-	-
R. glutinis		18	1	6	60	12	2	-
R. toruloides		24.3	1.1	7.7	54.6	2.1	-	-
Fungi								
M. circinelloides	[214]	20	2.3	2	37	14.3	18.5	2
Bacteria								
R. opacus	[230]	16.8	5.9	2.8	73.8	-	-	-
Algae								
B. braunii	[230]	19.1	0.9	4.8	24.4	8.4	19.0	15.4
C. sorokiniana	[159]	40	4.0	-	5	36	23	32
Tallow	[23]	26	3.5	19.5	40	4.5	-	3
Soybean oil	[66]	11.8	-	4	25	55.4	3.8	Trace

is dictated mainly by two critical regulatory enzymes: malic enzyme and ATP:citrate lyase (ACL) [133]. Although malic enzyme can be found in both oleaginous and nonoleaginous microorganisms, it is considered to be essential in generating an abundant supply of reductants (NADPH) required for fatty acid biosynthesis via the action of fatty acid synthase (FAS) [163]. Oleaginous microorganisms are differentiated from nonoleaginous strains by the presence of ACL, which is a cytosolic enzyme whose action yields an increased cytosolic pool of acetyl-CoA precursors for enhanced fatty acid and TAG biosynthesis [46, 165].

10.6.3 WASTEWATER AS MEDIA FOR OLEAGINOUS MICROORGANISMS

A major cost factor in microbial oil production is the substrate required for the growth of microorganisms. Hence, using inexpensive waste resources as cultivation media for oleaginous microorganisms is extremely desirable. Wastewaters from municipal, agricultural, and industrial sources were investigated, and several of those wastewaters offered the potential for biodiesel production. Microbial oil or single-cell-oil production from industrial wastewaters has attracted a great deal of attention of researchers for the production of renewable biodiesel during the last two decades. Yeast treatment process, which involves removing pollutant from wastewater by oleaginous yeast for the production of yeast biomass and oil, is considered an attractive approach for both wastewater treatment and resource exploitation. Discovery of new oleaginous yeast species, understanding of the oleaginicity of the yeast species through their metabolic pathways, and optimization of the cultivation conditions have been implemented in recent years. To achieve higher rates of yeast biomass and oil production, enhanced pollutant removal, lower requirement of nutrient supplement, and minimized production cost, highly adaptive oleaginous yeast for the appropriate wastewater substrate is required. However, the selected oleaginous yeast must be capable of using variety of carbon sources with strong ability to tolerate different type of pollutants (organic and inorganic materials in the wastewater) to produce oils with similar fatty acid composition to plant oils.

Based on the information provided by U.S. Congressional Budget Office, the annual cost expenditures for wastewater treatments was estimated to be in average between $13.0–$20.9 billion for the years

2000–2019 [121]. Manipulation of wastewater treatment scenarios by ole-aginous yeast to produce microbial oil could lead to a generation of an alternative renewable feedstock for biodiesel manufacturing. To that aim, two purposes are fulfilled, the generation of alternative feedstock for the production of renewable biodiesel and the treatment of industrial wastewa-ter. Oleaginous yeast species that have been used for industrial wastewa-ter treatment purposes include *Lipomyces starkeyi* [10, 92], *Cryptococcus curvatus* [37, 76], *Rhodotorula glutinis* [6, 36, 79, 218, 219], *Trichosporon dermatis* CH007 [160], *Trichosporon coremiiforme* [34], *Rhodosporidium toruloides* [121, 191]. Among these oleaginous yeasts, *Rhodotorula glu-tinis* is favorable for biodiesel production due to high lipid productivity from industrial wastewater and high pollutant removal efficiency. Table 10.7 shows a summary of the various studies involving the growth of lipid-producing oleaginous microorganisms in different types of municipal and industrial wastewaters.

Most of industrial wastewaters are highly acidic with pH levels lower than 5, which necessitated pH adjustment prior to activated sludge treat-ment process. Yeast treatment process is considered profitable for high-organic- strength wastewaters, due to their high tolerance to acidity and salinity. Yeasts are able to metabolize various carbon sources, mainly sugars such as glucose, xylose, mannose, galactose, sucrose and maltose. Oleaginous yeasts have short doubling times, high lipid content (up to 80 wt.% of their dry biomass), and can produce different classes of lipids from various carbon sources [122, 196]. Oleaginous yeasts are effective in degradation of organic substances [chemical oxygen demand (COD) reduction as high as 68–86%] and have shown a significant growth and lipid productivity in high strength industrial effluents with initial COD levels of 15,000–50,000 mg/L in a comparatively short cultivation time compared to microalgae [120].

High organic strength industrial wastewaters used as a substrates for cultivation of oleaginous yeasts include those from starch processing [124, 168, 217], potato, fruit juice and lettuce processing [186], butanol fermenta-tion [34, 160], glutamate production [218, 219], brewery and distillery [181, 187], palm oil mill [131, 183], olive oil mill [224], pulp and paper mill [6, 162]), etc. (see Table 10.7), with levels of carbon residues described indi-rectly by the COD.

TABLE 10.7 Production of Biomass and Lipid Accumulation Using Various Oleaginous Yeasts from Different Industrial Wastewaters

Yeast strain	Wastewater	Supplement source	Biomass (g/L)	Lipid content (wt.% of dry biomass)	Initial COD (mg/L)	COD Removal (%)	Fermentation mode	References
Cryptococcus curvatus	Brewery wastewater	Crude glycerol	50.4	37.7	-	-	Flask	[181]
Cryptococcus curvatus	Distillery wastewaters from tequila production	No supplement	5.19	25.2	23,125	78.98	Flask	[76]
Rhodotorula glutinis	Starch wastewater	Less than 5% waste syrup	40	35	50,000	80	Pilot-scale 300-L fermenter	[217]
Rhodotorula glutinis	Starch wastewater	No supplement	60	30	50,000	55	5-L fermenter	[217]
Rhodotorula glutinis	Monosodium glutamate wastewater	No supplement	2.44	9.1	10,000	85	Flask	[219]
Rhodotorula glutinis	Monosodium glutamate wastewater	Glucose	25	20	40,000	45	5-L fermenter	[218]
Rhodotorula glutinis	Brewery wastewater	No supplement	4.5	11	36,000	-	Flask	[187]

Rhodotorula glutinis	Palm oil mill effluent	Ammonium sulfate + Tween 20	9.15	60.62	25,000	69.6	2-L fermenter	[183]
Rhodotorula glutinis TISTR 5159	Palm oil mill effluent	No supplement	2.06	36.89	37,211	68.7	Flask	[33]
Rhodotorula glutinis	Pulp and paper wastewater	Glycerol + $(NH_4)2SO_4$	19	15	-	-	3-L fermenter	[162]
Rhodotorula glutinis	Distillery wastewaters from tequila production	No supplement	6.06	27.02	23,125	84.44	Flask	[76]
Y. lipolytica TISTR 5151	Palm oil mill effluent	No supplement	3.5	48	37,211	47.84	Flask	[128]
Trichosporon coremiiforme	Wastewater after butanol fermentation	No supplement	5.8	19.1	23,560	68	Flask	[34]
Rhodosporidium toruloides	Distillery wastewater	No supplement	8.12	43.65	52,900	86.11	Flask	[122]
Rhodosporidium toruloides Y2	Bioethanol wastewater	Glucose	3.8	34.9	-	72.3	Flask	[231]
Lipomyces starkeyi	Potato starch wastewater	Glucose + $(NH_4)2SO_4$	2.59	8.88	-	-	Flask	[124]

TABLE 10.7 (Continued)

Yeast strain	Wastewater	Supplement source	Biomass (g/L)	Lipid content (wt.% of dry biomass)	Initial COD (mg/L)	COD Removal (%)	Fermentation mode	References
Lipomyces starkeyi	Olive oil mill wastewaters	No supplement	11	22.4	43,000	-	Flask	[224]
Lipomyces starkeyi HL	Fishmeal wastewater	Glucose	17.6	-	-	43.4	Flask	[92]
Yarrowia lipolytica TISTR 5151	Palm oil mill effluent	4% crude glycerol	3.21	68	86,826	-	Flask	[33]

10.6.3.1 Carbohydrate-Rich Wastewaters

Carbohydrate-rich wastewaters from food processing have attracted the attention of researchers for bioconversion to microbial oils. Starch wastewater is one of the most polluting wastewaters in food industries. Traditional starch wastewater treatments such as aerobic, anaerobic, and biological treatment processes are only for the purpose of removing pollutants from the wastewaters without considering a system to recover valuable products. In addition to carbohydrate, starch wastewater contains nitrogen, phosphorus and minerals such as Fe, Mg, Zn [168] which makes it suitable for simultaneous production of energy and wastewater treatment by oleaginous yeasts. The study on pilot-scale production of microbial oil using oleaginous yeast *Rhodotorula glutinis* by Xue and colleagues [217], demonstrated the potential industrialization of microbial oil production using starch wastewater. Their study resulted to a biomass production of 40 g/L containing 35 wt.% (dry biomass) of lipid with 40,000 mg/L of COD removed. All these were achieved without nutrient addition, pH adjustment, or sterilization.

Wastewaters produced by postbutanol fermentation distillation process contain high levels of organic acids and residual sugars with high COD (usually >20,000 mg/L). Chen and co-workers [34] showed that this wastewater could be used as a substrate with no need for nutrient and trace mineral addition. The cultivation of oleaginous yeast *Trichosporon coremiiforme* in butanol fermentation wastewater resulted in 68% of COD degradation, biomass and lipid content of 5.8 g/L and 19.1 wt.% (dry biomass), respectively.

Wastewaters from the beverage industry normally have high organic contents, recognized by a high chemical (COD) and biological (BOD) oxygen demand. The COD of brewery wastewaters ranges between 2000 and 6000 mg/L. Schneider and colleagues [187] examined low cost brewery effluents as growth media to cultivate *Rhodotorula glutinis* for lipid and carotenoid production. They observed that brewery wastewater is a suitable fermentation substrate for lipid production since it serves as a sole nitrogen source and contains substantial amounts of residual sugars (sucrose, maltose, glucose, and fructose) as carbon source. The potential utilization of organic waste from brewery industry was also studied using *Cryptococcus curvatus*, which led to 37 wt.% (dry biomass) lipid content [181]. The wastewater contained essential nutrients for the growth of oleaginous yeast; thus, no pretreatment and additional nutrient was needed.

Utilization of raw distillery wastewater without addition of external nutrients, sterilization and pH adjustment was investigated for enhanced lipid production by *Rhodosporidium toruloides*. Relatively high lipid production, and high COD, total nitrogen and phosphorus removal was achieved in the presence of indigenous microorganisms in distillery wastewater [122].

10.6.3.2 Oil-Rich Wastewaters

The food processing industries are responsible for the majority of the wastewater discharges with high quantities of oily wastewaters (e.g., oil and diary mills). Palm oil mill effluent (POME), and olive oil mill wastewater, which both contain high amount of free fatty acids, are usually discarded as oil-rich industrial wastewater. POME contains 0.6–0.7 oils and 4–5 wt.% solids in water. The large amount of fatty acids, carbohydrates, proteins, and mineral salts in palm oil mill wastewater can stimulate the growth of oleaginous microorganism for the production of oil-rich biomass. It is estimated that the wastewater discharge for the production of each ton of crude palm oil is approximately 2.5 tones [131]. In addition to high organic carbon content, POME is rich in mineral salts, proteins, and vitamins that could stimulate the growth of oleaginous microorganisms for the production of oil-rich biomass. Cheirsilp and Louhasakul [33] have investigated the potential utilization of palm oil mill industrial wastes for low-cost production of microbial oil through microbial fermentation of several oleaginous yeasts. They showed that *Y. lipolytica* TISTR 5151 could effectively grow in POME and produce relatively high lipid production (1.6 g/L) corresponding to a lipid content of (48 wt.% of dry biomass) in POME. The lipid content in *Y. lipolytica* has improved to 68 wt.% (dry biomass), when 4% crude glycerol was added to POME.

Biological treatment of olive oil mill wastewater is challenging due to antimicrobial activity of its phenolic compounds. Yousuf and colleagues [224] showed that oleaginous yeast *Lipomyces starkeyi* was able to survive in untreated olive oil mill wastewater and produce lipids without addition of organic supplements while significantly reducing both total organic carbons and phenol content.

10.7 ENHANCEMENT OF OIL ACCUMULATION BY ACTIVATED SLUDGE MICROFLORA

10.7.1 INTRODUCTION

The amount of extractable lipids for biofuels production from raw activated sludges is limited due to the fact that these sludges are typically generated under low C/N conditions, which are not conducive to increased storage lipid biosynthesis and accumulation. In addition, the dominant microbial population in the activated sludge consortia might not have the metabolic capacities for lipid accumulation under these conditions. Attempts to incorporate oleaginous yeast species into the heterotrophic microbial consortium in wastewater treatment and generation of "enhanced" activated sludge biomass with increased lipid content and biodiesel production yield were unsuccessful as the oleaginous species were eventually outcompeted by the indigenous microorganisms during typical cultivation in WWTPs [82]. Successful proliferation of the oleaginous consortia in wastewater was only made possible after disinfection of the wastewater influent stream via ozonation [142]. A low dose ozone treatment reduced heterotrophic bacterial populations but at the same time partially oxidized recalcitrant organic materials into biodegradable materials, which supplied a portion of the carbon and nutrients that supported the growth of an oleaginous yeast consortium in the wastewater. However, the prospect of adding a preozonation step prior to the aerobic bio-oxidation process in order to replace the heterotrophic microbial population with specialized oil accumulating yeasts could add significant process costs.

It is hypothesized that subjecting the activated sludge microorganisms to high carbon-to-nitrogen ratio (C/N) conditions in wastewater can elicit the same stress response of generating lipid storage materials within specific constituents of the heterotrophic consortium in a similar fashion as with oleaginous yeasts. Formation of intracellular storage materials and population shifts within the activated sludge microbiota may result from metabolic stress conditions such as alternating increasing or decreasing organic loading of the influent wastewater towards specific microbial groups producing PHA biopolymers [18, 167]. However, typical municipal/domestic wastewaters have low C/N ratios, which hinder the proliferation of these specialized microbial groups. Therefore, an innovative approach for enhancing lipid contents of activated sludge is to increase the C/N ratio of the wastewater through the supplementation of carbon such as sugars obtained through hydrolysis of waste lignocellulosic biomass (see Figure 10.7), short chain fatty acids (SCFAs) from anaerobic digestion of sewage sludge (see Section 10.8), or high organic wastewater streams (see Section 10.6). Studies have shown that this technique can trigger lipid accumulation among potentially oleaginous constituents of the activated sludge microflora and allow them to proliferate and dominate the mixed culture.

A significant amount of research efforts were conducted by the authors of this text on this research area with the aim of integrating microbial oil production into conventional wastewater treatment operations using the existing wastewater influent streams and heterotrophic microbial population within the activated sludge. In this section, studies on the utilization of lignocellulosic biomass hydrolyzate sugars as supplemental carbon sources for enhanced lipid accumulation by activated sludge microflora is discussed. The use of SCFAs from anaerobic digestion as carbon source for lipid accumulation is discussed in Section 10.8.

10.7.2 LIGNOCELLULOSIC BIOMASS AS CARBON SOURCE FOR ENHANCED ACTIVATED SLUDGE OIL ACCUMULATION

Since enhanced oil accumulation in oleaginous microorganisms requires the supplementation of high amounts of carbon relative to nutrients, it is critical that the selected carbon source for such process be obtained from abundant and low cost sources. Lignocellulosic biomass from agricultural wastes, forestry residues, nonfood energy crops, and municipal solid wastes has been typically used as renewable source of sugars for bioconversion to biofuels such as bioethanol. These have been similarly applied as carbon source for lipid accumulation by specialized oleaginous yeasts [35,

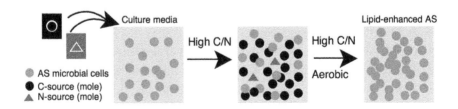

FIGURE 10.7 Generalized schematic for the enhancement of oil content of activated sludge (AS) microflora.

44, 91, 116]. Most studies on sugar bioconversion to biofuel compounds focused on utilization of glucose for microbial growth and production of biofuel compounds as it has the most direct biochemical route through glycolysis. However, the processes for liberating fermentable sugars from the heterogeneous polymeric carbohydrate structures of lignocellulosic biomass not only yield glucose but also other hexose (i.e., galactose, mannose, etc.) and pentose (i.e., xylose, arabinose, etc.) sugars. Chemical hydrolysis processes using high temperature dilute acid treatment also generate lignocellulose breakdown byproducts such as organic acids (i.e., acetic acid) and furans (i.e., furfural, hydroxymethylfurfural), which have been known to exert inhibitory effects on microbial growth and metabolism [153]. Therefore, the activated sludge microorganisms must be able to use different sugar components of lignocellulosic biomass hydrolyzates towards lipid accumulation and withstand the inhibitory effects of the nonsugar hydrolysis byproducts during lipid accumulation.

10.7.2.1   Glucose as Sole Carbon Source

The study conducted by Mondala and colleagues [141] demonstrated for the first time that cultivating activated sludge microorganisms in a high C/N ratio (70:1) synthetic wastewater medium using glucose (60 g/L) as sole carbon source produced activated sludge biomass with significantly increased total lipid content (17.5 wt.% of dry sludge) and higher biodiesel yield (10.2 wt.% of dry sludge). These yields were higher compared to raw activated sludge from the WWTP and sludge biomass grown at low C/N ratios (10:1 and 40:1) under the same initial glucose level. Changing the initial glucose concentration at a constant high C/N ratio did not appear to significantly affect the total lipid and biodiesel yield from the enhanced activated sludge biomass, but were consistently higher than those of raw activated sludges. Additionally, cultivation of activated sludge microorganisms in glucose-rich media resulted in a shift in the FAME profile from saturated fatty acid-dominant (C16:0, palmitate) in raw activated sludge, to one with an unsaturated fatty acid component majority, with oleate (C18:1) comprising up to 40 wt.% of the esterifiable lipid fraction. This change was speculated to be indicative of a dynamic shift in the activated sludge microbial population towards components with high amounts of storage lipids, possibly TAG with oleate residues. Findings stemming from analysis of the dynamics of the activated sludge microbial community composition resulting from cultivation in oleaginous-selecting wastewater media are discussed in Section 10.7.4. The results of this seminal study demonstrated the proof-of-concept of the proposed WWTP biorefinery approach of enhancing lipid contents of activated sludge through the application of techniques for triggering storage lipid production within a component of the activated sludge heterotrophic microbial population.

10.7.2.2   Co-Utilization of Glucose and Xylose

Lignocellulosic biomass sugars produced under mild hydrolysis conditions typically contain higher levels of the pentose sugar xylose than glucose due to the fact that hemicelluloses which contain a mixture of pentose and hexose sugars are easier to hydrolyze than cellulose, which is composed of pure glucose. The microbial co-utilization of all sugars in lignocellulose hydrolyzate is considered to be one of the hurdles for achieving high economic competitiveness of biomass-based products such as microbial oils for biodiesel feedstock use from oleaginous microorganisms [45, 60, 110, 229]. Although xylose is usually the most abundant sugar in the hemicellulose fraction of biomass, it considered to be the most difficult to ferment [152]. Most microorganisms lack the genes encoded for xylose reductase (XR) and xylitol dehydrogenase (XH) enzymes, hence cannot use xylose directly (Chung and Lee, 1985). Even so, xylose has to be shuttled through additional metabolic steps such as the pentose phosphate pathway to generate glycolysis intermediates before being used in lipid biosynthesis Papanikolaou and Aggelis, 2011; [165]. Xylose utilization capabilities of oleaginous microorganisms such as *Candida curvata, Rhodotorula glutinis,* and *Lipomyces starkeyi* and the fungi *Cunninghamella echinulata* and *Mortierella isabelina* have been investigated and these have all been shown to use xylose by itself or as a co-substrate with glucose for lipid accumulation [60, 61, 229].

Using glucose and xylose as sole carbon sources or as co-substrates for enhanced lipid accumulation by activated sludge showed that using xylose as sole carbon source or in combination with glucose resulted in almost twice the biomass and lipid conversion yields (i.e., mass of biomass or lipids produced per mass of sugar consumed) than when using glucose as the sole carbon source [139]. This higher conversion yield could be attributed to the slower uptake rate of xylose compared to glucose by the proliferating oil-producing subpopulation of the activated sludge microflora. The microbial sugar consumption trends exhibited a diauxic pattern; in which xylose was only consumed at a higher rate by the culture after glucose levels have been depleted. The total gravimetric lipid and biodiesel yields (in dry sludge mass basis) from the generated oily sludge biomass were not significantly different across the treatments (i.e., type of sugar/s used as carbon source) investigated. Similar to glucose-fed activated sludge cultures, the dominant fatty acyl residue found in the FAMEs generated from transesterification of the extracted lipids from xylose- and glucose/xylose mixture-grown sludges was oleate (C18:1), which comprised up to 40–45 wt.% of total FAMEs. Given the highly diverse nature of the activated sludge microflora, it is not a surprise that certain members of the microflora could possess xylose utilization capabilities for microbial storage lipid biosynthesis that can be triggered under stress conditions. The results demonstrated that xylose can be efficiently used by activated sludge microbial cultures along with glucose for enhanced oil accumulation for increased biodiesel yield from sludge biomass. Further studies on using other hexose and pentose sugars present in lignocellulose hydrolyzates or actual lignocellulosic biomass hydrolyzates are needed to fully assess the capability of oil-accumulating activated sludge microbial cultures using sugars from renewable biomass substrates.

10.7.2.3 Effect of Lignocellulose Hydrolysis By-Products

Furfural and acetic acid were chosen as representative compounds for furans and organic acids, respectively that are commonly generated during dilute acid hydrolysis of lignocellulosic biomass. Ideally, biomass hydrolyzates can be detoxified to remove these compounds prior to being fed to microbial cultures. However, this approach can further add costs to microbial lipids and biodiesel production from enhanced activated sludge grown using cellulosic sugars. Studies were conducted to determine the effects of acetic acid and furfural on activated sludge microflora growing on high C/N ratio wastewater medium with glucose as sole carbon source [136, 138].

Mondala [136] showed that 1.5 g/L of furfural in wastewater media was toxic to activated sludge microflora and resulted in very little cell growth and lipid accumulation. Glucose was fully consumed in this culture, most likely for maintenance of existing viable cells in the sludge inoculum. A furfural level of 0.5 g/L resulted in a slight increase in the lipid content but because of the very small cell concentration, did not produce any appreciable amount of extractable oils that could be practically harnessed for biodiesel production. However, the cultures demonstrated *in situ* furfural uptake to significantly reduce furfural levels and detoxify the cultivation medium.

Addition of 10 g acetic acid per L of wastewater medium led to an overall increase in cell growth, most likely due to the additional carbon source provided into the medium in the form of acetate ions [138]. However, lipid and biodiesel yields from activated sludge grown in the presence of acetic acid were lower than in glucose media with no acetic acid present. Similar to glucose grown enhanced oil-rich sludges, oleate (C18:1) was observed to be the dominant fatty acyl residue present in their lipidic fraction. The observed high sugar uptake rates in these cultures with acetic acid could be attributed to high ATP production coupled to the high activity of the microbial cell membrane proton pump as a countermeasure to maintain intracellular pH and prevent acid buildup. Moreover, a combination of furfural and acetic acid in the wastewater medium resulted in increased cell growth but significantly reduced lipid and biodiesel yields from activated sludge biomass [136]. In summary, these findings imply the potential of directly using lignocellulosic biomass hydrolyzates as carbon sources for growth by activated sludge microorganisms without prior detoxification necessary. The activated sludge microflora demonstrate the capacity for *in situ* furfural and acetic acid detoxification as well as using acetate as an additional carbon source of cell growth. Cultivation conditions and strategies must then be optimized in order to improve storage lipid biosynthesis in activated sludge cultures using these complex carbon sources.

10.7.2.4 Utilizing Actual Biomass Hydrolyzates as Complex Carbon Source

Mondala and co-workers [137] tested sugarcane bagasse hydrolyzate containing different sugars (in g/L: xylose – 63.34, dimers – 12.87, glucose – 3.28, galactose – 2.72, arabinose – 3.95) and inhibitors (in g/L: acetic acid – 4.55, furfural – 1.69, and formic acid – 1.63) as carbon substrate for activated sludge as lipid accumulation cultures. The investigators produced enhanced activated sludges with the highest lipid contents (40–47 wt.% of dry sludge) reported so far but was made only possible after prior xylose acclimation of the activated sludge inoculum and supplementation of nutrients in the wastewater medium during bagasse hydrolyzate fermentation. Biodiesel consisting mostly of C_{16} and C_{18} FAME at yields of up to 20 wt.% (dry sludge) were also achieved during the xylose accumulation phase but declined to around 12.5 wt.% (dry sludge) during the actual bagasse fermentation phase. Based on the outcomes of the study, the investigators proposed using a sequential batch feeding and sludge biomass harvesting cultivation process with alternating low and high nutrient levels in order to first acclimate the activated sludge microflora to the hydrolyzate, especially with regards to the levels of inhibitory byproducts present, and consistently maintain a viable microbial cell concentration in the culture with enhanced oil accumulation capacities. Overall, the study demonstrates the feasibility of enhancing activated sludge biomass oil contents and biodiesel yields by supplementing wastewater media with renewable biomass-derived carbon sources. Studies using hydrolyzates from other types of biomass materials as carbon source are essential to demonstrate the robustness of the technology in handling a wide variety of lignocellulosic biomass materials as sugars sources to be used in the process.

10.7.3 BIOPROCESSING MODES FOR ENHANCED ACTIVATED SLUDGE LIPID ACCUMULATION

In addition to the basic batch fermentation, other cultivation modes such as fed-batch or sequential batch, semicontinuous and continuous were also tested for feeding lignocellulosic biomass hydrolyzates to activated sludge cultures for enhanced oil accumulation [136]. An artificial biomass hydrolyzate based on corn stover hydrolyzate containing 26.7% glucose, 59.2% xylose, 12.8% acetic acid, and 1.3% furfural (percentage based on total mass of carbon compounds) was used in the experiments. The findings shown in Figure 10.8 showed that the semicontinuous fermentation mode resulted in the highest lipid yield achieved during the initial stages of the cultivation while a continuous fermentation mode resulted in a more consistent lipid content greater than 1 wt.% (dry sludge) throughout the duration of the cultivation run. Unlike the batch and fed-batch modes, the gradual addition of the hydrolyzate in the semicontinuous mode resulted in lower instantaneous concentrations of acetic acid and furfural, which then lessened the inhibitory effect on growth and lipid accumulation of the activated sludge microflora.

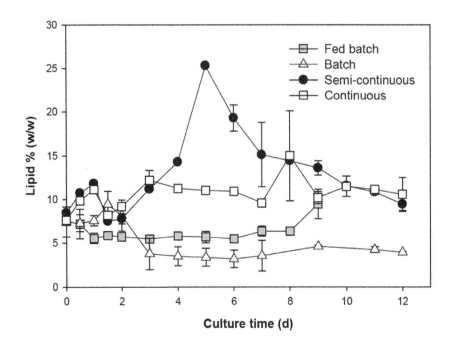

FIGURE 10.8 Comparison of lipid yields from enhanced activated sludge fed with artificial biomass hydrolyzate using different fermentation modes. Data were obtained from Mondala [136]. (Reprinted with permission from Mondala, A., (2010). *Enhanced Lipid Production and Biodiesel Yields from Activated Sludge via Fermentation of Lignocellulose Hydrolyzate.* Ph.D. Dissertation, Dave C. Swalm School of Chemical Engineering, Mississippi State University.)

The gradual buildup of carbon levels also contributed to the higher lipid accumulation in this culture. However, since the withdrawing cycle was only done batch-wise, the buildup of inhibitory compounds from the hydrolyzate and microbial metabolic byproducts could have also contributed to the observed gradual decline of the lipid contents of the activated sludge biomass after the maximum level was achieved. On the other hand, a continuous fermentation mode resulted in a more consistent lipid yield profile because of the gradual addition of substrate combined with continuous withdrawal of the spent culture. A hybrid or alternating sequence of semicontinuous with continuous processing with optimized dilution rates can be an appropriate configuration for the enhanced activated sludge accumulation process to maximize sludge oil and biodiesel yields.

10.7.4 ACTIVATED SLUDGE MICROBIAL COMMUNITY DYNAMICS DURING ENHANCED LIPID ACCUMULATION

DNA extraction and 16s rRNA sequencing techniques were employed by Mondala and co-workers [141] to explore the microbial community composition dynamics in activated sludge lipid accumulation cultures. Figure 10.9 shows significant shifts in activated sludge microbial community composition cultivated in wastewater media with high C/N ratio of 70:1 using glucose as carbon source after three and seven days of cultivation to Betaproteobacteria (90.4% of sequences) and Alphaproteobacteria (99.5% of sequences), respectively. At the seventh day when high lipid accumulation has been achieved, the Alphaproteobacteria were composed almost entirely of *Rhodospirillales* bacteria, which has been previously shown to be able to generate PHA biopolymers [12]. In addition to PHAs, this microbial group also produces intracellular TAGs, which can then be converted to biodiesel or renewable diesel. A deeper understanding of the underlying microbial population dynamics within a complex mixed culture such as activated sludge under lipid accumulation conditions can be exploited for engineering microbial consortia with enhanced lipid accumulation capabilities in conjunction with wastewater organic pollutant degradation capabilities.

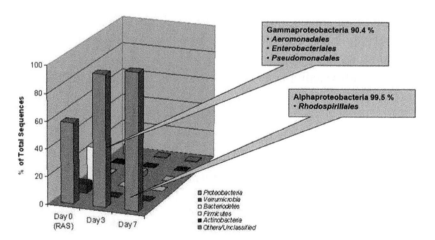

FIGURE 10.9 Microbial community population shift in activated sludge cultures lipid accumulation cultures relative to raw activated sludge (RAS). Data were obtained from [141]. (Reprinted with permission from Mondala, A. H., Hernandez, R., French, T., McFarland, L., Santo Domingo, J. W., Meckes, M., Ryu, H., & Iker, B. (2012b). Enhanced lipid and biodiesel production from glucose-fed activated sludge: Kinetics and microbial community analysis. *AIChE J., 58*(4), 1279–1290. © 2011 John Wiley and Sons.)

10.7.5   ECONOMIC ESTIMATES

In 2010, a study conducted by Mondala et al. [140] on the biodiesel production from raw activated sludge through *in situ* transesterification was extended for enhanced activated sludge. This was done to have an initial estimate of the economic viability of the proposed sludge enhancement technology. The estimates included the costs of lipid production generating activated sludge with increased lipid content via cultivation in wastewater media supplemented with biomass sugars. For this study, a biodiesel break-even price of $4.06 per gallon was estimated which was higher than that of biodiesel produced from raw activated sludge ($3.23/gallon). With the cost of biomass sugars as the only factor differentiating the two estimates, it was concluded that reduction of sugars cost to $0.10 per lb. could drop the biodiesel price below $3.00 per gallon [136].

10.8   COUPLED ANAEROBIC DIGESTION AND ACTIVATED SLUDGE LIPID ACCUMULATION

10.8.1   INTRODUCTION

The concept of coupling of anaerobic digestion and activated sludge lipid accumulation via SCFAs platform is motivated by the need to design not only an economical lipid accumulation but also a structurally compatible integrated subsystem. Figure 10.10 illustrates this concept. SCFAs include

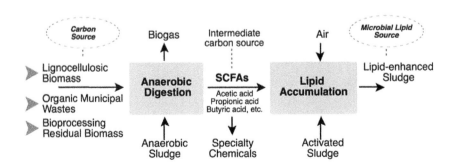

FIGURE 10.10 Generalized schematic for the integration of anaerobic digestion and aerobic lipid accumulation to produce lipid-enhanced sludge using SCFAs as substrate: short chain fatty acids (SCFAs).

acetic, propionic, butyric, iso-butyric, valeric, and iso-valeric acids. Several reviewers suggested the potential of these acids as carbon sources for fuels and chemical production owing an advantage for less operating cost and more stable microbial system compared to that of pure cultures [31, 157]. These acids are produced through anaerobic digestion of organics such as carbohydrates, proteins, and lipids in pretreated or untreated organic wastes [2, 15, 105]. Recent experimental results show that these SCFAs can act as carbon sources for the lipid accumulation of activated sludge.

10.8.2 SHORT CHAIN FATTY ACIDS PLATFORM

The SCFAs platform has been viewed as an alternative conversion pathway for organic wastes to fuels and chemicals [31]. This conversion pathway takes advantage of the spontaneity of breaking organic wastes into constituent monomers, which are then converted to SCFAs via anaerobic microbial consortia [115]. Then, the SCFAs are converted to value-added materials. A SCFAs downstream application that has been extensively studied is the thermochemical processing MixAlco, which requires separation of the SCFAs from the spent liquor prior to thermochemical conversion to alcohols [87, 88]. The separation is achieved by salting out the SCFAs followed by dewatering and drying. This separation of the SCFAs from the spent liquor is a significant cost that a trade-off between the digestion cost and dewatering cost were optimized in order to find a suitable operating SCFAs concentration in the final digestion stream is necessary [78, 88]. Another possible SCFAs downstream application that has been speculated [31], but has not been extensively studied yet is biochemical conversion such as the coupling of anaerobic digestion with the lipid accumulation process described previously in Section 10.7 using SCFAs as the platform chemical. This application uses the SCFAs as carbon sources for the lipid accumulation of activated sludge microbial consortia. This process emulates the single cell oils (SCO) technology by using high C/N ratio as physiological trigger to lipid content enhancement. The works of Holtzapple et al. [88] and Taco Vasquez et al. [197] are comprehensive literatures for the state-of-the-art of thermochemical application called MixAlco process. This section focuses on the biochemical conversion of organic wastes to SCFAs then to microbial lipids.

10.8.3 PRODUCTION OF SCFAS FROM ANAEROBIC DIGESTION

Studies on anaerobic digestion of organic matter have established that SCFAs are intermediate carbon carriers or some of the end-products [5]. Lee et al. [115] published a recent extensive review on the production of SCFAs via anaerobic digestion of organic wastes. The reader is referred to this publication for comprehensive discussion of the topic and for references of additional literature.

Various solid and liquid wastes have been used as feedstocks for anaerobic SCFAs. The solid wastes include primary sludge (PS) [130, 212, 213], waste activated sludge (WAS) [128, 133], organic fraction of municipal wastes (OFMSW) [24, 185], food wastes [58, 119], and kitchen wastes [226]. The liquid wastes include POME [89], olive oil mill effluent [51], wood mill effluent [16], paper mill effluent [17, 100], cheese whey [17], dairy wastewater [48], pharmaceutical wastewater [148], and gelatin-rich proteinaceous wastewater [225]. Also used were mixtures of solid and liquid wastes such as PS with WAS [98]. PS with starch-rich wastewater [14], WAS with food wastes [65], and sugar industry wastewater with pressed beet pulp [3].

The conversion of organic wastes to SCFAs involves hydrolysis of the complex polymers followed by acidogenesis of the monomers to SCFAs [115]. Hydrolysis is the rate-limiting step and it has been the focus of some pretreatment studies. Some of the pretreatment techniques used were acid [50, 58], alkaline [58, 126], ozone [26, 30], hydrogen peroxide [189], biological [62, 220], microwave [189], ultrasound [26], and thermal [26, 58]. Combinations of these techniques were also used: acid plus ultrasound [58], alkaline plus ultrasound [58], thermal plus ultrasound [58], ozone plus ultrasound [215], thermochemical [62], alkaline plus microwave [52], thermal plus biological [104], and hydrogen peroxide plus microwave [189]. Some operational implementations of anaerobic digestion, however, do not include pretreatment. Most municipal WWTPs in the U.S. anaerobically digest WAS without any chemical or physical pretreatment [207]. The typical anaerobic digesters used for SCFAs production are upflow anaerobic sludge blanket reactor (UASB), continuous stirred tanked reactor (CSTR), packed bed reactor, and fluidized bed reactor [115]. The main operational factors that significantly affect the production of SCFAs are pH, temperature, hydraulic retention time (HRT), solids retention time (SRT), and organic loading rate (OLR) [5, 48,

115]. Summaries of production performance and composition of SCFAs from digestion of organic wastes are shown in Tables 10.8 and 10.9, respectively.

10.8.4 LIPID ACCUMULATION BY ACTIVATED SLUDGE MICROORGANISMS USING SCFAS AS CARBON SOURCE

Unlike sugars, SCFAs are toxic to many microorganisms at concentrations greater than 5–10 g/L [194]. Nonetheless, their potential as practical and economical carbon carriers motivated several studies on their use for microbial lipid accumulation. Most of these early studies used pure microbial cultures and they proved true the hypothesis that SCFAs can function as alternative carbon sources for lipid accumulation [37, 63, 64, 67, 108]. Though majority of these studies used chemical grade SCFAs [39, 63, 64, 67], the work of Chi et al. [37] demonstrated that actual waste-derived SCFAs are successfully assimilated for lipid content enhancement in oleaginous yeast. This work also showed that the SCFAs could be fed for lipid accumulation without separation from the digestion liquor, a feature not present in the counterpart thermochemical conversions. At almost the same time, a work by Mondala and colleagues [138] has been testing the effect of acetic acid on glucose-fed activated sludge microbial consortia dedicated for enhanced lipid and biodiesel production. The study found that acetic acid enhanced biomass production but reduced lipid content. Though the objective of this study was to evaluate the possible effects of using lignocellulosic hydrolyzate as feedstock, which typically contains organic acids in addition to sugar monomers and other pretreatment by-products, the study hinted the potential of using SCFAs as sole carbon sources of activated sludge. Then, experiments were focused on testing the hypothesis that activated sludge microbial consortia can use SCFAs as sole carbon sources for lipid accumulation [68–70].

Figure 10.11 shows results from lipid accumulation of activated sludge feeding on SCFAs after 24 h growth in glucose cultivated in shake flasks. Glucose was initially fed to the microbial consortia to stimulate growth. The nominal initial SCFAs concentration for each acid and their mixture (1:1:1 mass ratio) was set to 1.25 g/L. The acids were consumed with corresponding increase in solids concentration (measure of microbial biomass) and lipid content during the first 24 hours. Complete consumption of the

TABLE 10.8 Empirical Results on the SCFAs Production Performance from Various Studies on Digestion of Organic Wastes

SCFA Production Parameter	Empirical Results	Reference
Total SCFAs concentration (in mg/L)	18,700	[202]
	16,000	[201]
	15,110	[179]
	18,400–26,300	[143]
	17,200–23,000	[75]
	13,260–14,690	[74]
	14,600–56,100	[71]
	16,800–20,200	[53]
	16,290–25,990	[2]
	11,780–23,110	[185]
Total SCFAs concentration (in mg-COD/L)	2,070–3,960	[17]
	9,700–16,900	[58]
Total SCFAs yield (in mg/g VS fed)	581	[202]
	550	[201]
	360	[179]
	230–360	[143]
	180–370	[71]
	100–420	[53]
	175–276	[2]
Total SCFAs yield (in mg-COD/g VS fed)	91.5–319.9	[212]
	298–368	[228]
Total SCFAs productivity(in mg/L-d)	2,490	[202]
	1,810	[201]
	840	[75]
	1,260–1,400	[143]
	799–824	[75]
	798–1,070	[74]
	760–1,270	[71]
	800–1,400	[53]
	829–1,360	[202]
	1,710–1,830	[119]
Total SCFAs productivity (in mg/g VS-d)	30.6–45.3	[130]
	8–57	[14]

VS-volatile solids, COD-chemical oxygen demand

TABLE 10.9 Mass Distribution of Individual Acid in Total SCFAs Produced from Various Studies on Digestion of Organic Wastes

Acetic acid (%)	Propionic acid (%)	Butyric acid (%)	i-Butyric acid (%)	Valeric acid (%)	i-Valeric acid (%)	Reference
34–48	25–38	9–17	1–5	3–5	2–10	[213]
56–74	24–35	9–19	–	0–6	–	[130]
38–58	12–19	7–9	7–9	14–16	0–5	[133]
35.7–37.5	30–31.5	16.1–17	–	15.1–17.1	–	[119]
57–93	2–10	4–20	0–4	0–5	1–7	[179]
74–90	1.5–5.5	7.4–19.3	–	0.23–1.23	–	[143]
33–42	36.7–46.6	5.2–7	–	7.2–13.9	–	[75]
65.9–90.6	1.87–3.50	6.7–31.1	–	0.25–0.76	–	[71]
39–57	11.4–19	12–30	–	6–9	–	[53]

acids occurred after 72 hours, but the solids concentration and lipid content decreased from the levels at 24-hours sampling. Acetic acid was easily assimilated as indicated by complete utilization within 24 hours. This preference for acetic acid to the other acids was also observed in pure oleaginous cultures [64]. Cultivation at higher SCFAs loading (2.5 g/L and 5 g/L) did not change solids concentration and lipid content levels, which implies inhibition (data not shown). Fed-batch feeding of the SCFAs can be done to improve lipid accumulation.

Several studies proved that regulation of SCFAs loading via fed-batch operation minimizes inhibition while still allowing high molar C/N ratio in the culture media resulting to lipid accumulation [63, 67, 118]. Figure 10.12 shows the cultivation performance by feeding acetic acid every 12-hour interval at 1.5 g/L loading per feeding. The solids concentration significantly increased during the cultivation from around 14 g/L to around 20 g/L. On the other hand, the lipid content did not increase for the first 48 hours, but continuously increased afterwards resulting to a change from around 8 wt.% (dry sludge) to 12.5 wt.% (dry sludge) lipid content. The lipid accumulation pattern is comparable to that of glucose-fed activated sludge studied by Mondala et al. [141].

So far, lipid accumulation of activated sludge feeding on waste-derived SCFAs has not been extensively studied even though there is already a comprehensive literature on the upstream anaerobic production of SCFAs.

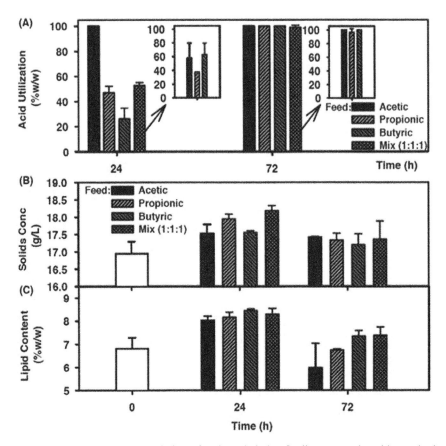

FIGURE 10.11 Lipid accumulation of activated sludge feeding on acetic acid, propionic acid, and butyric acid cultivated in 500-mL shake flasks after 24-h growth in glucose. Operating conditions: 25°C, and 180 rpm benchtop shaker. Glucose was completely depleted prior to the addition of the SCFAs. The nominal initial SCFAs concentration was set to 1.25 g/L for each acid including the Mix at 1:1:1 mass ratio of the three acids. Initial molar C/N for each treatment was set to 70 using ammonium sulfate. (A) Acid utilization calculated as the reduction of acid concentration relative to the initial concentration. (B) Solids concentration as a measure of the microbial biomass concentration since majority of activated sludge is composed of active microbial cells. (C) Lipid content calculated as the extracted lipid from the dry solids measured gravimetrically.

Nonetheless, recent few experimental results showed the potential of the technology as alternative conversion pathway of organic wastes to fuels and chemicals. Moreover, existing infrastructures might reduce the challenges in scaling-up the process. Anaerobic digesters are used in most WWTPs in the

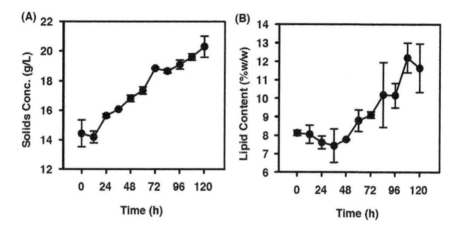

FIGURE 10.12 Fed-batch lipid accumulation of activated sludge feeding on acetic acid cultivated in 5-L (4-L working volume) bioreactor. Acetic acid was fed every 12-hour interval at a concentration 1.5 g/L buffered by equimolar amount of acetate (sodium acetate). Initial molar C/N was set to 70 using ammonium sulfate. Operating conditions: 25°C, 300 rpm, 1vvm air and no pH control. (A) Solids concentration as a measure of the microbial biomass concentration since majority of activated sludge is composed of active microbial cells. (B) Lipid content calculated as the extracted lipid from the dry solids measured gravimetrically.

U.S. while sequencing batch reactors (SBRs) operate on the principle of the fed-batch mode [135, 207].

10.9 CONCLUDING REMARKS AND FUTURE PERSPECTIVES

By the turn of the twenty first century, wastewaters have been widely viewed as sources of energy, and value-add materials in addition to being sources of potable water [200]. This evolution of wastewater treatment has been embraced not only by researchers, but also by communities via the implementation of several mature technologies in large-scale operations. Most of these technologies use wastewater sludges, which are the sinks of carbon, nitrogen, and nutrients from wastewater [200].

The successful utilization of activated sludge as feedstock for biofuel production is hindered by the several factors including water removal, inconsistent extract properties and composition, and low biodiesel yield. Water removal is critical for efficient extraction of materials from this feedstock which contains ~98 wt.% water. The literature proposes two water-tolerant extraction techniques namely, BD and reactive extraction (*in situ* transesterification). The choice of which technique to use depends on the targeted product for the extract. BD will recover the main compounds in activated sludge such as those shown in Table 10.2, while the *in situ* transesterification will result to an extract containing mainly biodiesel.

Inconsistent extract properties and low biodiesel yield could be addressed by fattening the microorganisms by adding carbon sources in a nitrogen-limited media, which is the focus of Sections 10.6–10.8 of this chapter. According to Mondala [136], the cost of the additional carbon substrate is a limiting factor for enhanced sludge to be economically competitive. Consequently, the suggested strategy will require the cost of the carbon substrate at around $0.10 per lb. With abundant lignocellulosic biomass that can be sustainably harvested in the US (~1.3 billion tons per year) [111] as well as different high – C containing industrial wastewater streams, this could be easily addressed.

Catalytic cracking of activated sludge with or without prior extraction, presents another route to convert these unwanted waste materials into useful compounds. Catalytic cracking of activated sludge extract might need some pretreatment to remove phosphorus from PLs as well as possible metals which are catalyst poisons. These could be accomplished by simple hydrolysis reaction, followed by extraction to remove the unwanted components.

Fluidized bed catalytic cracking of activated sludge (raw and enhanced) seems to be the more promising thermochemical conversion option due to its possible integration with existing processes within WWTPs. However, severe coke formation over ZSM5 suggests the need for a more suitable catalyst for this process [172]. Activated sludge microorganisms have PL-containing cell membranes, which are the first point of contact during fluidized bed catalysis [176]. Thus, the targeted catalyst must have high tolerance to phosphorus poisoning (or that it can recover from it) in addition to high water-tolerance.

The technologies presented in this chapter were studied with the goal of achieving energy and environmental sustainability simultaneously through the integrated WWTP biorefinery platform. The key aspects highlighted here are the utilization of wastewater and sewage sludge/biosolids streams as biofuel production substrates either through thermochemical or biochemical processes and the use of existing WWTP infrastructures such as aeration ditches, sedimentation/clarification, anaerobic digestion, and dewatering/drying operations for simultaneous treatment and resource recovery from these waste streams. Currently, the commonly used technology for resource recovery from activated sludge is through anaerobic digestion to produce biogas (methane + carbon dioxide). The biogas produced is either burned for thermal energy or used for electrical energy generation while the residual solids are disposed through landfilling. In comparison to anaerobic digestion, the technologies presented in this chapter have the following advantages: (i) production of fuels which have higher energy density than methane (i.e., biodiesel and renewable diesel), (ii) reduction of the amount of material going into anaerobic digestion of WWTPs (i.e., extraction and *in situ* transesterification of raw activated sludge), and (iii) reduction or potential complete elimination of anaerobic digestion in WWTPs (i.e., catalytic cracking). On the other hand, the main disadvantage of these technologies is the lack of more complete techno-economic analyses. In addition, the enhancement strategy could potentially increase the amount of materials to be stabilized by anaerobic digestion, which is not entirely a bad thing since methane generation could also potentially increase.

Among the technologies presented, economic viability has been estimated for biodiesel production from raw and enhanced activated sludges through the *in situ* transesterification process. However, pilot scale studies must be carried out to improve these initial estimates. Once a more accurate economic assessment is completed, it can be easily extended for lipid accumulation through activated sludge enhancement using high strength wastewater or SCFAs followed by biodiesel production. In addition, pilot and demonstration scale implementations must be considered for a more comprehensive techno-economic improvements and infrastructure integration. Furthermore, studies on the dynamics of heterotrophic microbial communities in wastewater and sludge must be conducted to identify the mechanisms that lead towards enhanced oil accumulation in natural wastewater microflora in order to develop engineered microbial consortia for enhanced wastewater treatment and oil production capabilities. With respect to the thermochemical conversion of activated sludges (both raw and enhanced), the technology is still in its infancy and will require a lot of work on optimization and catalyst development to obtain an initial cost estimates. For all the technologies presented in this chapter, the authors believe that the basic knowledge and theoretical foundation to convert existing WWTPs into a biorefinery have been presented. The prospect of re-engineering WWTP systems to incorporate renewable energy production is a research area worth pursuing well into the future as fuel and water resources become more deficient while world population continues to increase in the years to come.

KEYWORDS

- activated sludge
- biodiesel
- in-situ transesterification
- lipids
- wastewater

REFERENCES

1. Adjaye, J. D., Katikaneni, S. P. R., & Bakhshi, N. N., (1996). Catalytic conversion of a biofuel to hydrocarbons: effect of mixtures of HZSM-5 and silica-alumina catalysts on product distribution. *Fuel Process. Technol.*, *48*(2), 115–143.
2. Aiello-Mazzarri, C., Agbogbo, F. K., & Holtzapple, M. T., (2006). Conversion of municipal solid waste to carboxylic acids using a mixed culture of mesophilic microorganisms. *Bioresour. Technol.*, *97*(1), 47–56.
3. Alkaya, E., & Demirer, G. N., (2011). Anaerobic acidification of sugar-beet processing wastes: Effect of operational parameters. *Biomass Bioenergy*, *35*(1), 32–39.
4. Alvarez, H. M., & Steinbüchel, A., (2002). Triacylglycerols in prokaryotic microorganisms. *Appl. Microbiol. Biotechnol.*, *60*(4), 367–376.
5. Amani, T., Nosrati, M., & Sreekrishnan, T. R., (2010). Anaerobic digestion from the viewpoint of microbiological, chemical, and operational aspects — a review. *Environ. Rev.*, *18*(NA), 255–278.
6. Amirsadeghi, M., Shields-Menard, S., French, W. T., & Hernandez, R., (2015). Lipid Production by *Rhodotorula glutinis* from Pulp and Paper Wastewater for Biodiesel Production. *Journal of Sustainable Bioenergy Systems*, *5*(3), 114–125.
7. Anderson, A. J., & Dawes, E. A., (1990). Occurrence, metabolism, metabolic role, and industrial uses of bacterial polyhydroxylakanoates. *Microbiol. Rev.*, *54*(4), 450–472.
8. Anderson, S., (2004). Soxtec: Its Principles and Applications. in: *Oil Extraction and Analysis: Critical Issues and Comparative Studies*, (Ed.) D. L. Luthria, AOCS Press. Champaigne, Ill., pp. 11–24.

9. Angelé, B., & Kirchner, K., (1980). The poisoning of noble metal catalysts by phosphorus compounds—I chemical processes, mechanisms and changes in the catalyst. *Chem. Eng. Sci.*, *35*(10), 2089–2091.

10. Angerbauer, C., Siebenhofer, M., Mittelbach, M., & Guebitz, G. M., (2008). Conversion of sewage sludge into lipids by *Lipomyces starkeyi* for biodiesel production. *Bioresour. Technol.*, *99*(8), 3051–3056.

11. Ardern, E., & Lockett, W. T., (1914). Experiments on the oxidation of sewage without the aid of filters. *Journal of the Society of Chemical Industry*, *33*(10), 523–539.

12. Asrar, J., & Hill, J. C., (2002). Biosynthetic processes for linear polymers. *J. Appl. Polym. Sci.*, *83*(3), 457–483.

13. Bamgboye, A. I., & Hansen, A. C., (2008). Prediction of cetane number of biodiesel fuel from the fatty acid methyl ester (FAME) composition. *International Agrophysics*, *22*(1), 21–29.

14. Banerjee, A., Elefsiniotis, P., & Tuhtar, D., (1999). The effect of addition of potato-processing wastewater on the acidogenesis of primary sludge under varied hydraulic retention time and temperature. *J. Biotechnol.*, *72*(3), 203–212.

15. Batstone, D. J., Keller, J., Angelidaki, I., Kalyuzhnyi, S. V., Pavlostathis, S. G., Rozzi, A., Sanders, W. T. M., Siegrist, H., & Vavilin, V. A., (2002). *Anaerobic Digestion Model No. 1 (ADM1)*. IWA Publishing, Cornwall, UK.

16. Ben, M., Mato, T., Lopez, A., Vila, M., Kennes, C., & Veiga, M. C., (2011). Bioplastic production using wood mill effluents as feedstock. *Water Sci. Technol.*, *63*(6), 1196–1202.

17. Bengtsson, S., Hallquist, J., Werker, A., & Welander, T. (2008a). Acidogenic fermentation of industrial wastewaters: Effects of chemostat retention time and pH on volatile fatty acids production. *Biochem. Eng. J.*, *40*(3), 492–499.

18. Bengtsson, S., Werker, A., Christensson, M., & Welander, T. (2008b). Production of polyhydroxyalkanoates by activated sludge treating a paper mill wastewater. *Bioresour. Technol.*, *99*(3), 509–516.

19. Benson, T., (2008). *Elucidation of Reaction Pathways for Catalytically Cracked Unsaturated Lipids*. Ph.D. Dissertation, Dave C. Swalm School of Chemical Engineering, Mississippi State University.

20. Benson, T. J., Hernandez, R., French, W. T., Alley, E. G., & Holmes, W. E., (2009). Elucidation of the catalytic cracking pathway for unsaturated mono-, di-, and triacylglycerides on solid acid catalysts. *J. Mol. Catal. A: Chem.*, *303*(1–2), 117–123.

21. Benson, T. J., Hernandez, R., White, M. G., French, W. T., Alley, E. E., Holmes, W. E., & Thompson, B., (2008). Heterogeneous cracking of an unsaturated fatty acid and reaction intermediates on H⁺ZSM-5 catalyst. *Clean - Soil Air Water*, *36*(8), 652–656.

22. Bligh, E. G., & Dyer, W. J., (1959). A rapid method of total lipid extraction and purification. *Can. J. Biochem. Physiol.*, *37*(8), 911–917.

23. Bockisch, M., (1993). *Fats and Oils Handbook*. AOCS Press, Champaign, IL.

24. Bolzonella, D., Fatone, F., Pavan, P., & Cecchi, F., (2005). Anaerobic Fermentation of Organic Municipal Solid Wastes for the Production of Soluble Organic Compounds. *Ind. Eng. Chem. Res.*, *44*(10), 3412–3418.

25. Boocock, D. G. B., Konar, S. K., Leung, A., & Ly, L. D., (1992). Fuels and chemicals from sewage sludge. 1. The solvent extraction and composition of a lipid from a raw sewage sludge. *Fuel*, *71*(11), 1283–1289.

26. Bougrier, C., Albasi, C., Delgenès, J. P., & Carrère, H., (2006). Effect of ultrasonic, thermal and ozone pretreatments on waste activated sludge solubilization and anaerobic biodegradability. *Chemical Engineering and Processing: Process Intensification*, *45*(8), 711–718.

27. Bozaghian, M., (2014). *Characterization and Synthesis of Biodiesel from Sludge Available in the Umeå Region*. Degree Project in Engineering Chemistry, Department of Chemistry, Umeå Universitet.

28. Brennan, P. J., (1988). Mycobacterium and other actinomycetes. in: *Microbial Lipids, vol. 1*, (Eds.) C. Ratledge, S. G. Wilkinson, Academic Press. London, pp. 203–298.

29. Bringe, N. A., (2005). Soybean oil composition for biodiesel. 1st ed. in: *The Biodiesel Handbook*, (Eds.) G. Knothe, J. Krahl, J. H. Van Gerpen, AOCS Press. Champaign, Illinois, pp. 161–164.

30. Cesaro, A., & Belgiorno, V., (2013). Sonolysis and ozonation as pretreatment for anaerobic digestion of solid organic waste. *Ultrason. Sonochem.*, *20*(3), 931–936.

31. Chang, H. N., Kim, N.-J., Kang, J., & Jeong, C. M., (2010). Biomass-derived volatile fatty acid platform for fuels and chemicals. *Biotechnol. Bioprocess Eng.*, *15*(1), 1–10.

32. Charusiri, W., Yongcharoen, W., & Vitidsant, T., (2006). Conversion of used vegetable oils to liquid fuels and chemicals over HZSM-5, sulfated zirconia and hybrid catalysts. *Korean J. Chem. Eng.*, *23*(3), 349–355.

33. Cheirsilp, B., & Louhasakul, Y., (2013). Industrial wastes as a promising renewable source for production of microbial lipid and direct transesterification of the lipid into biodiesel. *Bioresour. Technol.*, *142*, 329–337.

34. Chen, X.-F., Huang, C., Xiong, L., Chen, X.-D., Chen, Y., & Ma, L.-L., (2012). Oil production on wastewaters after butanol fermentation by oleaginous yeast *Trichosporon coremiiforme*. *Bioresour. Technol.*, *118*, 594–597.

35. Chen, X., Li, Z., Zhang, X., Hu, F., Ryu, D. D. Y., & Bao, J., (2009). Screening of oleaginous yeast strains tolerant to lignocellulose degradation compounds. *Appl. Biochem. Biotechnol.*, *159*, 591–604.

36. Chi, Z., Zheng, Y., Jiang, A., & Chen, S., (2011a). Lipid Production by Culturing Oleaginous Yeast and Algae with Food Waste and Municipal Wastewater in an Integrated Process. *Appl. Biochem. Biotechnol.*, *165*(2), 442–453.

37. Chi, Z., Zheng, Y., Ma, J., & Chen, S., (2011b). Oleaginous yeast *Cryptococcus curvatus* culture with dark fermentation hydrogen production effluent as feedstock for microbial lipid production. *Int. J. Hydrogen Energy*, *36*(16), 9542–9550.

38. Choi, O. K., Song, J. S., Cha, D. K., & Lee, J. W., (2014). Biodiesel production from wet municipal sludge: Evaluation of *in situ* transesterification using xylene as a cosolvent. *Bioresour. Technol.*, *166*, 51–56.

39. Christophe, G., Deo, J. L., Kumar, V., Nouaille, R., Fontanille, P., & Larroche, C., (2012). Production of Oils from Acetic Acid by the Oleaginous Yeast *Cryptococcus curvatus*. *Appl. Biochem. Biotechnol.*, *167*(5), 1270–1279.

40. Chung, I., & Lee, Y., (1985). Ethanol fermentation of crude acid hydrolyzate of cellulose using high-level yeast inocula. *Biotechnol. Bioeng.*, *27*, 308–315.

41. Coker, A. T., (2013). *Evaluation of Catalytic and Noncatalytic Production of Biodiesel from Wet Microbial Media and Reaction Schemes*. Ph.D. Dissertation, Dave C. Swalm School of Chemical Engineering, Mississippi State University.

42. Corma, A., Huber, G. W., Sauvanaud, L., & O'Connor, P., (2008). Biomass to chemicals: Catalytic conversion of glycerol/water mixtures into acrolein, reaction network. *J. Catal.*, *257*(1), 163–171.

43. Corma, A., Huber, G. W., Sauvanaud, L., & O'Connor, P., (2007). Processing biomass-derived oxygenates in the oil refinery: Catalytic cracking (FCC) reaction pathways and role of catalyst. *J. Catal.*, *247*(2), 307–327.

44. Dai, C.-C., Tao, J., Xie, F., Dai, Y.-J., & Zhao, M., (2007a). Biodiesel generation from oleaginous yeast *Rhodotorula glutinis* with xylose assimilating capacity. *Afr. J. Biotechnol.*, *6*(18), 2130–2134.

45. Dai, C., Tao, J., Zhao, M., & Jiang, B., (2007b). Energetic Efficiency and Environmental, Economic, Societal Benefits of Microdiesel from Biowastes. *Energy Exploration & Exploitation*, *25*(3), 219–225.

46. Davies, R. J., & Holdsworth, J. E., (1992). Synthesis of lipids in yeasts: biochemistry, physiology, production. in: *Advances in Applied Lipid Research*, (Ed.) F. B. Padley, JAI Press Ltd. Greenwich, CT, pp. 119–159.

47. de Andrés, C., Espuny, M. J., Robert, M., Mercadé, M. E., Manresa, A., & Guinea, J., (1991). Cellular lipid accumulation by *Pseudomonas aeruginosa* 44T1. *Appl. Microbiol. Biotechnol.*, *35*(6), 813–816.

48. Demirel, B., & Yenigün, O., (2004). Anaerobic acidogenesis of dairy wastewater: the effects of variations in hydraulic retention time with no pH control. *J. Chem. Technol. Biotechnol.*, *79*(7), 755–760.

49. Demirel, B., & Yenigün, O., (2002). Two-phase anaerobic digestion processes: a review. *J. Chem. Technol. Biotechnol.*, *77*(7), 743–755.

50. Devlin, D. C., Esteves, S. R. R., Dinsdale, R. M., & Guwy, A. J., (2011). The effect of acid pretreatment on the anaerobic digestion and dewatering of waste activated sludge. *Bioresour. Technol.*, *102*(5), 4076–4082.

51. Dionisi, D., Carucci, G., Papini, M. P., Riccardi, C., Majone, M., & Carrasco, F., (2005). Olive oil mill effluents as a feedstock for production of biodegradable polymers. *Water Res.*, *39*(10), 2076–2084.

52. Doğan, I., & Sanin, F. D., (2009). Alkaline solubilization and microwave irradiation as a combined sludge disintegration and minimization method. *Water Res.*, *43*(8), 2139–2148.

53. Domke, S. B., Aiello-Mazzarri, C., & Holtzapple, M. T., (2004). Mixed acid fermentation of paper fines and industrial biosludge. *Bioresour. Technol.*, *91*(1), 41–51.

54. Du, J., Wang, H., Jin, H., Yang, K., & Zhang, X., (2007). Fatty acids production by fungi growing in sweet potato starch processing waste water. *Chin J Bioprocess Eng.*, *5*(1), 33–36.

55. Dufreche, S., Hernandez, R., French, T., Sparks, D., Zappi, M., & Alley, E., (2007). Extraction of lipids from municipal wastewater plant microorganisms for production of biodiesel. *J. Am. Oil Chem. Soc.*, *84*(2), 181–187.

56. Dufreche, S. T., (2008). *Effect of Phosphorus Poisoning on Catalytic Cracking of Lipids for Green Diesel Production*. Ph.D. 3297818, Dave C. Swalm School of Chemical Engineering, Mississippi State University.

57. Easterling, E. R., French, W. T., Hernandez, R., & Licha, M., (2009). The effect of glycerol as a sole and secondary substrate on the growth and fatty acid composition of *Rhodotorula glutinis*. *Bioresour. Technol.*, *100*(1), 356–361.

58. Elbeshbishy, E., Hafez, H., Dhar, B. R., & Nakhla, G., (2011). Single and combined effect of various pretreatment methods for biohydrogen production from food waste. *Int. J. Hydrogen Energy*, *36*(17), 11379–11387.

59. Energy Information Administration (2016). *Gasoline and Diesel Fuel Update*, https://www.eia.gov/petroleum/gasdiesel/, (accessed: March 2, 2016).

60. Evans, C. T., & Ratledge, C., (1983). A comparison of the oleaginous yeast, *Candida curvata*, grown on different carbon sources in continuous and batch culture. *Lipids*, *18*(9), 623–629.

61. Fakas, S., Papanikolaou, S., Batsos, A., Galiotou-Panayotou, M., Mallouchos, A., & Aggelis, G., (2009). Evaluating renewable carbon sources as substrates for single cell oil production by *Cunninghamella echinulata* and *Mortierella isabellina*. *Biomass Bioenergy*, *33*(4), 573–580.

62. Fdez.-Güelfo, L. A., Álvarez-Gallego, C., Sales, D., & Romero, L. I., (2011). The use of thermochemical and biological pretreatments to enhance organic matter hydrolysis and solubilization from organic fraction of municipal solid waste (OFMSW). *Chem. Eng. J.*, *168*(1), 249–254.

63. Fei, Q., Chang, H. N., Shang, L., & Choi, J.-D.-R. (2011a). Exploring low-cost carbon sources for microbial lipids production by fed-batch cultivation of *Cryptococcus albidus*. *Biotechnol. Bioprocess Eng.*, *16*(3), 482–487.

64. Fei, Q., Chang, H. N., Shang, L., Choi, J.-D.-R., Kim, N., & Kang, J. (2011b). The effect of volatile fatty acids as a sole carbon source on lipid accumulation by *Cryptococcus albidus* for biodiesel production. *Bioresour. Technol.*, *102*(3), 2695–2701.

65. Feng, L., Yan, Y., & Chen, Y., (2011). Co-fermentation of waste activated sludge with food waste for short-chain fatty acids production: effect of pH at ambient temperature. *Frontiers of Environmental Science & Engineering in China*, *5*(4), 623–632.

66. Ferrari, R. A., Oliveira, V. D. S., & Scabio, A., (2005). Oxidative stability of biodiesel from soybean oil fatty acid ethyl esters. *Scientia Agricola*, *62*, 291–295.

67. Fontanille, P., Kumar, V., Christophe, G., Nouaille, R., & Larroche, C., (2012). Bioconversion of volatile fatty acids into lipids by the oleaginous yeast *Yarrowia lipolytica*. *Bioresour. Technol.*, *114*, 443–449.

68. Fortela, D. L., Hernandez, R., French, W. T., Mondala, A., Holmes, W., Revellame, E., & Egede, E., (2013). Integration of Anaerobic Digestion of Cellulose Into Lipid Accumulation By a Mixed Microbial Consortium. *American Institute of Chemical Engineers (AIChE) Annual Meeting*, November 8, San Francisco, CA, USA.

69. Fortela, D. L., Hernandez, R., Zappi, M., French, W. T., Bajpai, R., Chistoserdov, A., & Holmes, W., (2015). Microbial oil accumulation capability of activated sludge microorganisms feeding on short chain fatty acids. *American Institute of Chemical Engineers (AIChE) Annual Meeting*, Salt Lake City, UT, USA.

70. Fortela, D. L., Hernandez, R., Zappi, M., Holmes, W., Revellame, E., Dufreche, S., Subramaniam, R., & French, W. T., (2014). Refining the concept of integrating anaerobic-aerobic microbial systems to produce chemicals and lipids for fuels. *American Institute of Chemical Engineers (AIChE) Annual Meeting*, Atlanta, GA, USA.

71. Fu, Z., & Holtzapple, M. T., (2010). Consolidated bioprocessing of sugarcane bagasse and chicken manure to ammonium carboxylates by a mixed culture of marine microorganisms. *Bioresour. Technol.*, *101*(8), 2825–2836.

72. Gary, J. H., & Handwerk, G. E., (2001). *Petroleum Refining: Technology and Economics. 4th ed*. Marcel Dekker, New York.

73. Gassiot-Matas, M., & Juliá-Danés, E., (1972). Pyrolysis gas chromatography of some sterols. *Chromatographia*, *5*(9), 493–501.

74. Golub, K. W., Forrest, A. K., Wales, M. E., Hammett, A. J. M., Cope, J. L., Wilkinson, H. H., & Holtzapple, M. T., (2013). Comparison of three screening methods to select mixed-microbial inoculum for mixed-acid fermentations. *Bioresour. Technol.*, *130*, 739–749.

75. Golub, K. W., Smith, A. D., Hollister, E. B., Gentry, T. J., & Holtzapple, M. T., (2011). Investigation of intermittent air exposure on four-stage and one-stage anaerobic semicontinuous mixed-acid fermentations. *Bioresour. Technol.*, *102*(8), 5066–5075.

76. Gonzalez-Garcia, Y., Hernandez, R., Zhang, G., Escalante, F. M. E., Holmes, W., & French, W. T., (2013). Lipids accumulation in *Rhodotorula glutinis* and *Cryptococcus curvatus* growing on distillery wastewater as culture medium. *Environmental Progress & Sustainable Energy, 32*(1), 69–74.

77. Gouveia, L., & Oliveira, A. C., (2009). Microalgae as a raw material for biofuels production. *J. Ind. Microbiol. Biotechnol., 36*(2), 269–274.

78. Granda, C. B., Holtzapple, M. T., Luce, G., Searcy, K., & Mamrosh, D. L., (2009). Carboxylate Platform: The MixAlco Process Part 2: Process Economics. *Appl. Biochem. Biotechnol., 156*(1–3), 107–124.

79. Granger, L.-M., Perlot, P., Goma, G., & Pareilleux, A., (1993). Effect of various nutrient limitations on fatty acid production by *Rhodotorula glutinis*. *Appl. Microbiol. Biotechnol., 38*(6), 784–789.

80. Gunstone, F. D., & Harwood, J. L., (2007). Occurrence and characterization of oils and fats. 3rd ed. in: *The Lipid Handbook with CD-ROM*, (Eds.) F. D. Gunstone, J. L. Harwood, A. J. Dijkstra, CRC Press/Taylor & Francis. Boca Raton, FL, pp. 37–142.

81. Haas, M. J., & Foglia, T. A., (2005). Alternative feedstocks and technologies for biodiesel production. 1st ed. in: *The Biodiesel Handbook*, (Eds.) G. Knothe, J. Krahl, J. H. Van Gerpen, AOCS Press. Champaign, IL, pp. 42–61.

82. Hall, J., Hetrick, M., French, T., Hernandez, R., Donaldson, J., Mondala, A., & Holmes, W., (2011). Oil production by a consortium of oleaginous microorganisms grown on primary effluent wastewater. *J. Chem. Technol. Biotechnol., 86*(1), 54–60.

83. Hanif, M., Atsuta, Y., Fujie, K., & Daimon, H., (2010). Supercritical fluid extraction of microbial phospholipid fatty acids from activated sludge. *J. Chromatogr. A., 1217*(43), 6704–6708.

84. Hara, A., & Radin, N. S., (1978). Lipid extraction of tissues with a low-toxicity solvent. *Anal. Biochem., 90*(1), 420–426.

85. Harrison, E. Z., Oakes, S. R., Hysell, M., & Hay, A., (2006). Organic chemicals in sewage sludges. *Sci. Total Environ., 367*(2–3), 481–497.

86. Hoang, T. Q., Zhu, X., Danuthai, T., Lobban, L. L., Resasco, D. E., & Mallinson, R. G., (2010). Conversion of Glycerol to Alkyl-aromatics over Zeolites. *Energy Fuels, 24*(7), 3804–3809.

87. Holtzapple, M., & Granda, C., (2009). Carboxylate Platform: The MixAlco Process Part 1: Comparison of Three Biomass Conversion Platforms. *Appl. Biochem. Biotechnol., 156*(1–3), 95–106.

88. Holtzapple, M. T., Davison, R. R., Ross, M. K., Aldrett-Lee, S., Nagwani, M., Lee, C.-M., Lee, C., Adelson, S., Kaar, W., Gaskin, D., Shirage, H., Chang, N.-S., Chang, V. S., & Loescher, M. E., (1999). Biomass conversion to mixed alcohol fuels using the MixAlco process. *Appl. Biochem. Biotechnol., 79*(1), 609–631.

89. Hong, S. K., Shirai, Y., Aini, A. R. N., & Hassan, M. A., (2009). Semi-Continuous and Continuous Anaerobic Treatment of Palm Oil Mill Effluent for the Production of Organic Acids and Polyhydroxyalkanoates. *Research Journal of Environmental Sciences, 3*(5), 552–559.

90. Hu, Q., Sommerfeld, M., Jarvis, E., Ghirardi, M., Posewitz, M., Seibert, M., & Darzins, A., (2008). Microalgal triacylglycerols as feedstocks for biofuel production: perspectives and advances. *PlJ, 54*(4), 621–639.

91. Huang, C., Zong, M.-H., Wu, H., & Liu, Q.-P., (2009). Microbial oil production from rice straw hydrolysate by *Trichosporon fermentans*. *Bioresour. Technol., 100*(19), 4535–4538.

92. Huang, L., Zhang, B., Gao, B., & Sun, G., (2011). Application of fishmeal wastewater as a potential low-cost medium for lipid production by *Lipomyces starkeyi* HL. *Environ. Technol.*, *32*(16), 1975–1981.

93. Huynh, L.-H., Kasim, N. S., & Ju, Y.-H., (2010). Extraction and analysis of neutral lipids from activated sludge with and without subcritical water pretreatment. *Bioresour. Technol.*, *101*(22), 8891–8896.

94. Huynh, L. H., Tran Nguyen, P. L., Ho, Q. P., & Ju, Y.-H., (2012). Catalyst-free fatty acid methyl ester production from wet activated sludge under subcritical water and methanol condition. *Bioresour. Technol.*, *123*, 112–116.

95. Idem, R. O., Katikaneni, S. P. R., & Bakhshi, N. N., (1997). Catalytic conversion of canola oil to fuels and chemicals: roles of catalyst acidity, basicity and shape selectivity on product distribution. *Fuel Process. Technol.*, *51*(1–2), 101–125.

96. Illman, A. M., Scragg, A. H., & Shales, S. W., (2000). Increase in Chlorella strains calorific values when grown in low nitrogen medium. *Enzyme Microb. Technol.*, *27*(8), 631–635.

97. Jardé, E., Mansuy, L., & Faure, P., (2005). Organic markers in the lipidic fraction of sewage sludges. *Water Res.*, *39*(7), 1215–1232.

98. Ji, Z., Chen, G., & Chen, Y., (2010). Effects of waste activated sludge and surfactant addition on primary sludge hydrolysis and short-chain fatty acids accumulation. *Bioresour. Technol.*, *101*(10), 3457–3462.

99. Jia, C.-J., Liu, Y., Schmidt, W., Lu, A.-H., & Schüth, F., (2010). Small-sized HZSM-5 zeolite as highly active catalyst for gas phase dehydration of glycerol to acrolein. *J. Catal.*, *269*(1), 71–79.

100. Jiang, Y., Marang, L., Tamis, J., van Loosdrecht, M. C. M., Dijkman, H., & Kleerebezem, R., (2012). Waste to resource: Converting paper mill wastewater to bioplastic. *Water Res.*, *46*(17), 5517–5530.

101. Kargbo, D. M., (2010). Biodiesel Production from Municipal Sewage Sludges. *Energy Fuels*, *24*(5), 2791–2794.

102. Katikaneni, S. P. R., Adjaye, J. D., & Bakhshi, N. N., (1995). Studies on the Catalytic Conversion of Canola Oil to Hydrocarbons: Influence of Hybrid Catalysts and Steam. *Energy Fuels*, *9*(4), 599–609.

103. Katikaneni, S. P. R., Adjaye, J. D., Idem, R. O., & Bakhshi, N. N., (1996). Catalytic Conversion of Canola Oil Over Potassium-Impregnated HZSM-5 Catalysts: C_2-C_4 Olefin Production and Model Reaction Studies. *Ind. Eng. Chem. Res.*, *35*(10), 3332–3346.

104. Kim, H. J., Choi, Y. G., Kim, D. Y., Kim, D. H., & Chung, T. H., (2005). Effect of pretreatment on acid fermentation of organic solid waste. *Water Sci. Technol.*, *52*(1–2), 153–160.

105. Kim, N.-J., Park, G. W., Kang, J., Kim, Y.-C., & Chang, H. N., (2013). Volatile fatty acid production from lignocellulosic biomass by lime pretreatment and its applications to industrial biotechnology. *Biotechnol. Bioprocess Eng.*, *18*(6), 1163–1168.

106. Kinast, J. A., (2003). *Production of Biodiesels from Multiple Feedstocks and Properties of Biodiesels and Biodiesel/Diesel Blends* National Renewable Energy Laboratory http://www.nrel.gov/docs/fy03osti/31460.pdf, Accessed).

107. Knothe, G., (2005). Introduction: What is biodiesel? 1st ed. in: *The Biodiesel Handbook*, (Eds.) G. Knothe, J. Krahl, J. H. Van Gerpen, AOCS Press. Champaign, IL, pp. 1–3.

108. Kolouchová, I., Schreiberová, O., Sigler, K., Masák, J., & Řezanka, T., (2015). Biotransformation of volatile fatty acids by oleaginous and nonoleaginous yeast species. *FEMS Yeast Res.*, *15*(7).

109. Konar, S. K., Boocock, D. G. B., Mao, V., & Liu, J., (1994). Fuels and chemicals from sewage sludge: 3. Hydrocarbon liquids from the catalytic pyrolysis of sewage sludge lipids over activated alumina. *Fuel*, *73*(5), 642–646.

110. Kong, X.-L., Liu, B., Zhao, Z.-B., & Feng, B., (2007). Microbial production of lipids by cofermentation of Glucose and xylose with *Lipomyces starkeyi* 2#. *Chin. J. Bioproc. Eng.*, *5*(2), 36–41.

111. Kosa, M., & Ragauskas, A. J., (2011). Lipids from heterotrophic microbes: advances in metabolism research. *Trends Biotechnol.*, *29*(2), 53–61.

112. Kurosawa, K., Boccazzi, P., de Almeida, N. M., & Sinskey, A. J., (2010). High-cell-density batch fermentation of *Rhodococcus opacus* PD630 using a high glucose concentration for triacylglycerol production. *J. Biotechnol.*, *147*(3–4), 212–218.

113. Kwon, E. E., Kim, S., Jeon, Y. J., & Yi, H., (2012). Biodiesel Production from Sewage Sludge: New Paradigm for Mining Energy from Municipal Hazardous Material. *Environ. Sci. Technol.*, *46*(18), 10222–10228.

114. Lam, M. K., Lee, K. T., & Mohamed, A. R., (2010). Homogeneous, heterogeneous and enzymatic catalysis for transesterification of high free fatty acid oil (waste cooking oil) to biodiesel: A review. *Biotechnol. Adv.*, *28*(4), 500–518.

115. Lee, W. S., Chua, A. S. M., Yeoh, H. K., & Ngoh, G. C., (2014). A review of the production and applications of waste-derived volatile fatty acids. *Chem. Eng. J.*, *235*, 83–99.

116. Li, Q., Du, W., & Liu, D., (2008). Perspectives of microbial oils for biodiesel production. *Appl. Microbiol. Biotechnol.*, *80*(5), 749–756.

117. Li, Q., & Wang, M., (1997). Use food industry waste to produce microbial oil. *Sci. Technol. Food Ind.*, *6*, 65–69.

118. Li, Y., Zhao, Z., & Bai, F., (2007). High-density cultivation of oleaginous yeast *Rhodosporidium toruloides* Y4 in fed-batch culture. *Enzyme Microb. Technol.*, *41*(3), 312–317.

119. Lim, S.-J., Kim, B. J., Jeong, C.-M., Choi, J.-D.-R., Ahn, Y. H., & Chang, H. N., (2008). Anaerobic organic acid production of food waste in once-a-day feeding and drawing-off bioreactor. *Bioresour. Technol.*, *99*(16), 7866–7874.

120. Ling, J., Nip, S., Cheok, W. L., de Toledo, R. A., & Shim, H., (2014). Lipid production by a mixed culture of oleaginous yeast and microalga from distilery and domestic mixed wastewater. *Bioresour. Technol.*, *173*(0), 132–139.

121. Ling, J., Nip, S., de Toledo, R. A., Tian, Y., & Shim, H., (2015). Evaluation of specific lipid production and nutrients removal from wastewater by *Rhodosporidium toruloides* and biodiesel production from wet biomass via microwave irradiation. *Energy*, doi: 10.1016/j.energy.2015.05.141.

122. Ling, J., Nip, S., & Shim, H., (2013). Enhancement of lipid productivity of *Rhodosporidium toruloides* in distillery wastewater by increasing cell density. *Bioresour. Technol.*, *146*, 301–309.

123. Liu, B., & Zhao, Z., (2007). Biodiesel production by direct methanolysis of oleaginous microbial biomass. *J. Chem. Technol. Biotechnol.*, *82*(8), 775–780.

124. Liu, J.-X., Yue, Q.-Y., Gao, B.-Y., Wang, Y., Li, Q., & Zhang, P.-D., (2013). Research on microbial lipid production from potato starch wastewater as culture medium by *Lipomyces starkeyi*. *Water Sci. Technol.*, *67*(8), 1802–1808.

125. Liu, Z.-Y., Wang, G.-C., & Zhou, B.-C., (2008). Effect of iron on growth and lipid accumulation in *Chlorella vulgaris*. *Bioresour. Technol.*, *99*(11), 4717–4722.

126. López Torres, M., & Espinosa Lloréns, M. D. C., (2008). Effect of alkaline pretreatment on anaerobic digestion of solid wastes. *Waste Manage. (Oxford)*, *28*(11), 2229–2234.

127. Losel, D. M., (1988). Fungal lipids. in: *Microbial Lipids, Vol. 1*, (Eds.) C. Ratledge, S. G. Wilkinson, Vol. 1, Academic Press. London, pp. 699–806.

128. Louhasakul, Y., & Cheirsilp, B., (2013). Industrial Waste Utilization for Low-Cost Production of Raw Material Oil Through Microbial Fermentation. *Appl. Biochem. Biotechnol.*, *169*(1), 110–122.

129. Luthria, D. L., Vinjamoori, D., Noel, K., & Ezzell, J., (2004). Accelerated Solvent Extraction. in: *Oil Extraction and Analysis: Critical Issues and Comparative Studies*, (Ed.) D. L. Luthria, AOCS Press. Champaigne, IL, pp. 25–38.

130. Maharaj, I., & Elefsiniotis, P., (2001). The role of HRT and low temperature on the acid-phase anaerobic digestion of municipal and industrial wastewaters. *Bioresour. Technol.*, *76*(3), 191–197.

131. Marjakangas, J. M., Lakaniemi, A.-M., Koskinen, P. E. P., Chang, J.-S., & Puhakka, J. A., (2015). Lipid production by eukaryotic microorganisms isolated from palm oil mill effluent. *Biochem. Eng. J.*, *99*, 48–54.

132. Melero, J. A., Sánchez-Vázquez, R., Vasiliadou, I. A., Martínez Castillejo, F., Bautista, L. F., Iglesias, J., Morales, G., & Molina, R., (2015). Municipal sewage sludge to biodiesel by simultaneous extraction and conversion of lipids. *Energy Convers. Manage.*, *103*, 111–118.

133. Meng, X., Yang, J., Xu, X., Zhang, L., Nie, Q., & Xian, M., (2009). Biodiesel production from oleaginous microorganisms. *Renewable Energy*, *34*(1), 1–5.

134. Mengmeng, C., Hong, C., Qingliang, Z., Shirley, S. N., & Jie, R., (2009). Optimal production of polyhydroxyalkanoates (PHA) in activated sludge fed by volatile fatty acids (VFAs) generated from alkaline excess sludge fermentation. *Bioresour. Technol.*, *100*(3), 1399–1405.

135. Metcalf & Eddy, I., Tchobanoglous, G., Stensel, H. D., Tsuchihashi, R., & Burton, F., (2014). *Wastewater Engineering: Treatment and Resource Recovery*. McGraw-Hill, New York.

136. Mondala, A., (2010). *Enhanced Lipid Production and Biodiesel Yields from Activated Sludge via Fermentation of Lignocellulose Hydrolyzate*. Ph.D. Dissertation, Dave C. Swalm School of Chemical Engineering, Mississippi State University.

137. Mondala, A., Hernandez, R., French, T., Green, M., McFarland, L., & Ingram, L., (2015). Enhanced microbial oil production by activated sludge microorganisms from sugarcane bagasse hydrolyzate. *Renewable Energy*, *78*, 114–118.

138. Mondala, A., Hernandez, R., French, T., McFarland, L., Sparks, D., Holmes, W., & Haque, M. (2012a). Effect of acetic acid on lipid accumulation by glucose-fed activated sludge cultures. *J. Chem. Technol. Biotechnol.*, *87*(1), 33–41.

139. Mondala, A., Hernandez, R., Holmes, W., French, T., McFarland, L., Sparks, D., & Haque, M., (2013). Enhanced microbial oil production by activated sludge microorganisms via cofermentation of glucose and xylose. *AIChE J.*, *59*(11), 4036–4044.

140. Mondala, A., Liang, K., Toghiani, H., Hernandez, R., & French, T., (2009). Biodiesel production by *in situ* transesterification of municipal primary and secondary sludges. *Bioresour. Technol.*, *100*(3), 1203–1210.

141. Mondala, A. H., Hernandez, R., French, T., McFarland, L., Santo Domingo, J. W., Meckes, M., Ryu, H., & Iker, B. (2012b). Enhanced lipid and biodiesel production from

glucose-fed activated sludge: Kinetics and microbial community analysis. *AIChE J.*, *58*(4), 1279–1290.

142. Mondala, A. H., Hernandez, R., French, W. T., Estévez, L. A., Meckes, M., Trillo, M., & Hall, J., (2011). Preozonation of primary-treated municipal wastewater for reuse in biofuel feedstock generation. *Environmental Progress & Sustainable Energy*, *30*(4), 666–674.

143. Nachiappan, B., Fu, Z., & Holtzapple, M. T., (2011). Ammonium carboxylate production from sugarcane trash using long-term air-lime pretreatment followed by mixed-culture fermentation. *Bioresour. Technol.*, *102*(5), 4210–4217.

144. National Biodiesel Board (2009). *Benefits of Biodiesel*, http://biodiesel.org/docs/ffs-basics/benefits-of-biodiesel.pdf?sfvrsn=4, (accessed: February 29, 2016).

145. National Biodiesel Board (2016). *Biodiesel Production Rises in 2015 as Consumers Seek Cleaner Fuels*, http://nbb.org/news/nbb-press-releases/press-release-display/2016/01/25/biodiesel-production-rises-in-2015-as-consumers-seek-cleaner-fuels, (accessed: February 26, 2016).

146. Ngo, T.-A., Kim, J., Kim, S. K., & Kim, S.-S., (2010). Pyrolysis of soybean oil with H-ZSM5 (Proton-exchange of Zeolite Socony Mobil #5) and MCM41 (Mobil Composition of Matter No. 41) catalysts in a fixed-bed reactor. *Energy*, *35*(6), 2723–2728.

147. O'Leary, W. M., & Wilkinson, S. G., (1988). Gram-positive bacteria. in: *Microbial Lipids, Vol. 1*, (Eds.) C. Ratledge, S. G. Wilkinson, Vol. vol. 1, Academic Press. London, pp. 117–202.

148. Oktem, Y. A., Ince, O., Donnelly, T., Sallis, P., & Ince, B. K., (2006). Determination of optimum operating conditions of an acidification reactor treating a chemical synthesis-based pharmaceutical wastewater. *Process Biochem.*, *41*(11), 2258–2263.

149. Olkiewicz, M., Caporgno, M. P., Fortuny, A., Stüber, F., Fabregat, A., Font, J., & Bengoa, C., (2014). Direct liquid–liquid extraction of lipid from municipal sewage sludge for biodiesel production. *Fuel Process. Technol.*, *128*, 331–338.

150. Olkiewicz, M., Fortuny, A., Stüber, F., Fabregat, A., Font, J., & Bengoa, C., (2015). Effects of pretreatments on the lipid extraction and biodiesel production from municipal WWTP sludge. *Fuel*, *141*, 250–257.

151. Olkiewicz, M., Fortuny, A., Stüber, F., Fabregat, A., Font, J., & Bengoa, C., (2012). Evaluation of Different Sludges from WWTP as a Potential Source for Biodiesel Production. *Procedia Engineering*, *42*, 695–706.

152. Olsson, L., & Hahn-Hägerdal, B., (1993). Fermentative performance of bacteria and yeasts in lignocellulose hydrolysates. *Process Biochem.*, *28*(4), 249–257.

153. Palmqvist, E., & Hahn-Hägerdal, B., (2000). Fermentation of lignocellulose hydrolysates. II: Inhibitors and mechanisms of inhibition. *Bioresour. Technol.*, *74*, 25–33.

154. Pan, J. G., Kwak, M. Y., & Rhee, J. S., (1986). High density cell culture of *Rhodotorula glutinis* using oxygen-enriched air. *Biotechnol. Lett.*, *8*(10), 715–718.

155. Papanikolaou, S., & Aggelis, G., (2011). Lipids of oleaginous yeasts. Part I: Biochemistry of single cell oil production. *Eur. J. Lipid Sci. Technol.*, *113*(8), 1031–1051.

156. Papanikolaou, S., Fakas, S., Fick, M., Chevalot, I., Galiotou-Panayotou, M., Komaitis, M., Marc, I., & Aggelis, G., (2008). Biotechnological valorisation of raw glycerol discharged after bio-diesel (fatty acid methyl esters) manufacturing process: Production of 1,3-propanediol, citric acid and single cell oil. *Biomass & Bioenergy*, *32*(1), 60–71.

157. Park, G. W., Fei, Q., Jung, K., Chang, H. N., Kim, Y. C., Kim, N. J., Choi, J. D., Kim, S., & Cho, J., (2014). Volatile fatty acids derived from waste organics provide an eco-

nomical carbon source for microbial lipids/biodiesel production. *Biotechnol. J, 9*(12), 1536–1546.

158. Pastore, C., Lopez, A., Lotito, V., & Mascolo, G., (2013). Biodiesel from dewatered wastewater sludge: A two-step process for a more advantageous production. *Chemosphere, 92*(6), 667–673.

159. Patterson, G. W., (1970). Effect of culture temperature on fatty acid composition of *Chlorella sorokiniana. Lipids, 5*(7), 597–600.

160. Peng, W.-F., Huang, C., Chen, X.-F., Xiong, L., Chen, X.-D., Chen, Y., & Ma, L.-L., (2013). Microbial conversion of wastewater from butanol fermentation to microbial oil by oleaginous yeast *Trichosporon dermatis. Renewable Energy, 55,* 31–34.

161. Pham, P. J., Hernandez, R., Revellame, E. D., & French, W. T., (2013). Activated Sludge Oil: Identification and Characterization of Components. *Journal of Biobased Materials and Bioenergy, 7*(5), 626–638.

162. Poudel, S. R., Marufuzzaman, M., Ekşioğlu, S. D., AmirSadeghi, M., & French, T., (2015). Supply Chain Network Model for Biodiesel Production via Wastewaters from Paper and Pulp Companies. in: *Handbook of Bioenergy: Bioenergy Supply Chain - Models and Applications*, (Eds.). D. S. Eksioglu, S. Rebennack, M. P. Pardalos, Springer International Publishing. Cham, pp. 143–162.

163. Ratledge, C., (2002). Regulation of lipid accumulation in oleaginous microorganisms. *Biochem. Soc. Trans., 30*(Pt 6), 1047–1050.

164. Ratledge, C., (2005). Single Cell Oils for the 21st Century. in: *Single Cell Oils*, (Eds.) Z. Cohen, C. Ratledge, AOCS Press. Champaign, IL, pp. 1–20.

165. Ratledge, C., & Wynn, J. P., (2002). The biochemistry and molecular biology of lipid accumulation in oleaginous microorganisms. *Adv. Appl. Microbiol., 51,* 1–51.

166. Rattray, J. B. M., (1988). Yeasts. in: *Microbial Lipids*, (Eds.) C. Ratledge, S. G. Wilkinson, Vol. 1, Academic Press. London; San Diego, pp. 555–698.

167. Reddy, S. V., Thirumala, M., Reddy, T. V. K., & Mahmood, S. K., (2008). Isolation of bacteria producing polyhydroxyalkanoates (PHA) from municipal sewage sludge. *World J. Microbiol. Biotechnol., 24*(12), 2949–2955.

168. Ren, H.-Y., Liu, B.-F., Kong, F., Zhao, L., & Ren, N., (2015). Hydrogen and lipid production from starch wastewater by coculture of anaerobic sludge and oleaginous microalgae with simultaneous COD, nitrogen and phosphorus removal. *Water Res., 85,* 404–412.

169. Réveillé, V., Mansuy, L., Jardé, É., & Garnier-Sillam, É., (2003). Characterization of sewage sludge-derived organic matter: lipids and humic acids. *Org. Geochem., 34*(4), 615–627.

170. Revellame, E., Hernandez, R., French, W., Holmes, W., & Alley, E., (2010). Biodiesel from activated sludge through *in situ* transesterification. *J. Chem. Technol. Biotechnol., 85*(5), 614–620.

171. Revellame, E., Hernandez, R., French, W., Holmes, W., Alley, E., & Callahan II, R., (2011). Production of biodiesel from wet activated sludge. *J. Chem. Technol. Biotechnol., 86*(1), 61–68.

172. Revellame, E., Holmes, W., Hernandez, R., & French, W. T. (2012a). Production of Renewable Fuel From Enhanced Activated Sludge Through a Fluidized-Bed Catalytic Cracking (FCC) Process. *AIChE Annual Meeting*, Pittsburgh, PA.

173. Revellame, E. D., (2011). *Activated Sludge as Renewable Fuels and Oleochemicals Feedstock*. Ph.D. Dissertation, Dave C. Swalm School of Chemical Engineering, Mississippi State University.

174. Revellame, E. D., Hernandez, R., French, W., Holmes, W. E., Benson, T. J., Pham, P. J., Forks, A., & Callahan II, R. (2012b). Lipid storage compounds in raw activated sludge microorganisms for biofuels and oleochemicals production. *RSC Adv.*, *2*(5), 2015–2031.

175. Revellame, E. D., Hernandez, R., French, W. T., Holmes, W. E., Forks, A., & Callahan II, R., (2013). Lipid-enhancement of activated sludges obtained from conventional activated sludge and oxidation ditch processes. *Bioresour. Technol.*, *148*, 487–493.

176. Revellame, E. D., Holmes, W. E., Benson, T. J., Forks, A. L., French, W. T., & Hernandez, R. (2012c). Parametric Study on the Production of Renewable Fuels and Chemicals from Phospholipid-Containing Biomass. *Top. Catal.*, *55*(3–4), 185–195.

177. Richter, B. E., Jones, B. A., Ezzell, J. L., Porter, N. L., Avdalovic, N., & Pohl, C., (1996). Accelerated Solvent Extraction: A Technique for Sample Preparation. *Anal. Chem.*, *68*(6), 1033–1039.

178. Rittman, B. E., & McCarty, P. L., (2001). *Environmental Biotechnology: Principles and Applications*. McGraw-Hill, New York.

179. Rughoonundun, H., Mohee, R., & Holtzapple, M. T., (2012). Influence of carbon-to-nitrogen ratio on the mixed-acid fermentation of wastewater sludge and pretreated bagasse. *Bioresour. Technol.*, *112*, 91–97.

180. Rushdi, A. I., Ritter, G., Grimalt, J. O., & Simoneit, B. R. T., (2003). Hydrous pyrolysis of cholesterol under various conditions. *Org. Geochem.*, *34*(6), 799–812.

181. Ryu, B.-G., Kim, J., Kim, K., Choi, Y.-E., Han, J.-I., & Yang, J.-W., (2013). High-cell-density cultivation of oleaginous yeast *Cryptococcus curvatus* for biodiesel production using organic waste from the brewery industry. *Bioresour. Technol.*, *135*, 357–364.

182. Sadrameli, S. M., Green, A. E. S., & Seames, W., (2009). Modeling representations of canola oil catalytic cracking for the production of renewable aromatic hydrocarbons. *J. Anal. Appl. Pyrolysis*, *86*(1), 1–7.

183. Saenge, C., Cheirsilp, B., Suksaroge, T. T., & Bourtoom, T., (2011). Efficient concomitant production of lipids and carotenoids by oleaginous red yeast *Rhodotorula glutinis* cultured in palm oil mill effluent and application of lipids for biodiesel production. *Biotechnol. Bioprocess Eng.*, *16*(1), 23–33.

184. Sangaletti-Gerhard, N., Cea, M., Risco, V., & Navia, R., (2015). *In situ* biodiesel production from greasy sewage sludge using acid and enzymatic catalysts. *Bioresour. Technol.*, *179*, 63–70.

185. Sans, C., Mata-Alvarez, J., Cecchi, F., Pavan, P., & Bassetti, A., (1995). Volatile fatty acids production by mesophilic fermentation of mechanically sorted urban organic wastes in a plug-flow reactor. *Bioresour. Technol.*, *51*(1), 89–96.

186. Schneider, T., Graeff-Hönninger, S., French, W. T., Hernandez, R., Claupein, W., Holmes, W. E., & Merkt, N., (2012). Screening of Industrial Wastewaters as Feedstock for the Microbial Production of Oils for Biodiesel Production and High-Quality Pigments. *J. Combust.*, doi: 10.1155/2012/153410.

187. Schneider, T., Graeff-Hönninger, S., French, W. T., Hernandez, R., Merkt, N., Claupein, W., Hetrick, M., & Pham, P., (2013). Lipid and carotenoid production by oleaginous red yeast *Rhodotorula glutinis* cultivated on brewery effluents. *Energy*, *61*, 34–43.

188. Schweizer, E., (1989). Biosynthesis of fatty acids and related compounds. in: *Microbial Lipids, Vol. 2*, (Eds.) C. Ratledge, S. G. Wilkinson, Vol. Vol. 2, Academic Press. London, pp. 3–50.

189. Shahriari, H., Warith, M., Hamoda, M., & Kennedy, K. J., (2012). Anaerobic digestion of organic fraction of municipal solid waste combining two pretreatment modalities,

high temperature microwave and hydrogen peroxide. *Waste Manage. (Oxford)*, *32*(1), 41–52.

190. Sheik, A. R., Muller, E. E. L., & Wilmes, P., (2014). A hundred years of activated sludge: time for a rethink. *Frontiers in Microbiology*, *5*, 1–7.

191. Shen, H., Gong, Z., Yang, X., Jin, G., Bai, F., & Zhao, Z. K., (2013). Kinetics of continuous cultivation of the oleaginous yeast *Rhodosporidium toruloides*. *J. Biotechnol.*, *168*(1), 85–89.

192. Shields-Menard, S. A., Amirsadeghi, M., Sukhbaatar, B., Revellame, E., Hernandez, R., Donaldson, J. R., & French, W. T., (2015). Lipid accumulation by *Rhodococcus rhodochrous* grown on glucose. *J. Ind. Microbiol. Biotechnol.*, *42*(5), 693–699.

193. Siddiquee, M. N., & Rohani, S., (2011). Experimental analysis of lipid extraction and biodiesel production from wastewater sludge. *Fuel Process. Technol.*, *92*(12), 2241–2251.

194. Sijtsma, L., Anderson, A. J., & Ratledge, C., (2010). Alternative carbon sources for heterotrophic production of docosahexaenoic acid by the marine alga *Crypthecodinium cohnii*. in: *Single Cell Oils*, (Eds.) Z. Cohen, C. Ratledge, AOCS Press. Champaign, IL, pp. 131–150.

195. Smith, A. D., & Holtzapple, M. T., (2011). Investigation of the optimal carbon–nitrogen ratio and carbohydrate–nutrient blend for mixed-acid batch fermentations. *Bioresour. Technol.*, *102*(10), 5976–5987.

196. Subramaniam, R., Dufreche, S., Zappi, M., & Bajpai, R., (2010). Microbial lipids from renewable resources: production and characterization. *J. Ind. Microbiol. Biotechnol.*, *37*(12), 1271–1287.

197. Taco Vasquez, S., Dunkleman, J., Chaudhuri, S. K., Bond, A., & Holtzapple, M. T., (2014). Biomass conversion to hydrocarbon fuels using the MixAlco™ process at a pilot-plant scale. *Biomass Bioenergy*, *62*, 138–148.

198. Taufiqurrahmi, N., & Bhatia, S., (2011). Catalytic cracking of edible and nonedible oils for the production of biofuels. *Energy & Environmental Science*, *4*(4), 1087–1112.

199. Tchobanoglous, G., Burton, F. L., & Stensel, H. D., (2003). *Wastewater Engineering: Treatment and Reuse. 3rd ed.* McGraw-Hill, New York.

200. Tchobanoglous, G., Stensel, H. D., Tsuchihashi, R., Burton, F., Abu-Orf, M., Bowden, G., Pfrang, W., Metcalf & Eddy (2014). *Wastewater Engineering: Treatment and Resource Recovery*. McGraw-Hill, New York.

201. Thanakoses, P., Black, A. S., & Holtzapple, M. T. (2003a). Fermentation of corn stover to carboxylic acids. *Biotechnol. Bioeng.*, *83*(2), 191–200.

202. Thanakoses, P., Mostafa, N. A. A., & Holtzapple, M. T. (2003b). Conversion of Sugarcane Bagasse to Carboxylic Acids Using a Mixed Culture of Mesophilic Microorganisms. in: *Biotechnology for Fuels and Chemicals: The Twenty-Fourth Symposium*, (Eds.) B. H. Davison, J. W. Lee, M. Finkelstein, J. D. McMillan, Humana Press. Totowa, NJ, pp. 523–546.

203. Tran-Nguyen, P. L., Go, A. W., Ismadji, S., & Ju, Y.-H., (2015). Transesterification of activated sludge in subcritical solvent mixture. *Bioresour. Technol.*, *197*, 30–36.

204. Tsigie, Y. A., Wang, C.-Y., Truong, C.-T., & Ju, Y.-H., (2011). Lipid production from *Yarrowia lipolytica* Po1g grown in sugarcane bagasse hydrolysate. *Bioresour. Technol.*, *102*(19), 9216–9222.

205. U.S. EPA., (1999). *Biosolids Generation, Use, and Disposal in The United States*, https://www.epa.gov/sites/production/files/2015-07/documents/biosolids_generation_ use_disposal_in_u.s_1999.pdf, (accessed: February 23, 2016).

206. U.S. EPA., (2016). *Clean Watersheds Needs Survey*, https://www.epa.gov/cwns, (accessed: February 23, 2016).

207. U.S. EPA., (2006). *Emerging Technologies for Biosolids Management*, http://nepis.epa.gov/Exe/ZyPDF.cgi/P1006DGM.PDF?Dockey=P1006DGM.PDF, (accessed:March 10, 2016).

208. Vicente, G., Bautista, L. F., Rodríguez, R., Gutiérrez, F. J., Sádaba, I., Ruiz-Vázquez, R. M., Torres-Martínez, S., & Garre, V., (2009). Biodiesel production from biomass of an oleaginous fungus. *Biochem. Eng. J.*, *48*(1), 22–27.

209. Wagner, J. L., Ting, V. P., & Chuck, C. J., (2014). Catalytic cracking of sterol-rich yeast lipid. *Fuel*, *130*, 315–323.

210. Wilkinson, S. G., (1988). Gram-negative bacteria. in: *Microbial Lipids, Vol. 1*, (Eds.) C. Ratledge, S. G. Wilkinson, Academic Press. London, pp. 299–488.

211. Wood, B. J. B., (1988). Lipids of algae and protozoa. in: *Microbial Lipids, Vol. 1*, (Eds.) C. Ratledge, S. G. Wilkinson, Vol. vol. 1, Academic Press. London, pp. 807–868.

212. Wu, H., Yang, D., Liu, W., Zhou, Q., & Gao, J. (2009a). The Production of Short-Chain Fatty Acids and Constituents with Primary Sludge as Fermentation Substrate under Different pHs. *International Conference on Energy and Environment Technology, ICEET*, 16–18 Oct., (2009). pp. 645–648.

213. Wu, H., Yang, D., Zhou, Q., & Song, Z. (2009b). The effect of pH on anaerobic fermentation of primary sludge at room temperature. *J. Hazard. Mater.*, *172*(1), 196–201.

214. Wynn, J. P., Hamid, A. A., Li, Y. H., & Ratledge, C., (2001). Biochemical events leading to the diversion of carbon into storage lipids in the oleaginous fungi *Mucor circinelloides* and *Mortierella alpina*. *Microbiology-SGM*, *147*(10), 2857–2864.

215. Xu, G., Chen, S., Shi, J., Wang, S., & Zhu, G., (2010). Combination treatment of ultrasound and ozone for improving solubilization and anaerobic biodegradability of waste activated sludge. *J. Hazard. Mater.*, *180*(1–3), 340–346.

216. Xu, H., Miao, X., & Wu, Q., (2006). High quality biodiesel production from a microalga *Chlorella protothecoides* by heterotrophic growth in fermenters. *J. Biotechnol.*, *126*(4), 499–507.

217. Xue, F., Gao, B., Zhu, Y., Zhang, X., Feng, W., & Tan, T., (2010). Pilot-scale production of microbial lipid using starch wastewater as raw material. *Bioresour. Technol.*, *101*(15), 6092–6095.

218. Xue, F., Miao, J., Zhang, X., Luo, H., & Tan, T., (2008). Studies on lipid production by *Rhodotorula glutinis* fermentation using monosodium glutamate wastewater as culture medium. *Bioresour. Technol.*, *99*(13), 5923–5927.

219. Xue, F., Zhang, X., Luo, H., & Tan, T., (2006). A new method for preparing raw material for biodiesel production. *Process Biochem.*, *41*(7), 1699–1702.

220. Yang, Q., Luo, K., Li, X.-M., Wang, D.-B., Zheng, W., Zeng, G.-M., & Liu, J.-J., (2010). Enhanced efficiency of biological excess sludge hydrolysis under anaerobic digestion by additional enzymes. *Bioresour. Technol.*, *101*(9), 2924–2930.

221. Yoda, E., Ootawa, A., (2009). Dehydration of glycerol on H-MFI zeolite investigated by FT-IR. *Appl. Catal., A*, *360*(1), 66–70.

222. Yoon, J. J., (2011). *What's the Difference Between Biodiesel and Renewable (Green) Diesel*, http://advancedbiofuelsusa.info/wp-content/uploads/2011/03/11–0307-Biodiesel-vs-Renewable_Final-_3_-JJY-formatting-FINAL.pdf, (accessed: March 9, 2016).

223. You, Y.-D., Shie, J.-L., Chang, C.-Y., Huang, S.-H., Pai, C.-Y., Yu, Y.-H., & Chang, C. H., (2008). Economic cost analysis of biodiesel production: Case in soybean oil. *Energy Fuels*, *22*(1), 182–189.

224. Yousuf, A., Sannino, F., Addorisio, V., & Pirozzi, D., (2010). Microbial Conversion of Olive Oil Mill Wastewaters into Lipids Suitable for Biodiesel Production. *J. Agric. Food Chem.*, *58*(15), 8630–8635.

225. Yu, H. Q., & Fang, H. H. P., (2003). Acidogenesis of gelatin-rich wastewater in an upflow anaerobic reactor: influence of pH and temperature. *Water Res.*, *37*(1), 55–66.

226. Zhang, B., Zhang, L. L., Zhang, S. C., Shi, H. Z., & Cai, W. M., (2005). The Influence of pH on Hydrolysis and Acidogenesis of Kitchen Wastes in Two-phase Anaerobic Digestion. *Environ. Technol.*, *26*(3), 329–340.

227. Zhang, G., French, W. T., Hernandez, R., Hall, J., Sparks, D., & Holmes, W. E., (2011). Microbial lipid production as biodiesel feedstock from N-acetylglucosamine by oleaginous microorganisms. *J. Chem. Technol. Biotechnol.*, *86*(5), 642–650.

228. Zhang, P., Chen, Y., & Zhou, Q., (2009). Waste activated sludge hydrolysis and short-chain fatty acids accumulation under mesophilic and thermophilic conditions: effect of pH. *Water Res.*, *43*(15), 3735–3742.

229. Zhao, X., Kong, X., Hua, Y., Feng, B., & Zhao, Z., (2008). Medium optimization for lipid production through cofermentation of glucose and xylose by the oleaginous yeast *Lipomyces starkeyi*. *Eur. J. Lipid Sci. Technol.*, *110*(5), 405–412.

230. Zhila, N. O., Kalacheva, G. S., & Volova, T. G., (2005). Effect of Nitrogen Limitation on the Growth and Lipid Composition of the Green Alga *Botryococcus braunii* Kutz IPPAS H-252. *Russian Journal of Plant Physiology*, *52*(3), 311–319.

231. Zhou, W., Wang, W., Li, Y., & Zhang, Y., (2013). Lipid production by *Rhodosporidium toruloides* Y2 in bioethanol wastewater and evaluation of biomass energetic yield. *Bioresour. Technol.*, *127*, 435–440.

232. Zhu, F., Zhao, L., Jiang, H., Zhang, Z., Xiong, Y., Qi, J., & Wang, J., (2014). Comparison of the Lipid Content and Biodiesel Production from Municipal Sludge Using Three Extraction Methods. *Energy Fuels*, *28*(8), 5277–5283.

233. Zhu, L. Y., Zong, M. H., & Wu, H., (2008). Efficient lipid production with *Trichosporon fermentans* and its use for biodiesel preparation. *Bioresour. Technol.*, *99*(16), 7881–7885.

CHAPTER 11

BIOELECTROCHEMICAL SYSTEMS FOR BIOFUEL (ELECTRICITY, HYDROGEN, AND METHANE) AND VALUABLE CHEMICAL PRODUCTION

MOBOLAJI SHEMFE, KOK SIEW NG, and JHUMA SADHUKHAN

Centre for Environmental Strategy, University of Surrey, Guildford, UK

CONTENTS

ABSTRACT

The production of electricity from microbes was first demonstrated in the early 1900s when scientific enquiries were made about the nature of the electrical effects associated with the decomposition of organic compounds due to the influence of microorganisms. This discovery inspired further investigations into the use of electrochemical devices to harvest electrical energy from the microbial decomposition of organic substrates, thus leading to the concept of a bioelectrochemical system. As the search for sustainable alternatives to fossil fuels has intensified, this area of research has been generating significant interest in the scientific community. The renewed interest in this research domain is mainly driven by its prospective application for the production of sustainable energy, along with other synergetic benefits, including wastewater treatment and resource recovery. This chapter offers perspective on the production of fuels, electricity, and chemicals using bioelectrochemical systems. As the production of biofuels and valuable chemicals is the main emphasis of this chapter, the following subheadings shed light on the working principles of bioelectrochemical systems, the integration of biorefineries with bioelectrochemical systems for the enhanced production of biofuels and valuable chemicals, state-of-the-art thermodynamic feasibility models and methods for evaluating the economic viability of the integrated systems. The major challenges be setting the commercialization of bioelectrochemical systems and the future direction of the technology are also covered in this chapter.

11.1   INTRODUCTION

Mounting scientific evidence indicates that the rise in global mean temperatures is due to the increase in anthropogenic greenhouse gas emissions, as a consequence of cumulative fossil fuel combustion since the start of the industrial revolution [11]. Fossil fuels remain the primary source of energy globally, accounting for about 80% of total energy supply. In 2015, global efforts to mitigate the effects of possible run-off climate change led to the Paris agreement, bringing together nations, corporations, and various stakeholders to make a commitment towards limiting the increase in global mean temperatures to 1.5°C above preindustrial levels [36]. This commitment has given more momentum to research, development, and deployment of sustainable renewable energy sources. While the roadmap to the implementation of sustainable energy sources has gradually begun to shape up, the transition to a low-carbon global economy will take considerable effort before fossil fuels can be displaced as the primary source of energy (fuels, chemicals, heat, and power). Several attractive renewable alternatives to fossil fuels, such as biomass, solar, wind, geothermal, and tidal are currently being deployed globally, to reduce the carbon footprint of global energy use. Nevertheless, reconciling energy supply from these alternative renewable sources with the present global energy demand, along with projected growth in the world's population, remains a challenge due to various factors. These include variability in energy efficiencies of renewable energy platforms due to external factors, such as solar irradiance and wind speed, and their limited energy efficiencies and polygeneration potentials in comparison with fossil fuels. At present, biomass is the only source of renewables available in sufficient quantities with a polygeneration upside. As the fourth largest source of energy on the planet, after coal, oil and gas, biomass has the potential to complement or even replace the supply of different forms of energy presently sourced from fossil fuels. Biomass feedstocks can be converted into various forms of energy through a combination of physical, chemical, biochemical and thermochemical processes in biorefineries [28]. Biorefineries comprise various processing stages, including feed preprocessing, biofuel conversion platforms, product conditioning, and waste management, which result in a plethora of waste that impairs their energy and conversion efficiencies. Nevertheless, the energy and conversion efficiencies of biorefineries can be enhanced by their integration with a resource recovery system. One of such technologies that is generating significant interest in research is bioelectrochemical systems (BESs). BESs can enhance the polygeneration potential of biorefineries by converting low-value waste streams and pollutants into high-value products. Moreover, the recovery of valuable products from biorefineries wastes using BESs offers significant environmental benefits by synergetic waste reduction and reuse.

11.2 BIOELECTROCHEMICAL SYSTEMS

Electrochemistry is the mechanism for cellular energy storage, transfer and release in all living things and the basis for photosynthesis and cellular respiration. All living organisms gain or release energy *via* biochemical redox reactions (electron transfer through cellular protein complexes) and proton transfer across the mitochondrial membranes of cells to generate an electrochemical gradient (difference in charge). This difference in charge along with several cellular redox reactions is used by mitochondrial enzymes to synthesize ATP and NADPH, which are essential bioorganic molecules for the release and storage of cellular energy and the sustenance of life [35]. Pioneering scientific probes into the nature of electron transfer within living cells in the early 20th century revealed that all microorganisms are indeed capable of generating electrons through their metabolism [20]. More interestingly, it was discovered that certain groups of microbes can achieve extracellular electron transfer (electron transfer in and out of the cell) to electron acceptors, such as metals in their environment [20]. This discovery prompted further investigations into the interactions between certain microorganisms and electrodes of electrochemical cells, leading to the concept of a BES, where whole microbes or their isolated enzymes are used as biocatalysts to drive redox reactions in fuel cells [5, 13]. At the most fundamental level, a BES is an electrochemical system, aided by pure cultures or bacteria communities, or isolated enzymes to catalyze redox reactions of biodegradable organic compounds (substrates) to generate electricity, fuels, and chemicals. Thus, the electrodes in BESs are called bioelectrodes, comprising a bioanode, where microorganisms or their enzymes catalyze the oxidation of substrates and a cathode/biocathode, where reduction occurs electrochemically/bioelectrochemically. The biocatalysts in BESs can either synthesize organic substrates through cellular metabolism or enhance electron transfer from substrate to the electrode. Similar to their conventional counterparts, a BES consists of bioanode and biocathode compartments, connected through their bioelectrodes by an external electric circuit to allow the flow of electrons and separated by a membrane to allow proton/cation exchange. Table 11.1 shows a comparison between conventional electrochemical systems and BESs.

BESs can be broadly classified based on four main criteria: (i) the type of biocatalysts employed in the system, (ii) use of mediators to enhance electron transfer from the biocatalysts to the electrodes, (iii) mode of operation in terms of the application of a load or external voltage, and (iv) type of physical configuration. The classifications mentioned above are not mutually

TABLE 11.1 Comparison Between Conventional Electrochemical Fuel Cells and BESs

Electrochemical systems	Bioelectrochemical systems
Electrodes	Bioelectrodes
Metal Catalyst: Pt, Pt-Ru alloy, Pd, metal porphyrins	Biocatalysts: microbes, enzymes
Electrodes separated by electrolyte layer	Bioelectrodes separated by membrane or liquid electrolyte
Operating temperatures: 30–1000°C	Ambient temperature: 25°C

exclusive, as there are overlaps between particular groups of BESs. Figure 11.1 depicts the various classification of BESs based on the criteria mentioned above.

The first grouping is based on the type of biocatalyst employed to catalyze the redox reactions occurring in the system, namely microbial BESs and enzymatic BESs. As the name implies, microbial BESs use microbial biocatalysts, specifically metal reducing/oxidizing bacteria to catalyze redox reactions of biodegradable substrates. In contrast to microbial BESs, enzymatic BESs uses isolated enzymes rather than whole organisms to catalyze the redox reactions of organic substrates. While all BESs use microbes or enzymes that can oxidize or reduce organic substrates, only a few microbes/enzymes can efficiently transfer electrons to an anode or receive electrons from a cathode. Many microbes/enzymes require the addition of a mediator to aid the transfer of electrons to and fro electrodes. The difference between biocatalysts that are capable and incapable of exoelectron transfer suggests another classification of BESs: mediated BESs and mediator-free BESs. Mediated BESs uses mediators to aid the transfer of electrons. The main mediators used for mediated BESs include thionine, methyl viologen, methyl blue, humic acid, and neutral red [21]. On the other hand, mediator-free BESs

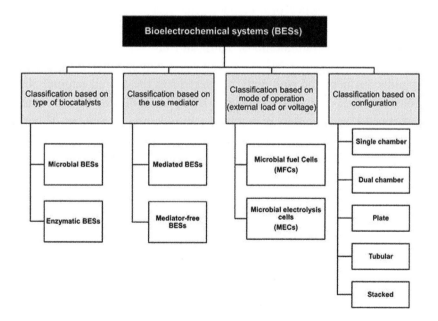

FIGURE 11.1 Classification of Bioelectrochemical systems.

uses electrochemically active bacteria that are capable of extracellular electron transfer to and fro electrodes. The mediators used in mediated BESs are expensive to manufacture, making them economically unattractive in comparison with mediator-free types. Depending on the mode of operation of microbial BESs, in terms of the application of a load or an external voltage, they can be grouped into two major types, namely microbial fuel cells (MFCs) and microbial electrolysis cells (MECs). MFCs are configured to generate electricity through the direct/indirect electron transfer of electrons from organic substrates, metabolically oxidized by bacteria, to the anode. The electrons released from the substrate then go through an electric circuit to do work and recombines at the cathode to reduce oxygen into water in an open-air system. MECs also employ electrons transferred from the anodic oxidation of substrates but differ from MFCs regarding the application of an external voltage to the circuit, which in combination with the electrons generated at the anode produces hydrogen at the cathode under anaerobic conditions. Lastly, BESs can be classified based on the physical configuration of the system. The configurations of BESs currently available are single chamber BESs, dual chamber BESs, tubular BESs, plate BESs and stacked BESs [14]. As the name suggests, a single chamber BES, has a single chamber, usually an anodic chamber, coupled with a cation exchange membrane, conjoined with the cathode. The absence of a cathodic chamber makes this configuration very simple to design and operate. Moreover, they are cost effective and more efficient than other configurations. Thus, they are very attractive for power generation applications in MFCs, as they can function without the need for a cathodic chamber and catholyte, which reduces the overall internal ohmic resistance of the system. Dual chambers BESs have both anodic and cathodic compartments, separated by a cation/proton exchange membrane. This configuration of BESs is more prevalent than single chamber BESs, as they can be used for applications that require the operational modes in MFCs and MECs. Tubular BESs have a cylindrical profile, where the anodic chamber is located at the center of the cylinder, encircled by a proton/cation exchange membrane to separate the cathodic chamber. Plate BESs have a flat profile, with two rectangular plates, separated by a membrane and engraved with flow channels to allow the movement of substrates at the anode or cathode or air at the cathode. The different configurations of BESs can be cascaded or stacked up in parallels like conventional electrochemical fuel cells, in order to maximize their productivity. The next subheadings will focus on the working principles of MFCs and MECs.

11.2.1 MICROBIAL FUEL CELLS

MFCs converts chemical energy, locked within the bonds of organic substrates, into electrical energy using electrochemically active microbes. The working principle involves the oxidation of organic substrates by the metabolism of bacteria in the anodic compartment of the MFC, which results in the release of electrons and protons/cations. The electrons can be transferred to the anode either by direct electron transfer by the bacteria or by the aid of an electron transfer enhancer (a mediator). The electrons generated at the anode generates electric power, when passed through an external electric circuit (wire), before they subsequently go into the cathodic chamber to reduce an oxidant, such as oxygen in open-air MFCs. The reduction at the cathode can be catalyzed by either a chemical catalyst or by microbes. The protons/cations generated in the anodic chamber migrate towards the cathodic chamber via a membrane, which separates the two compartments. Figure 11.2 illustrates the schematic of a typical MFC.

Since the inception of MFCs in the 1910s, significant advancements have been made in research of the technology towards its commercialization. MFCs can be used for various applications, including the generation of alternative energy in remote locations, resource recovery from industrial effluents, wastewater treatment and desalination [9, 18]. Due to the limited electrical power and thus the economic value that can be produced from MFCs, recent research efforts are focused on the recovery of products of higher value from organic substrates [21].

11.2.2 MICROBIAL ELECTROLYSIS CELLS

MECs are a relatively new concept compared with MFCs. A MEC works using the same principle as an MFC, except an external voltage is applied to the electric circuit, and the cathodic compartment operates under anaerobic conditions. The introduction of an external voltage to the circuit propagates the production of hydrogen at the cathode through the reduction of protons. This approach was first illustrated in the early 2000s, when an electrical voltage was applied to an MFC, thereby reducing the cathode potential sufficiently to allow the electrolysis of water to produce hydrogen gas. This approach has two major advantages in terms of lower energy requirements for hydrogen production than conventional electrolysis and the generation of

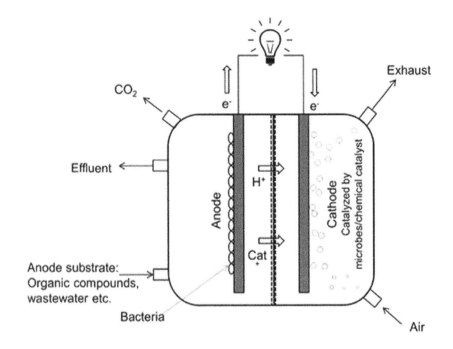

FIGURE 11.2   Schematic of a dual chamber microbial fuel cell.

high-value hydrogen gas from any low-value organic substrates. Figure 11.3 shows the schematic of an MEC.

Subsequently, in 2010, the reduction of CO_2 in the cathode chamber to produce methane was demonstrated via microbial electrosynthesis. Since 2010, research efforts in microbial electrosynthesis systems (MESs) have rapidly gathered momentum to demonstrate the generation of medium aliphatic and aromatic compounds from organic wastes.

11.3   BES BIOCATALYSTS

As shown in Figure 11.1, the redox reactions that occur in the anodic chambers and, or the cathodic chambers of BESs can be either catalyzed by electrogenic bacteria or isolated enzymes. Despite the fact that several species of electrogenic bacteria have been discovered that can catalyze the oxidation or reduction of organic substrates, only a few groups of bacteria are capable of extracellular transfer. These exoelectrogenic bacteria can transfer electrons via three main mechanisms: (i) direct electron transfer

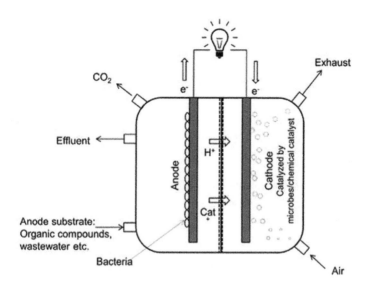

FIGURE 11.3 Schematic of a dual chamber microbial electrolysis cell.

via the outer membrane cytochromes; (ii) conductive pili/nanowires; and (iii) indirect electron transfer via electron shuttle secreted by the bacteria. Some bacteria are capable of using all three methods of electron transfer, such as *Shewanella oneidensis*, while others only have the ability to transfer electrons via one or two mechanisms. The operational mode of a BES in terms of harvesting electricity as in the case of MFCs or generating hydrogen gas as in the case of MECs places limits on the type of microbial communities that can be used for each mode of operation. This limitation is due to the variations in the growth of various microbes under aerobic conditions. There are fewer microbes that can operate exclusively under anaerobic conditions as required in MECs. Thus, the bacteria species used in MECs are less diverse than those employed in MFCs.

The second category of BES biocatalysts is enzymatic biocatalysts. In comparison to microbial catalyzed BESs, enzyme catalyzed BESs are less stable, have a limited lifetime and electron transfer rates, and results in partial oxidation of organic substrates [17]. Furthermore, they are not self-generating like microbes and have limited adaptation to various types of substrates. Recent efforts have been made to improve the stability and extend their lifetime using some novel polymers. Nevertheless, enzymes offer some benefits over using whole microbes, as they can target specific organic compounds, through their selectivity towards particular products by using relatively defined reaction pathways. Moreover, the requirement for a membrane for separating the two compartments of the BES can be eliminated in enzymatic BESs.

11.4   INTEGRATED BIOREFINERY BIOELECTROCHEMICAL SYSTEMS

Wastes streams from biorefineries can be used as substrates for BESs to produce products of higher economic value. Biorefineries wastes streams contain considerable concentrations of biodegradable organic compounds, which can be readily oxidized by microbes, or enzymes in the anode of MFCs to generate electric power, or reduced at the cathode with the addition of external voltage to obtain chemicals and fuels of higher economic and energetic values as in MECs and MESs. Biorefinery waste streams that can be integrated with BESs are summarized in Table 11.2.

In order to appreciate the range of plausible products from biorefineries integrated with BESs, it is important to understand the chemical composition of typical biomass feedstocks. Figure 11.4 shows the composition of biomass feedstocks, biorefinery preprocessing and conversion technologies, conversion mechanisms and products.

The symbiotic integration of biorefineries with BESs have the potential to enhance the overall sustainability of biorefineries, regarding economic, environmental and societal benefits [28]. In terms of economic and environmental benefits, an integrated biorefinery bioelectrochemical system offers the advantage of producing clean energy, while also contributing to waste and pollution reduction. Furthermore, the flexibility of BESs highlights the potential of this integration to enable the recovery of products including electricity, biofuels, and biochemicals, and thus can increase the overall energy efficiency of the system significantly. As the production of fuels and chemicals using bioelectrochemistry is a thriving new field, it will create more collaboration between scientist, engineers, microbiologists and electrochemists, and hence create a new discipline with prospective benefits to the society regarding generation of new knowledge, skills, and jobs, as well as improvement of health and safety in local communities.

TABLE 11.2   Feeds and Potential Products of Various Biorefineries Integrated with BES

Biorefinery type	Biorefinery feed	Biorefinery product	Biorefinery byproducts (Feed to BES)	Potential products from BESs
1G and 2G bioethanol plants	Lignocellulosic biomass, corn, sugarcane, energy crops	Bioethanol		
Ethanol 2G	CO_2, acetate, C_6 and C_5 sugars.	MFC: Electricity; MEC/MES: H_2, CH_4, glutamate, propionate, butanol		
1G biodiesel plants	Oils, oily seeds, wastes oils, oily residues	Biodiesel vegetable oils	Glycerol, waste oils	MFC: electricity; MEC/MES: H_2, ethanol
Anaerobic digestion	Organic wastes	Biomethane	Digestate	MFC: electricity; MEC/MES: H_2, ammonia, potassium, water
Fast pyrolysis and bio-oil hydroprocessing	Lignocellulosic biomass (wood, grasses, shrubs)	Biohydrocarbons: gasoline and diesel range products	Aqueous wastes containing carbohydrates, organic acids, alcohols, and aldehydes	MFC: electricity; MEC: H_2
Gasification	Lignocellulosic biomass, waste wood, MSW, dried sewage sludge	Synfuels (F-T) heat, electricity (CHP), methane (Sabatier), producer gas, methanol, hydrogen	CO_2	MFC: electricity; MES methane (CO_2 reduction at cathode)

11.4.1   INTEGRATED BIOETHANOL AND BIOELECTROCHEMICAL SYSTEMS

Bioethanol presently accounts for 80% of liquid biofuel supply globally. In 2011, The United States, Brazil and China were the main producers of bioethanol, and produced 63%, 24% and 2.5% of the total production,

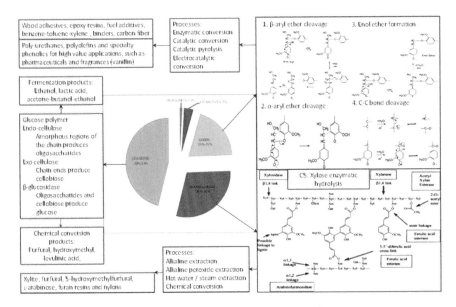

FIGURE 11.4 Biorefinery preprocessing and processing technologies, mechanisms, and products [27]. (Reprinted with permission from Sadhukhan, J., Ng, K. S., & Hernandez, E. M. (2014). *Biorefineries and Chemical Processes: Design, Integration and Sustainability Analysis,* © 2014 John Wiley.)

respectively. These include first generation bioethanol produced from corn mainly in the US and sugarcane in Brazil. The integration of BESs with waste streams generated in bioethanol plants offers significant advantages for the recovery of valuable products, as biomass to fuel conversion of most operational bioethanol plants are very low. For example, in Brazil, only 38% of the sugarcane feedstock is converted into fuel, while the remainder is disposed of as liquid effluent and solid wastes in the form of vinasse and bagasse, respectively. Vinasse is a potential feedstock for BESs, as it contains organic substrates, including waste ethanol and glycerol, which can be oxidized by microorganisms at the anode of BESs. Also, in the United States, where corn is being used as a feedstock for the extraction of sugars for subsequent conversion into bioethanol, some wastes and by-products are also generated that can be converted into higher value products. These include residues generated from dry and wet mills, containing a high concentration of carbohydrates, glycerol, and ethanol. There are two plausible routes for the recovery of higher value compounds from the integration of wastes products in bioethanol plants with BESs as shown in Figure 11.5 [28].

In the first route, a fraction of pretreated lignocellulosic feedstock (pretreatment involves size reduction and steam pretreatment) is used for *in-situ* production of enzyme and yeast, which is subsequently used for solid-state fermentation of the remaining fraction of the pretreated feed-stock to produce bioethanol. This approach has been proven to reduce the operating cost of bioethanol plants, thereby offering significant improvements to their economic viability. A near purity ethanol product is obtained downstream of the solid-state fermentation process in the bioethanol purification section, consisting of distillation, molecular sieve adsorption, and dehydration operations. The liquid by-products from the purification stage, comprising residual C6 and C5 sugars can be used as substrate in the anode compartment of a BES, while the solid by-products, mainly consisting of

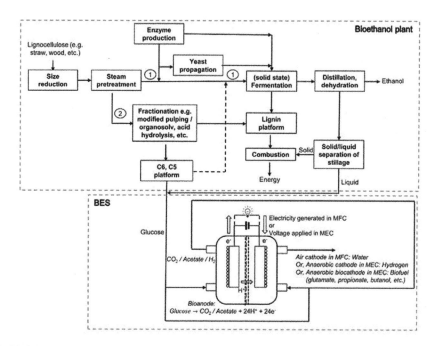

FIGURE 11.5 Integrated bioethanol and BES process flow diagram [28]. (Reprinted with permission from Sadhukhan, J., Lloyd, J. R., Scott, K., Premier, G. C., Yu, E. H., Curtis, T., & Head, I. M. (2016). A Critical Review of Integration Analysis of Microbial Electrosynthesis (MES) Systems with Waste Biorefineries for the Production of Biofuel and Chemical from Reuse of CO₂. *Renew. Sustain. Energy Rev.*, *56*, 116–132. © 2016 Elsevier.)

lignin can be either be combusted for combined heat and power generation (CHP), or upgraded into high-value chemicals via catalytic hydroprocessing. In the scenario, where lignin is upgraded into high-value chemicals, part of the hydrogen required for the hydroprocessing operation can be sourced from an MEC, which uses liquid by-products as a substrate to generate hydrogen with the addition of an external voltage to the system. Thus, this scenario reduces the additional operating cost, regarding purchasing hydrogen off-site. The alternative scenario for lignin postprocessing via combustion for CHP generation also offers significant benefits, as no external electricity is needed onsite and any excess electricity generated can be exported to the grid. The second route entails the processing of pretreated lignocellulosic feeds via organosolv, hydrolysis, and fractionation to obtain C6 and C5 sugars and lignin. The C6 and C5 sugars are fermented into bioethanol, while lignin can be converted into high-value chemicals or electricity using the postprocessing methods in route 1. Alternatively, C6 sugars can be separated before the fermentation process and metabolized in the anode compartment of a BES into CO_2, protons, and electrons. The cathode, either chemically or microbially catalyzed, can generate electricity and water under aerobic conditions as in the case of MFCs, or generate hydrogen under anaerobic condition in MECs. Equations 1 and 2 illustrate the oxidation of glucose in the anode and reduction of oxygen at the cathode of an MFC, respectively, with their corresponding cell potentials.

$$\text{Anode:} \qquad C_6H_{12}O_6 + 6H_2O \rightarrow 6CO_2 + 24H^+ + 24e^- E^0 = 0.014V \qquad (1)$$

$$\text{Cathode:} \qquad 24H^+ + 24e^- + 6O_2 \rightarrow 12H_2O E^0 = 1.2V \qquad (2)$$

11.4.2 INTEGRATED BIODIESEL AND BIOELECTROCHEMICAL SYSTEMS

Biodiesel accounts for 20% of the global supply of liquid biofuels. The largest producers of biodiesel in the order of market dominance include the EU (43%), South America (26%) and the United States (15%), comprising oils derived from plant seeds and animal fats. Biodiesel is produced by the catalytic reaction of triglycerides, found in vegetable oils or animal fats with alcohol, typically methanol or ethanol to produce fatty acids and methyl esters and glycerol. Several research studies have shown that the conversion processes of oils and fats into biodiesel are energy intensive. For example, 5.3 kg of oily waste and 10.7 kg of glycerol are produced, and 466 MJ of energy is consumed for every 100 kg of biodiesel produced. This apparent loss of energy in the conventional biodiesel process indicates opportunities for waste recovery using BESs. Experimental trials have shown that glycerol, which forms a large proportion of organic waste from diesel plants can be employed as a substrate in an MEC [12, 30]. Figure 11.6 shows the plausible integration of biodiesel plants with BESs [28].

Glycerol can be oxidized in the anode compartment of BESs by *Enterobacteriaceae species* to generate ethanol, along with the release of electrons and protons. The cathode, either chemically or microbially catalyzed, can produce electricity and water in open-air configurations of MFCs or generate hydrogen by application of additional voltage to the circuit under anaerobic conditions in an MEC. Alternatively, carbon dioxide and hydrogen ions generated

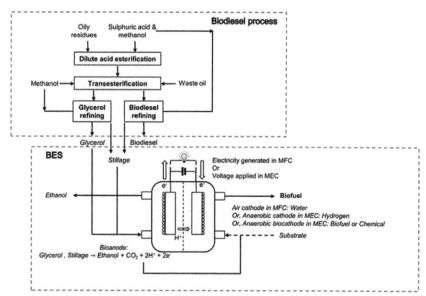

FIGURE 11.6 Integrated biodiesel and BES process flow diagram [28]. (Reprinted with permission from Sadhukhan, J., Lloyd, J. R., Scott, K., Premier, G. C., Yu, E. H., Curtis, T., & Head, I. M. (2016). A Critical Review of Integration Analysis of Microbial Electrosynthesis (MES) Systems with Waste Biorefineries for the Production of Biofuel and Chemical from Reuse of CO_2. *Renew. Sustain. Energy Rev., 56,* 116–132. © 2016 Elsevier.)

at the anode can be used, with or without additional waste streams sourced from other industrial effluents, to generate biofuels or chemicals in MECs.

11.4.3 INTEGRATED ANAEROBIC DIGESTION AND BIOELECTROCHEMICAL SYSTEMS

Anaerobic digestion (AD) is a matured technology used for waste management and biogas production from organic wastes. AD involves the anaerobic fermentation of organic wastes, including sewage effluent, animal wastes, and food processing wastes to produce biogas, mainly consisting of methane and carbon dioxide, and trace quantities of ammonia and hydrogen sulfide. The biogas produced from AD, after undergoing acid scrubbing to remove pollutants, is primarily used for the production of electricity and heat *via* CHP. The by-products from AD include a solid digestate residue and a nutrient-rich liquid with low chemical oxygen demands. BESs can offer complementary benefits to the AD process by broadening the spectrum of products that can be produced from the process. Various products can be generated from an AD integrated BES, depending on the mode of operation of the BES. For an AD integrated with an MFC, electricity can be generated, while ammonia is simultaneously recovered from the AD effluent (substrate), which can then be recycled back to the AD reactor, or discharged, or applied for secondary applications, including the production of fertilizer and clean water [19]. Otherwise, products, including hydrogen, amines, carboxylates and alcohols can be produced from an AD integrated with an MEC/MES either by using ammonia, or CO_2 recovered from acid gas scrubbing of biogas. The conceptual model for the integration of AD with BESs is depicted in Figure 11.7.

11.4.4 INTEGRATED FAST PYROLYSIS AND BIOELECTROCHEMICAL SYSTEMS

Fast pyrolysis is one of the thermochemical conversion technologies earmarked for the production of second-generation biofuels. It involves the anaerobic and thermal degradation of biomass at temperatures between 450 and 600°C to produce bio-oil, noncondensable gasses and char [2, 3]. The bio-oil product is a viscous liquid and an energy carrier that can be upgraded into gasoline and diesel range products either by hydroprocessing or fluid

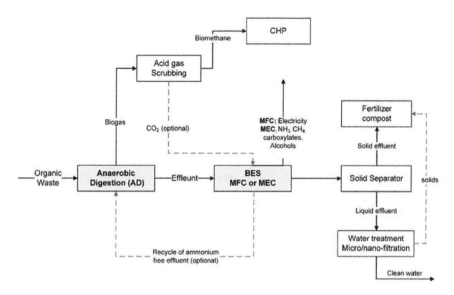

FIGURE 11.7 Integrated AD and BES process flow diagram.

catalytic cracking over zeolites (analogous to conventional petroleum refining operations) [4]. Of the two upgrading methods, hydroprocessing has been the most employed bio-oil upgrading technique and have shown acceptable results in terms of techno-economic viability [31, 32, 37] and environmental performance [33]. Bio-oil hydroprocessing involves two hydrogen intensive operations, namely hydrodeoxygenation and hydrocracking. Hydrodeoxygenation involves the stabilization and rejection of oxygen from bio-oil through its catalytic reaction with hydrogen over alumina-supported, sulfided CoMo or NiMo catalysts or noble metal catalysts, while hydrocracking involves the simultaneous scission and hydrogenation of heavy aromatic and naphthenic molecules in the organic phase of bio-oil into lighter aliphatic and aromatic molecules [6, 8]. Hydrodeoxygenated bio-oil readily separates into an aqueous phase and an organic phase under gravity [7]. The aqueous phase of bio-oil composes of carbohydrates, furans, aldehydes, phenols and carboxylic acids that can be used as a substrate for BESs. Particularly, the aqueous phase can be fed to an MEC to generate hydrogen required for hydroprocessing. Generating hydrogen from an MEC offers advantages over alternative hydrogen generation routes, such as steam reforming and gasification, in terms of replacing expensive catalysts with nonexpensive biocatalysts, lower energy consumption, and high conversion efficiency. Figure 11.8 shows the schematic of fast pyrolysis and bio-oil hydroprocessing integrated with an MEC. The compounds of interest in the aqueous phase of fast pyrolysis derived bio-oil that are plausible MEC substrates include levoglucosan, furfurals, and organic acids.

11.4.5 INTEGRATED GASIFICATION AND BIOELECTROCHEMICAL SYSTEMS

Gasification is a well-established thermochemical conversion technology for volatilizing biomass into producer gas or syngas under temperatures of about 700°C in oxygen and/or steam controlled operating environments. The resultant producer gas or syngas from the gasification process can be used to power gas turbines in biomass-integrated gasification combined cycles (BIGCC) for CHP generation. Alternatively, the producer gas or syngas can be used for the production of renewable fuels and chemicals via methanol hydration into dimethyl ether, Sabatier reaction into methane and the Fischer-Tropsch process to produce synfuels. Recent advancements in electrochemistry and fuel cells have impelled the integration of solid oxide fuel cells (SOFC) with the gasification process to enhance the relative CHP generation efficiency of the gasification process in comparison with BIGCC. SOFC operates effectively at elevated temperatures, up to 1,000°C, making them suitable candidates

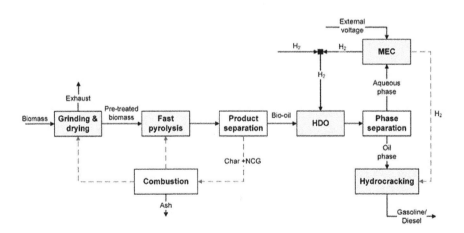

FIGURE 11.8 Integrated fast pyrolysis, bio-oil hydroprocessing, and MES process flow diagram.

for integration with the gasification process. A hot-gas cleanup process is integrated into the gasification process to remove pollutants and particulates that can contaminate the SOFC, or reduce its efficiency. Figure 11.9 shows the block flow diagram of an integrated biomass gasification fuel cell (BGFC) system.

The electrochemical reactions of H_2 and CO gas in the cleaned gasification syngas are illustrated in Eqs. (3)–(7).

Anode:
$$H_2 + O^{2-} \rightarrow H_2O + 2e^- \tag{3}$$

$$CO + O^{2-} \rightarrow CO_2 + 2e^- \tag{4}$$

Cathode:
$$O_2 + 2e^- \rightarrow O^{2-} \tag{5}$$

Net reaction:
$$2H_2 + O_2 \leftrightarrow 2H_2O \tag{6}$$

$$2CO + O_2 \leftrightarrow 2CO_2 \tag{7}$$

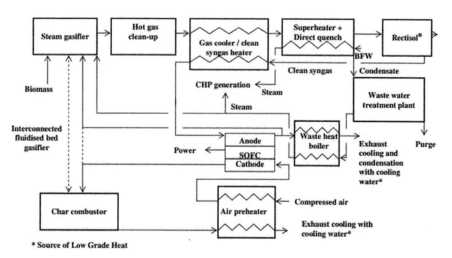

FIGURE 11.9 Block diagram of an integrated BGFC system [27]. (Reprinted with permission from Sadhukhan, J., Ng, K. S., & Hernandez, E. M. (2014). *Biorefineries and Chemical Processes: Design, Integration and Sustainability Analysis*, © 2014 John Wiley.)

The need for CO_2 capture from the exhaust gasses of the BGFC process presents an interesting proposition for the plausible integration of BESs. Cooled and particulate free CO_2 generated from SOFC can be fixated in the cathode of an MES through the cathode reduction of CO_2 to generate high-value chemicals, such as methane or other mid-ranged organic compounds. The techno-economic and sustainability appraisal of this symbiotic integration is subject to further research.

11.5 THERMODYNAMIC FEASIBILITY MODEL FOR MFCS AND MECS

Several attempts have been made to develop mathematical models for BESs towards predicting the performance and behavior of the system [15]. The two common approaches available in the open literature for modeling BESs are mechanistic and empirical modeling methods. These modeling methods have specific advantages and disadvantages. Mechanistic models include the underpinning phenomena, conservation laws, and mathematical relations occurring in the system, which require information about the system from the perspective of allied disciplines, including microbiology, biochemistry, chemical engineering, and electrochemistry. Typically, a mechanistic model will entail mathematical relationships about cell thermodynamics, bioelectrochemical reaction kinetics, mass, energy, momentum, and charge transport of species and growth rate of microbes/ stability of enzymes. Mechanistic models differ in complexity depending on the number of dimensions considered. Given the nonideal nature of BESs, it is challenging to implement multidimensional mechanistic models. Empirical models, on the other hand, uses measurements and statistical methods to model the complexity of the system, thus are relatively easy to implement. There is on-going research effort to develop standardized models for BESs. Nevertheless, a nondimensional model based on reaction stoichiometry [10, 23, 25, 26, 29, 34, 35, 38] that can determine the thermodynamic feasibility of BES reactions has been established [28]. The generalized model for the anodic oxidation of substrates of an MFC is described in Eq. (8).

$$C_xH_yO_z + (3x - z)H_2O \rightarrow xHCO_3^- + wH^+ + we^- + \frac{y + 5x - w - 2z}{2}H_2$$

$$\forall(3x - z) > 0, (y + 5x - w - 2z) \geq 0 \text{ and } w, x, y, x > 0$$

$$(8)$$

The Gibbs free energy of the generic anodic reaction given in Eq. (9) can be derived from Eq. (10) using the values of the Gibbs free energy of formation of the reacting species (see Table 11.3) under standard temperature and pressure (25°C and 1 atm), and neutral pH (pH [7]).

$$\Delta G^o_{r,anode} = x\Delta G^o_{f,HCO_3^-} + w\Delta G^o_{f,H^+} - (3x - z)\Delta G^o_{f,H_2O} - \Delta G^o_{f,C_xH_yO_z}$$

$$(9)$$

Equation (10) can be derived by substituting the values given in Table 14.3 into Eq. (9).

$$\Delta G^o_{r,anode} = 124.684x - 39.9w - 273.178z - \Delta G^o_{f,C_xH_yO_z}$$

$$(10)$$

The generic equation for the cathodic reduction of oxygen into water in an MFC is illustrated in Eq. (11).

$$\frac{w}{4}O_2 + wH^+ + we^- = \frac{w}{2}H_2O$$

$$(11)$$

Equation 12 shows the standard Gibbs free energy of the cathodic reaction in Eq. (11), by substituting values from Table 11.3.

$$\Delta G^o_{r,cathode} = 78.69w$$

$$(12)$$

TABLE 11.3 Gibbs Free Energy of Formation of Reacting Species

Species	ΔG^o_f(kJ/mol.substrate)
HCV_3^-	-586.85
H^+	-39.9
H_2O	-37.178

For an MEC, under anaerobic conditions, the generic model for the cathodic reduction of H⁺ and the Gibbs free energy of the cathode are given in Eqs. (13) and (14).

$$wH^+ + we^- = \frac{w}{2}H_2 \tag{13}$$

$$\Delta G^o_{r,cathode} = 39.9w \tag{14}$$

The net energy generated from an MFC and the net energy consumed in an MEC can be determined from Eq. (15) through the summation of Gibbs free energies of the anode and cathode reactions as shown in Eqs. (16) and (17).

$$\Delta G^o_{r,cell} = \Delta G^o_{r,anode} + \Delta G^o_{r,cathode} \tag{15}$$

$$\Delta G^o_{r,MFC} = 124.69x - 118.59w - 237.18z - \Delta G^o_{f,C_xH_yO_z} \tag{16}$$

$$\Delta G^o_{r,MEC} = 124.69x - 237.18z - \Delta G^o_{f,C_xH_yO_z} \tag{17}$$

Equations (16) and (17) can be expressed in terms of 1 eV of potential generation from an MFC and 1eV consumed by an MEC, respectively, as shown in Eqs. (18) and (19).

$$\Delta G^o_{r,MFC} = \frac{124.69x - 118.59w - 237.18z - \Delta G^o_{f,C_xH_yO_z}}{w} \left(\frac{kJ}{electron\ transfer} \right) \tag{18}$$

$$\Delta G^o_{r,MFC} = \frac{124.69x - 118.59w - \Delta G^o_{f,C_xH_yO_z}}{w} \left(\frac{kJ}{electron\ transfer} \right) \tag{19}$$

The Gibbs free energy of cathodic reactions in MECs involving the formation of products different from hydrogen can be derived by reversing Eq. (10) to a negative form as illustrated in Example 11.1.

EXAMPLE 11.1

Consider an MEC with the cathodic half-cell reaction given in Equation 20. Find the standard Gibbs free energy of the MEC cathode reaction.

$$HCO_3^- + H^+ + 4H_2 \rightarrow CH_4 + 3H_2O \tag{20}$$

Solution:
Using Equation (8), the values of w, x, y, and z in Eq. (20) are 1, 4, 1, and 0, respectively.

As the chemical reaction given in Equation 20 occurs at the cathode, the negative form of Eq. (10) is applied as follows:

$$\Delta G_{r,cathode}^o = -124.684 + 39.9 - \Delta G_{f,CH_4}^o \tag{21}$$

where $\Delta G_{f,CH_4}^o = -50.8 \dfrac{\text{kJ}}{\text{mol of hydrogen}}$

By substituting the value of $\Delta G_{f,CH_4}^o$ into Eq. (21):

$$\Delta G_{r,cathode}^o = -135.6 \dfrac{\text{kJ}}{\text{mol of hydrogen}}$$

The change in Gibbs free energy across an MFC under actual conditions can be derived from Eq. (22).

$$\Delta G_{r,MFC} = \Delta G_{r,MFC}^o = -RT \ln \dfrac{1}{\left([O_2]^{0.5} + [H^+]^2 \right)} \tag{22}$$

where, $\Delta G_{r,MFC}$ is the molar Gibbs free energy change as a function of temperature and pressure; R is the universal gas constant: 8.314 $Jmol^{-1}K^{-1}$; $[O_2]$ is the partial pressure of oxygen; $[H^+]$ is the concentration of protons, which is $10^{-7} M/L$.

The change in Gibbs free energy across an MEC, where the reduction of H^+ occurs under actual conditions can be derived from Eq. (23).

$$\Delta G_{r,MEC} = \Delta G^o_{r,MEC} - RT \ln(\frac{[H_2]}{[H^+]^2}$$

(23)

where $[H_2]$ is the partial pressure of hydrogen.

The change in Gibbs free energy of a multicomponent system can be estimated from Eq. (24).

$$\Delta G_{r,cell} = \Delta G^o_{r,cell} + \sum_{j=1}^{Nreact} n_j RT \ln\left(\frac{n_j}{n_T}\right) - \sum_{j=1}^{Nprod} n_{j'} RT \ln\left(\frac{n_j}{n_T}\right)$$

(24)

where n_j is the stoichiometric number of moles of reactant j in the overall reaction equation of the cell; n_T is the total number of moles of reactants and products in the overall reaction equation of the cell; n_j' is the stoichiometric number of moles of product j in the overall reaction equation of the cell; N_{react} is the total number moles of reactants in the overall reaction equation of the cell; and N_{prod} is the total number of moles of products in the overall reaction equation of the cell.

The maximum theoretical voltage corresponding to the Gibbs free energy change across the cell is given by the Nernst equation, as shown in Eq. (25).

$$E = -\frac{\Delta G_{r,cell}}{n_e F}$$

(25)

The Nernst equation gives the mathematical relationship between the maximum theoretical voltage (E), number of electrons transferred in the overall reaction (n_e), Faraday's constant (F), and the change in Gibbs free energy ($\Delta G_{r,cell}$). In actual operation, the operating voltage of the cell (V_{net}) will be lower than the value that can be derived from Equation 25, due to three main voltage losses: activation ($V_{activation}$), ohmic (V_{ohmic}) and concentration ($V_{concentration}$) losses. Thus, the net voltage of the cell can be derived from Eq. (26).

$$V_{net} = E - V_{activation} - V_{ohmic} - V_{concentration}$$

(26)

Activation losses ($V_{activation}$) is given in Eqs. (27)–(29).

$$V_{activation} = V_{activation,anode} + V_{activation,cathode} \qquad (27)$$

$$V_{activation,anode} = \frac{2RT}{\eta_e F} \sinh^{-1} \sinh^{-1} \left(\frac{i}{2i_{o,anode}} \right) \qquad (28)$$

$$V_{activation,cathode} = \frac{2RT}{\eta_e F} \sinh^{-1} \sinh^{-1} \left(\frac{i}{2i_{o,cathode}} \right) \qquad (29)$$

where $V_{activation,anode}$ is the voltage loss due to activation losses in the anode; $V_{activation,cathode}$ is the voltage loss due to activation losses in the cathode; $i_{o,anode}$ is the anode exchange density; and $i_{o,cathode}$ is the cathode exchange density.

The ohmic losses (V_{ohmic}) can be derived from Eqs. (30)–(32).

$$V_{ohmic} = i \left(\frac{L_{electrolyte}}{\sigma_{electrolyte}} + \frac{L_{anode}}{\sigma_{electrolyte}} + \frac{L_{cathode}}{\sigma_{cathode}} + \frac{L_{interconnect}}{\sigma_{interconnect}} \right) \qquad (30)$$

where L_k is the thickness of k; $\forall k \in$ electolyte,anode,cathode,interconnect; and σ_k is the electronic or ionic conductivity in k, which is a function of temperature (Kelvin).

$$\sigma_k = \frac{C1_k}{T} e \left(\frac{C2_k}{T} \right); \forall k \in \{anode, cathode, interconnect \qquad (31)$$

$$\sigma_k = C1_{electrolyte} e \left(\frac{C2_{electrolyte}}{T} \right) \qquad (32)$$

where $C1_k$, $C1_{electrolyte}$, $C2_k$ and $C2_{electrolyte}$ are constants.

Concentration losses ($V_{Concentration}$) resulting from mass transfer limitations of the substrate through the electrodes can be derived from Equations 33–35.

$$V_{concentration} = V_{concentration,anode} + V_{concentration,cathode} \qquad (33)$$

$$V_{concentration,anode} = -\frac{RT}{n_e F} \ln\left(1 - \frac{i}{i_{l,anode}}\right) \tag{34}$$

$$V_{concentration,cathode} = -\frac{RT}{n_e F} \ln\left(1 - \frac{i}{i_{l,cathode}}\right) \tag{35}$$

$$V_{net} = E - V_{activation} - V_{ohmic} - V_{concentration}$$

11.6 ECONOMIC EVALUATION OF INTEGRATED BIOREFINERY BESS

Concerns over the maturity and high capital investment of the novel integrated systems show the necessity of conducting an economic evaluation to justify the viability of introducing a new system and scaling-up the system. A comprehensive economic analysis should comprise of capital cost estimation (Section 11.6.1), operating cost evaluation (Section 11.6.2) and profitability analysis (Section 11.6.3).

11.6.1 CAPITAL COST

Open-source literature (e.g., technical reports, journal) provides the costs of equipment for a given size/capacity of that particular system under consideration. This piece of information for this system (known as a base system) can be adopted in other case studies for systems with different sizes, by applying Eq. (36) [27].

$$\frac{COST_{size2}}{COST_{size1}} = \left(\frac{SIZE_2}{SIZE_1}\right)^R \tag{36}$$

where $SIZE_1$ is the capacity of the base system, t/h or t/y; $SIZE_2$ is the capacity of the system after scaling up/down, t/h or t/y; $COST_{size1}$ is the cost of the base system; $COST_{size2}$ is the cost of the system after scaling up/down; and R is the scaling factor.

In addition, the costs given in literatures are only valid at the time of reporting. Each cost of equipment has to be updated to the present year using Equation 37, applying Chemical Engineering Plant Cost Index (CEPCI) [27]. CEPCI can be found in *Chemical Engineering Journal*.

$$C_{pr} = C_o \left(\frac{I_{pr}}{I_o} \right)$$

(37)

where C_{pr} is the present cost of equipment; C_o is the original cost of equipment; I_{pr} is the present index value; and I_o is the original index value. The estimated purchased cost of equipment using Eqs. (36) and (37) has not taken into account the delivery cost, known as free-on-board (f.o.b.) cost. The delivered cost of equipment can be assumed to be 10% of the f.o.b. cost. Other direct costs, indirect costs and working capital can be estimated using Lang factor. As a general rule of thumb, Lang factors of 4.7 for solid processing system, 5.0 for solid-fluid processing system and 5.9 for fluid processing system can be adopted for estimation purposes [27].

Annual capital cost ($C_{PL}^{capital}$) is estimated by multiplying capital cost (*CC*) with annual capital charge (*ACC*), shown in Equation 38.

$$C_{PL}^{capital} = ACC \times CC$$

(38)

where *CC* is the summation of the direct costs, indirect costs, and working capital. The direct capital cost comprises the cost of equipment, installation, instrumentation and control, piping, electrical systems, building, yard improvements and service facilities. The cost of equipment can be estimated using cost and size correlation shown in Eq. (36). *ACC* is derived by the discounted cash flow (DCF) method.

In the DCF analysis, the cumulative DCF is expressed as the net present value (NPV), shown in Equation 39 subject to conditions in Eqs. (40) and (41) [27].

$$NPV_{yr} = \sum_{yr=-Y^c}^{Y} DCF_{yr} = \sum_{yr=-Y^c}^{0} DCF_{yr} + \sum_{yr=0}^{Y} DCF_{yr} = 0$$

(39)

where Y is the plant life; and Y^C is the start-up/construction period. Subject to constraints:

1. DCF in the years during construction period, $-Y^c \leq yr \leq 0$, assuming 0th year for the plant start-up, when the plant starts operating:

$$DCF_{yr} = \frac{SCF_{yr} \times CC}{\left(1 + \dfrac{IRR}{100}\right)^{yr}} \qquad (40)$$

where SCE_{Yr} is the fraction of CC invested in year (yr), during plant construction period ($-Y^c \leq yr \leq 0$).

where IRR is the internal rate of return.

2. DCF after plant start-up and before NPV is zero, $-0 \leq yr \leq Y$:

$$DCF_{yr} = \frac{ACC \times CC}{\left(1 + \dfrac{IRR}{100}\right)^{yr}} \qquad (41)$$

3. $0 \leq ACC \leq 1$.

11.6.2 OPERATING COST

Operating cost ($C_{PL}^{capital}$) evaluation includes fixed and variable costs. Fixed operating costs such as maintenance, capital charges, insurance, local taxes, and royalties are estimated based on percentage of indirect capital cost (except for the cost for personnel). Other fixed costs such as laboratory costs, supervision, and plant overheads are estimated based on the cost of personnel. Variable operating costs such as fuel, feedstock, electricity, catalyst and solvent can be estimated using the latest available price data from suppliers' quote (Table 11.4).

The cost of personnel can be estimated using Eq. (42) [27].

Cost of personnel = Number of personnel per shift × 5 shift
× 40 hours/week × 52 weeks/year × hourly wages   (42)

where the number of personnel requirement is related to the number of processing steps depending on the process, given in Eq. (43).

TABLE 11.4 Cost Estimation of Fixed Operating Cost [27]

No.	Specification	Cost Estimation
Fixed Operating Costs		
1	Maintenance	5–10% of indirect capital cost
2	Personnel	See below
3	Laboratory costs	20–23% of (2)
4	Supervision	20% of (2)
5	Plant overheads	50% of (2)
6	Capital charges	10% of indirect capital cost
7	Insurance	1% of indirect capital cost
8	Local taxes	2% of indirect capital cost
9	Royalties	1% of indirect capital cost
4	Supervision	20% of (2)
Direct Production Cost (DPC) = Variable + Fixed Operating Costs		
10	Sales expense	20–30% of DPC
11	General overheads	20–30% of DPC
12	Research and development	20–30% of DPC
Total operating cost = 1.2 or 1.3 times the DPC		

(Reprinted with permission from Sadhukhan, J., Ng, K. S., & Hernandez, E. M. (2014). *Biorefineries and Chemical Processes: Design, Integration and Sustainability Analysis*, © 2014 John Wiley.)

Number of personnel per shift

$$= \text{number of processing steps} \times \text{number of personnel per processing step} \quad (43)$$

11.6.3 PROFITABILITY ANALYSIS

Profitability analysis gives an indication of whether a project is feasible or not. This can be evaluated using payback time, return on investment and total annualized cost.

Payback time gives an indication of how fast the capital investment is recovered or break-even, calculated using Eq. (44), assuming constant annual cash flow. Intuitively, shorter payback time is preferred.

$$\text{Payback time (year)} = \frac{\text{Initial capital investment}}{\text{Cash flow per year}} \times 100\% \qquad (44)$$

Return on investment (ROI) provides an indication of the efficiency of investment being used, expressed in Eq. (45).

$$\text{ROI} = \frac{\text{Annual income}}{\text{Capital investment}} \times 100\% \qquad (45)$$

Total annualized cost includes capital and operating costs, shown in Eq. (46).

$$\text{Total annual cost} = C_{PL}^{capital} + C_{PL}^{operating} \qquad (46)$$

A more rigorous profitability analysis considering the time value of money may be needed considering that the plant life of the integrated systems is 15–30 years.

Economic potential (EP) can be evaluated using Eq. (47) if values of products, feed, capital cost and operating cost information are available.

$$\text{EP} = \text{Value of products} - (\text{Value of feed} + \text{Annualised capital cost} + \text{Annual operating cost}) \qquad (47)$$

Netback can be determined using Eq. (48) if values of products, capital cost and operating cost information are available. However, the value of feed is unknown. The netback thus indicates the value of a feedstock at which the product is sold at its market price. The netback also sets the maximum acceptable buy-in price of a feedstock. The market price of the feedstock thus must be less than the netback to result in an economic processing scenario.

$$\text{Netback} = \text{Value of products} - \text{Total annual cost} \qquad (48)$$

Cost of production can be employed when the value of product is not known especially when a new product is synthesized, or a conventional product is generated from a nonconventional feedstock. The cost of production is calculated using Eq. (49).

$$\text{Cost of production} = \frac{\text{Value of feed} + \text{Total annual cost}}{\text{Production rate}} \qquad (49)$$

11.6.4 LEARNING EFFECT

The cost of a new and developing technology such as microbial electrosynthesis and integrated technologies is usually very high at the beginning of the development stage. The cost of the technologies decreases as more plants are built and productivity increases due to more experience gained by the organization. This effect is known as learning curve/experience curve/progress curve/learning by doing the effect, illustrated in Figure 11.10 [27].

The trend of the learning curve can be described as in Eq. (50).

$$y = a\,x^{-b} \qquad (50)$$

where y is the cost of xth unit, a is the cost of the first unit, x is the cumulative number of units and b is a parameter in which $b = \log$ (progress ratio)/log 2.

The learning rate is shown in Eq. (51).

$$\text{Learning rate} = 1 - (\text{progress ratio}) \qquad (51)$$

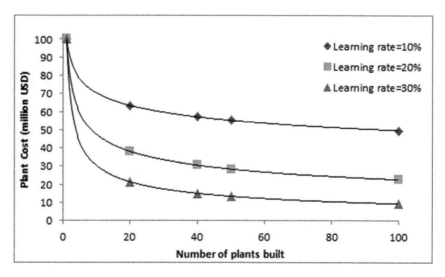

FIGURE 11.10 Learning curve effect [27]. (Reprinted with permission from Sadhukhan, J., Ng, K. S., & Hernandez, E. M. (2014). *Biorefineries and Chemical Processes: Design, Integration and Sustainability Analysis*, © 2014 John Wiley.)

The rates of learning are different and vary considerably across the different organization, even if they may be producing the same products.

11.7   VALUE ANALYSIS

Value analysis can be employed to examine the economic margins of individual streams and processing pathways in the integrated systems [16, 24, 27]. The objective is to identify which products are economically profitable to generate, how much value of materials is lost from the system and economic margins of individual processing streams. The value analysis methodology enables effective tracking and mapping of cost and value and thereby economic margin of each stream. Aggregation of economic margins of net mass flows gives the overall economic margin of the system. Thus, maximizing positive economic margins (profit) and minimizing negative economic margins (loss) of streams can ensure overall highest economic margin of the system. The Economic margin of a stream i, EM_i is calculated by multiplying the flowrate of the stream, F_i with the difference between its value on processing (VOP) and its cost of production (COP), shown in Eq. (52). The unit of F can be t/h and that of COP and VOP is €/t, and EM is €/h.

$$EM_i = F_i \times (VOP_i - COP_i)$$

(52)

The VOP of a stream is the prices of products that will ultimately be produced from it, subtracted by the costs of auxiliary raw materials, utilities and annualized capital cost of equipment that will contribute to its further processes into these final products.

The COP of a stream is the summation of all associated cost components, i.e., the costs of feedstocks, auxiliary raw materials, utilities and annualized capital cost that have contributed to the production of the stream. This means that only those fractional costs involved with the stream's production are included in its COP.

VOP of a feed f to a process unit k is calculated from the known values of the product streams p and the total costs of the process unit k, shown in Eq. (53).

$$VOP_f = \frac{\left[\sum_{p=1}^{q} VOP_p P_p - \bar{O}_k \right]}{\sum_{f=1}^{g} F_f}$$

(53)

where q is the number of products (excluding emissions/wastes); g is the number of feedstock considered as main material streams (excluding auxiliary raw materials); P_p and F_f correspond to the mass flow rates of product and feedstock, respectively.

COP of a product p from a process unit k is calculated from the known prices or costs of the feed streams f and the total costs of the process unit k, shown in Eq. (54).

$$COP_f = \frac{\left[\sum_{f=1}^{q} COP_f P_f + \bar{O}_k\right]}{\sum_{f=1}^{g} F_f} \tag{54}$$

11.8 CHALLENGES AND FUTURE DIRECTION

Although significant breakthroughs have been made in research and applications of BESs at lab-scale, there are still several hurdles to be crossed before they can gain parity with established sustainable energy production systems. The main challenge inhibiting the application of BESs for bioenergy production is the constraint imposed by their typical low power densities and power per unit electrode surface area [18]. Other performance issues associated with BES result from activation, ohmic, concentration and coulombic losses. Despite successful lab-scale demonstrations of BESs with encouraging results, the scaling up of the technology to industrial scale is still a difficult barrier to be yet overcome, as pilot scale demonstrations have shown poorer performance compared with lab-scale setups. The major challenge with scaling-up BESs stems from low system performance with increasing system scale due to incomplete technical comprehension of scale-up parameters [1]. Moreover, it is crucial to ensure that pilot and industrial-scale BES units are cost-effective and environmentally feasible to justify the upscaling of the technology. The use of expensive precious metal catalysts on the cathodes of BESs is another major challenge hindering the commercialization of the technology. Platinum and Palladium have been used extensively as catalysts at the cathode of BESs due to their excellent catalytic activity and resistance to fouling. However, the high costs of such metals make their utilization as catalysts on cathodes of BESs economically infeasible for commercial applications. While BESs are yet to be commercially viable, collaborative research efforts are ongoing to improve their performance at pilot and industrial scales at low production costs. Thus, the successful integration of BESs with biorefinery waste streams for enhanced bioenergy production will largely depend on the successful scale up of BESs towards commercial sustainability.

Several alternative electrode materials that are less expensive than precious metals have been developed to drive down the high cost of BESs systems. Materials such as polypyrroles macrocycles have been demonstrated as suitable electrode materials and have shown satisfactory results. Efforts are also being made to fully comprehend the mechanism of extracellular electron transfer in microbes used in BESs in order to identify ways of maximizing electron extraction from organic substrates. While previous research efforts have mainly concentrated on the bioanode of BESs, the exploration of potential applications at the biocathode of BESs is rapidly becoming more prevalent in research. An offshoot of this development is MESs, which involve the use of BES-generated electricity with or without additional of external supplied renewable electricity to synthesize biochemical production. One pathway for the application of microbial electrosynthesis systems that is gaining more prominence in laboratory tests is the reduction of CO_2 in the cathodic chamber of BESs into formate, acetate and other low carbon organic salts. With anticipated advances in scaling up and reducing the production cost of BESs, the cathodic reduction of CO_2 to produce biochemical and biofuels have the potential to become a viable CO_2 utilization technology.

KEYWORDS

- **biochemical**
- **bioelectricity**
- **bioelectrochemical systems**
- **biorefinery**
- **microbial electrosynthesis**
- **process integration**

REFERENCES

1 Borole, A. P. (2015). Microbial Fuel Cells and Microbial Electrolyzers. *The Electrochemical Society Interface*, pp. 55–59.

2. Bridgwater, A. V. (1999). Principles and Practice of Biomass Fast Pyrolysis Processes for Liquids. *J. Anal. Appl. Pyrolysis., 51*(1–2), 3–22.

3. Bridgwater, A. V., & Peacocke, G. V. C. (2000). Fast Pyrolysis Processes for Biomass. *Renew. Sustain. Energy Rev., 4*(1), 1–73.

4. Bridgwater, A. V. (2012). Review of Fast Pyrolysis of Biomass and Product Upgrading. *Biomass and Bioenergy, 38*, 68–94.

5. Chaudhuri, S. K., & Lovley, D. R. (2003). Electricity Generation by Direct Oxidation of Glucose in Mediatorless Microbial Fuel Cells. *Nat Biotechnol., 21*(10), 1229–1232.

6. Elliott, D. C. (2007). Historical Developments in Hydroprocessing Bio-Oils. - *Energy Fuels, 21*(3), 1792–1815.

7. Elliott, D. C., & Hart, T. R., (2009). Neuenschwander, G. G., Rotness, L. J., Zacher, A. H. Catalytic Hydroprocessing of Biomass Fast Pyrolysis Bio-Oil to Produce Hydrocarbon Products. *Environ. Prog. Sustain. Energy, 28*(3), 441–449.

8. Furimsky, E. (2012). Hydroprocessing Challenges in Biofuels Production. *Catal. Today,* No. 0.

9. Hamelers, H. V. M., Ter Heijne, A., Sleutels, T. H. J. A., Jeremiasse, A. W., Strik, D. P. B. T. B., & Buisman, C. J. N. (2010). New Applications and Performance of Bioelectrochemical Systems. *Applied Microbiology and Biotechnology,* pp. 1673–1685.

10. Haseli, Y., Dincer, I., & Naterer, G. F. (2008). Thermodynamic Modeling of a Gas Turbine Cycle Combined with a Solid Oxide Fuel Cell. *Int. J. Hydrogen Energy, 33*(20), 5811–5822.

11. IPCC. (2014). *Summary for Policymakers, In: Climate Change Mitigation of Climate Change. Contribution of Working Group III to the Fifth Assessment Report of the Intergovernmental Panel on Climate Change,* Cambridge University Press: Cambridge,United Kingdom and New York, NY, USA., (2014).

12. Ito, T., (2005). Nakashimada, Y., Senba, K., Matsui, T., Nishio, N. Hydrogen and Ethanol Production from Glycerol-Containing Wastes Discharged after Biodiesel Manufacturing Process. *J. Biosci. Bioeng., 100*(3), 260–265.

13. Kim, H. J., Park, H. S., Hyun, M. S., Chang, I. S., Kim, M., & Kim, B. H. (2002). A Mediator-Less Microbial Fuel Cell Using a Metal Reducing Bacterium, Shewanella Putrefaciens. *Enzyme Microb. Technol., 30*(2), 145–152.

14. Leong, J. X., Daud, W. R. W., Ghasemi, M., Liew, K., & Ben Ismail, M. (2013). Ion Exchange Membranes as Separators in Microbial Fuel Cells for Bioenergy Conversion: A Comprehensive Review. *Renew. Sustain. Energy Rev., 28*(August 2016), 575–587.

15. Luo, S., Sun, H., Ping, Q., Jin, R., & He, Z. (2016). A Review of Modeling Bioelectrochemical Systems: Engineering and Statistical Aspects. *Energies,* MDPI AG pp. 1–27.

16. Martinez-Hernandez, E., Campbell, G. M., & Sadhukhan, J. (2014). Economic and Environmental Impact Marginal Analysis of Biorefinery Products for Policy Targets. *J. Clean. Prod., 74*, 74–85.

17. Minteer, S. D., Liaw, B. Y., & Cooney, M. J. (2007). Enzyme-Based Biofuel Cells. *Curr. Opin. Biotechnol., 18*(3), 228–234.

18. Pant, D., Singh, A., Van Bogaert, G., Irving Olsen, S., Singh Nigam, P., Diels, L., & Vanbroekhoven, K. (2012). Bioelectrochemical Systems (BES) for Sustainable Energy

Production and Product Recovery from Organic Wastes and Industrial Wastewaters. *RSC Adv., 2* (4), 1248.

19. Pham, T. H., Rabaey, K., Aelterman, P., Clauwaert, P., De Schamphelaire, L., Boon, N., & Verstraete, W. (2006). Microbial Fuel Cells in Relation to Conventional Anaerobic Digestion Technology. *Eng. Life Sci., 6*(3), 285–292.

20. Potter, M. C. (1911). Electrical Effects Accompanying the Decomposition of Organic Compounds. *Proc. R. Soc. London, 84*(571), 260–276.

21. Rabaey, K., & Rozendal, R. A. (2010). Microbial Electrosynthesis - Revisiting the Electrical Route for Microbial Production. *Nat. Rev. Microbiol., 8*(10), 706–716.

22. Rabaey, K., Johnstone, A., Wise, A., Read, S., & Rozendal, R. A. (2010). Microbial Electrosynthesis: From Electricity to Biofuels and Biochemicals. *Bio Tech Int., 22*(3), 6–8.

23. Rubi, J. M., & Kjelstrup, S. (2003). Mesoscopic Nonequilibrium Thermodynamics Gives the Same Thermodynamic Basis to Butler–Volmer and Nernst Equations. *J. Phys. Chem. B., 107*(48), 13471–13477.

24. Sadhukhan, J., Mustafa, M. A., Misailidis, N., Mateos-Salvador, F., Du, C., & Campbell, G. M. (2008). Value Analysis Tool for Feasibility Studies of Biorefineries Integrated with Value Added Production. *Chem. Eng. Sci., 63*(2), 503–519.

25. Sadhukhan, J., Zhao, Y. R., Leach, M., Brandon, N. P., & Shah, N. (2010a). Energy Integration and Analysis of Solid Oxide Fuel Cell Based Microcombined Heat and Power Systems and Other Renewable Systems Using Biomass Waste Derived Syngas. *Ind. Eng. Chem. Res., 49*(22), 11506–11516.

26. Sadhukhan, J., Zhao, Y., Shah, N., & Brandon, N. P. (2010b).Performance Analysis of Integrated Biomass Gasification Fuel Cell (BGFC) and Biomass Gasification Combined Cycle (BGCC) Systems. *Chem. Eng. Sci., 65*(6), 1942–1954.

27. Sadhukhan, J., Ng, K. S., & Hernandez, E. M. (2014). *Biorefineries and Chemical Processes: Design, Integration and Sustainability Analysis*, Wiley.

28. Sadhukhan, J., Lloyd, J. R., Scott, K., Premier, G. C., Yu, E. H., Curtis, T., & Head, I. M. (2016). A Critical Review of Integration Analysis of Microbial Electrosynthesis (MES) Systems with Waste Biorefineries for the Production of Biofuel and Chemical from Reuse of CO_2. *Renew. Sustain. Energy Rev., 56*, 116–132.

29. Schirmer, A., Rude, M. A., Li, X., Popova, E., & del Cardayre, S. B. (2010). Microbial Biosynthesis of Alkanes. *Science, 329*(5991), 559–562.

30. Selembo, P. A., Perez, J. M., Lloyd, W. A., & Logan, B. E. (2009). High Hydrogen Production from Glycerol or Glucose by Electrohydrogenesis Using Microbial Electrolysis Cells. *Int. J. Hydrogen Energy, 34*(13), 5373–5381.

31. Shemfe, M. B. (2016).Performance Assessment of Biofuel Production via Biomass Fast Pyrolysis and Refinery Technologies, Cranfield University,

32. Shemfe, M. B., Fidalgo, B., & Gu, S. (2015). Heat Integration for Bio-Oil Hydroprocessing Coupled with Aqueous Phase Steam Reforming. *Chem. Eng. Res. Des.*

33. Shemfe, M. B., Whittaker, C., Gu, S., & Fidalgo, B. (2016). Comparative Evaluation of GHG Emissions from the Use of Miscanthus for Bio-Hydrocarbon Production via Fast Pyrolysis and Bio-Oil Upgrading. *Appl. Energy, 176*, 22–33.

34. Tan, X., Yao, L., Gao, Q., Wang, W., Qi, F., & Lu, X. (2011). Photosynthesis Driven Conversion of Carbon Dioxide to Fatty Alcohols and Hydrocarbons in Cyanobacteria. *Metab. Eng., 13*(2), 169–176.

35. Thauer, R. K. K., Jungermann, K., & Decker, K. (1977). Energy Conservation in Chemotrophic Anaerobic Bacteria - ERRATUM. *Microbiol. Mol. Biol. Rev., 41*, 100–180.

36. United Nations. (2015). *Adoption of the Paris Agreement*, Paris, France, Vol. 21932.

37. Wright, M. M., Daugaard, D., Satrio, J. A., Brown, R., & Hsu, D. (2010). *Techno-Economic Analysis of Biomass Fast Pyrolysis to Transportation Fuels*, NREL Golden, CO.

38. Zhao, Y., Sadhukhan, J., Lanzini, A., Brandon, N., & Shah, N. (2011). Optimal Integration Strategies for a Syngas Fuelled SOFC and Gas Turbine Hybrid. *J. Power Sources, 196*(22), 9516–9527.

PART IV

ENERGY BALANCE, TECHNO-ECONOMICS, AND LIFE-CYCLE INVENTORIES

CHAPTER 12

ENERGY BALANCE/EFFICIENCY AND ECONOMIC ANALYSIS OF BIOFUEL PRODUCTION

MARÍA GONZÁLEZ ALRIOLS, XABIER ERDOCIA,
MARÍA ANGELES ANDRES, and JALEL LABIDI

Biorefinery Processes Research Group (BioRP), Chemical and Environmental Engineering Department, University of the Basque Country UPV/EHU, Plaza Europa, 1, 20018, Donostia-San Sebastián, Spain

CONTENTS

ABSTRACT

To be a viable substitute for fossil fuels and be able to provide an actual alternative to the instable prices and supplies associated to the petroleum-based energy, biofuels need to be economically competitive to present environmental benefits and to ensure a stable production to cover the market energy demand. To evaluate whether biofuels provide a better alternative over the fossil fuels they displace, a complete set of parameters must be analyzed, including all the aspects related to their full production and use life cycles. In this chapter, the different biofuels industries energy balances are submitted to evaluation, considering their global inputs and outputs. As inputs, the requirements for the seed growing, the conversion of crops into biofuels, the transporting of the crops to the production facilities, or the productions plant efficiencies are considered. As outputs, the energetic potential of the biofuels and the obtained coproducts of the production process are included. Furthermore, the greenhouse gas emissions and other environmental effects associated to these production systems are also evaluated.

12.1   INTRODUCTION

Fulfilling an increasing energy demand and keeping the guidelines dictated in the United Nations Conference on Climate Change, COP 21 [1], recently celebrated in Paris, related to the mitigation of changing climate, is putting together governments, commercial organizations and academic communities with the aim of finding a way to face these two global challenges. It has been widely recognized that the solution lies in the development of economically rational, environmentally friendly, sustainable, and renewable energy [2]. In this context, biomass derived fuels are expected to play a leading role [3] and policies promoting the production and use of biofuels have been established in the main industrialized countries including the United States of America (USA), members of European Union, China, and Brazil [4]. The interest in the biofuel market is growing along with the inversions and research efforts of most of the major oil companies [5]. The share of renewables in transportation (biofuels and renewable electricity) is expected to reach around 11% in 2020 in all decarbonization scenarios and it is expected to rise to 19–20% in 2030 and up to 62–73% in 2050 [6]. Nevertheless, in order to represent an actual alternative over the fossil fuels, their use should be beneficial, under environmental and economical points of view. Furthermore, their production must be considerable and regular, in order to represent a meaningful impact on the energy market. For the evaluation of the mentioned parameters, it is necessary to consider both the direct and indirect inputs and outputs for their full production and use life cycles and include their energy balances [7].

In this chapter, the different variables implied in the production of the main biofuels (bioethanol, biodiesel, biobutanol and biogas) are evaluated, i.e., plants growing efficiencies, agrochemistry, conversion process technologies and yields, coproduct production, transport, energy balances, emissions and other environmental effects. The obtained results are related to gasoline and diesel, the fossil fuels they displace in the market.

12.2   BIOETHANOL

Bioethanol (ethyl alcohol, grain alcohol, $CH_3–CH_2–OH$ or ETOH) is a colorless volatile liquid and flammable biofuel with molecular weight of 46.07 g and density of 789 kg/m^3 at 294 K, that can be produced from several different biomass feedstocks and conversion technologies [8].

The main application of this product is to become an alternative transportation biofuel in response to the variable prices of fossil fuels, the instability in supplies and global warming [9]. It can be used in mixtures with gasoline up to 10% without modification of the engines and it also can be used in higher proportion, up to 85% alcohol in gasoline, in the so-called flexi-fuel vehicles. It is also possible to use 100% bioethanol in specially designed engines [10].

Bioethanol has a higher octane number, broader flammability limits, higher flame speeds and higher heats of vaporization than gasoline. These properties allow for a higher compression ratio, shorter burn time and leaner burn engine, which lead to theoretical efficiency advantages over gasoline in an internal combustion engine [11]. Disadvantages of bioethanol include its lower energy density than gasoline (bioethanol has 66% of the energy than gasoline), its corrosiveness, low flame luminosity, lower vapor pressure (making cold starts difficult), miscibility with water forming and azeotrope, toxicity to ecosystems and low flash point [8,12]. On the other hand, the cost of bioethanol production is higher when compared to the fossil fuels one.

The world bio-ethanol production in 2008 was 66.77 billion liters. It grew to 88.69 billion liters in 2013 [13] and it reached almost 93 billion liters in 2014 [14]. Worldwide total bioethanol production is expected to rise further to 100 billion liters in 2015 [15]. USA and Brazil are the two major bioethanol producing countries with 58.20% and 25.19% of the world production (Figure 12.1). The price is a significant factor for the large-scale extension of bioethanol production. Feedstocks contribute significantly (around 80–90%)

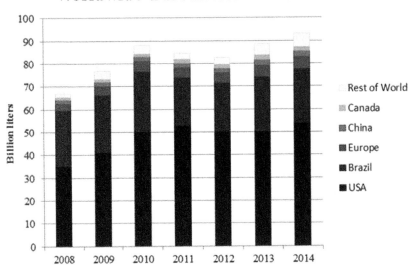

FIGURE 12.1   Worldwide bioethanol production (adapted from Ref. [7]).

in the total cost of biofuels [16]. Depending on the feedstock used for the bio-ethanol production, the biofuels are classified as first or second generation. The raw materials conversion process for bioethanol obtaining in the case of using first or second generation feedstock defers mainly in the pretreatments that have to be applied to biomass before submitting it to fermentation, espe-cially with second generation type raw materials. These pretreatments repre-sent a considerable part of the whole production process energy requirement and are responsible of a noteworthy percentage of greenhouse gas emissions (GHG). Thus, in the following sections the pretreatments that need to be applied to prepare the biomass in the case of first and second generations feedstocks is presented in detail.

12.2.1   FIRST GENERATION BIOETHANOL

First generation bioethanol is produced from feedstocks used for food and feed, such as cereals, tubers, high sugar content plants and agro-industrial processing coproducts [10]. Thus, there is a growing food vs. fuel debate among the concerned members of the civil societies and the stakeholders.

Many critics are arguing that increasing in land use for growing biofuel crops will result in shortage of land, water and other resources for growing food crops, which will contribute towards food shortage [17]. Nowadays almost all the bioethanol produced worldwide comes from these types of feedstocks. Among the main feedstocks, the most exploited ones are grain and sugar crops.

12.2.1.1 From Grain

Starch contained in grains is the major polymer used for bioethanol production all over the world [18]. Among all the grain types, corn grain is the major raw material, especially in the United States. Chemical structure of starch consists of long chain polymer of glucose units linked by glycosidic bonds. These chains can be linear (amylose) or branched (amylopectin). The macromolecular starch cannot be directly fermented to ethanol by conventional fermentation technology. The first step of the ethanol production from grains is the milling of the substrate and subsequent mixing with water to produce a mash typically containing 15–20% of starch. The mash is then cooked at or above its boiling point and subsequently treated with two enzyme types. The first enzymes, called amylases, hydrolyze starch molecules to short chains. This hydrolysis of the starch can also be achieved by chemical methods without any enzyme, under pressure and usually employing acid catalysts. Pressure-cooking is a very effective method for further fermentation of starchy materials but production costs are very elevated due to the high-energy consumption in the cooking process. In addition, nonpressure method allows obtaining high ethanol yields, while saving energy and reducing the further fermentation time [19].

At industrial scale, enzymatic starch hydrolysis is one of the most important enzymatic reactions that are carried out for bioethanol production [20]. Liquefaction is a key step in the starch hydrolysis process and it is commonly achieved through the dispersion of insoluble starch granules in an aqueous solution. Liquefaction, typically performed at temperatures around 90°C to gelatinize the starch making it hydrolysable by conventional amylases, requires the equivalent of 10–20% of the energy content of ethanol produced [21]. The aim of this liquefaction is to destroy the starch cristalinity (gelatinization) and thus make it easier for amylases to hydrolyze it [22]. The factors affecting starch liquefaction include the source and concentration of the starch; the source and activity of the α-amylase; the concentration of calcium ions, which are related to the activation and stability of α-amylase; and other reaction conditions, such as temperature and pH [19]. After the liquefaction of the starch, partial hydrolysis is carried out at a relatively high temperature using thermostable α-amylases, which are endoglucanases that catalyze the hydrolysis of internal α-1,4-glycosidic linkages in starch. Amylases liberate "maltodextrin" oligosaccharides by liquefaction process and they can hydrolyze both insoluble starch and starch granules held in aqueous suspension [23]. After this first hydrolysis step, the dextrin and oligosaccharides are further hydrolyzed by the second enzyme preparation, which generally is composed by pullulanases and glucoamylases in a process known as saccharification. Saccharification converts all dextrans to glucose, maltose and isomaltose [24]. Finally, the resulting sugar is fermented and the sugar monomers are converted into ethanol and carbon dioxide [25]. There are two basic types of fermentation: aerobic and (b) anaerobic depending on the presence or absence of oxygen in the process. The microorganisms employed for ethanol production are classified into three categories, viz., yeast (*Saccharomyces* species), bacteria (*Zymomonas* species), and mold *(Mycelium)*, being the former the most common one. In the bioethanol production from grains, *Saccharomyces cerevial*, *Saccharomyces uvarum*, *Schizosaccaharomyces pombe*, and *Kluyveromyces* species of yeast are used. Alternative to this methods, were saccharification and fermentation are separated, there are simultaneous saccharification and fermentation (SSF) methods or fermentation with stillage recycling [26].

Theoretically, the maximum conversion efficiency of glucose to ethanol is 51% on the weight basis, which comes from a stoichiometric calculation according to the Equation 1. The fermentation requires 48–72 h and has a final ethanol concentration of 10–12% [24]. The pH of the beer declines during the fermentation to pH values under 4, due to the carbon dioxide formed during the ethanol fermentation. The decrease in pH is important for increasing the activity of *Glucoamylase* and inhibiting the growth of contaminating bacteria [27].

$$C_6H_{12}O_6 \quad\quad \text{-->} \quad\quad 2C_2H_6O + 2CO_2 \quad\quad\quad\quad (1)$$
$$\text{(glucose)} \quad\quad\quad\quad\quad\quad \text{(ethanol)}$$

There are two principal methods for bioethanol production from grain, the so-called dry and wet mills (Figure 12.2). In the wet milling process,

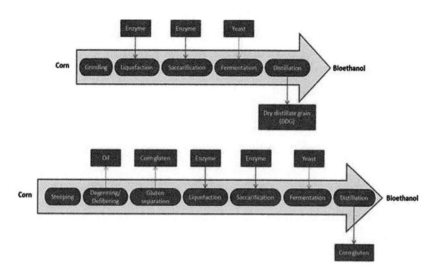

FIGURE 12.2 Dry and wet mill processes for bioethanol production from corn.

when corn is used for ethanol production, the main components of the grain are recovered. In this way, only starch enters to the process. The range of products that could be obtained from a modern biorefinery employing the wet milling technology includes bioethanol and many others of valuable coproducts such as nutraceuticals, pharmaceuticals, organic acids and solvents [28]. Modern wet milling plants are able to produce 3.785 liters bioethanol consuming 37,083 KJ of thermal energy and 2134 KWh of electricity. If molecular sieves are used, the thermal energy input drops to 8961 KJ/L [29]. When dry milling of corn is employed for bioethanol production, all components of the grain (starch, fiber, proteins, fats, minerals) are involved in the process. Thin stillage represents the liquid fraction obtained after centrifugation or pressing of the whole stillage. The solid fraction contains the remaining corn and fermentation solids. Thin stillage can be concentrated by evaporation in order to obtain a syrup of concentrated solubles that are mixed with the remaining solids. Dry grinding mill process is specially designed for ethanol production and animal feed [28].

The starch-based bioethanol industry has been commercially viable for about 30 years. In this time, tremendous improvements have been made in enzyme efficiency, reducing process costs and time, and increasing bioethanol yields [30]. Nowadays, in a typical biothanol biorefinery, were corn is used as feedstock, the usual method is the following: corn kernels are ground to 3–4 mm flour, wetted with water into slurry, and heated by steam at 110–120°C for 2 h to form the corn mash. Then, α-amylase is added in the liquefaction step, which occurs at 80–90°C. Afterwards, saccharification step is carried out at 30°C adding *Glucoamylase* as enzyme. The saccharified corn mash is then fermented at 32°C for 50 h with addition of yeast, yielding 8–12% ethanol by weight in the slurry. Ethanol is recovered from the slurry by distillation, de-watered by passing through molecular sieves, and denatured by mixing with 2–5% gasoline. Typically, 9.5–11.0 liters of bioethanol can be generated from 25.4 kg of corn grains [31].

12.2.1.2   From Sugar Crops

Besides grain, first generation bioethanol can also be obtained by another feedstock: sugar crops. Sugar cane, either in the form of cane juice or cane molasses, is the most important feedstock used in tropical and subtropical countries for ethanol producing. Since early 1970s Brazil has been the major fuel ethanol producer in the world depending on sugarcane as feedstock. Ethanol from sugarcane, with its bio-renewable nature and optimized production technology, has been proven to be a replacement for fossil fuels in Brazil [32]. Actually, in Brazil, gasoline is required to contain at least 22% of bioethanol [33]. Otherwise, in European countries, beet molasses are the most used sucrose-containing feedstock [28].

The first step in the bioethanol production from sugar crops is the obtaining of sugar-rich juices, which contain free sugars, specially, sucrose, glucose, and fructose [34]. The conversion of these sugars into bioethanol is easier compared to starchy materials because previous hydrolysis of the feedstock is not required, since these disaccharides can be broken down by the yeast cells [8]. After obtaining the juice, yeasts are added to convert these sugars into ethanol. *Saccharomyces cerevisiae* is the main specie of yeast employed for ethanol production at industrial level since this microorganism is easy to handle, shows no high nutritional needs and can produce ethanol concentrations above 15%. In addition, it tolerates high concentrations of sugars, is not expensive, produces low levels of by-products, is osmotolerant and presents high viability for recycling [35].

Currently, first-generation ethanol is produced either from sugarcane juice or molasses or a mixture depending on the processing plant: in autonomous distilleries, ethanol is produced from sugarcane juice, whereas in annexed plants, a fraction of the sugarcane juice is diverted for sugar production and the remaining fraction along with the molasses is used for ethanol production. In Brazil, 63.5% of the sugarcane processing units are annexed plants, 30.5% are autonomous plants and the remaining units produce only sugar. The prevalence of annexed plants in the country is related to its flexibility to produce more ethanol or more sugar depending on the market demands, which is part of the reason for the success of bioethanol production in Brazil [36].

12.2.2 SECOND GENERATION BIOETHANOL

Although corn-based and sugar based-ethanol are promising substitutes to gasoline, mainly in the transportation sector, they are not enough in volume to replace a considerable portion of the gallons of fossil fuel presently consumed annually worldwide [37]. Furthermore, the ethical concerns about the use of food as fuel raw materials have encouraged research efforts to focus on the potential of inedible feedstock alternatives. This way the second generation bioethanol, which is produced from non food raw material, such as woody species, tall grasses, crop and paper residues, agricultural and municipal wastes, and many other lignocellulosic materials, has raised considerable interest as a potential alternative to the fossil fuels [38]. Indeed, the worldwide potential annual bioethanol production, only from agricultural wastes, such as rice, wheat, corn straws, and baggase, is as high as 418.9 GL [39]. Although the mentioned feedstocks present considerable potential, due to their residual character, wide availability and low price, the second generation bioethanol production in many countries has been so far discouraging due to the costs associated to the technology required to the raw materials processing that make this type of bioethanol still prohibitively expensive to be used as transportation biofuel [40]. The reason for these high production costs is partly related to the characteristic of lignocellulosic feedstock. The lignocellulosic biomass is primarily composed by three different polymers, which are connected to each other mainly by hydrogen bonds but also by some covalent bonds: cellulose, hemicelluloses and lignin. In order to produce bioethanol it is necessary to separate the cellulose from the rest of the components and this first step, which is still under development, considerably raises the cost of the whole process. Overall, there are four stages in the production of lignocellulosic-based bioethanol: pretreatment (delignification), hydrolysis, fermentation and distillation (Figure 12.3) [37].

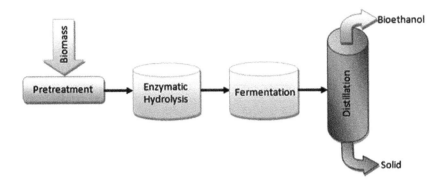

FIGURE 12.3   Second generation bioethanol production flow diagram.

Pretreatment is the first challenge for obtaining potential fermentable sugars susceptible of being digested from lignocellulosic biomass [41] and involves more than 40% of the total processing cost. The lignocellulosic biomass pretreatment consist of the disrupting of the hydrogen bonds in the crystalline cellulose, the breaking down of the cross-linked matrix of hemi-celluloses and lignin and the increase of the surface area and porosity of the substrate making the cellulose more accessible to hydrolytic enzymes (Figure 12.4) [42]. In order to achieve these goals, a number of pretreatment methods have been developed, which can be classified into physical, chemical, physicochemical and biological pretreatments [43].

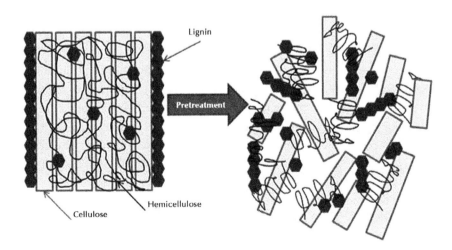

FIGURE 12.4   Pretreatment of lignocellulosic biomass.

Physical pretreatments of lignocellulosic biomass include milling, grinding, chipping, freezing or radiation, to increase the surface area enhancing mass and heat transfer in the subsequent treatments of the biomass. The efficiency in the later process is also contributed by the capability of the pretreatment process to reduce the degree of crystallinity and polymerization of cellulose and hemicellulose [44]. A drawback of physical pretreatments is the high-energy input required, which can seriously impair the energy obtained by the bioethanol produced. Chemical pretreatments comprise acidic, alkaline, organosolv, ozonolysis, and ionic liquid (IL) treatments of the lignocellulosic biomass. Depending on the chemical used, the pretreatment will has diverse effect on the structure of lignocellulosic materials [43].

Acid pretreatment is the most commonly employed chemical pretreatment for lignocellulosic biomass. Although sulfuric acid is, by far, the most used acid, nitric and hydrochloric acids are also used in the chemical pretreatments of biomass [45]. The acid pretreatment can be performed either under high temperatures and low acid concentrations (dilute-acid pretreatment), or under low temperatures and high acid concentrations (concentrated-acid pretreatment). Concentrate-acid processes enable the hydrolysis of both hemicelluloses and cellulose and have the advantage to allow operating at low/medium temperatures leading to the reduction of the operational costs [46]. However, toxicity, corrosiveness of equipment and acid recovery are important drawbacks that avoid the wide extend application of this method [47]. Diluted acid pretreatment is most commonly applied and appears as a more favorable method for industrial application. In light of that, numerous studies have been conducted employing this technique [48]. This pretreatment is performed at elevated temperatures (between 140–190°C), low acid concentrations (in a range of 0.5–1.5%) and can achieve high reaction rates significantly improving cellulose's susceptibility to enzymatic hydrolysis. Almost 100% hemicellulose removal is possible by dilute-acid pretreatment [49]. In numerous studies, sugar yields higher than 83% (even reaching values of 94%) were achieved after applying dilute acid pretreatment to different raw materials [50, 51]. However, this pretreatment also presents some drawbacks as the formation of some fermentation inhibitors like, furfural, 5-hydroxymethylfurfural (5-HMF) and further degradation products such as levulinic acid or formic acid. Phenolic compounds are also formed during pretreatment from the partial breakdown of lignin. All these compounds have negative effects on the downstream processes. Therefore, the removal of these compounds is essential, which along with the high temperature and pressure operation conditions, increases the process cost [52].

Alkaline pretreatment is one of the other extensively studied chemical pretreatment methods, which employs various alkali compounds such as sodium hydroxide, sodium carbonate, calcium hydroxide, potassium hydroxide, ammonia, hydrogen peroxide or their combination [52, 53]. Alkaline pretreatment is carried out under milder conditions than those needed for acid pretreatment. In addition, it provides the most effective method for lignin removal and the breaking of the ester bonds between lignin, hemicellulose and cellulose avoiding also fragmentation of the hemicellulose polymers [52]. During alkaline pretreatment, saponification reaction takes place, which causes the removal of crosslinks, acetyl group and various uronic acid substitutions in hemicelluloses. Furthermore, alkaline pretreatment leads to an increase of porosity and internal surface area, structural swelling, a decrease in the degree of polymerization and crystallinity, disruption of lignin structure, and a breakdown of links between lignin and carbohydrate polymers [54]. All these changes in the structure of biomass enhance the accessibility of cellulose to further hydrolytic enzymes. The effectiveness of alkaline pretreatment varies, depending on the substrate and treatment conditions. In general, alkaline pretreatment is more effective on hardwood, herbaceous crops, and agricultural residues with low lignin content than on softwood with high lignin content [55].

In organosolv pretreatments, lignin is extracted from lignocellulosic feedstock by lignin dissolution using organic solvents or their aqueous solutions. After this pretreatment, the remaining solid fraction is much enriched in cellulose, has lower quantity of lignin and presents higher accessibility toward hydrolytic enzymes [56]. The most commonly used solvents for organosolv delignification include alcohols such as methanol and ethanol (usually with at least 50% of concentration), organic acids such as formic and acetic acid, amines, ketones, phenols and mixed organic solvent–inorganic alkali chemicals [57]. The treatment can be carried out in a wide range of temperature (100–250°C) and, normally, under high pressures.

Another chemical pretreatment of lignocellulosic materials is the so-called ozonolysis which is carried out employing ozone. Due to ozone electron deficiency in the terminal oxygen, it attacks preferably lignin, an electron-rich substrate, than carbohydrates. This way, lignin is effectively degraded while cellulose and hemicelluloses suffer minimal effects [58]. The main advantages of the ozonolysis pretreatment are that it is usually carried out at room temperature, and does not lead to inhibitory compounds like furfural or 5-HMF [45]. However, the main drawback of the process is the ozone generation mainly due to two factors: its current production costs and the large amount of ozone that process needs. Technological advances are steadily reducing ozone production costs, which have decreased a 30% in the last four years. Nevertheless, currently 1.65MJ are required for producing only 100 g of ozone [58]. The main parameters in ozonolysis pretreatment are moisture content of the sample, biomass type, particle size, and ozone concentration in the gas flow. Among these parameters, moisture is a reaction controlling parameter for values below 30%. [59].

One of the newest chemical pretreatments consists of the use of ionic liquids. In the field of lignocellulosic biomass, ionic liquids have been used as lignocellulosic material solvents, as a greener alternative to classic fractionation processes. One of the advantage of ionic liquids is that are easily recovered and reused, so the amount of wastes generated on a process is considerably reduced. The combination of the reutilization with their low volatility is the reason why ionic liquids are considered as green solvents. The dissolution and reactivity of cellulose in ILs has been widely studied by many authors [60, 61]. Among the studied ILs for cellulose dissolution the most important ones are: 1-butyl-3-methylimidazolium cations ([Bmim]$^+$) with a range of anions, from small hydrogen-bond acceptors (Cl$^-$) to large, noncoordinating anions ([PF$_6$]$^-$) besides, Br$^-$, SCN$^-$ and [BF$_4$]$^-$ [60], 1,3-dialkylimidazolium formats, 1-ethyl-3-methylimidazolium methylphosphate, 1-N-Allyl-3-methylimidazolium chloride, or the less toxic and corrosive IL, 1-N-ethyl-3-methylimidazolium acetate [62–65]. The presence of water in the reaction media is also a very important issue, as the dissolution of the cellulose precise the absence of water because the mechanism of dissolution implies the formation of hydrogen bonds. When the water is present in the media, those hydrogen bonds are formed between water and IL decreasing solubility of wood. So that, the reaction has to be done on inert atmosphere and the ILs as well as the wood need to be dried before. In general, in order to have a successful solubility of wood into ionic liquids, the presence of water, particle size, and reaction time are the main factors to consider [66]. The cellulose dissolved in ILs can be reconstituted using rapid precipitation from its solution by the addition of different antisolvents including water [61], alcohols [67], supercritical CO$_2$ [68] or by using two immiscible ILs and sugar derivatives as water-IL solution additives [69]. Reconstituted cellulose could be obtained in different forms such as monoliths, fibers and films with the same degree of polymerization and polydispersity, but with lower crystallinity [70] and it is suitable for the enzymatic hydrolysis. On the other hand, studies of the dissolution of lignin on IL have shown the success of several ILs. This way, the remaining substrate is enriched in cellulose and can be derived to the next step of hydrolysis.

In physicochemical pretreatments, lignin and hemicellulose are removed and cellulose is disrupted by changing the operating conditions (pressure and temperature) in the presence or absence of a chemical. Steam explosion, ammonia fiber explosion, carbon dioxide explosion, and wet oxidation are the most common examples of this type of pretreatments [71]. Steam explosion is the most extensively investigated thermo-mechano-chemical method, which involves the breakdown of structural components by steam-heating, shearing, and auto-hydrolysis of glycosidic bonds. The process explodes biomass using pressurized steam (20–50 bar, 160–270°C) for several seconds to a few minutes by sudden decompression from high pressure and temperature conditions to improve accessibility of the cell wall material to hydrolysis by cellulases [41,72]. Ammonia fiber explosion retreatment is conducted by using liquid ammonia and based on the steam explosion process concept. Four parameters including ammonia loading, water loading, reaction temperature, and residence time can be varied in order to optimize the this pretreatment. Similarly, carbon dioxide explosion is based on the steam explosion concept but using super-critical CO_2 [73, 74]. Lastly, the wet oxidation physicochemical pretreatment involves the subcritical oxidation of organics or oxidizable inorganic components at elevated temperatures (125–320°C) and pressures (0.5–2 MPa) and in which oxygen or air is employed as a catalyst [75]. This pretreatment is very effective in the separation of the cellulosic fractions from lignin and hemicelluloses, and the most important parameters to take into account are the reaction temperature, time and oxygen pressure [76].

Finally, biological pretreatments use different fungi species such as white-rot, brown-rot, soft-rot and bacterias which degrade mostly lignin, hemicelluloses and very little of cellulose [77]. The main advantages of this pretreatment over physical/chemical pretreatments are the substrate and reaction specificity, low energy requirements, no generation of toxic compounds, and high yield of desired products [78]. Nevertheless, it also has some drawbacks such as long time requirements (from days to weeks), the need of a careful control of the growth conditions and large performing space [79].

After all these pretreatments, the cellulose contained in lignocellulosic biomass is ready for the enzymatic hydrolysis step. All the subsequent treatments applied to the pretreated lignocellulosic feedstock are essentially the same to those applied to the first generation bioethanol feedstock. Therefore, the main difference only resides in isolating the cellulose from the rest of the components. The hydrolysis of the pretreated lignocellulosic substrate is carried out employing cellulase enzyme, which hydrolyzes the cellulosic polymer into sugar monomers; this process is known to be a dominant factor in the overall cost of bioethanol production. The manufacture of this enzyme is expensive (0.12 € per liter) and energy intensive [39].

Once the hydrolysis of cellulose is completed, the fermentation of the released sugars into bioethanol takes place. The most common yeast used in this process is *Saccharomyces cerevisiae*, which only metabolizes hexoses (glucose) but it is not able to ferment pentoses such as xylose. In lignocellulosic biomass, xylose is an important fraction of the hemicelluloses accounting up to one-third of the sugars in the lignocelluloses. Consequently, xylose fermentation is a challenging subject to be overcome to increase the economic feasibility of the processes [10]. *Pichia stipitis, Pachysolen tannophilus,* and *Candida shehatae* microorganisms have been successfully employed to ferment xylose into bioethanol [13]. However, the fermentation of hexoses and pentoses at the same time is still under development. In the first approach, xylose-metabolizing genes have been engineered into wild-type *Ethanologens* such as yeast and the bacterium *Zymomonas mobilis* [80]. Otherwise, in order to reduce the cost of bioethanol production, as well as in the case of first generation bioethanol, the hydrolysis (saccharification) and fermentation processes can be carried out simultaneously in the so-called SSF process. Other configurations include simultaneous saccharification and cofermentation (SSCF) and consolidated biomass processing (CBP). Process integration reduces the capital costs [81]. Finally, in the last step of the whole process, the obtained bioethanol is distilled and purified. The lignocellulosic feedstock to produce second-generation bioethanol can be obtained from several sources. The most used and studied are woody crops, straw and energy grasses.

12.2.2.1   From Woody Crops

Fast growing species of trees constitutes a very abundant source of lignocellylosic biomass for bioethanol production. Several studies have been made employing different Eucalyptus species (*Eucalyptus globulus, Eucalyptus grandis*) [82, 83]. The pretreatment employed in this type of feedstock is usually steam explosion, which enhances the digestibility of cellulose. Romaní et al. [82] reported a recovery of 18.1 g sugars/100 g oven-dry raw material in liquor by SSF of solids reaching the concentration of 51 g ethanol/L. Pine wood chips have been used for bioethanol production as well, reaching a maximum yield of 10.60 g ethanol/100 g of raw dry material [84]. On the other hand, among perennial species like pine, short rotation woody crops (SRWC) provide a stable yield and there is a well-developed technology for their cultivation. The yield of willow and poplar can reach as much as 30 Mg ha^{-1} year^{-1} of dry matter of cellulose, when cultivated on good soils and under favorable weather conditions [85]. Afterwards, this high quantity of cellulose would be converted into bioethanol.

12.2.2.2   From Straw

A variety of lignocellulosic agricultural wastes are available for ethanol production such as sugarcane bagasse, rice hull, timber species, Willow, Salix, Switchgrass, softwood, rice straw, wheat straw, etc. Among all the lignocellulosic wastes, cereal straws are the most abundant, cheap, renewable and easily available. Rice straw is a promising alternative for bioethanol production [86]. Many studies have been carried, especially in India and Japan about the suitability of rice straw for bioethanol production and significant amounts of soft carbohydrates (62–200 g kg^{-1}, average 139 g kg^{-1}) were measured [87]. Wheat straw is another feedstock widely employed for the bioethanol production. Leitner et al. [88] achieved the production of 964 MJ of purified ethanol per ton of untreated straw, which corresponded to a share of approximately 55% of the lower heating value [88]. However, they concluded, as in other investigations in biorefinery frameworks, that it was more energetically efficient to produce a combination of different biofuels from straw, including biogas, than producing bioethanol only.

12.2.2.3   From Energy Grasses

Energy crops are crops grown primarily to provide a feedstock for energy production, included in this category are those generated from agricultural activities and forest log. Some energy crops, such as Miscanthus, Switchgrass, and sweet Sorghum, which are called C4 crops, can grow with high biomass yield even on poor land. Thus, these crops are used in energy farming. Furthermore, C4-type crops possess the features of resistance to aridity, high photosynthetic yield and a high rate of CO_2 capture when compared with C3 crops. In conclusion, C4 crops tend to produce more biomass than C3 crops [33]. All, these advantages makes energy grasses or crops very suitable for bioethanol production. Among all the energy grasses, Miscanthus and Switchgrass have been the most studied ones. When comparing these two feedstock, the difference between output energy obtained by ethanol and the input energy used in producing ethanol, is 12.41 MJ/L of ethanol for Miscanthus and 7.90 MJ/L of ethanol for Switchgrass [89]. Therefore, these two energy grasses were found to be very suitable for bioethanol production.

12.2.3 BIOETHANOL ENERGY BALANCE AND ENVIRONMENTAL EFFECTS

Once the core conversion processes to convert biomass in first and second generations bioethanol have been carefully described, putting especial emphasis in the pretreatments part, which entails the main difference among the mentioned conversion technologies, the rest of parameters that determines the net energy balance (NEB) of the biofuel should be considered for a proper estimation. Apart from the main conversion process of biomass into a biofuel, energy is required for other activities associated mainly to the crops growth (seed, fertilizers and pesticides production, farm machinery, feedstock collection, storage, drying, chipping…), plant construction and maintenance and the transport of the crops to the biofuel production facilities [7].

On the other hand, the outputs of biofuel production accounts for the potential energy of the biofuels and the generated coproducts. Corn grain, as the most representative first generation bioethanol raw material, will be the first considered example for the analysis of the NEB. In this case, the coproducts are distillers' dry grain with solubles (DDGS) and straw. The former is generally used as for animal feeding, but can also be used for power generation for the production process, as can straw [90].

Corn grain ethanol production has been reported to present a positive NEB in many studies [10], indicating that the energy contained in the biofuel exceeded the fossil energy required for its production. The average calculated NEBs was 1.25 both considering as outputs the coproduct and the biofuel or only the biofuel [7, 10, 91, 92]. The main contribution in the inputs part was the facility energy use, with the 50% of the energy require-ments. Fertilizers and pesticides consumption as well as the fossil fuel use supposed about a 10% each. Transportation, storage after harvest, which is often neglected although being very important, and household energy use demand entailed a 6% each. These results were calculated including all the above-mentioned inputs, specifically farm machinery production and pro-cessing facilities. Thus, they counter the assertion that including all ener-getic costs of producing causes negative NEB values for bioethanol [93, 94]. Nevertheless, what it can be highlighted the small NEB associated to this type of first generation ethanol, which provided about 25% more energy than the one required to produce it. This fact can be explained by the high-energy requirement associated to the corn production.

Other type of first generation bioethanol raw materials, from the sugar-type plants are the sugar beet, that has been reported to present NEB between 0.5 and 2.5 [95, 96] and the sugarcane, with a minimum NEB reported of 1.1 [97] and a maximum one of 11. This difference is explained by the use of cogeneration to improve the process efficiency and the use of the coproducts which, in this case are the pulp and leaves are used as animal feed or occa-sionally fertilizer [98].

Talking about second generation bioethanol, it is in most of the cases, the energy ratios are higher for lignocellulosic bioethanol than the ones for first generation bioethanol, due to use of lignin instead of fossil fuels for process energy. Other coproducts generated in this process are acetic acid, furfu-ral and xylitol, that are considered as high value coproducts for subsequent applications but they do not contribute in the potential energy and GHG emissions and, thus, have not been considered here [99].

Wheat straw presents a NEB of 2.5 without considering cogenera-tion and between 6.6 and 9.2 when cogeneration is included [100]. Wood species have been reported to have a NEB between 2 and 8 [101]; agri-cultural wastes an average NEB of 2.5, similar value than the one of the Switchgrass [10].

Regarding the emissions, in general, the published literature agrees in the significant reduction of bioethanol emissions compared to fossil fuels. Nevertheless, it is important to consider the N_2O emissions associated to the use of fertilizers. Regarding the environmental impacts of corn based first generation bioethanol, the fertilizer use, expressed as g per NEB in MJ, was found to be 7. In the case of pesticides, the quantity was 0.1 g/ NEB in MJ. The associated greenhouse gases emissions were 84.9 g CO_2

Eq./MJ, when the gasoline ones are 96.9 g CO_2 Eq/MJ [7, 94]. The comparison with this fossil fuel indicated that the production and use of corn grain ethanol releases about 87–88% of the net GHG emissions associated to the production and combustion of an energetically equivalent amount of gasoline [7, 102]. Nevertheless, the E85 fuel, a mixture of bioethanol and gasoline, 85/15% V/V, presents in its combustion, higher emission contents of carbon monoxide (CO), volatile organic compounds (VOCS), sulfur and nitrogen oxides and particulate matter with an aerodynamic diameter smaller than 10 μm (PM10) than gasoline per unit of energy released upon combustion [103].

Different raw materials present differences in GHG emissions at the same blend proportion. Agricultural residues, such as corn stover and wheat straw, offer the highest GHG reduction per distance traveled, with reductions between 82 and 91% for E100 [10]. Other second-generation bioethanol raw materials, such as switch grass and wood have been reported reductions between 53–93% and 50–62%, respectively, mainly due to the fact that these residues would be decomposed to CO_2 by natural processes. [10].

To sum up, it could be concluded that, excluding coproduct credits, first-generation ethanol, from corn-grain and sugar beet, produced greater GHG emissions and was less energy efficient than second-generation ethanol [7, 99].

12.3   BIODIESEL

Biodiesel, or fatty acid methyl ester, is a mixture of long-chain fatty acids monoalkyl esters obtained from different renewable lipid feedstocks, such as virgin or used vegetable oil (both nonedible and edible) and animal fats [104]. The similarity in its physical properties to diesel fuels allows its use in diesel engines, pure or mixed with diesel from fossil sources with little or no engine modifications [105]. This fact has pushed its commercial value in the automobile markets of many parts of the world as Europe, America (mainly in US, Brazil) or Asia (mainly in Japan and India) [106]. Numerous advantages are attributed to this biofuel, including its renewable nature, biodegradability [107], better combustion behavior (higher combustion efficiency, cetane number, flash point and better lubrication) [108, 109].

Biodiesel feedstocks are divided in different categories. First generation biodiesel is made from virgin edible oils, waste oils (oils already used in cooking and no longer suitable for human consumption [110]), animal fats and nonedible oils. Depending on the location characteristics (climate, soil conditions, etc.) the most used vegetal species of the virgin edible oils group are rapeseed and sunflower (used mainly in Europe), soybean (used mainly in America) and palm oil (used mainly in South Asia) [111], whereas the most commonly used nonedible oils are jatropha, neem castor or tall oils [110, 112]. Second generation biodiesel is obtained from lignocellulosic species, as woody crops, straw or energy grasses [99] and third generation biodiesel is made from microalgae [113].

Different technologies are used to obtain first, second and third generations biodiesel. First generation biodiesel is obtained via chemical processing by the transesterification reaction of the fatty acid methyl esters from vegetable oils, whereas second generation biodiesels are obtained via thermo-chemical conversion and third generation ones may be obtaind by both techno-routes. The thermo-chemical conversion, also known as biomass-to-liquids, BTL, includes a first step in which, via pyrolysis or gasification, a synthesis gas, composed mainly by CO and H_2, is produced. A subsequent Fischer–Tropsch conversion of the syngas allows the obtaining of synthetic diesel.

12.3.1   FIRST GENERATION BIODIESEL

To obtain fatty acid methyl esters from vegetable oils and, with the aim of reducing the density of the latter, transesterification, which involves the oil alcoholysis, is the widest used method. Triglycerides are firstly converted to diglycerides and then to monoglycerides, which are subsequently converted to glycerol [114]. Figure 12.5 presents a scheme of the overall reaction of transesterification for biodiesel production from vegetable oil.

In this process, excess of alcohol is used to shift the equilibrium of the reaction to the product side and increase the yield of biodiesel. Nevertheless, to limit alcohol consumption due to the higher production cost that bigger quantities would entail, different catalysts are used in the transesterification reactions. Catalyst is an important factor that may influence the economic feasibility and environmental impact of the entire biodiesel production process [115].

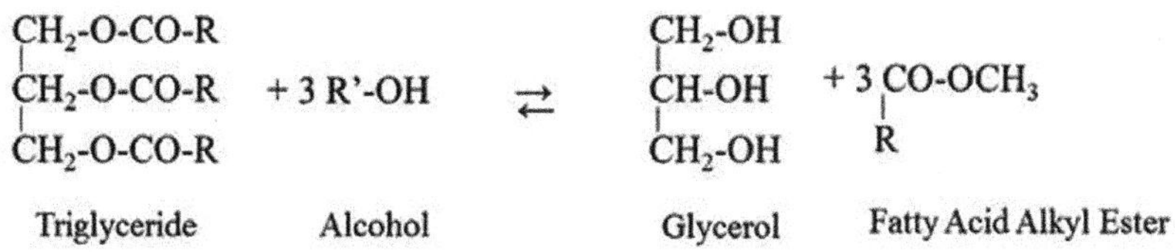

CH₂-O-CO-R   CH₂-OH
| |
CH₂-O-CO-R   + 3 R'-OH   ⇌   CH-OH   + 3 CO-OCH₃
| | |
CH₂-O-CO-R   CH₂-OH   R

Triglyceride   Alcohol   Glycerol   Fatty Acid Alkyl Ester

FIGURE 12.5 Overall reaction of transesterification for biodiesel production from vegetable oil.

The most common catalyst type is homogeneous alkaline catalyst, typically NaOH or KOH. Acid catalysts are also used but they need higher reaction temperatures and times. When working with alkaline catalysts in a transesterification reaction, it is very important not to have the presence of water, as its mixture with free fatty acids that are in the composition of the original vegetable oil could induce a saponification process in which the free fatty acid reacts with the alkaline catalyst to form soap and water. Furthermore, the triglyceride itself can also react with the alcohol to produce soap and glycerol. Figure 12.6 presents a scheme of the saponification reactions that may occur in the transesterification of vegetable oil in the presence of water and alkaline catalysts. The dissolved soap in the glycerol phase increases the solubility of the methyl ester in the glycerol and makes difficult the subsequent separation process [116].

Other less spread option would be enzymatic catalysis. The former is not yet commercially viable because of it is not economically competitive due to the high cost of the enzyme, long reaction times required as well as an unfavorable reaction yields in comparison to the alkaline catalyst [117]. Finally, an option that would allow avoiding the use of catalysts is the supercritical alcohol transesterification technology, that uses supercritical conditions to favor the mass transfer among the triglyceride and alcohol to obtain a homogeneous phase. Nevertheless, at the moment, the costs associated to this energy demanding technology cannot be faced at industrial scale [118].

After the transesterification reaction has finished, the mixture of biodiesel, glycerol and the excess of alcohol must be properly separated and the obtained products purified. In fact, ineffective biodiesel separation and purification may cause severe diesel engine problems, such as plugging of filters, coking on injectors, oil ring sticking, engine knocking and thickening of lubricant oil [115]. Separation and purification stages, including biodiesel

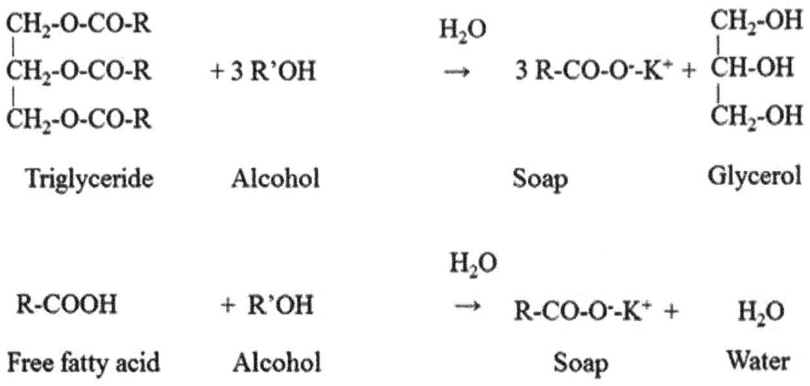

$$
\begin{array}{llll}
\text{CH}_2\text{-O-CO-R} & & \text{H}_2\text{O} & \text{CH}_2\text{-OH} \\
| & & & | \\
\text{CH}_2\text{-O-CO-R} & + 3 \text{ R'OH} & \rightarrow \quad 3 \text{ R-CO-O}^-\text{-K}^+ + & \text{CH-OH} \\
| & & & | \\
\text{CH}_2\text{-O-CO-R} & & & \text{CH}_2\text{-OH}
\end{array}
$$

| Triglyceride | Alcohol | Soap | Glycerol |

$$
\begin{array}{llll}
 & & \text{H}_2\text{O} & \\
\text{R-COOH} & + \text{ R'OH} & \rightarrow \quad \text{R-CO-O}^-\text{-K}^+ + & \text{H}_2\text{O} \\
\text{Free fatty acid} & \text{Alcohol} & \text{Soap} & \text{Water}
\end{array}
$$

FIGURE 12.6 Saponification reactions that may occur in the transesterification process of vegetable oil with an alkaline catalyst in presence of water.

purification, glycerol separation, alcohol recovery and catalyst neutralization entail over 60–80% of the total cost of a transesterification process plant [119]. The average energy used to produce a gallon of biodiesel from virgin vegetable oils is 3,184 BTUs. Energy use among plants that use blends of virgin oil and recycled or reclaimed fats and oils varies, as does the composition of these feedstocks. Taking into account all of these variations, the overall industry average for all feedstocks and all production technologies is 4,192 BTUs per gallon of biodiesel [120].

12.3.1.1 From Oil Seeds

In the biodiesel production process from oilseeds, the main generated coproducts are rapemeal (to be used as animal feed or for cofiring), glycerine and straw, that can be used for energy obtaining as well [121]. NEBs of first generation biodiesel increased substantially when coproduct credits were included, with average values improved by 35–50%. For soybeans made biodiesel, the average calculated NEB was 1.93 considering the coproducts and 3.67 considering only the biofuel energy balance [7]. The main contribution in the inputs part was the facility and household energy uses, which accounted for the 50% of the energy requirements. Oilseed rape biodiesel has been reported to present a NEB of 1.56 and 3.44 without considering the coproducts, and considering glycerine and rapemeal as coproducts, respectively [99].

In the case of palm oil, the composition of the fresh fruit bunches (FFB) is about 20% of palm oil and 1.7% of palm kernel oil. The generated coproducts are palm oil mill effluent (POME), with the 50%, empty fruit bunches (EFB), with a 22%, fibers (13%), shells (6% and kernel oil cake (3.5%) [122]. The use of these coproducts for steam and power generation allows palm oil refining to be self sufficient and to present a fossil inputs and their respective GHG emissions negligible [123]. The NEB associated to palm oil biodiesel production was found to be 5.4 [124].

Regarding the GHG emissions, 49 g/NEB in MJ where attributed to biodiesel from soybeans, when the diesel from fossil resources contributed with 82.3 g/NEB in MJ. This comparison entails that GHG emissions of soybean biodiesel are 59% those of diesel fuel [7]. Furthermore, low levels of soybeans made biodiesel blended into diesel reduce emissions of VOC, CO, PM10, and sulfur oxides during combustion, and biodiesel blends show reduced life-cycle emissions for CO, sulfur oxides relative to diesel [125]. The emissions associated to the combustion of this type of biodiesel presented lower contents in several major air pollutants, and a minimal impact on human and environmental health through N, P, and pesticide release [7]. Oilseed rape biodiesel GHG emissions where found to be in the range of 40 to 55 g CO_2 Eq./MJ, depending if coproducts where considered (lower emissions ratio) or not [99].

Palm oil biodiesel production resulted in low emissions due to the use of coproducts to produce power and the use of green manure. Due to the manual harvesting, low the diesel consumption was required for the bunches transportation to the processing unit, accounting for 14% of the total GHG emissions. The industrial and agricultural phases contributed with 21% and 64%, respectively, of the total LCA emissions, being the former main significant contribution the methanol production while the latter biggest contribution came from nitrogen. The total life cycle emissions associated to palm oil biodiesel production were 1437 kg CO_2 Eq. /ha·year considering coproducts allocation and 1900 kg CO_2 Eq. /ha·year if allocation was not considered [124].

12.3.1.2   From Recycled Vegetable Oil

Biodiesel made from used vegetable oil presents the lowest GHG emissions and the better NEB among all biodiesel types, due to its residual nature, as its production does not have emissions or energy input allocated. While this simple comparison tells a clear story, the impact of coproduct utilization on these production chains clearly needs to be investigated to provide a complete assessment [99]. In this case, the only coproduct generated is glycerine and it is not clear how the consideration or not of this by-product may influence its NEB and emissions [126]. The average calculated NEB was about 7, both considering and excluding the coproduct contribution. Regarding the emissions, 11.2 g CO_2 Eq./MJ where attributed to this type of biodiesel combustion [99].

12.3.2 SECOND GENERATION BIODIESEL

Second generation biodiesel, also known as synthetic diesel, obtained by the thermochemical technology, known as biomass to liquids (BTL) presents, in general, better properties than the first generation one, for example a higher cetane content, absence of sulfur and low aromatic compound content, which mean improved combustion behavior and fewer GHG emissions [127]. BTL process has two stages: biomass gasification and fuel synthesis from the resulting syngas, via Fischer Tropsch reaction. Depending on the selected synthesis method, different gaseous (dimethylether, methanol or ethanol) or liquid (diesel and kerosene) fuels may be produced. Figure 12.7 (adapted from Ref. [128]) presents the Fischer Tropsch synthesis (FTS) process for the obtaining of liquid biofuels from lignocellulosic biomass by thermochemical conversion.

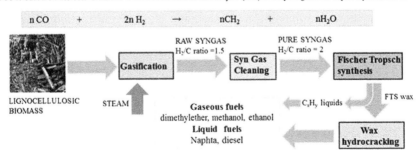

Fischer Tropsch synthesis (FTS)

FTS is based on the conversion of a misture of carbón monoxyde (CO) and hydrogen into liquid hydrocarbons.

FIGURE 12.7   Scheme of the Fischer Tropsch synthesis (FTS) process for the obtaining of liquid biofuels from lignocellulosic biomass by thermochemical conversion. Adapted from [128].

The thermochemical conversion process is a considerably mature technology that has been used for decades, focusing on coal-to-liquids and more recently natural gas-to-liquids. [129]. In the BTL process, all lignocellulosic biomass components (cellulose, hemicelluloses and lignin) are converted into synthesis gas, allowing the generation of 6.5 GJ/t of energy carrier in the form of biofuels per 1 dry Mgrn of biomass. Original biomass energy potential is about 20 GJ/Mgr, which means that the overall biomass to biofuel conversion efficiency is around 35% [130]. Although this efficiency may appear relatively low, the process overall efficiency is improved by including surplus heat, power and coproduct generation in the total system. Production of second-generation biodiesel does not generate any significant coproducts [99].

NEBs reported in this category include woody crops biodiesel, with about 2.5 and Miscanthus biodiesel with about 5, which are considerable higher than the values presented by first generation biodiesel, with an average value of 1.6. Published values of emissions associated to the combustion of these biodiesel types where 18.8 g CO_2 Eq./MJ in the case of woody crops, 37.4 g CO_2 Eq./MJ for Miscanthus [131], 29.6 and 6.9 g CO_2 Eq./MJ for short-rotation coppice willow and poplar, respectively and 4.8 g CO_2 Eq./MJ for forestry residue [132]. First generation biodiesel, in general, was found to be less energy efficient and responsible of the emission of greater GHG quantities than second-generation biodiesel when compared excluding coproduct credits. The former group produced average GHG emissions of 55 g CO_2 Eq/MJ, compared with 22 and 36 g CO_2 Eq/MJ, for biodiesel from woody crops and energy grasses, respectively [131].

12.3.3 THIRD GENERATION BIODIESEL

Third generation biodiesel is produced from microalgae crops. Some published works agrees in the good results presented by these raw materials as a source for renewable energy producing, based on their high growths rate, they quantities of polysaccharides (sugars) and triacylglycerides (fats) they can provide, depending on the species and the opportunity to develop a completely closed algae-to-biofuel cycle [133]. Nevertheless, other studies in the literature find that the production of biofuels from microalgae appears to be too costly as the process is quite energy and water demanding [134–136].

Microalgae can be converted into energy both by thermochemical processes (to generate oil and gas), and by using biochemical processes (to produce ethanol and biodiesel) [137].

Nevertheless, in order to represent an actual alternative for fuels obtaining at industrial scale, some aspects of microalgae production should be carefully analyzed: the energy and carbon balance, environmental impacts and the production cost [138]. Indeed, some studies report that the energy demand needed for the provision of biofuels from microalgae was found to be responsible for no significant reduction in GHG emissions compared with fossil fuels or even for a high increase in emissions [139].

There are two main systems for microalgae cultivating, raceway pond systems and photobioreactors (PBRs). The former is composed by a closed loop oval shallow channel (0.25–0.4 m deep) open to the air and mixed with a paddle wheel to circulate the water and prevent sedimentation. PBRs, a more expensive and energy demanding option, are designed as a closed transparent array of tubes or plates in which microalge circulates from a central reservoir. This technology allows a better control of the algae grow with about 4–5 times higher yields [138].

Algae production can be performed in marginal land, which is an advantage in terms of land use and location. In the case of raceway pond systems, as they have to be shallow to let the light in and keep the efficiency, they need relatively flat terrain, which limits the land availability [140].

Energy balances of third generation biodiesel will be determined by the energy used for cultivation, harvesting and drying operations. The cost and carbon footprint of electricity can significantly affect the economics and environmental footprints of algal diesel, respectively [141]. Thus, to achieve a positive energy balance, aspects that would need to be addressed include the energy required for pumping, the embodied energy required for construction, the embodied energy in fertilizer and the energy required for drying and dewatering. The last point is especially decisive due to the high-energy requirement of microalgae dewatering. To improve the energy balance of this step two different strategies are used: one is the dry route, based on using low energy consuming drying techniques to improve the dewatering efficiency; the other one is the wet route, in which no drying process is done and the oil extraction occurs in the water phase [142]. Figure 12.8 presents the schemes of the dry route (a) and the wet route (b). In the dry route, transesterification is used as the converting technology as it is commonly used in the production of the first generation biodiesels, while in the

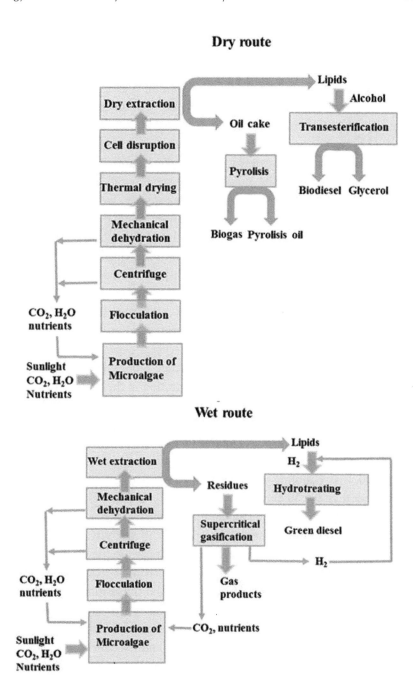

FIGURE 12.8 Third generation production from microalgae by (a) dry route and (b) wet route. Adapted from Ref. [138].

wet route, the supercritical gasification generates the hydrogen necessary for the hydrotreating process that produces the green diesel.

Energy balances for biodiesel, in the case of pond systems, have been reported to be between 1 and 2 [142–147]. In this case, the most important contributions to the energy demand in the cultivation came from the electricity required to circulate the culture (energy fraction 22%–79%) and the embodied energy in pond construction (energy fraction 8%–70%). Another important parameter observed was the energy embodied in the nitrogen fertilizer (energy fraction for the cultivation phase 6%–40%) [138].

The NEBs of the PBR systems, on the contrary, were all smaller than 1, meaning that these systems consume more energy than they produce [143–146]. The best performing PBR was found to be the flat-plate system, which outperformed the tubular configuration achieving a large illumination surface area and low oxygen build-up [139]. In the case of cultivation in PBR systems, the energy used to pump the culture medium and overcome frictional losses accounted for the majority of energy consumption (energy fraction for tubular PBRs: 86%–92%, energy fraction for flat plat PBRs: 22%) [138].

Results of pond systems using the dry route reported NEBs between 1.2 and 1.5, depending on the nutrients concentration in the media [147]. It was observed that culturing, dewatering and lipid conversion were the main the energy demanding steps of the dry route. In the wet route, NEBs between 1.2 and 1.4 were obtained [147]. In summary, compared to petroleum diesel and corn ethanol, microalgal fuels were found to be energy efficient with a NEB of 1.2–1.50, that, coupling waste heat into the process, could rise up to 2.38, value higher than the NEB of the first generation biodiesel [142]. This figure refers to open ponds technology and includes the recycling cost of nutrients.

Regarding the environmental impact of this activity, water management, carbon dioxide handling and nutrient supply are the main factors that could constrain the system viability. Algae cultivation requires the addition of nutrients, primarily nitrogen, phosphorus and potassium. Fertilization is compulsory as the dry algal mass fraction consists of about 7% nitrogen and 1% phosphorus. GHG emissions were mainly associated with electricity consumption for pumping and mixing and heat for the drying stage. Emissions associated with algal biomass production in raceway ponds are in most of the presented studies, comparable with the ones from the cultivation and production stages of rape methyl ester biodiesel (45 g CO_2 Eq./MJ) [140, 143, 144, 146]. Only one study has presented higher values of about

150 g CO_2 Eq./MJ [142]. Production in PBRs, however, presented emissions values comprised between 100 and 500 (45 g CO_2 Eq./MJ, greater than conventional fossil diesel ones (84 g CO_2 Eq./MJ) [138].

12.4   OTHER BIOFUELS

12.4.1   BIOBUTANOL

Biobutanol is an aliphatic saturated alcohol with the molecular formula of $C_4H_{10}O$ that can be used as an intermediate in chemical synthesis and as a solvent for a wide variety of chemical and textile industry applications. Moreover, it has been considered as a potential fuel or fuel additive as it can be used directly or blended with gasoline or diesel without any vehicle retrofit and supplied through the existing gasoline pipes [148]. Biobutanol is one of the second-generation biofuels, superior to bioethanol, due to higher energy content, lower Reid vapor pressure, easy blending with gasoline at any ratio and ease in transportation. Although bioethanol has acquired enough attention from the transportation industry as the current commercially available liquid fuel for transportation, biobutanol possesses has emerged as an attractive alternative biofuel and has the potential for replacing bioethanol and biodiesel in the fuel market estimated to be around $247 billion by 2020 [149, 150].

Biobutanol can be obtained from renewable resources (biomass) by the acetone-butanol-ethanol fermentation; this process is called the ABE production [151]. In 1861, Louis Pasteur discovered the bacterial butanol production and after that, the fermentative ABE production flourished specially in the beginning of the 20th century. At that time, the research was focused on producing acetone, amyl alcohol or butanol by fermentation to use them for the manufacture of synthetic rubber. However, the desired product of the fermentation process (especially during the First World War) was acetone, while butanol was considered only a byproduct [150]. It was during the oil crisis in the 70's and the rising costs of petrochemicals when the production of biobutanol as fuel grabbed the attention of researchers. Nevertheless, the efforts were most focused in bioethanol production because the popular yeast fermentation process produced 0.37 liters of ethanol whereas the ABE fermentation process managed only 0.19 liters of butanol from a kg of corn [152]. However, nowadays the use of modern fermentation processes has considerably improved the yield of butanol (see Figure 12.9).

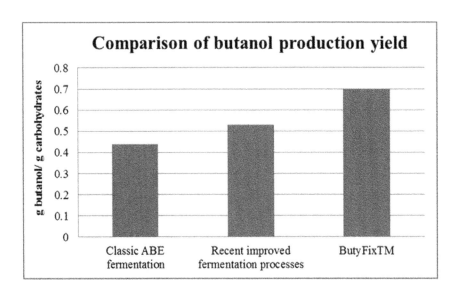

FIGURE 12.9 Comparison of biobutanol production yield by different fermentation processes [153, 154].

There are a number of biotechnology companies around the world dedicated to provide strains and process solutions for ABE fermentation for industrial customers. Various inventions have been reported as well for the biological production of butanol, maintaining its competitiveness in efficiency, economy, and production scale [152]. Butanol has been traditionally produced by anaerobic fermentation of sugar substrates using various species of *solventogenic clostridia* [153]. These species are known to have the capability of using simple and complex sugars, including both pentose and hexose, as well as CO_2, H_2 and CO [154]. However, butanol toxicity to the fermenting microorganisms limits its concentration in the fermentation broth, resulting in low butanol yields and a high cost for butanol recovery from the dilute solutions. Otherwise, although research on the genetics, fermentation, and downstream processing has progressed significantly in recent years, the solventogenic clostridia are not able to efficiently hydrolyze fiber-rich agricultural residues. For this reason, agricultural biomass must be pretreated and hydrolyzed to simple sugars using different methods [153]. The traditional biobutanol production process is shown in Figure 12.10.

Employing lignocellulosic biomass (which is much cheaper than corn or other food-feedstock), the cost of the biobutanol production process is

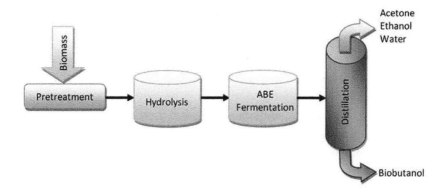

FIGURE 12.10   Simplified flow diagram of biobutanol production.

significantly reduced, so it can be more competitive. Thus, great deal of effort has been dedicated for the development of microorganisms that can efficiently hydrolyze starch and lignocellulosic substrates. This way, some studies have been carried out employing hyperamylolytic *Clostridium beijerinckii* BA101, which has the capability to use starch and accumulate higher concentrations of butanol (17–21 g/L) in the fermentation medium [155].

In addition, in order to improve the efficiency in butanol production by ABE fermentation process, some innovative strategies have been recently developed [156]. On the one hand, much research effort has been exerted to improve the batch performance of butanol fermentation by applying various fermentation strategies. One of those strategies is to perform the fermentation in continuous system constantly removing the inhibitory compounds produced. Furthermore, application of immobilized cell culture and cell recycle reactors is known to increase reactor productivity 40–50 times as compared to batch reactors. An increase in productivity results in the reduction of process volume and reactor size, thus improving process economics [157]. On the other hand, alternative economically feasible technologies to classic distillation-which is a very expensive process due to biobutanol low concentration-, have been developed to recover the produced biobutanol. Gas stripping, ionic liquids, liquid-liquid extraction, pervaporation and supercritical extraction are the new downstream technologies that are under research in order to improve and to reduce the cost of the biobutanol recovery [152, 158, 159].

Combining all the upstream and downstream new strategies, a highly efficient biobutanol production process can be developed. An efficient integration of all the process steps along with reduction in waste generation and water requirements will further promote the success of ligoncellulosic biomass butanol plant. The commercial exploitation of the by-products that are formed or can be produced during the whole process would provide a hand in increasing market incursion of butanol. Briefly summing up, bioscience and bioengineering together can set a step forward towards successful industrial biobutanol production [160].

The gas natural and electricity consumptions of the biobutanol production process are, respectively, 32.2 MJ/m^3 and 7 kWh/L. These quantities includes the requirements for the whole life cycle process: the manufacture of fertilizer and farming machinery, raw material farming operations, fertilizers, lime, herbicides and pesticides application, harvest, transport to the fuel production facilities, biochemical processing for fuel production and liquid fuel transportation to refueling stations [161]. The use of corn butanol could achieve substantial fossil energy savings (39%–56%) when compared with the use of gasoline. Biobutanol production presented a positive energy balance of about 3,6 [162].

GHG total emissions of biobutanol process are composed mainly by 58% in weight by CO_2, followed by N_2O with a 38% (associated with fertilizer application at the corn farming stage) and remaining CH_4 with less than 4%. The global emissions were found to be lower that the equivalent ones from gasoline combustion. Vehicles fueled by biobutanol achieved reductions of 32%–48% in GHG emissions relative to gasoline-fueled vehicles [163].

12.4.2   BIOGAS

Waste-to-bioenergy technologies involving biological treatment of livestock waste have been

longer used to convert organic wastes into methane biogas. Anaerobic digestion (AD) involves the breakdown of complex organic wastes by a community of anaerobic microorganisms to generate, mainly, methane (CH_4) and carbon dioxide (CO_2) and other minor components as water, hydrogen sulfide, nitrogen and oxygen, as well as ammonia and other organic components in very low quantities. AD process is formed by three stages: hydrolysis, fermentation and methanogenesis. During hydrolysis the present complex compounds are broken down into soluble components, to be susceptible of being fermented by acidogenic and acetogenic bacteria to be converted into intermediate products: alcohols, acetic acid, other volatile fatty acids, and gas containing H_2 and CO_2. In the following step, methanogens metabolize these intermediate products into CH_4 (65–75%), CO_2 (25–40%) and other associated gases [164]. The overall performance of an AD system is highly dependent on different variables as pH, temperature, the composition of feedstock, the organic loading rate or hydraulic retention time [165]. Temperature is a very sensitive parameter, as it deeply affects the metabolic activities of the microorganisms that control the rate of digestion and methane production. There are three common temperature ranges for anaerobic digestion: low temperature ranges, or psychrophilic, under 20°C; mesophilic range, with temperatures within 25–38°C; and a temperature range of 48–58°C, named thermophilic [164].

Traditionally, mainly sewage animal manure or sludge was used to generate biogas but these single sourced AD systems have been found to present low energy efficiency due to the structural and nutritional limitation of these feedstocks. Co-digestion of multiple sources was hence introduced to improve AD performance of biogas production. [166]. Many different substrates are susceptible of being used for this proposal: crops and grasses, harvest residues, manure, industrial organic waste, by-products and waste from horticulture and landscape management, municipal organic waste. In the biogas composition, the presence of carbon dioxide reduces significantly its calorific value, whereas the minor components, as NH_3 and H_2S, may lead to critical operational problems, like corrosion and clogging. This means that, in order to obtain a higher quality combustible gas, known as biomethane, a cleaning step is required for the removing of most of that carbon dioxide and of the minor components [167].

In most agricultural biogas plants, cogeneration is used to obtain heat and electricity from biogas. The heat consumption in the biogas plants is usually met with the own heat generation whereas electricity from the grid needs to be consumed, as the own produced electricity does not met the requirements. In Figure 12.11, a flow chart of the production of biogas and biomethane as well as the cogeneration of heat and electricity from the biogas is presented.

In the analysis of the NEB of the AD process, the highest energy consumption is associated to the heating of the digester, which is needed to generate favorable conditions for microbes. Published results of NEB vary between 3 and 6, which means that the obtained biogas presents a considerably higher energy potential than the energy required for its production

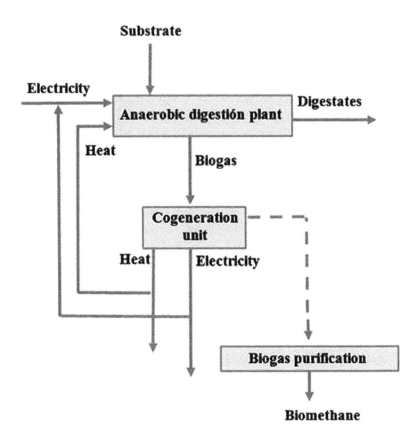

FIGURE 12.11   Simplified flow diagram of biogas production.

[94, 168]. The NEB associated to the use of organic waste as raw material should include the gas refinement stages (dehydration, removal of CO_2
and trace gases) and gas compression, which are highly energy consuming.
Furthermore, the yield and the composition of the obtained biogas varies
considerably, which makes its commercial use is difficult.

Regarding the GHG emissions of the two main gases produced in an AD
plant, carbon dioxide and methane, the latter is a highly potential greenhouse
gas and, thus, the release of methane during biogas production is of major
interest considering the environmental performance of biogas production.

The carbon footprint of the transport service with biogas from the new
established inventories amounts to between 95 g CO_2 Eq /km (biogas from
grass refinery) and 163 gCO_2 Eq /km (beet residues) [169]. The biggest carbon

footprint of biogas is comparable with natural gas fuels whereas those bio-gas types made form substrates with the lowest carbon footprint enable a reduction of 54% of GHG emissions compared to transportation with a petrol fuelled passen-ger car [169]. CO_2 emissions are the dominant participant in the carbon footprint of transportation with conventional fuels during the car operation; during the biogas production and purification steps, CH_4 is the main component of the emissions, whereas N_2O emissions prevail in the substrate cultivation step [169]. Beet residue was the raw material, which presented the highest emissions within the different biogas types, due to the low methane yield of this substrate, which results in a higher amount of beet residues that is required to produce one m^3 of biogas. This fact means that the electricity and heat consumption for its handling in the biogas plant and its transportation entails higher GHG emissions compared to biogas from other substrates [169].

12.5 CONCLUSIONS

Among all the biofuels, bioethanol is the most employed and studied one. The current most extended production of bioethanol usually involves starches and simple sugars derived from sources such as sugar cane and corn. The methodology of bioethanol production from these substrates is optimized and the fermentation is highly efficient. Thus, all the new efforts of are focused on employing new lignocellulosic substrates which are more abundant, cheaper and do not compete with the food supply. In the so-called second-generation bioethanol, pretreatment of the feedstock is the key-point, and different techniques (physical, chemical, physicochemical and biological pretreatments) are presently under development in order to increase the efficiency of the process.

Studies of ethanol and biodiesel NEBs suggest that, in general, biofuels would provide greater benefits if their biomass feedstocks production had a lower agricultural energy input as well as lower fertilizers and pesticides demand, and were converted into fuels by lower energy technologies. The biofuels cost competitiveness would improve by using low-input biomass or agricultural residues to provide energy for the biofuel conversion pro-cess. For second-generation ethanol, the use of the lignin fraction to pro-vide energy could improve the efficiency of biofuel-processing plants. This biofuel presents, in general, better NEB results than first generation one. In total, agricultural and forestry residues-based biofuels have the potential to provide much higher NEB ratios and much lower environmental impacts per net energy gain than food-based biofuels. On the other hand, the best case scenarios comparison for first and second-generation fuels indicated that the lowest calculated emissions processes were the second-generation fuels, with average emissions below 20 g CO_2 Eq./MJ, excepting in the case of biodiesel produced from straw/grasses where GHG emissions were relatively high and variable. Furthermore, options about coproduct use and heat and power cogeneration can have a significant impact on the overall GHG balance.

In the case of biobutanol, the new research is concentrated on upstream and downstream strategies to make its production process more competitive. On the one hand, new microorganisms that can efficiently hydrolyze starch and lignocellulosic substrates are being developed, like *Clostridium beijerinckii* BA101. On the other hand, more efficient ways of recovering the produced biobutanol are being studied, such as, gas stripping, ionic liquids, liquid-liquid extraction, pervaporation and supercritical extraction. It could be said that using biogas, especially when obtained from waste substrates, as vehicle fuels presents some benefits regarding the consumption of nonrenewable energy resources and the associated GHG emissions when compared to conventional fuels. In fact, new approaches on green chemistry era being developed for the use of excreting products which can be converted to final products without the cost of fertilization, mixing, extraction and refinement [170].

Finally, as a final conclusion, it must be said that the NEB values find in the literature and mentioned along this chapter, are usually calculated in optimal conditions, for example, they may not take into account that energy crops prevent land rotation and the fertility of the soils declines after long-term usage in mono culture, or that a perfect process control is not usually reached. This fact may entail that the mentioned values could be lower and, thus, when comparing their impact in the environment and the one associated to fossil fuels, the positive difference may be not so evident.

KEYWORDS

- **biobutanol**
- **biodiesel**
- **bioethanol**

- **biogas**
- **efficiency**
- **greenhouse gases emissions**
- **net energy balance**

REFERENCES

1. United Nations Conference on Climate Change, COP 21. http://www.cop21.gouv.fr/en/ (accessed February 2, 2016).

2. Mata, T., Martins, A., & Caetano, N., (2010). Microalgae for biodiesel production and other applications: a review. *Renew. Sust. Energ. Rev., 14*, 217–232.

3. Srirangan, K., Akawi, L., Moo-Young, M., & Chou, C., (2012). Towards sustainable production of clean energy carriers from biomass resources. *Appl. Energ., 100*, 172–186.

4. Butterbach-Bahl, K., & Kiese, R., (2013). Biofuel production on the margins. *Nature, 493*, 483–485.

5. Chu, S., & Majumdar, A., (2012)Opportunities and challenges for a sustainable energy future. *Nature, 488*, 294–303.

6. EC, Energy Road map 2050. Communication from the Commission to the European Parliament, the Council, the European Economic and Social Committee and the Committee of the Regions, COM (2011) 885 final. 2011. http://ec.europa.eu/smart-regulation/impact/ia_carried_out/ docs/ ia_2011/sec_2011_1565_en.pdf (accessed Feb. 5, 2016).

7. Hill, J., Nelson, E., Tilman, D., Polasky, S., & Tiffany, D., (2006). Environmental, economic, and energetic costs and benefits of biodiesel and ethanol biofuels. Proceedings of the National Academy of Science of the United States of America, PNAS. Online. *103*(30), 11206–11210. www.pnas.org/cgi/doi/10.1073/pnas.0604600103 (accessed January 23, 2016).

8. Balat, M., Balat, H., & Öz, C., (2008). Progress in bioethanol processing. *Prog. Energy Combust. Sci., 34*, 551–573.

9. Wiloso, E. I., Heijungs, R., & de Snoo, G. R., (2012). LCA of second generation bioethanol: A review and some issues to be resolved for good LCA practice. *Renewable Sustainable Energy Rev., 16*, 5295–5308.

10. Morales, M., Quintero, J., Conejeros, R., & Aroca, G., (2015). Life cycle assessment of lignocellulosic bioethanol: Environmental impacts and energy balance. *Renewable Sustainable Energy Rev., 42*, 1349–1361.

11. Balat, M., (2007). Global bio-fuel processing and production trends. *Energy Explor. Exploit, 25*, 195–218.

12. Baeyens, J., Kang, Q., Appels, L., Dewil, R., Lv, Y., & Tan, T., (2015). Challenges and opportunities in improving the production of bio-ethanol. *Prog. Energy Combust. Sci., 47*, 60–88.

13. Gupta, A., & Verma, J. P., (2015). Sustainable bio-ethanol production from agro-residues: A review. *Renewable Sustainable Energy Rev., 41*, 550–567.

14. U. S. Department of Energy. Energy Efficiency & Renewable Energy. Alternative Fuels Data Center. www.afdc.energy.gov/data/ (accessed February 24, 2016).

15. Karmee, S. K., (2016). Liquid biofuels from food waste: Current trends, prospect and limitation. *Renewable Sustainable Energy Rev., 53*, 945–953.

16. Chhetri, A. B., Watts, K. C., & Islam, M. R., (2008). Waste cooking oil as an alternate feedstock for biodiesel production. *Energies, 1*, 3–18.

17. Searchinger, T., Heimlich, R., Houghton, R. A., Dong, F., Elobeid, A., Fabiosa, J., et al., (2008). Use of, U. S. Croplands for Biofuels Increases Greenhouse Gases Through Emissions from Land-Use Change. *Science, 319*, 1238–1240.

18. Lennartsson, P. R., Erlandsson, P., & Taherzadeh, M. J., (2014). Integration of the first and second generation bioethanol processes and the importance of by-products. *Bioresour. Technol., 165*, 3–8.

19. Li, Z., Liu W, Gu Z, Li C, Hong Y, & Cheng, L., (2015). The effect of starch concentration on the gelatinization and liquefaction of corn starch. *Food Hydrocolloid. 18*, 189–96.

20. Presečki, A. V., Blažević, Z. F., & Vasić-Rački, D., (2013). Mathematical modeling of maize starch liquefaction catalyzed by α-amylases from Bacillus licheniformis: effect of calcium, pH and temperature. *Bioprocess. Biosyst. Eng., 36*, 117–126.

21. Edouard, Y., Nkomba, E. Y., van Rensburg, E., Chimphango, A. F. A., & Görgens, J. F., (2016). The influence of sorghum grain decortication on bioethanol production and quality of the distillers' dried grains with solubles using cold and conventional warm starch processing. *Bioresour. Technol., 203*, 181–189.

22. Blazek, J., & Gilbert, E. P., (2010). Effect of enzymatic hydrolysis on native starch granule structure. *Biomacromolec., 11*, 3275–3289.

23. Apar, D. K., & Özbek, B., (2005). α-Amylase inactivation during rice starch hydrolysis. *Process. Biochem., 40*, 1367–1379

24. Naik, S. N., Goud, V. V., Rout, P. K., & Dalai, A. K., (2010). Production of first and second generation biofuels: A comprehensive review. *Renewable Sustainable Energy Rev. 14*, 578–597.

25. Hahn-Hägerdal, B., Galbe, M., Gorwa-Grauslund, M. F., Lidén, G., & Zacchi, G., (2006). Bio-ethanol -the fuel of tomorrow from the residues of today. *Trends Biotechnol. 24*, 549–556.

26. Bialas, W., Szymanowska, D., & Grajek, W., (2010). Fuel ethanol production from granular corn starch using Saccharomyces cerevisiae in a long-term repeated SSF process with full stillage recycling. *Bioresour. Technol., 101*, 3126–3131.

27. Bothast, R. J., & Schlicher, M. A., (2005). Biotechnological processes for conversion of corn into ethanol. *Appl. Microbiol. Biotechnol., 67*, 19–25.

28. Cardona, C. A., & Sánchez, O. J., (2007). Fuel ethanol production: Process design trends and integration opportunities. *Bioresour. Technol., 98*, 2415–2547.

29. Shapouri, H., Duffield, J. A., & Graboski, M. S., (1995). Estimating the net energy balance of corn ethanol. U. S. Department of Agriculture, Agricultural Economic Report Number 721.

30. Pinzi, S., & Dorado, M. P., (2011). Vegetable-based feedstocks for biofuels production. In *Handbook of Biofuels Production: Processes and Technologies*; Luque, R., Campelo, J; Clark, J., Eds., Woodhead Publishing Limited: Cambridge, p. 61.

31. Guo, M., Song, W., & Buhain, J., (2015). Bioenergy and biofuels: History, status, and perspective. *Renewable Sustainable Energy Rev., 45*, 712–725.

32. Luo, L., van der Voet, E., & Huppes, G., (2009). Life cycle assessment and life cycle costing of bioethanol from sugarcane in Brazil. *Renewable Sustainable Energy Rev., 13,* 1613–1619.

33. Koçar, G., & Civaş, N., (2013). An overview of biofuels from energy crops: Current status and future prospects. *Renewable Sustainable Energy Rev., 28,* 900–916.

34. Dhaliwal, S. S., Oberoi, H. S., Sandhu, S. K., Nanda, D., Kumar, D., & Uppal, S. K., (2011). Enhanced ethanol production from sugarcane juice by galactose adaptation of a newly isolated thermotolerant strain of *Pichiakudriavzevii. Bioresour. Technol., 102,* 5968–5975.

35. Muruaga, M. L., Carvalho, K. G., Domínguez, J. M., Oliveira, R. P. S., & Perotti, N., (2016). Isolation and characterization of *Saccharomyces* species for bioethanol production from sugarcane molasses: Studies of scale up in bioreactor. *Renew. Energ., 85,* 649–656.

36. Moraes, B. S., Zaiat, M., & Bronomi, A., (2015). Anaerobic digestion of vinasse from sugarcane ethanol production in Brazil: Challenges and perspectives. *Renewable Sustainable Energy Rev., 44,* 888–903.

37. Limayem, A., & Ricke, S. C., (2012). Lignocellulosic biomass for bioethanol production: Current perspectives, potential issues and future prospects. *Prog. Energy Combust. Sci., 38,* 449–467.

38. Galadima, A., & Muraza, O., (2015). Zeolite catalysts in upgrading of bioethanol to fuels range hydrocarbons: A review. *J. Ind. Eng. Chem., 31,* 1–14.

39. Sarkar, N., Ghosh, S. K., Bannerjee, S., & Aika, K., (2012). Bioethanol production from agricultural wastes: An overview. *Renew. Energ., 37,* 19–27.

40. Wiloso, E. I., Heijungs, R., & de Snoo, G. R., (2012). LCA of second generation bioethanol: A review and some issues to be resolved for good LCA practice. *Renewable Sustainable Energy Rev., 16,* 5295–5308.

41. Hendriks, A., & Zeeman, G., (2009). Pretreatments to enhance the digestibility of lignocellulosic biomass. *Bioresour. Tehcnol., 100,* 10–18.

42. Mood, S. H., Golfeshan, A. H., Tabatabaei, M., Jouzani, G. S., Najafi, G. H., & Gholami, M., (2013). Lignocellulosic biomass to bioethanol, a comprehensive review with a focus on pretreatment. *Renewable Sustainable Energy Rev., 27,* 77–93.

43. Kubiceck, C. P., (2013). *Fungi and Lignocellulosic Biomass, 1st ed.,* Wiley-Blackwell: Ames.

44. Harun, M. Y., Radiah, A. B. D., Abidin, Z. Z., & Yunus, R., (2011). Effect of physical pretreatment on dilute acid hydrolysis of water hyacinth (*Eichhornia crassipes*). *Bioresour. Technol., 102,* 5193–5199.

45. Taherzadeh, M. J., & Karimi, K., (2008). Pretreatment of Lignocellulosic Wastes to Improve Ethanol and Biogas Production: A Review. *Int. J. Mol. Sci., 9,* 1621–1651.

46. Gírio, F. M., Fonseca, C., Carvalheiro, F., Duartem, L. C., Marques, S., & Bogel-Lukasik, R., (2010). Hemicelluloses for fuel ethanol: A review. *Bioresour. Technol., 101,* 4775–4800.

47. Alvira, P., Tomás-Pejó, E., Ballesteros, M., & Negro, M. J., (2010). Pretreatment technologies for an efficient bioethanol production process based on enzymatic hydrolysis: A review. *Bioresour. Technol., 101,* 4851–4861.

48. Noparat, P., Prasertsan, P., Thong, O-S., & Pane, X., (2015). Dilute Acid Pretreatment of Oil Palm Trunk Biomass at High Temperature for Enzymatic Hydrolysis. *Energy Procedia., 79,* 924–929.

49. Wyman, C. E., Dale, B. E., Elander, R. T., Holtzapple, M., Ladisch, M. R., & Lee, Y. Y., (2005). Coordinated development of leading biomass pretreatment technologies. *Bioresour. Technol., 96*, 1959–1966.

50. Hsu, T. C., Guo, G. L., Chen, W. H., & Hwang, W. S., (2010). Effect of dilute acid pretreatment of rice straw on structural properties and enzymatic hydrolysis. *Bioresour. Technol., 101*, 4907–4913.

51. Redding, A. P., Wang, Z., Keshwani, D. R., & Cheng, J. J., (2011). High temperature dilute acid pretreatment of coastal Bermuda grass for enzymatic hydrolysis. *Bioresour. Technol., 102*, 1415–1424.

52. Behera, S., Arora, R., Nandhagopal, N., & Kumar, S., (2014). Importance of chemical pretreatment for bioconversion of lignocellulosic biomass. *Renewable Sustainable Energy Rev., 36*, 91–106.

53. Kim, J. S., Lee, Y. Y., & Kim, T. H., (2016). A review on alkaline pretreatment technology for bioconversion of lignocellulosic biomass. *Renewable Sustainable Energy Rev., 199*, 42–48.

54. Zheng, Y., Zhao, J., Xu, & F., Li, Y., (2014). Pretreatment of lignocellulosic biomass for enhanced biogas production. *Prog. Energy Combust. Sci., 42*, 35–53.

55. Zheng, Y., Pan, Z., & Zhang, R., (2009). Overview of biomass pretreatment for cellulosic ethanol production. *Int. J. Agric. & Biol. Eng., 2*, 51–68.

56. Toledano, A., Alegría, I., & Labidi, J., (2013). Biorefining of olive tree *(Olea europea)* pruning. *Biomass BioEnergy, 59*, 503–511.

57. González-Alriols, M., Tejado, A., Blanco, M., Mondragon, I., & Labidi, J., (2009). Agricultural palm oil tree residues as raw material for cellulose, lignin and hemicelluloses production by ethylene glycol pulping process. *Chem., Eng., J. 148*, 106–114.

58. Travaini, R., Martín-Juárez, J., Lorenzo-Hernando, A., & Bolado-Rodríguez, S., (2016). Ozonolysis: An advantageous pretreatment for lignocellulosic biomass revisited. *Bioresour. Technol., 199*, 2–12.

59. García-Cubero, M. T., González-Benito, G., Indacoechea, I., Coca, M., & Bolado, S., (2009). Effect of ozonolysis pretreatment on enzymatic digestibility of wheat and rye straw. *Bioresour. Technol., 100*, 1608–1613.

60. Swatloski, R. P., Spear, S. K., Holbrey, J. D., & Rogers, R. D., (2002). Dissolution of Cellose with Ionic Liquids. *J. Am. Chem., Soc., 124*, 4975–4976.

61. Sun, N., Rahman, M., Qin, Y., Maxim, M. L., Rodríguez, H., & Rogers, R. D., (2009). Complete dissolution and partial delignification of wood in the ionic liquid1-ethyl-3-methylimidazolium acetate. *Green Chem., 11*, 646–655.

62. Fukaya, Y., Hayashi, K., Wadab, M., & Ohno, H., (2008). Cellulose dissolution with polar ionic liquids under mild conditions: required factors for anions. *Green Chem., 10*, 44–46.

63. Fukaya, Y., Sugimoto, A., & Ohno, H., (2006). Superior Solubility of Polysaccharides in Low Viscosity, Polar, and Halogen-Free 1, 3-Dialkylimidazolium Formates. *Biomacromolecules, 7*, 3295–3297.

64. Cao, Y., Wu, J., Zhang, J., Li, H., Zhang, Y., & He, J., (2009). Room temperature ionic liquids (RTILs): A new versatile platform for cellulose procesing and derivatization. *Chem., Eng. J., 147*, 13–21.

65. Hermanutz, F., Gähr, F., Uerdingen, E., Meister, F., & Kosan, B., (2008). New developments in dissolving and processing of cellulose in ionic liquids. *Macromol. Symp., 262*, 23–27.

66. Prado, R., Erdocia, X., & Labidi, J., (2014). *Ionic Liquid Application for Lignin Extraction and Depolymerization.* In Ionic Liquids: Synthesis, Characterization and Applications; Brooks, A., Ed., Nova Publishers: New York, 43.

67. Crosthwaite, J. M., Aki, S., Maginn E J., & Brennecke, J. F., (2004). Liquid Phase Behavior of Imidazolium-Based Ionic Liquids with Alcohols. J. *Phys. Chem., B., 108,* 5113–5119.

68. Aki, S. N. V. K., Mellein, B. R., Saurer, E. M., & Brennecke, J. F., (2004). High-Pressure Phase Behavior of Carbon Dioxide with Imidazolium-Based Ionic Liquids. *J. Phys. Chem., B., 108,* 20355–20365.

69. Wu, B., Liu, W., Zhang, Y., & Wang, H., (2009). Do We Understand the Recyclability of Ionic Liquids?. *Chem., Eur. J., 15,* 1804–1810.

70. Lee, S. H., Doherty, T. V., Linhardt, R. J., & Dordick, J. S., (2009). Ionic liquid-mediated selective extraction of lignin from wood leading to enhanced enzymatic cellulose hydrolysis. *Biotechnol. Bioeng. 102,* 1368–1376.

71. Shirkavand, E., Baroutian,S., Gapes, D. J., & Young, B. R., (2016). Combination of fungal and physicochemical processes for lignocellulosic biomass pretreatment -A review. *Renewable Sustainable Energy Rev., 54,* 217–234.

72. Zhao, X., Moates, G. K., Wilson, D. R., Ghogare, R. J., Coleman, M. J., & Waldron, K. W., (2015). Steam explosion pretreatment and enzymatic saccharification of duckweed (*Lemna minor*) biomass. *Biomass BioEnergy, 72,* 206–215.

73. Bals, B., Wedding, C., Balan, V., Sendich, E., & Dale, B., (2011). Evaluating the impact of ammonia fiber expansion (AFEX) pretreatment conditions on the cost of ethanol production. *Bioresour. Tehcnol., 102,* 1277–1283.

74. Srinivasan, N., & Ju, L. K., (2010). Pretreatment of guayale biomass using supercritical carbon dioxide based method. *Bioresour. Technol., 101,* 9785–9791.

75. Amarasekara, A. S., (2014). *Handbook of Cellulosic Ethanol, 1st ed., S*crivener Publishing: Salem.

76. Martin, C., Marcet, M., & Thomsen, A. B., (2008). Comparison between wet oxidation and steam explosion as pretreatment methods for enzymatic hydrolysis of sugarcane bagasse. *Bioresour., 3,* 670–683.

77. Saritha, M., Arora, A., & Lata., (2012). Biological Pretreatment of Lignocellulosic Substrates for Enhanced Delignification and Enzymatic Digestibility. *Indian, J. Microbiol., 52,* 122–130.

78. Sindhu, R., Binod, P., & Pandey, A., (2016). Biological pretreatment of lignocellulosic biomass-An overview. *Bioresour. Technol., 199,* 76–82.

79. Anwar, Z., Gulfraz, M., & Irshad, M., (2014). Agro-industrial lignocellulosic biomass a key to unlock the future bio-energy: A brief review. *J. Radiat. Res. Appl. Sci., 7,* 163–173.

80. Gray, K. A., Zhao, L., & Emptage, M., (2006). Bioethanol. *Curr. Opin. Chem., Biol., 10,* 141–146.

81. Menon, V., & Rao, M., (2012). Trends in bioconversion of lignocellulose: Biofuels, platform chemicals & biorefinery concept. *Prog. Energy Combust. Sci., 38,* 522–550.

82. Romaní, A., Garrote, G., Ballesteros, I., & Ballesteros, M., (2013). Second generation bioethanol from steam exploded *Eucalyptus globulus* wood. *Fuel., 111,* 66–74.

83. Park, J. Y., Kang, M., Kim, J. S., Lee, J. P., Choi, W. I., & Lee, J. S., (2012). Enhancement of enzymatic digestibility of *Eucalyptus grandis* pretreated by NaOH catalyzed steam explosion. *Bioresour. Technol., 123,* 707–712.

84. Cotana, F., Cavalaglio, G., Gelosia, M., Nicolini, A., Coccia, V., & Petrozzi, A., (2014). Production of Bioethanol in a Second Generation Prototype from Pine Wood Chips. *Energy Procedia.*, *45*, 42–51.

85. Stolarski, M. J., Krzyzaniak, M., Michał Łuczynski, M., Załuski, D., Szczukowski, S., Tworkowski, J., et al., (2015). Lignocellulosic biomass from short rotation woody crops as a feedstock for second-generation bioethanol production. *Ind. Crops Prod., 75*, 66–75.

86. Singh, R., Srivastava, M., & Shuklab, A., (2016). Environmental sustainability of bio-ethanol production from rice straw in India: A review. *Renewable Sustainable Energy Rev., 54*, 202–216.

87. Jeung-yil Park, J. Y., Kanda, E., Akira Fukushima, A., Motobayashi, K., Nagata, K., Kondo, M., et al., (2011). Contents of various sources of glucose and fructose in rice straw, a potential feedstock for ethanol production in Japan. *Biomass BioEnergy, 35*, 3733–3735.

88. Leitner, V., & Lindorfer, J., (2016). Evaluation of technology structure based on energy yield from wheat straw for combined bioethanol and biomethane facility. *Renew. Energ., 87*, 193–202.

89. Koçar, G., & Civaş, N., (2013). An overview of biofuels from energy crops: Current status and future prospects. *Renewable Sustainable Energy Rev., 28*, 900–916.

90. Woods, J., Brown, G., Gathorne-Hardy, A., Sylvester-Bradley, R., Kindred, D., Mortimer, N., (2008). Facilitating carbon (GHG) accreditation schemes for biofuels: feedstock production. HGCA Project No. MD-0607-0033.

91. Farrell, A. E., Plevin, R. J., Turner, B. T., Jones, A. D., O'Hare, M., & Kammen, D. M., (2006). Ethanol can contribute to energy and environmental goals. *Science, 311*, 506–508.

92. Shapouri, H., Duffield, J., McAloon, A., & Wang, M., (2004). The 2001 Net Energy Balance of Corn-Ethanol. U. S. Dept. of Agriculture, Office of the Chief Economist, Office of Energy Policy and New Uses, Washington, DC. 1–6.

93. Pimentel, D., & Patzek, T. W., (2005). Ethanol Production Using Corn, Switchgrass, and Wood; Biodiesel Production Using Soybean and Sunflower. *Nat. Resources Res., 14*, 65–76.

94. Pimentel, D., (2003). Ethanol fuels: energy balance, economics, and environmental impacts are negative: *Natural Resources Research., 12*(2), 127–134.

95. Fromentin, A., Biollay, F., Dauriat, A., Lucas-Porta, H., Marchand, J.-D., & Sarlos, G., (2000). Caractérisation de filières de production de bioéthanol dans le contexte helvétique. Lausanne: Laboratory de Systemes Energetiques and École Polytechnique Fédérale de Lausanne, 1–99.

96. Elsayed, M. A., Matthews, R., & Mortimer, N. D., (2003). Carbon and energy balances for a range of biofuels options. UK: Sheffield Hallam University, Project no. B/B6/00784/REP URN 03/386.

97. Vitousek, P. M., Aber, J. D., Howarth, R. W., Likens, G. E., Matson, P. A., Schindler, D. W., et al., (1997). Human alteration of the global nitrogen cycle: sources and consequences. *Ecol. Appl., 7*, 737–750.

98. Brinkman, N., Wang, M., Weber, T., & Darlington, T., (2005). Well-to-Wheels Analysis of Advanced Fuel/Vehicle Systems: A North American Study of Energy Use, Greenhouse Gas Emissions, and Criteria Pollutant Emissions. Argonne Natl. Lab., Argonne, IL.

99. Whitaker, J., Ludley, K. E., Rowe, R., Taylor, G., & Howard, D. C., (2010). Sources of variability in greenhouse gas and energy balances for biofuel production: a systematic review. *GCB BioEnergy, 2*, 99–112.

100. Rosenberger, A., Kaul, H. P., Senn, T., & Aufhammer, W., (2001). Improving the energy balance of bioethanol production from winter cereals: the effect of crop production intensity. *Appl. Energy, 68*, 51–67.

101. Huang, J., (2007). Life cycle analysis of hybrid poplar trees for cellulosic ethanol. Massachusetts: Massachusetts Institute of Technology. Doctoral Thesis

102. Macedo, I., (1998). Greenhouse gas emissions and energy balances in bio-ethanol production and utilization in Brazil. *Biomass BioEnergy, 14*, 77–81.

103. García, C., Fuentes, A., Hennecke, A., Riegelhaupt, E., Manzini, F., & Masera, O., (2011). Life-cycle greenhouse gas emissions and energy balances of sugar cane ethanol production in Mexico. *Appl. Energy, 88*, 2088–2097.

104. Agarwal, A. K., (2007). Biofuels (alcohols and biodiesel) applications as fuels for internal combustion engines. *Prog. Energy Combust. Sci., 33*, 233–271.

105. Lapuerta, M., Armas, O., & Rodríguez-Fernández, J., (2008). Effect of biodiesel fuels on diésel engine emissions. *Prog. Energy Combust. Sci., 34*, 198–223.

106. Janaun, J., & Ellis, N., (2010). Perspectives on biodiesel as a sustainable fuel. *Renewable Sustainable Energy Rev., 14*, 1312–1320.

107. Wardle, D. A., (2003). Global sale of green air travel supported using biodiesel. *Renewable Sustainable Energy Rev., 7*, 1–64.

108. Fazal, M. A., Haseeb, A. S. M. A., & Masjuki, H. H., (2011). Biodiesel feasibility study: an evaluation of material compatibility, performance, emission and engine durability. *Renewable Sustainable Energy Rev., 15*, 1314–1324.

109. Lin, L., Cunshan, Z., Vittayapadung, S., Xiangqian, S., & Mingdong, D., (2011). Opportunities and challenges for biodiesel fuel. *Appl. Energy, 88*, 1020–1031.

110. Lam, M. K., Lee, K. T., & Mohamed, A. R., (2010). Homogeneous, heterogeneous and enzymatic catalysis for transesterification of high free fatty acid oil (waste cooking oil) to biodiesel: a review. *Biotechnol Adv., 28*, 500–518.

111. Demirbas, A., (2008). New liquid biofuels from vegetable oils via catalytic pyrolysis. *Energy Educ.Sci. Technol., 21*, 1–59.

112. Shuit, S. H., Lee, K. T., Kamaruddin, A. H., & Yusup, S., (2010). Reactive extraction of Jatropha curcas, L. seed for production of biodiesel: process optimization study. *Environ. Sci. Technol., 44*, 4361–4367.

113. Ahmad, A. L., Yasin, N. H. M., Derek, C. J. C., & Lim, J. K., (2011). Microalgae as a sustainable energy source for biodiesel production: a review. *Renewable Sustainable Energy Rev., 15*, 584–593.

114. Sharma, Y. C., & Singh, B., (2009). Development of biodiesel: current scenario. *Renewable Sustainable Energy Rev., 13*, 1646–1651.

115. Shuit, S. H., Ong, Y. T., Lee, K. T., Subhash, B., & Tan, S. H., (2012). Membrane technology as a promising alternative in biodiesel production: A review. *Biotechnology Advances, 30*, 1364–1380.

116. Vicente, G., Martínez, M., & Aracil, J., (2004). Integrated biodiesel production: a comparison of different homogeneous catalysts systems. *Bioresour. Technol., 92*, 297–305.

117. Marchetti, J. M., Miguel, V. U., & Errazu, A. F., (2007). Possible methods for biodiesel production. *Renewable Sustainable Energy Rev., 11*, 1300–1311.

118. Pinnarat, T., & Savage, P. E., (2008). Assessment of noncatalytic biodiesel synthesis using supercritical reaction conditions. *Ind. Eng. Chem., Res., 47*, 6801–6808.

119. Tai-Shung, N. C., (2007). Development and purification of biodiesel. *Sep. Purif. Technol., 20*, 377–381.

120. National Biodiesel Board. http://biodiesel.org/docs/ffs-production/comprehensive-survey-on-energy-use-for-biodiesel-production.pdf?sfvrsn=4. (accessed, June 2, 21016).

121. DeWulf, J., van Langenhove, H., & van de Velde, B., (2005). Energy based efficiency and renewability assessment of biofuel production. *Environ. Sci. Technol., 39*, 3878–3882.

122. Gutiérrez, L. F., Sánchez, Ó. J., & Cardona, C. A., (2009). Process integration possibilities for biodiesel production from palm oil using ethanol obtained from lignocellulosic residues of oil palm industry. *Biores. Technol., 100*, 1227–1237.

123. Husain, Z., Zainal, Z. A., & Abdullah, M. Z., (2003). Analysis of biomass-residue-based cogeneration system in palm oil mills. *Biomass and BioEnergy, 24*, 117–124.

124. de Souza, S. P., Pacca, S., Turra de Ávila, M., & Borges, J. L. B., (2010). Greenhouse gas emissions and energy balance of palm oil biofuel. *Renewable Energy, 35*, 2552–2561.

125. Sheehan, J., Camobreco, V., Duffield, J., Graboski, M., & Shapouri, H., (1998). Life Cycle Inventory of Biodiesel and Petroleum Diesel for Use in an Urban Bus (Natl. Renewable Energy Lab., Golden, CO), NREL Publ. No. SR-580-24089.

126. Woods, J., & Bauen, A., (2003). Technology status review and carbon abatement potential of renewable transport fuels in the UK. DTI. Project no. B/U2/00785/REP URN 03/982.

127. Boerrigter, H., & den Uil, H., (2002). Green Diesel from Biomass via Fischer-Tropsch synthesis: New Insights in Gas Cleaning and Process Design. Paper presented at: Pyrolysis and Gasification of Biomass and Waste, Expert Meeting, 30 September – 1 October 2002. Strasbourg, France, page 1.

128. Tijmensen, M. J. A., Faaij, A. P. C., Hamelinck, C. N., & van Hardeveld, M. R. M., (2002). Exploration of the possibilities for production of Fischer Tropsch liquids and power via biomass gasification. *Biomass and BioEnergy, 23*, 129–152.

129. Sims, R. E. H., Mabee, W., Saddler, J. N., & Taylor, M., (2010). An overview of second generation biofuel technologies. *Biores. Technol., 101*, 1570–1580.

130. Mabee, W. E., & Saddler, J., (2007). Deployment of 2nd-generation biofuels. Technology Learning and Deployment Workshop, International Energy Agency, Paris, 11–12. June. http://www.iea.org/textbase/work/2007/learning/agenda.pdf.

131. Jungbluth, N., Tuchschmid, M., Frischknecht, R., Emmenegger, M. F., Steiner, R., & Schmutz, S., (2016). Life Cycle Assessment of BTL-fuel production. 2008. Final report. http://www.esu-services.ch/ fileadmin/download/jungbluth-2007-Del_5– 2-10_07–07–30_ESU.pdf (accessed February 20).

132. Departe, A., & Ollivier, T., (2011). A prospective study of second-generation biofuels: an analysis of their economic and environmental efficiency TRÉSOR-ECONOMICS, *89*, 1–8.

133. Mata, T. M., Martins, A. A., & Caetano, N. S., (2010). Microalgae for biodiesel production and other applications: a review. *Renew. Sust. Energy Rev., 14*, 217–232.

134. Wijffels, R. H., & Barbosa, M. J., (2010). An outlook on microalgal biofuels. *Science, 329*(5993), 796–799.

135. Norsker, N. H., Barbosa, M. J., Vermue, M. H., & Wijffels, R. H., (2011). Microalgal production – a close look at the economics. *Biotechnol. Adv., 29*(1), 24–27.

136. Delrue, F., Setier, P. A., Sahut, C., Cournac, L., Roubaud, A., Peltier, G., et al., (2012). An economic, sustainability, and energetic model of biodiesel production from microalgae. *Bioresource Technol., 111*, 191–200.

137. Amin, S., (2009). Review on biofuel oil and gas production processes from microalgae. *Energy Convers. Manage., 50*, 1834–1840.

138. Slade, R., & Bauen, A., (2013). Micro-algae cultivation for biofuels: Cost, energy balance, environmental impacts and future prospects. Biomass BioEnergy, *53*, 29–38.

139. Weinberg, J., Kaltschmitt, M., & Wilhelm, C., (2012). Biofuels from Microalgae – an environmental analysis. *Biomass Conversion and Biorefinery.*, *2*, 179–194.

140. Kadam, K. L., (2002). Environmental implications of power generation via coal-microalgae cofiring. *Energy, 27*(10), 905–922.

141. Brownbridge, G., Azadi, P., Smallbone, A., Bhave, A., Taylor, B., & Kraf, M., (2014). The future viability of algae-derived biodiesel under economic and technical uncertainties. *Bioresource Technology, 151*, 166–173.

142. Xu, L., Brilman, D. W. F., Withag, J. A. M., Brem, G., & Kersten, S., (2011). Assessment of a dry and a wet route for the production of biofuels from microalgae: Energy balance analysis. *Biores. Technol., 102*, 5113–5122.

143. Jorquera, O., Kiperstok, A., Sales, E. A., Embirçu, M., & Ghirardi, M. L., (2010). Comparative energy life-cycle analyzes of microalgal biomass production in open ponds and photobioreactors. *Bioresour. Technol., 101*(4), 1406–1413.

144. Campbell, P. K., Beer, T., & Batten, D., (2011). Life cycle assessment of biodiesel production from microalgae in ponds. *Bioresour. Technol., 102*(1), 50–56.

145. Sander, K., & Murthy, G. S., (2010). Life cycle analysis of algae biodiesel. *Int. J. Life Cycle Assess., 15*, 704–714.

146. Stephenson, A. L., Kazamia, E., Dennis, J. S., Howe, C. J., Scott, S. A., & Smith, A. G., (2010). Life-cycle assessment of potential algal biodiesel production in the United Kingdom: a comparison of raceways and air-lift tubular bioreactors. *Energ. Fuel., 24*(7), 4062–4077.

147. Lardon, L., Helias, A., Sialve, B., Steyer, J. P., & Bernard, O., (2009). Life-cycle assessment of biodiesel production from microalgae. *Environ. Sci. Technol., 43*(17), 6475–6481.

148. Lee, S. Y., Park, J. H., Jang, S. H., Nielsen, L. K., Kim, J., & Jung, K. S., (2008). Fermentative butanol production by clostridia. *Biotechnol. Bioeng., 101*, 209–228.

149. Morone, A., & Pandey, R. A., (2014). Lignocellulosic biobutanol production: Gridlocks and potential remedies. *Renewable Sustainable Energy Rev., 37*, 21–35.

150. Nanda, S., Azargohar, R., Dalai, A. K., & Kozinski, J. A., (2015). An assessment on the sustainability of lignocellulosic biomass for biorefining. *Renewable Sustainable Energy Rev., 50*, 925–941.

151. García, V., Päkkilä, J., Ojamo, H., Muurinena, E., & Keiski, R. L., (2011). Challenges in biobutanol production: How to improve the efficiency? *Renewable Sustainable Energy Rev., 15*, 964–980.

152. Kumar, B. R., & Saravanan, S., (2016). Use of higher alcohol biofuels in diesel engines: A review. *Renewable Sustainable Energy Rev., 60*, 84–115.

153. Huang, W. C., Ramey, D. E., & Yang, S. T., (2004). Continuous Production of Butanol by Clostridium acetobutylicum Immobilized in a Fibrous Bed Bioreactor. *Appl. Bio. Chem., Biotechnol., 115*(1), 887–898.

154. ITRI introduces ButyFix to make biobutanol from biomass. *Focus on Catalysts* (2014). *1*(7).

155. Jin, C., Yao, M., Liu, H., Lee, C. F., & Ji, J., (2011). Progress in the production and application of n-butanol as a biofuel. *Renewable Sustainable Energy Rev., 15*, 4080–4106.

156. Ezeji, T. C., Qureshi, N., & Blaschek, H. P., (2007). Bioproduction of butanol from biomass: from genes to bioreactors. *Curr. Opin. Biotech., 18*, 220–227.

157. Tracy, B. P., Jones, S. W., Fast, A. G., Indurthi, D. C., & Papoutsakis, E. T., (2012). Clostridia: the importance of their exceptional substrate and metabolite diversity for biofuel and biorefinery applications. *Curr. Opin. Biotech., 23*, 364–381.

158. Sun, Z. H., & Ni, Y., (2009). Recent progress on industrial fermentative production of acetone-butanol-ethanol by *Clostridium* acetobutylicum in China. *Appl. Microbiol. Biotechnol., 83*, 415–423.

159. Jang, Y. S., Malaviya, A., Cho, C., Lee, J., & Lee, S. Y., (2012). Butanol production from renewable biomass by clostridia. *Bioresour. Technol., 123*, 653–663.

160. Ezeji, T. C., Qureshi, N., & Blaschek, H. P., (2004). Butanol Fermentation Research: Upstream and Downstream Manipulations. *Chem., Rec., 4*, 305–314.

161. Ezeji, T. C., Qureshi, N., & Blasche, H. P., (2007). Production of acetone butanol (AB) from liquefied corn starch, a commercial substrate, using *Clostridium beijerinckii* coupled with product recovery by gas stripping. *J. Ind. Microbiol. Biotechnol., 34*, 771–777.

162. Morone, A., & Pandey, R. A., (2014). Lignocellulosic biobutanol production: Gridlocks and potential remedies. *Renewable Sustainable Energy Rev., 37*, 21–35.

163. Wu, M., Wang, M., Liu, J., & Huo, H., (2008). Assessment of Potential Life-Cycle Energy and Greenhouse Gas Emission Effects from Using Corn-Based Butanol as a Transportation Fuel. *Biotechnol. Prog., 24*, 1204–1214.

164. Cantrell, K. B., Kyoung, T. D., Ro, K. S., & Hunt, P. G., (2008). Livestock waste-to-bioenergy generation opportunities. *Biores. Technol., 99*, 7941–7953.

165. Chen, C. C., Lin, C. Y., & Lin, M. C., (2002). Acid-base enrichment enhances anaerobic hydrogen production process. *Appl. Microbiol. Biot., 58*, 224–228.

166. Carucci, G., Carrasco, F., Trifoni, K., Majone, M., & Beccari. M., (2005). Anaerobic digestion of food industry wastes: effect of codigestion on methane yield. *J. Environ. Eng., 131*(7), 1037–1045.

167. Mata-Alvarez, J., Dosta, J., Romero-Guza, M. S., Fonoll, X., Peces, M., & Astals, S., (2014). A critical review on anaerobic codigestion achievements between 2010 and 2013. *Renew. Sustain. Energy Rev., 36*, 412.

168. Prade, T., Svensson, S. E., & Mattsson, J. E., (2012). Energy balances for biogas and solid biofuel production from industrial hemp. *Biomass and BioEnergy, 40*, 36–52.

169. Jungbluth, N., Chudacoff, M., Dauriat, A., Dinkel, F., Doka, G., Faist Emmenegger, et al., (2007). Life Cycle Inventories of Bioenergy Eecoinvent report No. 17, v2.0. ESU-services, Uster, C. H., retrieved from: www.ecoinvent.org (accessed June 2, 2016).

170. Günther, A., Jakob, T., Goss, R., König, S., Spindler, D., Räbiger, N., et al., (2012). Methane production from glycolate excreting algae as a new concept in the production of biofuels. *Bioresource Technology, 121*, 454–457.

CHAPTER 13

TECHNO-ECONOMIC ANALYSIS OF MICROALGAE AND ALGAL BIOFUEL PRODUCTION (AS A TOOL FOR DRIVING R&D EFFORTS)

FLORIAN DELRUE

CEA Cadarache, Groupe Biomasse 3G, Cité des Energies, Saint-Paul-lez-Durance, F-13108 France

CONTENTS

ABSTRACT

The industrial production of microalgae is profitable for specific applications, either very high-value molecules such as nutraceuticals (e.g., omega 3, carotenoids) or whole microalgae produced using a low-cost process such as fish larva feed for aquaculture or *Spirulina* as a dietary supplement. However, producing biofuel or building block molecules for the chemical industry with microalgae is not economically viable at the moment.

For this kind of nonmature technology, techno-economic analyzes (TEA) can be of great help regarding two main ambitions: (i) many process options are to be explored especially for microalgae biofuel production and TEA is a practical tool for comparing them on similar bases. The process pathways with the best potential can then be specified, and (ii) sensitivity analyzes of TEA can identify key parameters and processes on which research efforts need to be addressed in order to decrease the production cost or improve the energetic and environmental balances.

The first TEAs on microalgae biofuel production have pointed out the drying as the most energy intensive step in the process. Since then, wet conversion processes such as hydrothermal liquefaction or wet lipid extraction have been preferred. Microalgae cultivation is the step with the highest impact on the economics of the whole biofuel production process. Reducing its cost is a major and crucial challenge. Sensitivity analyzes have shown that microalgae productivity is the most important factor for economically and energetically viable microalgae biofuel production. This validates the actual research efforts on screening and selecting highly efficient microalgae strain.

In the context of a difficult economic viability, the use of waste streams (i.e., wastewaters for nutrients and flue gases for CO_2) and the recycling of process waters are strongly recommended. The biorefinery concept needs to be applied to the microalgae biofuel production process.

Similarly, the valorization of the entire biomass is needed. Co-products such as pigments or omega 3 can be of great help to make the process profitable, especially now, at an early stage of the microalgae biofuel industry. However, when the full-scale of microalgae biofuel production will be reached, the market sizes of biofuel and these high-value molecules will not be compatible. At that time, animal feed, human food and bioremediation will emerge as serious covalorization opportunities.

13.1 INTRODUCTION

Microalgae have multiple potential applications, of which the most promising future objective on a large-scale is their use as a biofuel [50]. In 1978, the US

Department of Energy launched the Aquatic Species Program (ASP, 1978–1996) with a budget of $25 million dollars. The ASP was led by the National Renewable Energy Laboratory and it was focused on microalgae biofuel [41]. The researches were first dedicated to biohydrogen production (from 1978 till 1982) and they rapidly moved to biodiesel. Another large project was conducted in Japan by the New Energy Development Organization and Research for Innovative Technology of the Earth from 1990 until 2000 for a budget of $250 million dollars. The objective was to develop an Optical Fiber Reactor. Unfortunately the project was not successful [41].

At the end of the twentieth century, the effects of the competitive fossil fuels costs were decisive on these microalgae research program. Therefore after a short hiatus on this research, the interest over microalgae and especially microalgae biofuel has significantly grown over the recent years. For example, the number of publications on the subject has increased from 10 in 2007 up to 528 in 2015 (Scopus search using "microalgae biofuel" as keywords).

Microalgae for biodiesel production have many advantages in comparison with other feedstock. They can be cultivated on wastewater and exhaust fumes from combustion units and can grow almost anywhere requiring only sunlight and some simple nutrients [29].

Apart from biofuels, numerous microalgae-based products are already well established in high-value markets, for example as cosmetics, human dietary supplements (nutraceuticals) or components in animal feed [31]. However, the production costs are still too high in comparison to petroleum diesel (ex-tax price of $0.474/L in December 2015, IEA). Considerable advances in the field of biology and substantial processing improvements are required to achieve economic, environmental, and energetic sustainability in the production of microalgae biofuels [11]. Figure 13.1 shows most of the process pathways leading to microalgae biofuel (direct secretion of alkanes or lipids is not represented, and biohydrogen production has not been considered in this chapter since its level of maturity is still very low).

The evaluation of the cost of production of biofuel through techno-economic assessment (TEA) has given guidance to the research since the beginning of the microalgae biofuel adventure in the early 1980's (e.g., see Ref. [15]). The benefits of performing such TEAs are numerous: to evaluate the potential of microalgae biofuel, to identify the most promising pathways, and to determine the key process or biological parameters, which should concentrate the research and development efforts.

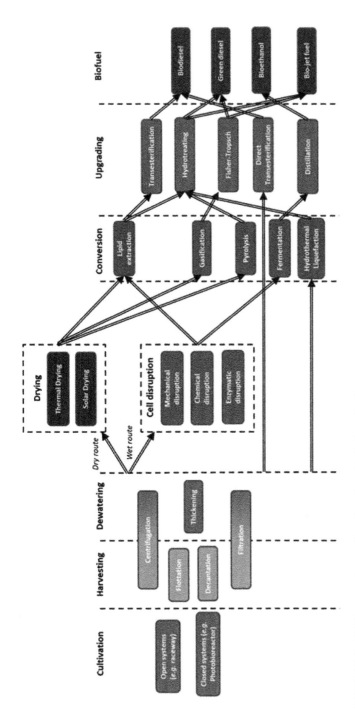

FIGURE 13.1 Different pathways for microalgae biofuel production.

This chapter will first present the evolution of TEA's result of the three most promising microalgae biofuel production pathways: lipid extraction, hydrothermal liquefaction and fermentation to bioethanol. Then, the improvement of TEA through the use of energy balance and the calculation of the Net Energy Ratio will be discussed. The biorefinery concept will be considered through the necessities of recycling fluxes within the process and of using waste streams for making microalgae biofuel viable. Lastly, the interest of coproducts will be discussed.

13.2 PRODUCTION COST FOR MICROALGAE BIOFUEL FOR DIFFERENT PATHWAYS

Actual costs for microalgae production are in the order of magnitude of €100/kg of biomass nowadays. For example, Acién et al. [1] have estimated the production cost of a real microalgae production plant of 30 m³ of tubular photobioreactors growing *Scenedesmus almeriensis* to be €69/kg of dry weight (DW) (or $79/kg-DW in 2015 $) using data collected during 2 years of continuous operation. In France, *Spirulina*, a well-known low-cost cyanobacteria, is usually sold at a price of $150–€200/kg-DW (or $160–$220/kg-DW in 2015 $). Microalgae from the genus *Chlorella* are sold at a price between €50 and $150/kg (up to €500/kg in some cases, between $55 and 160/kg-DW up to $550/kg-DW in 2015 $).

Production costs have been estimated to be between $15 and $40/kg (in 2015 $) for *Spirulina*, *Chlorella* and *Dunaliella* (grown in raceways, [6] and around $100/kg (in 2015 $) for *Haematococcus* (grown in photobioreactors, Li et al., 2011). These costs are significantly higher than any existing techno-economic analysis would produce. The two main reasons for this difference are the unoptimized processes employed as well as the small-scale operations (economies of scale). Techno-economic analyzes are based on extrapolations for large-scale and optimized production processes.

At first, the pathway to produce biofuel from microalgae has been designed based on the biodiesel process from first and second-generation biofuels. Since microalgae can accumulate high amount of neutral lipids up to 45–65% of DW [30], the first considered microalgae biofuel production processes were based on a dry lipid extraction step. By analogy with first and second-generation biodiesel, hexane is used as the lipid extraction solvent. However, dry biomass is needed for this process and drying was therefore included in the pathway. The microalgae lipids can then be converted into biodiesel by transesterification or hydrotreated to produce green diesel. Both process are efficient and give similar TEA results [11]. Therefore, both biodiesel and green diesel will be named indiscriminately "biodiesel" throughout this chapter.

Centrifugation is the current most used process for harvesting biomass in the microalgae industry. The reasons are that centrifugation is an easy-to-use and efficient technology for harvesting microalgae. For microalgae cultivation, high-rate ponds called raceways were the first systems to industrialize microalgae production. Their lower operational and capital costs and their readiness for scale-up have given them a decisive advantage over closed cultivation systems or photobioreactors (PBRs). The cost of PBRs is much higher and it is not counterbalanced yet by their better productivity. However, due to their vulnerability to contamination, raceways are not flexible for the strains that can be cultivated. Raceways have been mainly used for the cultivation of marine strains, very robust freshwater strains (such as *Chlorella sp.*) or for *Spirulina*, the common name of a cyanobacteria, *Arthrospira platensis*, cultivated under high pH conditions. .

In 1984, Feinberg estimated that microalgae could be produced at a cost of \$436/ton (\$995/ton in 2015 \$) using raceways for their culture, and microstrainer and centrifugation for their harvesting. This cost could be reduced to \$224/ton (\$511/ton in 2015 \$) if a series of improvements was to be done (increased salinity tolerance, photosynthetic yield and lipid content, and decreased losses from water evaporation and CO_2 outgassing). As a complement to this study, Neenan et al. [32] compared various microalgae biofuel production pathways: pseudo vegetable oil (degummed oil extracted from microalgae), ester fuel (transesterified microalgae oil), a gasoline-like fuel obtained through the M-Gas process from Mobil and ethanol through microalgae carbohydrates fermentation. The microalgae production system was the same than the previous study [15]: raceway, microstrainer, and centrifugation. For the pseudo vegetable oil and ester fuel processes, by analogy with terrestrial plants (first and second-generation biofuels), the solvent used for the lipid extraction step is assumed to be hexane. The calculated production costs were \$2.4/gal (or \$0.63/L and \$1.36/L in 2015 \$) for Pseudo Vegetable Oil, \$1.65/gal (or \$0.44/L and \$0.95/L in 2015 \$) for Ester Fuel, \$1.70/gal (or \$0.45/L and \$0.97/L in 2015 \$) for gasoline-like fuel and \$2.75/gal (or \$0.73/L and \$1.58/L in 2015 \$) for ethanol (20% starch content). This report particularly contributed to the success of the lipid extraction pathway.

Various other studies were dedicated to the evaluation of raw microalgae production cost at large scale in the 1980s. Tapie and Bernard (1987) made a review showing that the evaluated production cost of raw microalgae ranged from $0.15 to $4.00/kg (or $0.32 to $8.65 in 2015 $). In these analyzes, the microalgae were assumed to be produced in raceways. For microalgae grown in tubular reactors, Tapie and Bernard [46] estimated the cost to range from $3.70 to $4.50/kg for a productivity of 60 tons/ha/yr (or from $8.00 to $9.73 in 2015 $).

Until the year 2010, there was no significant breakthrough in the TEA analyzes of the lipid extraction pathway.

Lundquist et al. [26] designed a 400 ha production facility where microalgae are cultivated in 400 ha of high-rate ponds, harvested by clarifies, thickeners and drying beds, then dried in flash dryers and the microalgae lipids are extracted using hexane. The residual biomass is converted into biogas in an anaerobic digester to produce power. The microalgae unrefined oil production cost was estimated to be $1.90/L ($2.07/L in 2015 $). This analysis was very well detailed but the conversion of microalgae oil into biofuel was not considered.

Davis et al. [9] have compared the production of biodiesel using raceways and PBRs. In their system, the biomass is harvested using settling, dissolved air flotation (DAF) and centrifugation reaching a biomass concentration of 20%DW (200 g/L); then the cells are lysed using high pressure homogenizers, and the lipids are extracted with butanol as the solvent. Lysing the microalgae cells by a mechanical pretreatment allows the oil to be extracted without the needs for drying the microalgae. Then, the oil is converted into a mixture of biodiesel (78%) and naphta (2%) by hydrotreating. The residual biomass is sent to anaerobic digestion to produce biogas for power production.

The authors estimated the biodiesel production cost depending on the cultivation system: $2.60/gal ($0.69/L or $0.73/L in 2015 $) for raceways and more than twice higher for PBR at $5.42/gal ($1.43/L or $1.51/L in 2015 $). Since then, the number of TEA on microalgae biofuel have been constantly increasing from 22 studies in 2010 to 89 in 2015 (results of a Scopus search). The biodiesel production cost is significantly varying from one study to the other (from $0.43 to $24.60/L, or $0.44 to $25.03/L in 2015 $ [39]. However, most of them concluded that microalgae biodiesel was more expensive than petroleum diesel (ex-tax price of $0.474/L in December 2015, IEA).

Promising routes for biofuel production from microalgae are the direct secretion of energetic molecules such as oils [24] or even alkanes as drop-in fuel [2]. These processes would advantageously overcome the need for lipid extraction and even conversion to biofuel in the case of alkane secretion. Unfortunately, the biomass would probably have to be harvested in order to have a continuous lipid production (biomass that can be valorized through anaerobic digestion, for example) and the cultivation would have to be done in PBR in order to avoid contaminations and consumption of the secreted molecules. These constraints lead to slightly higher production costs in comparison to the wet lipid extraction pathway [12]. However, if the microalgae could be "milked" indefinitely without the need for harvesting and valorizing the biomass, the production costs would drop by 25% to 50%. In any case, the energy balance is much more interesting (see Section 13.3 for more details).

In addition to the lipid extraction pathway, alternative pathways have been investigated of which the most promising are the hydrothermal liquefaction (HTL) pathway and the bioethanol pathway. HTL is a thermochemical process that convert biomass into a biocrude (heavy oil, yields between 20 and 87%) [47], gas (>95% of CO_2 that can be recycle to the cultivation step) [17], some residual solids and an aqueous phase that contains large amount of nutrients. The biocrude can be directly burned in a boiler or upgraded through hydrotreating into a biofuel (a mix of naphta, gasoline and jetfuel, [9]). The main advantage of HTL is that it converts the whole biomass with moisture content up to 50% [35]. The TEAs dedicated to the HTL pathway are not as numerous as for the lipid extraction pathway. Using a Monte-Carlo based model for simulating various process conditions and parameters (e.g., raceway and/or PBR for cultivation or various biomass productivities), Delrue et al. [12] found a production cost of $2.77 to $4.30 (in 2015 $) for biodiesel obtained by microalgae HTL. A practical case was then simulated using experimental data from the hydrothermal conversion of *Chlamydomonas reinhardtii* [17] assuming microalgae cultivation in raceways and harvesting by centrifugation. A production cost of $3.67/L (in 2015 $) was found. Davis et al. [10] simulated a HTL pathway using raceways for cultivation, DAF and centrifugation for harvesting. They found a minimum fuel selling price of $2.59/L (in 2015 $). Ou et al. (2015) also performed a TEA of the HTL process but the perimeter of their study was focused on the HTL of defatted biomass (residue of lipid extraction). They found a production cost of $0.68/L (in 2015 $) assuming free of charge defatted biomass.

The bioethanol pathway is also a potential alternative since microalgae can accumulate large amounts of carbohydrate (e.g., up to 60% for *Chlorella vulgaris*, Brányiková et al., 2011. However, the fermentation of these carbohydrates into ethanol requires an additional step of pretreatment to be feasible. Biochemical, chemical, thermal or mechanical pretreatments have been considered [19] and research on microalgae bioethanol are now focusing on this step. Very few TEAs exist on the bioethanol pathway. As previously mentioned, one of the first TEA on microalgae biofuel Neenan et al. (1986) estimated the cost to be $2.75/gal (or $0.73/L or $1.58/L in 2015 $) for bioethanol. The main hypothesis was that the starch content of the microalgae was set at 20%, which is a very conservative figure.

Laurens et al. [22] have also performed a TEA on a modified lipid extraction pathway where the residual biomass is converted into ethanol. An acid-catalyzed pretreatment is performed to convert the residual biomass into fermentable soluble sugars. The bioethanol that is then produced by fermentation increases the total fuel yield by 54% and the production cost is reduced by 18 to 33% compared to a classic lipid extraction pathway. These promising results are giving credits for the research on microalgae carbohydrates conversion to bioethanol. Table 13.1 presents the results of recent TEAs for different scenarios of microalgae biofuel production processes. The results vary greatly between studies depending on the process options and the value chosen for the key parameters (such as lipid productivity). On average, the estimated production cost of microalgae biodiesel is in the range $3.09–$3.79/L [37]. Still, these costs are too high to address the current energy market (ex-tax price of $0.474/L in December 2015, IEA) and not competitive enough to convince the petrochemical industry that microalgae could become a valuable feedstock even in the long-term.

Production costs still need to be reduced by approximately an order of magnitude in order to obtain economically viable microalgae biofuel. The cultivation step is responsible for most of the biofuel production cost (83% if PBRs are used and 15% if raceways are used for Ref. [9]; 58% if PBRs are used and 29% if raceways for Ref. [11]). Sensitivity analyzes [9, 11, 17, 44] have also shown that productivities are the most influencing parameters (lipid productivity for the lipid pathways, biomass productivity and bio-oil yield for the HTL pathway, starch productivity for the bio-ethanol pathway).

TABLE 13.1 Results of Recent TEAs for Different Microalgae Biofuel Production Pathways

Cultivation	Harvesting	Conversion	Biomass aerial productivity (g/m²/d)	Lipid content (%)	Production cost (2015 $/L)	Reference
Raceway	Clarifier and bed drying	Lipid extraction	22	25	1.64a	[26]
Raceway	DAF – centrifugation	Wet lipid extraction	25	25	2.74	[9]
PBR	DAF – centrifugation	Wet lipid extraction	1.25 kg/m3/d	25	5.72	[9]
Raceway	Centrifugation	Dry Lipid Extraction	20–30	20–50	1.86–2.92	[11]
PBR	Belt Filter Press	Wet lipid extraction	20–30	20–50	2.90–5.01	[11]
Raceway and PBR	Clarifier and Belt Filter Press	Oil secretion	20–30	20–50	3.23–5.70	[12]
Raceway and PBR	Clarifier and Belt filter Press	Alkane secretion	20–30	20–50	3.08–5.51	[12]
Raceway and PBR	Clarifier and Belt Filter Press	HTL	20–30	–	2.77–4.30	[12]
Raceway	DAF – centrifugation	HTL	Model	–	2.59	[10]
Raceway and PBR	Natural settling + Filter press	Wet thermochemical extraction	23	38	3.02b	[4]
Raceway and PBR	Natural settling + Filter press	HTL	23	38	2.45b	[4]

Directly from defatted microalgae					0.68	
Raceway	Flocculation and belt filter Press	HTL	25	—	3.67	[17]
Raceway	Flocculation and belt filter Press	Pyrolysis	25	—	3.83	[17]
Not detailed	Not detailed	Wet lipid extraction and fermentation of the residues	30	40.9	2.11	[22]

(a) Cost of production for the bio-oil, not the biofuel.

(b) Biocrude production cost.

13.3 THE ENERGY RETURN ON INVESTMENT (EROI)

Energy balances are a side-product of TEAs. A dedicated model needs to be developed for their calculation but for biofuel production system, it is necessary to evaluate the energetic sustainability of the process. The energy return on investment (EROI) [28], or energy returned on energy invested (EROEI or ERoEI) or net energy ratio (NER) [38] is the ratio of the amount of usable energy delivered from the process to the amount of nonrenewable energy used to obtain that energy resource.

In the case of biofuels, nonmanmade and renewable energy inputs are not taken into account in the calculations. Solar energy is not accounted for an energy used in the process. It will give very low EROI since photosynthetic yields are no more than 6.3% for the best case for microalgae but rather 2.6–2.7% in reality [49]. Nevertheless, the energy needed to produce the nutrients for the cultivation step or chemicals that are used in the process (solvents, flocculants, …) is included in the calculations. The first objective is to have EROI (or NER) higher than 1 meaning that the process produces more energy than it consumes. However, Hall et al. [18] introduced the "law of minimum EROI" for a system. They evaluated that in order for the system to survive, it must gain substantially more energy than it consumes. This minimum EROI has been estimated to be 3:1 for biofuels to be considered as a prominent fuel. A review has been performed by Slade and Bauen [44] showing the discrepancy among the studies that have been calculated EROI for microalgae biofuel. However, EROI above 1 seems difficult to achieve. The first energy analyzes were quite optimistic. Lardon et al. [21] have shown that compared to dry lipid extraction, wet lipid extraction would increase the EROI by nearly a factor of 4 (from 1.25 to 4.34). This was confirmed by other studies. Indeed, a Monte Carlo-based sensitivity analysis has shown that wet lipid extraction and low-energy demanding process for harvesting (such as flocculation and belt-filter press) have significant impacts on the EROI [11].

The first energy balance of the HTL process was performed by Sawayama et al. [40], they estimated the energy needed for the HTL process at 6.69 MJ/kg of oil for *B. braunii* and 11.94 MJ/kg of oil for *D. tertiolecta*. This energy accounted for heating the water, the microalgae and for some heat loss during the heating and heat recovery was assumed to be 50%. A constant value of 4.18 kJ/kg/K was set for the specific heat capacity of water. However, its value varies significantly with temperature and has a huge influence on the energy balance (e.g., 14.6 kJ/kg/K at 360°C). The energy used during the HTL process is very difficult to evaluate despite its importance for an accurate estimation of the EROI.

Various results can be obtained depending on the processes that are taken into account (heating the medium, heat losses, energy needed by the reaction, ... Liu et al. [25] estimated the HTL reaction energy demand as the energy needed for heating the water (4.2 kJ/kg/K between 25°C and 150°C and 4.8 kJ/kg/K between 150°C and 300°C) leading to a consumption of less than 0.5 kWh/kg of biomass (or 1.8 MJ/kg of biomass). Therefore they evaluated EROIs between 1 and 3 for the whole process. For Bennion et al. [5], the HTL reaction energy consumption was calculated as the energy needed to heat the reactor, 1.65 kWh/kg of biomass (or 5.94 mJ/kg of biomass). The corresponding EROI was estimated to be 1.23. Then, when a thermochemical model of the HTL reaction is included, the energy demand of the HTL process is significantly higher (4.9 kWh/kg of biomass or 17.6 MJ/kg of biomass, [17]), leading to a EROI of 1.08. 50% of the heat of the products was assumed to be recovered using a tubular heat exchanger between the inlet and outlet of the HTL process. However, the energetic model of the HTL reaction was not even complete in this study (the heat losses were not accounted for).

The integration of renewable energy can significantly help in reaching the goal of a EROI of 3:1. Tredici et al. [48] have shown that the EROI of a PBR-based microalgae cultivation system can be doubled (from 0.82 to 1.73) if photovoltaic solar panels are used. The benefits of secreting the components of interest directly into the cultivation medium have been recently demonstrated [12]. The EROI is increased by about 50% in comparison to wet lipid extraction and 200% in comparison to dry lipid extraction. Luo et al. [27] have performed an energy balance on a bioethanol production system where ethanol is excreted by the microalgae. Based on their results, EROI from 1.82 up to 5.0 can be calculated, validating the benefits of secretion of the molecules of interest into the cultivation medium. In conclusion, EROI calculations and sensibility analyzes can lead to process choice for improving the energy balance. For example, wet processes and low-energy demanding harvesting processes have to be preferred. EROI analyzes can also help in evaluating the interest of future microalgae biofuel production pathways such as the direct secretion of the component of interest (ethanol, lipid or alkane). Finally, the energetic models (especially for HTL) have to be improved for more accurate EROI calculations.

TABLE 13.2 EROI for Different Microalgae Biofuel Production Scenarios

Cultivation	Harvesting	Conversion	Biomass productivity (g/ m²/d)	Lipid content (%)	Energy Return On Investment	Reference
Raceways	Flocculation	Dry lipid extraction	19.25	38.5	1.25	[21]
Raceways	Flocculation	Wet lipid extraction	19.25	38.5	4.34	[21]
Flexible film PBR	Ethanol secretion in the medium and separation by VCSS(a)		0.5–5% in the cultivation medium		1.82–5.0	[27]
Raceway	Centrifugation	Dry Lipid Extraction	20–30	20–50	0.93–1.20	[11]
PBR	Belt Filter Press	Wet lipid extraction	20–30	20–50	1.81–2.42	[11]
Raceway and PBR	Clarifier and Belt filter Press	Oil secretion	20–30	20–50	2.61–3.28	[12]
Raceway and PBR	Clarifier and Belt filter Press	Alkane secretion	20–30	20–50	3.09–4.18	[12]
Raceway and PBR	Clarifier and Belt filter Press	HTL	20–30	–	1.75–2.22	[12]
Raceway	Flocculation and centrifugation	Wet Lipid Extraction	20	45.7	1.07	[8]
Raceway and PBR	Natural settling + Filter press	Wet thermochemical extraction	23	38	1.16b	[4]
Raceway and PBR	Natural settling + Filter press	HTL	23	38	1.39b	[4]
Raceway	Flocculation and belt filter Press	HTL	25	–	1.08	[17]
Raceway	Flocculation and belt filter Press	Pyrolysis	25	–	0.75	[17]

Raceway	Filtration and centrifugation	HTL	13	—	1.23	[5]
Raceway	Filtration and centrifugation	Pyrolysis	13	—	2.27	[5]
Flat-panel PBR	Centrifugation	No conversion	21.5	—	0.59	[48]
Flat-panel PBR	Centrifugation	No conversion	39.4	—	0.82	[48]
Flat-panel PBR + solar panels	Centrifugation	No conversion	39.4	—	1.73	[48]

(a) VCSS: vapor compression steam stripping.

(b) EROI for biocrude.

13.4 IMPORTANCE OF RECYCLING AND USING WASTE STREAMS: THE BIOREFINERY CONCEPT

In analogy to the petroleum refinery, biorefinery is a facility that produces multiple fuels and products integrates from biomass. In a biorefinery, energy (fuel, heat, power) and matter are optimized leading to multiple recycling of streams. In addition for the microalgae industry, biorefineries use waste streams as input for its processes. This concept of biorefinery has to be fully implemented in the microalgae biofuel production process in order to reach positive economic, energetic and environmental balances.

Wastewater can effectively be used as a medium for microalgae cultivation since it contains all the major nutrients that microalgae need for their growth (nitrogen and phosphorus) [34]. Delrue et al. [11] have shown that wastewater can bring between 3 and 30% of the nitrogen and phosphorus needs of microalgae. Other sources of nitrogen and phosphorus have to be found (such as agricultural and industrial wastewaters and wastes). Also, wastewater would probably not be accounted in the water footprint (WF) calculations since reusing it will not impact the available water stocks (marine or freshwater). In this case, the WF will be reduced by 75% on average if wastewater is used as the medium for microalgae cultivation. Water scarcity is a global problem [16] inducing the urge to reduce our water consumption. Therefore, WF is an important metric for evaluating microalgae biofuel production systems. Yang et al. [43] have estimated a WF of 3726 kg/kg of biodiesel (or 93.2 L/MJ with a reasonable assumption for the High Heating Value of biodiesel at 40 MJ/kg). However, no recycling of process waters was assumed. Supernatant from coagulation-flocculation, clarified from centrifugation and other process waters still contains high amount of nutrients and need to be recycled. Nevertheless, recycling these process waters is a major challenge since it can contains growth inhibitors [13].

Then, Subhadra et al. [45] found WFs between 23–62 L/MJ using a recycling factor of 80%. Delrue et al. [12] assumed a recycling rate varying between 80% and 99% in a Monte-Carlo based model leading to WFs between 2.8 and 8.5 L/MJ for various biodiesel production pathways (lipid extraction, HTL, direct secretion of lipid or alkane). These WFs are blue WFs in the sense that they account for the direct water withdrawal of a process, for either consumptive or nonconsumptive use [3]. Lifecycle WF is a more comprehensive metric accounting for the direct water consumption in the process, the water consumed in materials and energy production that are needed by the process, and the water credits that are returned to the accounting due to the displacement of marketable products by the coproducts generated in the biofuel production process. Using this concept, Batan et al. [3] estimated lifecycle WFs between 80 and 291 L/MJ for different microalgae biofuels. Also, the carbon dioxide that is needed for microalgae to grow can be brought by flue gases [36] from coal or gas power stations, cement factories, distilleries or any CO_2 emitting industry. Using waste streams can have a significant impact on the production cost and also the environmental impact of microalgae biofuel. Based on the model by Delrue et al. [11], the microalgae biofuel production cost is reduced by 5% on average if a carbon credit between €10 and €50/ton is assumed for CO_2 from an industrial origin ($11 to $58/ton in 2015 $).

WF is an important metric for evaluating microalgae biofuel production pathways. However, similarly to the other indicators (production cost, NER), WF needs detailed models validated by full-scale data to be more accurate. Also high CO_2 credits could have a significant impact on the microalgae biofuel industry.

13.5   CO-VALORIZATION

As detailed in Section 13.2, microalgae biofuels are not yet economically viable. However, microalgae can also be a source for high-value molecules. Scenarios of covalorization of biofuels and high-value products such as omega 3, carotenoids, pigments are of great economic interest. For example, a simulation has been performed based on the model by Delrue et al. [11], where *Nannochloropsis* was used for producing biodiesel and eicosapentaenoic acid (EPA, range of 2 to 5%DW) [14, 42]. Assuming selling price between $330 and $1100/kg EPA, the production cost of biodiesel becomes negative (–$28 up to –$50/L of biodiesel, unpublished results). However, for a facility producing 100 tons of biomass per day (reasonable scale for a full-scale microalgae biofuel production system), the EPA extracted from the microalgae would represent 10% of the world omega 3 market (unpublished results). The market sizes of omega 3 and biofuel are not compatible. However such high-value molecules can help the microalgae biofuel industry to become economically viable in its early stage. Then, it would have to change to other coproducts with markets of similar size than biofuels. Feed and food are potential candidates. Valorization of the microalgae residue after lipid extraction as animal feed (selling prices between \$330 and \$550/ton) could lead to an average 15% drop of the biodiesel production cost (unpublished simulation based on the model by Ref. [12]). In their sensitivity analysis for a similar process, Beal et al. [4] found that reducing the cost of animal feed from \$600/ton to \$300/ton would lead to an increase of 15% of the biocrude production cost. However, the concept of feed or food covalorization would have to overcome the expected consumers' concerns and the legislative constraints if wastewaters are used for microalgae cultivation.

The use of microalgae as feedstock for a bio-based chemistry is also a potential covalorization pathway, which has not been much investigated yet. However, since the industrial chemistry will have to be decarbonized in the future years, there will certainly be an opportunity for microalgae.

13.6 CONCLUSION

TEAs are powerful tools for evaluating the various microalgae biofuel processes. It can effectively point at the most promising pathways and within these pathways, it can identify the critical steps, processes or parameters. TEAs have been able to identify the three most promising pathways for producing microalgae biofuel: the wet lipid extraction, HTL and bioethanol production. In the long-term, the direct secretion of the molecule of interest (lipid, alkane, alcohol) presents many advantages over the other pathways, but research efforts are still needed in order to find the appropriate microalgae strain through engineering and strain selection.

Biofuel production cost is the most common indicator of TEAs. Since microalgae biofuels are still one order-of-magnitude away from competing with petroleum fuels, reducing its production cost is a major challenge. TEAs have helped to identify the need for low-cost but efficient cultivation systems and high productivity yields giving avenues for future research. Then, the NER is another important indicator for evaluating microalgae biofuel production processes. The first objective of a EROI higher than 1 has been achieved. However, to be fully sustainable, the EROI of microalgae biofuel production systems has to be higher than 3. For that, higher productivity yields, wet processes (in order to limit the use of energy intensive drying) and low energy demanding harvesting processes are needed. In the long-term, secretion of the molecule of interest directly into the microalgae medium will certainly also play a major role in increasing the NER. The WF is crucial since water scarcity will be more and more pregnant in the future. In order to reduce the WF, the use of wastewaters and the recirculation of all the process waters have to be prioritized.

Finally, microalgae have a great potential in term of valorization, from very high-value molecules to commodities (fuel, feed, food). Co-valorization has to be considered in order to make the microalgae biofuel industry more profitable. This could be done in two steps. High-value molecules (such as carotenoids or omega 3) have to be targeted first in the early stage of the microalgae biofuel industry. But since the market sizes of these molecules are not compatible with the biofuel market size, covalorization will have to switch to feed, food or green chemistry. Microalgae biofuels potential as an alternative to fossil fuels has been demonstrated for a long time now, but research and development are still needed in order to make microalgae biofuel economically, environmentally and energetically competitive.

KEYWORDS

- **biorefinery**
- **coproducts**
- **microalgae biofuel**
- **net energy ratio**
- **production cost**
- **water footprint**

REFERENCES

1. Acién, F. G., Fernández, J. M., Magán, J. J., & Molina, E. (2012). Production cost of a real microalgae production plant and strategies to reduce it. *Biotechnol. Adv.,* 30, 1344–1353.
2. Bachofen, R., (1982). The production of hydrocarbons by Botryococcus braunii. *Experentia., 38*, 47–49.
3. Batan, L., Quinn, J. C., & Bradley, T. H. (2013). Analysis of water footprint of a photobioreactor microalgae biofuel production system from blue, green and lifecycle perspectives. *Algal Res., 2*, 196–203.

4. Beal, C. M., Gerber, L. N., Sills, D. L., Huntley, M. E., Machesky, S. C., Walsh, M. J., Tester, J. W., Archibald, I., Granados, J., & Greene, C. H. (2015). Algal biofuel production for fuels and feed in a 100-ha facility: A comprehensive techno-economic analysis and life cycle assessment. *Algal Res., 10*, 266–279.

5. Bennion, E. P., Ginosar, D. M., Moses, J., Agblevor, F., & Quinn, J. C. (2015). Lifecycle assessment of microalgae to biofuel: Comparison of thermochemical processing pathways. *Appl. Energ., 154*, 1062–1071.

6. Borowitzka, M. A. (1999). Commercial production of microalgae: ponds, tanks, tubes and fermenters. *J. Biotechnol., 70*, 313–321.

7. Brányiková, I., Maršálková, B., Doucha, J., Brányik, T., Bišová, K., Zachleder, V., & Vítová, M. (2011). Microalgae—Novel Highly Efficient Starch Producers. *Biotechnol. Bioeng., 108*, 766–776.

8. Collet, P., Lardon, L., Hélias, A., Bricout, S., Lombaert-Valot, I., Perrier, B., Lépine, O., Steyer, J-P., & Bernard, O. (2014). Biodiesel from microalgae – Life cycle assessment and recommendations for potential improvements. *Renew. Energ., 71*, 525–533.

9. Davis, R., Aden, A., & Pienkos, P. T. (2011). Techno-economic analysis of autotrophic microalgae for fuel production. *Appl. Energ., 88*, 3524–3531.

10. Davis, R. E., Fishman, D. B., Frank, E. D., Johnson, M. C., Jones, S. B., Kinchin, C. M., Skaggs, R. L., Venteris, E. R., & Wigmosta, M. S. (2014). Integrated Evaluation of Cost, Emissions, and Resource Potential for Algal Biofuels at the National Scale. *Environ. Sci. Technol., 48*, 6035–6042.

11. Delrue, F., Setier, P-A., Sahut, C., Cournac, L., Roubaud, A., & Peltier, G. (2012). An economic, sustainability, and energetic model of biodiesel production from microalgae. *Bioresource Technol., 111*, 191–200.

12. Delrue, F., Li-Beisson, Y., Setier, P-A., Sahut, C., Roubaud, A., Froment, A-K., & Peltier, G. (2013). Comparison of various microalgae liquid biofuel production pathways based on energetic, economic and environmental criteria. *Bioresour. Technol., 136*, 205–212.

13. Delrue, F., Imbert, Y., Fleury, G., Peltier, G., & Sassi, J-F. (2015). Using coagulation–flocculation to harvest Chlamydomonas reinhardtii: Coagulant and flocculant efficiencies, and reuse of the liquid phase as growth medium. *Algal Res., 9*, 283–290.

14. Fang, X., Wei, C., Zhao-Ling, C., & Fan, O. (2004). Effects of organic carbon sources on cell growth and eicosapentaenoic acid content of *Nannochloropsis sp. J. Appl. Phycol., 16*, 499–503.

15. Feinberg, D. A. (1984). Technical and Economic Analysis of Liquid Fuel Production from Microalgae. Solar Energy Research Institute, Prepared for the US Department of Energy, Contract No. DE-AC02-83CH10093, Golden, Colorado.

16. Gosling, S. N., & Arnell, N. W. (2013). A global assessment of the impact of climate change on water scarcity. *Clim. Chang.*, 1–15.

17. Hognon, C., Delrue, F., & Boissonnet, G. (2015). Energetic and economic evaluation of *Chlamydomonas reinhardtii* hydrothermal liquefaction and pyrolysis through thermochemical models. *Energy, 93*, 31–40.

18. Hall, C. A. S., Balogh, S., & Murphy, D. J. R. (2009). What is the Minimum EROI that a Sustainable Society Must Have? *Energies, 2*, 25–47.

19. Ho, S-H., Huang, S-W., Chen, C-Y., Hanusuma, T., Kondo, A., & Chang, J-S. (2013). Bioethanol production using carbohydrate-rich microalgae biomass as feedstock. *Bioresour. Technol., 135*, 191–198.

20. International Energy Agency. Monthly Prices Statistics. December (2015). http://www. iea.org/statistics/monthlystatistics/monthlyoilprices/ (accessed on the Feb 11, (2016)).

21. Lardon, L., Hélias, A., Sialve, B., Steyer, J. P., & Bernard, O. (2009). Life-cycle assessment of biodiesel production from microalgae. *Environ. Sci. Technol., 43*, 6475–6481.

22. Laurens, L. M. L., Nagle, N., Davis, R., Sweeney, N., Van Wychen, S., Lowell, A., & Pienkos, P. T. (2015). Acid-catalyzed algal biomass pretreatment for integrated lipid and carbohydrate-based biofuels production. *Green Chem., 17*, 1145–1158.

23. Li, J., Zhu, D., Shen, S., & Wang, G. (2011). An economic assessment of astaxanthin production by large scale cultivation of *Haematococcus pluvialis. Biotechnol. Adv., 29*, 568–574.

24. Liu, X., Sheng, J., & Curtiss III, R. (2011). Fatty acid production in genetically modified cyanobacteria. *PNAS* 108, 6899–6904.

25. Liu, X., Saydah, B, Eranki, P., Colosi, L. M., Mitchell, B. G., Rhodes, J., & Clarens, A. F. (2013). Pilot-scale data provide enhanced estimates of the life cycle energy and emissions profile of algae biofuels produced via hydrothermal liquefaction. *Bioresour. Technol., 148*, 163–171.

26. Lundquist, T. J., Woertz, C., Quinn, N. W. T., & Benemann, J. R. (2010). *A Realistic Technology and Engineering Assessment of Algae Biofuel Production.* Energy Biosciences Institute, Berkeley, California,

27. Luo, D., Hu, Z., Choi, D. G., Thomas, V. M., Realff, M. J., & Chance, R. R. (2010). Life Cycle Energy and Greenhouse Gas Emissions for an Ethanol Production Process Based on Blue-Green Algae. *Environ. Sci. Technol., 44*, 8670–8677.

28. Hammerschlag, R. (2006). Ethanol's Energy Return on Investment: A Survey of the Literature 1990-Present. *Environ. Sci. Technol., 40*, 1744–1750.

29. Mata, T. M., Martins, A. A., & Caetano, N. S. (2010). Microalgae for biodiesel production and other applications: a review. *Renew. Sustain. Energy Rev., 14*, 217–232.

30. Merchant, S. S., Kropat, J., Liu, B., Shaw, J., & Warakanont, J. (2012). TAG, You're it! Chlamydomonas as a reference organism for understanding algal triacylglycerol accumulation. *Curr. Opin. Biotech., 23*, 352–363.

31. Milledge, J. (2011). Commercial application of microalgae other than as biofuels: a brief review. *Rev. Environ. Sci. Biotechnol., 10*, 31–41.

32. Neenan, B., Feinberg, D., Hill, A., McIntosh, R., & Terry, K. (1986). Fuels from Microalgae: Technology Status, Potential, and Research Requirement. Solar Energy Research Institute, Prepared for the US Department of Energy, Contract No. DE-AC02–83CH10093, Golden, Colarado,

33. Ou, L., Thilakaratne, R., Brown, R. C., & Wright, M. M. (2015). Techno-economic analysis of transportation fuels from defatted microalgae via hydrothermal liquefaction and hydroprocessing. *Biomass Bioenerg, 72*, 45–54.

34. Park, J. B. K., Craggs, R. J., & Shilton, A. N. (2011). Wastewater treatment high rate algal ponds for biofuel production. *Bioresour. Technol., 102*, 35–42.

35. Pavlovíc, I., Knez, Z., & Skerget M. (2013). Hydrothermal reactions of agricultural and food processing wastes in sub and supercritical water: a review of fundamentals, mechanisms, and state of research. *J. Agric. Food Chem., 61*, 8003–8025.

36. Pires, J. C. M., Alvim-Ferraz, M. C. M., Martins, F. G., & Simões, M. (2012). Carbon dioxide capture from flue gases using microalgae: Engineering aspects and biorefinery concept. *Renew. Sust. Energ. Rev., 16*, 3043–3053.

37. Quinn, J. C., & Davis, R. (2015). The potentials and challenges of algae based biofuels: A review of the techno-economic, life cycle, and resource assessment modeling. *Bioresour. Technol., 184*, 444–452.

38. Razon, L. F., & Tan, R. R. (2011). Net energy analysis of the production of biodiesel and biogas from the microalgae: *Haematococcus pluvialis* and *Nannochloropsis*. *Appl. Energ., 88*, 3507–3514.

39. Ribeiro, L. A., & Silva, P. P. (2013). Surveying techno-economic indicators of microalgae biofuel technologies. *Renew. Sustain. Energy Rev., 25*, 89–96.

40. Sawayama, S., Minowa, T., & Yokoyama, S-Y. (1999). Possibility of renewable energy production and CO$_2$ mitigation by thermochemical liquefaction of microalgae. *Biomass Bioenerg., 17*, 33–39.

41. Sheehan, J., Dunahay, T., Benemann, J., & Roessler, P. (1998). A Look Back at the U.S. Department of Energy's Aquatic Species Program—Biodiesel from Algae. National Renewable Energy Laboratory Under Contract No. DE-AC36-83CH10093. Prepared for: U.S. Department of Energy's Office of Fuels Development.

42. Tonon, T., Harvey, D., Laron, T. R., & Graham, I. A., (2002). Long chain polyunsaturated fatty acid production and partitioning to triacylglycerols in four microalgae. *Phytochemistry, 61*, 15–24.

43. Yang, J., Xu, M., Zhang, X., Hu, Q., Sommerfeld, M., & Chen, Y. (2011). Life-cycle analysis on biodiesel production from microalgae: Water footprint and nutrients balance. *Bioresour. Technol., 102*, 159–165.

44. Slade, R., & Bauen, A. (2013). Micro-algae cultivation for biofuels: Cost, energy balance, environmental impacts and future prospects. *Biomass Bioenerg., 53*, 29–38.

45. Subhadra, B. G., & Edwards, M. (2011). Coproduct market analysis and water footprint of simulated commercial algal biorefineries. *Appl. Energ., 88*, 3515–3523.

46. Tapie, P., & Bernard, A. (1988). Microalgae Production: Technical and Economic Evaluations. *Biotechnol. Bioeng., 32*, 873–885.

47. Tian, C., Li, B., Liu, Z., Zhang, Y., & Lu, H. (2014). Hydrothermal liquefaction for algal biorefinery: A critical review. *Renew. Sust. Energ. Rev., 38*, 933–950.

48. Tredici, M. R., Bassi, N., Prussi, M., Biondi, N., Rodolfi, L., Chini Zitelli, G., & Sampietro, G. (2015). Energy balance of algal biomass production in a 1-ha "Green Wall Panel" plant: How to produce algal biomass in a closed reactor achieving a high Net Energy Ratio. *Appl. Energ., 154*, 1103–1111.

49. Weyer, K. M., Bush, D. R., Darzin, A., & Willson, B. D. (2010). Theoretical Maximum Algal Oil Production. *Bioenerg. Res., 3*, 204–213.

50. Wijffels, R. H., Kruse, O., & Hellingwerf, K. J. (2013). Potential of industrial biotechnology with cyan obacteria and eukaryotic microalgae. *Curr. Opin. Biotechnol., 24*, 405–413.

CHAPTER 14

MISMATCH OF LIFE-CYCLE INVENTORIES FOR BIOENERGY, FOSSIL FUEL, AND AGRICULTURAL RESOURCE PRODUCTION

SARAH C. DAVIS, KAITLIN C. STRAKER, ABBEY RODJOM, ESTHER GROSSMAN, ALEXANDER JONES, and KIM E. MILLER

Voinovich School of Leadership and Public Affairs, Ohio University, Athens, OH (45701), USA

CONTENTS

ABSTRACT

With growing concerns about climate change and energy demands, the need for alternatives to fossil fuels persists. Bioenergy has the potential to offset greenhouse gas (GHG) emissions from fossil fuel, but requires expansion, intensification, or repurposing of agricultural land. Complexities associated with land use change have fueled controversy around bioenergy, even while land development and environmental impacts for other energy industries are poorly described. Agriculture, bioenergy, and fossil fuels might instead be viewed as part of a multiuse landscape to promote optimized production of all resources and decrease environmental impacts of energy and agricultural sectors of the economy. Optimization requires complimentary analyses of bioenergy, agriculture and fossil fuel production systems, but currently there is a lack of standardization in the life-cycle analyzes (LCAs) of these production systems. In this chapter, we compare the GHG emissions estimated in published LCAs for each of these resources, analyzing differences in the system boundaries and associated effects of life-cycle GHG emissions. Systems for handling wastes and recycling or disposing chemical byproducts are also compared. System boundaries differ across production systems, with assessments of bioenergy consistently using larger system boundaries than assessments of fossil fuel energy and other agriculture. Differing system boundaries limit the ability to make direct comparisons of the environmental impacts of resource production systems. Standardized analyses of resource production systems would better inform policies that can incentivize efficient production of *all* resources, reduce wastes, and increase the opportunities for climate change mitigation.

14.1   INTRODUCTION

The production of both agricultural products and fossil fuels causes a large proportion of greenhouse gas (GHG) emissions globally. Sixty eight percent of all anthropogenic GHG emissions since 1750 were caused by fossil fuel use and 32% were the result of land use and land use changes (IPCC, 2013). Current industrial policies do not adequately address these causes of climate change despite the clear risks that have been identified [48]. There is however increasing interest in alternative energy systems. One debated avenue for reducing emissions from fossil fuels is the development of bioenergy, estimated in aggregate to have the potential to meet 10 to 100% of global energy demand depending on policy and behavioral changes that occur concomitantly with bioenergy development (e.g., see Ref. [87]).

Bioenergy production depends on agricultural/forestry systems as well as energy systems. Agricultural emissions, while smaller in magnitude than fossil fuel derived emissions, are also globally important. Worldwide, there are almost 5 billion ha of crop and pasture land in use [90] to support many commodities (including food, fiber, medicine, and other bioproducts), and cropland for biofuel feedstocks has emerged as the most controversial. Much of this controversy, as it relates to GHG emissions, revolves around the life-cycle emissions associated with land use change (LUC) for the production of bioenergy (e.g., see Refs. [33, 85]).

Advanced bioenergy production systems (defined by the U.S. Environmental Protection Agency as systems that have at least 50% lower GHG emissions than fossil fuels) have lower life-cycle emissions, greater energy return on investment, and potentially greater environmental benefits than first-generation biofuels (e.g., see Refs. [24, 88]), even when the most detailed life cycle assessment (LCA) of these production systems is applied [98]. Yet, these advanced systems are operating at a smaller scale than the first-generation biofuels like corn ethanol that have lesser environmental benefits. The introduction of novel bioenergy crops to the global agricultural landscape has attracted scrutiny rarely applied to conventional agricultural commodities (i.e., food, feed, and fiber).

Evaluations of agricultural resource production efficiencies are commonly completed in isolation from the energy sector, in spite of debates about competition for land to grow food or fuel. Yet developing global economies are increasing demands for all agricultural resources; and, as a result, efficient land use practices are needed to reduce environmental impacts associated with the production of any commodity. Bioenergy may be a resource to help support growing energy demands while mitigating GHG emissions, but bioenergy feedstock crops must be managed along with growing demands for other agricultural commodities.

Recent estimates indicate that without policy changes, there will be a 40% increase (relative to 2012) in fossil fuel demands by 2030 [48], which will increase GHG emissions beyond targets that have been set in international agreements (i.e., Kyoto Protocol, Cancun Agreements, Paris Agreement). Policy options for optimizing individual resource production systems must be considered within a broader multiuse landscape where there is a need to increase many goods while also decreasing environmental impacts. Although the current estimates of GHG emissions associated with bioenergy systems are highly variable, efficient agricultural management can in some cases enhance the feedstock production per unit land area and thereby increase the GHG mitigation potential [21] and spare land for other uses.

Evaluations of the GHG mitigation resulting from bioenergy development depends on the reference against which a production system is compared. Even though estimates of GHG emissions are positive for many bioenergy production systems, a review of LCA studies for bioenergy grasses indicated that 56% of these LCAs estimate negative life-cycle GHG emissions, or a net sink of GHG [20]. The differences that do exist among studies are sometimes explained by different definitions for the baseline condition (for example using fossil fuels or prior land use as a reference condition). The highly variable results from LCA studies frequently can also be attributed to differences in system boundaries [15, 20, 21], and the system boundary of LCAs for a reference energy production system are often not consistent with those used when calculating life-cycle emissions for bioenergy [15].

Here, we review the life-cycle impacts of agriculture and energy resource production systems to identify the different assumptions that influence estimates of GHG emissions from different industrial sectors. We review LCA studies of bioenergy, food, feed, and fossil fuel production systems; and compared the life-cycle inventories used to calculate GHG emissions for each of these resources. We also compare the system boundaries used to evaluate bioenergy products, other agricultural products, and fossil fuel production. A more detailed review is provided of certain stages in the production pathway for bioenergy, with a focus on (a) waste management strategies built into anaerobic digestion systems for biogas production, and (b) green chemistry solutions for liquid biofuel production. The final section of this chapter provides policy-relevant perspective on the potential for assessing environmental impacts of production systems that relate to both the agriculture and energy sectors.

14.2 DATA AND METHODOLOGY

Peer-reviewed articles that describe life-cycle analyses of bioenergy, other agricultural products, and fossil fuels were collected using Google Scholar and Web of Science as the primary search engines. Keywords used in the literature search include the scientific and common name of the crops, fuel types, and "life cycle analysis," "life cycle assessment," life cycle inventory," "feedstock production LC (A/I)," "LCA," "GHG," "energy input," "energy output," "GWP," "management," "life cycle," and "bioenergy CO_{2eq}," as search terms. For each search term, the results generated from each database were screened until the majority of the results were no long relevant (usually after the first 50 outputs). Only peer reviewed journal articles were used with the exception of five studies on fossil fuel and one on soy biodiesel published by the U.S. government that provided transparent calculations.

From each study retained after the search and filter process, the inventories used in the life-cycle analysis were recorded. The energy input, energy output, and GHG emissions per inventory were summarized and compared. Only studies with units that could be converted to $CO_{2\,eq}\,MJ^{-1}$ or $CO_{2eq}\,ha^{-1}$ were used for the discussion here. All values for energy associated with human labor were excluded because very few studies estimated GHG emissions of labor [71, 73].

Literature detailing LCA of anaerobic digestion (AD) systems was reviewed separately because these bioenergy production systems can involve a wide range of different feedstocks (not necessarily agricultural crops), systems designs, and products. Search engines used for this review included Google Scholar and the ALICE database maintained by the library at Ohio University that also accesses the Web of Science. Keywords include "anaerobic" "digestion" or "biogas" or "methane" separately and in combination with "life cycle analysis," "LCA," and "life cycle inventory."

To compare the life-cycle inventories used in analyses of different resource production systems, each inventory item list was simplified into broader categories that could be applied generally to most life-cycle frameworks: (1) upstream manufacturing, (2) direct inputs for cultivation, (3) harvest/baling/transport, (4) processing, (5) conversion, (6) coproducts, (7) end-use/fossil fuel displacement, (8) land-use change for the bioenergy and agricultural crops. Upstream manufacturing includes the emissions associated with engineering and delivering agricultural inputs like fertilizers. Direct inputs for cultivation include emissions at the time of application of agrochemicals and other cultivation practices. Processing, conversion, and transport refer to postfarm changes and transport of the crop. End use refers to emissions associated with the use of the final product by consumers. Parallel categories were defined for fossil fuel production, including (1) exploration, (2) infrastructure for extraction, (3) extraction, (4) processing, (5) conversion,

(6) transport, (7) coproducts, and (8) end use for fossil fuels. Exploration includes emissions involved in finding a fuel source. Infrastructure includes emissions from building and preparing to extract the fuel. Extraction includes the emissions at the time of obtaining the fuel. Processing, conversion, and transport include all emissions after the raw material has been collected. End use is the direct emissions from the fuel in its final form.

To compare GHG emissions of different resource production systems, the life-cycle inventory values were summed, converted to a common unit ($CO_{2\,eq}$ MJ^{-1} or $CO_{2eq}ha^{-1}$) and then averaged for each crop or fuel. To convert energy inputs from MJ ha^{-1} to CO_{2eq}, an emissions factor of 74.9 gCO_2 MJ^{-1} was used when coal was the primary energy source (e.g., for manufacturing fertilizer, pesticide, and seed), and an emissions factor of 84.8 gCO_2 MJ^{-1} was used when diesel was the primary energy source (*e,g,* harvesting and baling). For the bioenergy crops, if the total GHG emissions was reported in CO_{2eq} ha^{-1} and the yield per ha and energy density of the biofuel were provided, these estimates were used to calculate $CO_{2\,eq}$ MJ^{-1}.

14.3   COMPARING SYSTEM BOUNDARIES ACROSS ENERGY AND AGRICULTURAL INDUSTRIES

For all bioenergy and agricultural crops, GHG emissions during upstream manufacturing of plant production were estimated and included in the life-cycle inventory (Table 14.1). In the case of fossil fuel LCAs reviewed, only the study of natural gas included a comparable upstream exploration value in the life-cycle inventory. Emissions from direct agricultural inputs were accounted for in all bioenergy crop systems and 80% of agricultural crops, while only 1 in 4 of the fossil fuels (natural gas) were evaluated with extraction infrastructure in the life-cycle inventory (the upstream category that is most analogous to agricultural inputs). Processing, conversion, transportation, coproducts, and end use were accounted for in all fossil fuel types and many of the bioenergy crops. Agriculture production systems however consistently were evaluated with a smaller system boundary that did not include any downstream processing, manufacturing, transportation, coproducts, or end uses (Table 14.1).

Of all the studies reviewed (Tables 14.2 and 14.3), the average life-cycle GHG emission per unit energy produced were lowest for sugarcane and miscanthus bioenergy production (-15 gCO_{2eq} MJ^{-1} and -10 gCO_{2eq} MJ^{-1},

TABLE 14.1 Comparison of Life-Cycle Inventories of Bioenergy Crops[a], Other Agricultural Crops[b], and Fossil Fuels[c],*

Life Cycle Inventories	Bioenergy Crops								Other Agricultural Crops								
	Miscanthus (2)	Maize (10)	Sugarcane (3)	Switchgrass (4)	Soy (3)	Agave (1)	Sweet Sorghum (3)	Oil Palm (3)	Maize (4)	Soybean (3)	Wheat (4)	Wheat-fallow (2)	Grain sorghum (2)	Sweet sorghum (1)	cotton (4)	Range-land (1)	Alfalfa (4)
Upstream manufacturing costs	✓	✓	✓	✓	✓	✓	✓	✓	✓	✓	✓	✓	✓	✓	✓	✓	✓
Direct inputs for cultivation	✓	✓	✓	✓	✓	✓	✓	✓	✓	✓	✓	✓	✓	✓	✓		✓
Harvest/baling/transport	✓	✓	✓	✓	✓	✓	✓	✓	✓	✓	✓	✓	✓	✓	✓	✓	✓
Processing		✓		✓	✓	✓	✓	✓									
Conversion		✓	✓	✓	✓	✓	✓										
Transport		✓	✓	✓		✓	✓	✓									
Coproducts		✓		✓	✓		✓	✓									
End use/fossil fuel displacement	✓	✓	✓	✓			✓										
Land use change	✓	✓	✓	✓			✓										

Life Cycle Inventories	Fossil Fuels			
	Coal (3)	Natural Gas (1)	Gasoline (2)	Diesel (4)
Exploration		✓		
Infrastructure for extraction		✓		
Extraction	✓	✓	✓	✓
Processing	✓	✓	✓	✓
Conversion	✓	✓	✓	✓
Transport	✓	✓	✓	✓
Coproducts	✓	✓	✓	✓
End use	✓	✓	✓	✓
Land use change	✓	✓	✓	✓

[a] Detailed in Table 14.2.

[b] Refs. [2, 10, 19, 53, 50, 55, 56, 65, 72, 74, 76, 86, 92, 99, 103, 104].

[c] Refs. [38, 49, 51, 89].

* A check indicates a component of the inventory that was included in at least one of the LCA studies reviewed. The number in parentheses next to each species or fuel type name indicates the number of studies reviewed.

TABLE 14.2 GHG Estimates and Major Assumptions of Studies Evaluating Bioenergy Production Systems (Not Including anaerobic Digestion Systems)

Crop	Major Assumptions	GHG gCO$_2$ MJ^{-1}	GHG MgCO$_2$ ha^{-1}	Reference
Maize	Includes biomass and soil emissions and coproduct credits	-13.8	-1.2	[33]
	Cradle to grave study that includes surplus electricity returned to the grid	20.6	1.7	[54]
	Includes crop production and biorefinery emissions along with coproduct credits	31.1	2.3	[101]
	Includes crop production and biorefinery emissions along with coproduct credits	42	4.0	[59]
	Includes agricultural phase, transport, conversion, and fossil fuel displacement	70.3	5.0	[27]
	Includes crop cultivation, fuel production, transport, distribution, and end use	85	5.1	[26]
	Includes crop production through transport to end location and includes coproduct credits	96.9	1.6	[43]
	Includes cultivation, fuel production, transportation, distribution, and use in automobile engines	131	8.0	[68]
	Includes, crop and biofuel production, carbon sequestration by plants, and land use change	135	8.7	[85]
	Includes crop production, local processing, transport, fermentation, and distillation	241	7.9	[100]

Crop	Description			Ref.
Switchgrass	Includes crop and biofuel production, transport, and end use	20.8	1.3	[82]
	Includes crop cultivation, fuel production, transport, distribution, and end use	32.7	2.3	[26]
	Includes crop production, fuel production, and end use	69	–1.7	[1]
	Includes crop and biofuel production, carbon sequestration by plants, and land use change	138	9.6	[85]
Miscanthus	Includes crop production, on farm transport, land use change, and fossil fuel offset	–32.4	–4.4	[44]
	Includes biomass, biorefinery, and transportation	11.8	n/a	[84]
Oil Palm	Includes biomass and soil emissions and coproduct credits	–51.6	–7.2	[33]
	Includes agricultural phase, transport, and coproduct credit	0.784	1.9	[25]
	Includes agricultural phase, conversion, coproducts, and end-use	33.2	4.5	[17]
Sugarcane	Includes biomass, soil emissions, and coproduct credits	–71.3	–9.8	[33]
	Includes agricultural phase	0.16	0.027	[78]
	Includes agricultural phase, transport, conversion, and fossil fuel displacement	25.9	3.9	[27]
Soy	Includes biomass, soil emissions, and coproduct credits	–45.8	–0.90	[33]
	Includes crop production through transport to end location and includes coproduct credits	82.3	0.55	[43]
	Includes crop cultivation, fuel production, transport, distribution, and end use	110	1.3	[68]

TABLE 14.2 (Continued)

Crop	Major Assumptions	GHG gCO$_2$ MJ^{-1}	GHG MgCO$_2$ ha^{-1}	Reference
Sweet Sorghum	Includes crop production and biorefinery emissions along with coproduct credits	45.9	2.4	[101]
	Includes crop production, local processing, transport, fermentation, and distillation	107	3.3	[100]
	Includes crop cultivation, fuel production, transport, distribution, and end use	145	0.42	[68]
Agave	Includes cultivation, harvest, and transport and ethanol production also includes coproduct credit	3.1	1.6	[102]

TABLE 14.3 Life-Cycle Assessments of Anaerobic Digestion (AD) Reviewed with Brief Description

Description	Reference
Energy balances based on 8 raw materials	[9]
Fuel-cycle emissions of GHGs, SO_2, hydrocarbons, and particles from biogas systems based on six different raw materials.	[11]
Overall environmental impacts of biogas systems that replace traditional energy generation, waste management, and agricultural production.	[12]
Biogas cogeneration and tri-generation units	[16]
Evaluates AD of solid waste relative to landfilling, incineration, recycling, and composting.	[36]
AD of manure/maize in different combinations on small farms	[6]
AD for municipal solid waste in landfills	[28]
AD of manure for transportation fuel	[40]
AD of food waste from large grocery stores	[69a]
Farm-greenhouse system that digests manure, includes evaluation of toxicity of digestate fertilizer	[105]
Household food waste for AD compared with impacts of incineration	[62]
Compares AD with three other methods of managing residual municipal solid waste	[8]
Cradle to farm gate evaluation of manure management with variable cow diets	[4]
Evaluates 18 different methods of solid waste management including AD.	[75]
Comparison of 3 technologies to 4 sludge treatment methods, one of which is digestion.	[14]
AD applied after source separation of municipal solid waste	[29]
Compares AD systems with grass, hay, or silage feedstock	[67]
Compares farmscale AD of livestock waste, manure, olive waste, and silage	[91]

TABLE 14.3   (Continued)

Description	Reference
Comparison of batch and continuous feed with codigested and separate digestion of pig slurry and maize	[58]
Energy analysis of AD	[66]
Comparison of GHG emissions from heat, electricity, and transportation fuels generated from different crops/wastes including for AD systems	[30]

respectively) and highest for coal (245 gCO$_{2eq}$ MJ^{-1}) (Figure 14.1). Despite the smaller system boundary applied to coal, which excludes potentially large sources of GHG (e.g., land use change), this energy system has the greatest GHG emissions. The larger system boundaries applied to bioenergy systems result in greater variation in estimates of GHG emissions because more statistical error is introduced with the larger number of variables considered in the system. Although the mean GHG emissions estimated by all

[top]

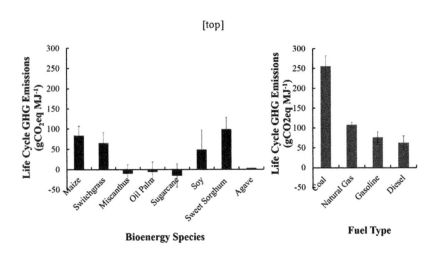

FIGURE 14.1   Average life cycle greenhouse gas emissions (gCO$_{2eq}$) per megajoule (MJ) of energy for bioenergy production from different crop species (left), and fossil fuel production from dominant fuels (right).

LCAs for AD systems was 27 g gCO_{2eq} MJ^{-1}, some estimates were negative and as low as -258 gCO_{2eq} MJ^{-1} [6].

Agriculture GHG emissions can be compared on an area basis and, on average, the greatest area-based emissions for a nonbioenergy agricultural cropping system was 3 $MgCO_{2eq}$ ha^{-1}, estimated for cotton, and for bioenergy systems was over 4 $MgCO_{2eq}$ ha^{-1} for maize (Figure 14.2). Despite the smaller system boundaries applied in LCA of nonbioenergy agricultural production systems, all of the systems had net positive emissions (net source of GHG to the atmosphere). None of the traditional agricultural crops are perennial, and there is wide consensus in the literature that perennial crops have greater potential for carbon sequestration (e.g., see Refs. [24, 81]). Average GHG estimates were negative for 37.5% of bioenergy crops (including perennial crops) and 38% of AD systems, suggesting that a subset of these production systems act as net sinks for GHG.

14.4 GHG AND ENERGY BALANCES OF ANAEROBIC DIGESTION SYSTEMS

Anaerobic digestion systems are the most variable of all the energy or agricultural systems reviewed. This is due to different feedstocks, processing technologies, and end uses for products that all affect both the GHG emissions and net energy balances of these systems. On average, AD was estimated to have 74% lower mean GHG emissions relative to the reference fossil fuel energy production systems, qualifying them as advanced bioenergy under the Renewable Fuel Standard in the United States.

The collection, transport, and digestion of feedstock and subsequent transport of effluent result in the highest GHG emissions relative to other inventory categories, making these critical inventory items for any LCA of AD [11]. The values assigned to these parameters depend largely on the system analyzed. More rarely included in life-cycle inventories were the GHG emissions from biogas storage and transportation, effluent treatment, digester inoculum, or construction of machinery and facilities (Table 14.4). Just two studies extended their LCA boundaries to include the construction of machinery and facilities [14, 28]. When reported, these emissions represented a very small fraction of the total emissions. The loss of carbon and nitrogen from digestate, as CO_2 and N_2O, respectively, are also included in very few analyses, but have potentially large impacts on GHG emissions [40].

TABLE 14.4 Percentage of 116 Anaerobic Digestion Systems Analyzed in 27 Studies* that Describe Inventory Items for GHG Emissions**

Life cycle inventory categories	Subcategories for AD systems	% of LCIs that estimate GHG emissions for this category
Upstream manufacturing		0
Direct inputs for cultivation	Cultivation	41%
Harvest/baling/ transport	Harvest	36%
	Collection/aggregating	73%
	Residue recovery/ supplements	64%
	Innoculum/manure	3%
	Transport	91%
Processing	Pretreatment	41%
	Preseparation	34%
	Loading/mixing	75%
Conversion	Digestion	86%
	Filtration/treatment of biogas	36%
	Effluent treatment	11%
	Effluent storage	21%
Transport	Effluent transportation	82%
	Biogas storage	7%
	Biogas transportation	8%
	Water treatment	29%
Coproducts	Co-products	81%
End use/fossil fuel displacement	End use transportation	33%
	End use heat	88%
	End use electricity	51%
Land use change		0

*Additional studies, which are not described in Table 14.1 include Refs. [7, 37, 41, 57, 60, 61, 77, 93, 106].

** The first column corresponds to the life-cycle inventories reviewed in Table 14.1.

One of five feedstock types were used in each AD system reviewed: (1) dedicated crops, (2) crop residues or wastes, (3) manure or livestock waste, (4) organic fraction of MSW, and (5) household food wastes. All of these systems have vastly different collection and transportation schemes, causing variation in emissions savings. Within these systems, digester specifications such as temperature, size, and location, as well as the fuel being replaced, influence biogas production and efficiency. Leakage from digestion and biogas upgrading equipment can drastically lower system efficiency and should be accurately reported, yet most literature cites overall methane loss as a conservative 1–5% [13].

Four studies reviewed [8, 9, 11, 14] also estimated net energy balances (ratio of energy out to energy input), and each of these examined several variations on AD systems. The analysis by Berglund and B rjesson [9] estimated the largest net energy outputs from AD systems even though similar feedstocks were evaluated. The most notable differences in this study were the estimates of transportation energy inputs [9]. Belboom et al. [8] and Chai et al. [14] both evaluated human waste, but the former analyzes the processing of municipal solid wastes from landfills and the latter evaluates the processing of wastewater treatment plant sludge. Upstream transportation requirements for the feedstocks are included in both of these studies, something that arguably is not an energy requirement specific to the AD since waste removal has inherent transport costs already.

Fifteen of the AD studies reviewed included energy inventories (even if they did not conclude a net energy balance), but there was no study that accounted for energy at all life cycle stages identified, nor was there an inventory item that was accounted for in all studies (Table 14.5). The most common energy life-cycle inventory item was a metric for potential energy lost or recovered from heat produced by the system. Food wastes can yield the greatest energy per unit of energy invested (at a ratio of 6.7:7.7), but the energy output per Mg of biomass can be relatively low (1.3 GJ Mg^{-1}). If the food waste is primarily grease, however, energy yields per unit of biomass can be larger than most other bioenergy systems reviewed here (22 GJ Mg^{-1}). Municipal organic waste yields the second highest energy return on investment in AD with four times the energy input produced, followed by livestock waste and crop residues (3.0–3.1).

TABLE 14.5 Percentage of 15 Life-Cycle Assessment Studies of Anaerobic Digestion Systems that Included Inventory Items to Estimate Life-Cycle Energy Balances

Life cycle inventory categories	Subcategories for AD systems	% of LCIs that estimate energy for this category
Upstream manufacturing		0
Direct inputs for cultivation	Cultivation	27%
Harvest/baling/ transport	Harvest	27%
	Collection/aggregating	20%
	Residue recovery/ supplements	13%
	Innoculum/manure	0
	Transport	40%
Processing	Pretreatment	40%
	Preseparation	7%
	Loading/mixing	27%
Conversion	Digestion	47%
	Filtration/treatment of biogas	40%
	Effluent treatment	0
	Effluent storage	27%
Transport	Effluent transportation	47%
	Biogas storage	7%
	Biogas transportation	20%
	Water treatment	13%
Coproducts	Co-products	27%
End use/fossil fuel displacement	End use transportation	33%
	End use heat	60%
	End use electricity	40%
Land use change		0

* The first column corresponds to the life-cycle inventories reviewed in Table 14.1.

14.5 WASTE REDUCTION SYSTEMS FOR BIOENERGY

There are wastes associated with every production system reviewed here. Wastes from both traditional energy systems and traditional agricultural systems have a legacy of impacts on air and water quality. As novel energy production systems (e.g., bioenergy) are developed, there is justifiable reason for additional scrutiny to reduce the risk of such impacts; this explains the more extensive system boundaries that have been applied in life-cycle assessments of bioenergy relative to those used in assessments of fossil fuels. It is clear that traditional crops with expanded production for bioenergy are frequently associated with excess runoff and high GHG emissions (i.e., palm oil, corn) when best management practices are not adopted [21]. New production systems however also have the potential to improve efficiencies and minimize environmental impacts, sometimes reaping environmental benefits [69], in part by recycling wastes and developing value added by-products [23].

The sustainability of traditional agricultural production systems and bioenergy systems could be enhanced by using waste streams as the raw feedstock for energy generation. Anaerobic digestion, the decomposition of organic materials without oxygen present, can be a complementary energy and fertilizer production system that is integrated with the other agricultural production systems reviewed here. In anaerobic conditions, microbes convert organic materials into methane-rich biogas, which can be used as a biofuel comparable with compressed natural gas. The residual organic matter after digestion, commonly called digestate, can be used directly or after slight processing as a soil amendment and fertilizer for agricultural systems. Thus, the residues of agricultural and/or bioenergy cropping systems can become the raw materials for AD systems, and products of AD can cycle back and be used to enhance productivity in agricultural and bioenergy systems.

Integrating AD into agricultural and bioenergy systems can lower the net environmental impact relative to those resulting from separately managed systems. Waste from cropping systems can generate fuel to replace fossil fuel natural gas, offsetting GHG emissions from both the disposal of the waste materials and the extraction, processing, and use of fossil fuels. The most common alternative fate for organic wastes is landfilling, where they generate and release GHGs like methane and nitrous oxide to the atmosphere. According to the latest report on waste generation and disposal conducted by the United States Environmental Protection Agency [95], Americans discarded 254 million tons of solid waste in 2013, not including agricultural or bioenergy system wastes; of the 254 million tons, 87 million tons was recovered and recycled or composted, leading to an annual reduction of 186 million tons of CO_2-equivalent emissions. Organic materials are the largest component of municipal solid waste, comprising over 60% of waste generated [95], much of which could be recovered and diverted into AD streams along with agricultural and bioenergy feedstock wastes. Anaerobic digestion of organic waste streams offers a way to combine multiple sustainability efforts, namely the goals of reducing landfill waste, decreasing fossil fuel consumption, and offsetting GHG emissions.

As AD is a relatively recently adopted technology in the U.S., LCAs of biogas systems have been treated most comparably to other bioenergy systems, with broader system boundaries included in the assessments (see Tables 14.3 and 14.4), and detailed reports of both upstream and downstream terms. One interesting difference in biogas LCAs that distinguishes them from conventional agriculture and energy LCAs is that waste streams are consistently internalized in the system and biogas production is sometimes inclusive of another agricultural production system or municipal waste treatment system. In other words, it can be truly integrated with other productions systems.

While all advanced bioenergy production systems strive to internalize waste, there are still chemical and organic loads that must be treated and/ or disposed of in most biofuel production systems. There are examples of bagasse and vinasse from sugarcane ethanol production that is recycled back to fields as a fertilizer, but there is also evidence of biological toxicity associated with this practice [18]. AD digestates can be recycled as soil amendment and fertilizer and are biologically stable [79], have been shown to improve overall soil health and water retention [97], and can replace commercial inorganic fertilizers, thereby offsetting environmental impacts of these fertilizers. There are also other potential uses for AD digestate wastes, including processing to create a fossil diesel replacement fuel, but the sustainability of this process technology is still being evaluated [45].

Global atmospheric levels of methane, a powerful GHG, have been on the rise. A recent survey found that U.S. methane emissions increased by more than 30% between 2002 and 2014, and the current emission rates from the U.S. alone could account for 30–60% of the rise in global atmospheric methane [94]. For that same time period, the bottom-up estimates for anthropogenic methane emissions reported in the U.S. EPA Greenhouse Gas Inventory attribute 30–32% to oil and gas fossil fuel use, 21–22% of emissions to landfills, and 31–34% to livestock systems which include enteric fermentation and manure management [96]. The GHG emissions from both landfills and livestock management could be dramatically decreased by integrating AD into waste management systems [31, 64]. The replacement of fossil natural gas with renewable biogas would further reduce net GHG emissions while also decreasing the amount of waste. In summary, biogas is a renewable energy source that uses organic waste materials and generates fertilizers that can be cycled back into cropping systems and increase net sustainability of multiple systems.

14.6 OPPORTUNITIES FOR GREEN CHEMISTRY SOLUTIONS

Chemical inputs and residual wastes in the production chain of bioenergy result in undesirable environmental impacts and costs in the system that might be reduced by the development of green chemistry solutions. The waste processing components of AD systems serve as an example of "greener" chemistry than some other bioenergy production systems, but there are still components that can be improved in AD. For example, there is a constant need to both buffer the acidity of an AD slurry and filter hydrogen sulfide.

In advanced cellulosic biofuel production, even when using crops with relatively low GHG emissions, the chemical loads required for pretreatment carry an environmental cost that could be eliminated if replaced with alternative green chemistry solutions. One approach is to mimic nature. Plant biomass and cell wall biopolymers are metabolized and recycled in a "green" manner within the terrestrial ecosystem via the synergistic action of microorganisms and macromycetous fungi.

Fungi, mostly in the phylum Basidiomycota within the subkingdom Dikarya, exude enzymes that are able to degrade wood and other cell wall components in one of three distinct manners; white-rot, brown-rot, and soft-rot. In the case of white and brown-rot, the species decompose mostly lignin or cellulose respectively, or unselectively degrade cell wall components as in the case of soft-rot. Many of these enzymes have recently become available commercially (e.g., Novozymes).

A combination of enzymes is required to release fermentable sugars from lignocellulosic biomass. Many fungal species exude extracellular enzymes, generally known as glycosidic hydrolases (GH), that also degrade cellulose by hydrolysis of the β-1,4-glycosidic bonds; specifically, endoglucanases (EC 3.2.1.4) hydrolyze cellulose to glucooligosaccharides, and cellobiohydrolases (EC 3.2.1.91) convert cellulose polymers to the glucose dimer cellobiose. This presents the need for further enzymatic hydrolysis, in the case of lignocellulosic biofuel conversion, via hydrolysis by β-glucosidases (EC 3.2.1.21) to achieve soluble glucose. These enzymes have been cataloged based upon protein structure and amino acid sequence according to work by Henrissat et al. [42], and were later termed "carbohydrate active enzymes," or CAZymes (http://www.cazy.org; http://www.CAZypedia.org).

Fungal species are able to delignify substrates via the powerful oxidation potential of laccases and peroxidases coupled with metallic cofactors. Interestingly, these enzymes have also been found to degrade organopollutants, such as Azure B [5]. However, there may be a similar mechanism by which complete conversion of cellulose to glucose may be possible. Cellobiose dehydrogenase, as described by Phillips et al. [70], has been shown to enhance cellulose degradation through metal-dependent catalyzed reactions. Metals, such as iron (Fe) and copper (Cu), are important in cellulose degradation, because they act as electron acceptors and therefore react with H_2O_2 to form hydroxyl radicals [3, 5, 70]. The formation of these radicals initiates a Fenton-like reaction that can further degrade cell wall biopolymers [5, 34, 35, 39].

There are many chemical pathways to convert biomass to fuel. Enzymatic routes for pretreatment of biomass and depolymerization are viable examples, but require infrastructure and energy to maintain supplies in a biofuel production chain. The implementation of these and other green chemistry solutions would affect life-cycle impacts. Enzymatic pathway that replace thermochemical treatments have the potential to reduce energy requirements, GHG emissions, and wastes associated with advanced cellulosic biofuel production.

14.7 SUMMARY OF POLICY IMPLICATIONS

There are clear differences in life-cycle inventories of the different industries analyzed in this study. At present, the life-cycle studies of bioenergy systems account for a larger system boundary and more extensive life-cycle inventory than life-cycle emissions of other energy or agricultural systems (Table 14.1). This may in part be fueling some of the controversy around bioenergy production. Environmental impacts associated with land use change from an expanding bioenergy industry are more widely recognized than similar impacts associated with other industries that often serve as the baseline or "business-as-usual" scenario against which bioenergy systems are compared.

System boundaries used in a life-cycle study are frequently subject to the objectives of the researchers. These differing system boundaries prevent clear comparisons between resources within a given industry and between resources from different industries. In cases where the same material is being used for different industries, this comparison is important. For example, maize has been estimated to have greater GHG emissions if produced for biofuel than it does if produced for feed. It is unclear whether this difference is due to differing life-cycle system boundaries or to differences in the production systems (Figure 14.2), and discrepancies like this may be preventing effective policies that would optimize land use, increase commodity and energy production, and decrease negative environmental impacts from both agriculture and energy systems.

The EPA has introduced standards for LCA studies of energy systems in the US, and the International Reference Life Cycle Data System (ILCD) Handbook provides international standards for life-cycle studies [32]. Neither of these guidelines have specifically addressed agriculture not in use for bioenergy. Future research using standardization will be necessary to allow for unbiased comparisons between agriculture and energy production systems. Such research will help determine the environmental impacts and benefits of bioenergy production and contribute to a resolution of the food versus fuel debate.

Anaerobic digestion systems are well suited for integration with agricultural production systems. The use of wastes, whether from crops or livestock or postconsumer, as feedstock provides an opportunity for improving the

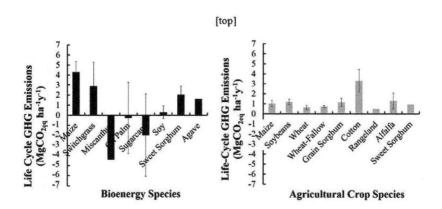

FIGURE 14.2 Average annual life cycle greenhouse gas emissions ($MgCO_{2eq}$) per hectare from bioenergy production using different feedstock crops (left) and from traditional agricultural crop production (right).

efficiency of agriculture and energy systems. The energy yields and GHG mitigation of AD frequently exceeds that of other bioenergy systems, but underscores the necessity of assessing innovative opportunities at the intersection of industrial systems [23].

As the world's demand for energy and agricultural products increases, it will be important to have policies that encourage the best land use practices. Optimization of landscapes to simultaneously increase resource production and reduce environmental impacts requires balanced analyses of all agricultural resources [22, 52] and other resource extraction from the land. Holistic life-cycle approaches can also be used to assess impacts on social welfare of differing agriculture and energy industries. LCA standardization across resource production systems would better inform policies that can incentivize efficient agricultural production of *all* resources (including feed, materials, and energy) and thereby increase the opportunities for mitigation of climate change.

ACKNOWLEDGMENTS

This work was partially funded by the Energy Biosciences Institute, a research institute that is sponsored by BP, University of California at Berkeley, and the University of Illinois at Urbana-Champaign. This work was also supported by the Voinovich School of Leadership and Public Affairs at Ohio University.

KEYWORDS

- **advanced biofuel**
- **anaerobic digestion**
- **biofuel**
- **biogas**
- **GHG**
- **greenhouse gas**
- **land use change**
- **LCA**
- **LCI**
- **life-cycle analysis**

REFERENCES

1. Adler, P. R., Del Grosso, S. J. & Parton, W. J. (2007). Life-cycle assessment of net greenhouse-gas flux for bioenergy cropping systems. *Ecological Applications, 17,* 675–691.
2. Adviento-Borbe, M. A. A., Haddix, M. L., Binder, D. L., Walters, D. T. & Dobermann, A. (2007). Soil greenhouse gas fluxes and global warming potential in four high-yielding maize systems. *Global Change Biology, 13,* 1972–1988.
3. Aguiar, A., Gavioli, D., & Ferraz, A. (2014). Metabolite secretion, Fe3+-reducing activity and wood degradation by the white-rot fungus Trametes versicolor ATCC 20869. *Fungal Biology, 118,* 935–942. http://doi.org/10.1016/j.funbio.2014.08.004.
4. Aguirre-Villegas, H. A., Passos-Fonseca, T. H., Reinemann, D. J., Armentano, L. E., Wattiaux, M. A., Cabrera, V. E., Norman, J. M., & Larson, R. (2015). Green cheese: Partial life cycle assessment of greenhouse gas emissions and energy intensity of integrated dairy production and bioenergy systems. *Journal of Dairy Science, 98,* 1571–1592.
5. Arantes, V., & Milagres, A. M. F. (2007). The synergistic action of ligninolytic enzymes (MnP and Laccase) and Fe3+-reducing activity from white-rot fungi for degradation of Azure B. *Enzyme and Microbial Technology, 42,* 17–22.
6. Bacenetti, J., & Fiala, M. (2015). Carbon Footprint of Electricity from Anaerobic Digestion Plants in Italy. *Environmental Engineering and Management Journal, 14,* 1495–1502.
7. Barbanti, L., Di Girolarno, G., Grigatti, M., Bertin, L., & Ciavatta, C. (2014). Anaerobic digestion of annual and multiannual biomass crops. *Industrial Crops and Products, 56,* 137–144.
8. Belboom, S., Digneffe, J. M., Renzoni, R., Germain, A., & Leonard, A. (2013). Comparing technologies for municipal solid waste management using life cycle assessment methodology: a Belgian case study. *International Journal of Life Cycle Assessment, 18,* 1513–1523.
9. Berglund, M., & Borjesson, P. (2006). Assessment of energy performance in the life-cycle of biogas production. *Biomass & Bioenergy, 30,* 254–266.
10. Biswas, W. K., Barton, L. & Carter, D. (2008). Global warming potential of wheat production in Western Australia: a life cycle assessment. *Water and Environment Journal, 22,* 206–216.
11. Börjesson, P., & Berglund, M. (2006). Environmental systems analysis of biogas systems—Part I: Fuel-cycle emissions. *Biomass and Bioenergy, 30,* 469–485.
12. Börjesson, P., & Berglund, M. (2007). Environmental systems analysis of biogas systems—Part II: The environmental impact of replacing various reference systems. *Biomass and Bioenergy, 31,* 326–344.
13. Bruun, S., Jensen, L. S., Vu, V. T. K., & Sommer, S. (2014). Small-scale household biogas digesters: An option for global warming mitigation or a potential climate bomb? *Renewable & Sustainable Energy Reviews, 33,* 736–741.
14. Chai, C. Y., Zhang, D. W., Yu, Y. L., Feng, Y. J., & Wong, M. S. (2015). Carbon Footprint Analyses of Mainstream Wastewater Treatment Technologies under Different Sludge Treatment Scenarios in China. *Water, 7,* 918–938.
15. Cherubini, F., Bird, N., Cowie, A., Jungmeier, G., Schlamadinger, B., & Woess-Gallasch, S. (2009). Energy- and greenhous gas-based LCA of biofuel and bioenergy sys-

tems: key issues, ranges and recommendations. *Resources, Conservation and Recycling, 53,* 434–447.

16. Chevalier, C., & Meunier, F. (2005). Environmental assessment of biogas co or trigeneration units by life cycle analysis methodology. *Applied Thermal Engineering, 25,* 3025–3041.

17. Choo, Y. M., Muhamad, H., Hashim, Z., Subramaniam, V., Puah, C. W. & Tan, Y. (2011). Determination of GHG contributions by subsystems in the oil palm supply chain using the LCA approach. *The International Journal of Life Cycle Assessment, 16,* 669–681.

18. Christofoletti, C. A., Escher, J. P., Correia, J. E., Urbano Marinho, J. F., & Fontanetti, C. S. (2013). Sugarcane vinasse: Environmental implications of its use. *Waste Management, 33,* 2752–2761.

19. Dalgaard, R., Schmidt, J., Halberg, N., Christensen, P., Thrane, M. & Pengue, W. A. (2007). LCA of soybean meal. *The International Journal of Life Cycle Assessment, 13,* 240–254.

20. Davis, S. C., Anderson-Teixeira, K. J., & Delucia, E. H. (2009). Life-cycle analysis and the ecology of biofuels. *Trends Plant Science, 14,* 140–146.

21. Davis, S. C., Boddey, R., Alves, B., Cowie, A., George, B., Ogle, S. M., Smith, P., Van Noordwijk, M., & Van Wijk, M. T. (2013). Management swing potential for bioenergy crops. *Global Change Biology Bioenergy, 5,* 623–638, doi: 10.1111/gcbb.12042.

22. Davis, S. C., House, J. I., Diaz-Chavez, R. A., Molnar, A., Valin, H., & Delucia, E. H. (2011). How can land-use modeling tools inform bioenergy policies? Journal of the Royal Society *Interface Focus, 1,* 212–223. doi:10.1098/rsfs.2010.0023.

23. Davis, S. C., Kauneckis, D., Kruse, N. A., Miller, K. E., Zimmer, M., & Dabelko, G. D. (2016). Closing the loop: integrative systems management of waste in food, energy, and water systems. *Journal of Environmental Studies and Sciences, 6,* 11–24.

24. Davis, S. C., Parton, W. J., Del Grosso, S. J., Keough, C., Marx, E., Adler, P., & Delucia, E. H. (2012). Impacts of second-generation biofuel agriculture on greenhouse gas emissions in the corn-growing regions of the US. *Frontiers in Ecology and the Environment, 10,* 69–74. *doi:10.1890/110003.*

25. De Souza, S. P., Pacca, S., De Ávila, M. T., & Borges, J. L. B. (2010). Greenhouse gas emissions and energy balance of palm oil biofuel. *Renewable Energy, 35,* 2552–2561.

26. Delucchi, M. A. (2006). Life-Cycle Analysis of Biofuels. Institute of Transportation Studies, University of California, Davis.

27. Dias De Oliveira, M. E., Vaughan, B. E., & EJ, R. J. (2005). Ethanol as Fuel: Energy, Carbon Dioxide Balances, and Ecological Footprint. *BioScience, 55,* 593–604.

28. Distefano, T. D., & Belenky, L. G. (2009). Life-cycle analysis of energy and greenhouse gas emissions from anaerobic biodegradation of municipal solid waste. *Journal of Environmental Engineering, 135,* 1097–1105.

29. Dong, J., NI, M. J., Chi, Y., Zou, D. A., & Fu, C. (2013). Life cycle and economic assessment of source-separated MSW collection with regard to greenhouse gas emissions: a case study in China. *Environmental Science and Pollution Research, 20,* 5512–5524.

30. Dubrovskis, V., & Plume, I. (2009). Forecasting of Ghg Emissions from Biomass Energy Usage in Latvia. International Scientific Conference: *Engineering for Rural Development,* 14–20.

31. Ebner, J. H., Labatut, R. A., Rankin, M. J., Pronto, J. L., Gooch, C. A., Williamson, A. A., & Trabold, T. A. (2015). Lifecycle Greenhouse Gas Analysis of an Anaerobic Codi-

gestion Facility Processing Dairy manure and Industrial Food Waste. *Environmental Science & Technology, 49,* 11199–111208. doi: 10.1021/acs.est.5b01331.

32. European Commission - Joint Research Centre - Institute for Environment and Sustainability: International Reference Life Cycle Data System (ILCD) Handbook – General Guide for Life Cycle Assessment—Detailed guidance. First edition March 2010. EUR 24708EN. Luxembourg. Publications Office of the European Union; (2010).

33. Fargione, J., Hill, J., Tilman, D., Polasky, S. & Hawthorne, P. (2008). Land clearing and the biofuel carbon debt. *Science, 319,* 1235–1238.

34. Fenton, H. J. H. (1894). Oxidation of tartaric acid in the presence of iron. *J. Chem. Soc., 65,* 899–910.

35. Fenton, H. J. H. (1899). Oxidation of certain organic acids in the presence of ferrous salts. *Proc. Chem. Soc., 15,* 224–228.

36. Finnveden, G., Johansson, J., Lind, P., & Moberg, A. (2005). Life cycle assessment of energy from solid waste—part *1,* general methodology and results. *Journal of Cleaner Production, 13,* 213–229.

37. Gebrezgabher, S. A., Meuwissen, M. P. M., Prins, B. A. M., & Lansink, A. G. J. M. O. (2010). Economic analysis of anaerobic digestion-A case of Green power biogas plant in The Netherlands. *Njas-Wageningen Journal of Life Sciences, 57,* 109–115.

38. Gerdes, K. J. (2009). Netl's Capability to Compare Transportation Fuels GHG Emissions and Energy Security Impacts. US Department of Energy.

39. Goldstein, S., Meyerstein, D., & Czapski, G. (1993). The Fenton reagents. *Free Radical Biology and Medicine, 15,* 435–445.

40. Han, J., Mintz, M., & Wang, M. (2011). Waste-to-wheel analysis of anaerobic-digestion-based renewable natural gas pathways with the Greet model. Argonne National Laboratory (ANL).

41. Haraldsen, T. K., Andersen, U., Krogstad, T., & Sorheim, R. (2011). Liquid digestate from anaerobic treatment of source-separated household waste as fertilizer to barley. *Waste Management & Research,* 0734242X11411975.

42. Henrissat, B., Claeyssens, M., Tomme, P., Lemesle, L., & Mornon, J.-P. (1989). Cellulase families revealed by hydrophobic cluster analysis. *Gene, 81,* 83–95.

43. Hill, J., Nelson, E., Tilman, D., Polasky, S. & Tiffany, D. (2006). Environmental, economic, and energetic costs and benefits of biodiesel and ethanol biofuels. *Proc Natl Acad Sci, 103,* 11206–11210.

44. Hillier, J., Whittaker, C., Dailey, G., Aylott, M., Casella, E., Richter, G. M., Riche, A., Murphy, R., Taylor, G. & Smith, P. (2009). Greenhouse gas emissions from four bioenergy crops in England and Wales: Integrating spatial estimates of yield and soil carbon balance in life cycle analyzes. *GCB Bioenergy, 1,* 267–281.

45. Hossain, A. K., Serrano, C., Brammer, J. B., Omran, A., Ahmed, F., Smith, D. I., & Davies, P. A., (2016). Combustion of fuel blends containing digestate pyrolysis oil in a multicylinder compression ignition engine. *Fuel, 171,* 18–28. doi: 10.1016/j.fuel.2015.12.012.

46. IEA (International Energy Agency). (2002). *World Energy Outlook* [Online]. Available: http://www.worldenergyoutlook.org/publications/2008–1994/ 2012].

47. IEA (International Energy Agency). (2012). *FAQs: Renewable Energy* [Online]. Available: http://www.iea.org/aboutus/faqs/renewableenergy/ 2012].

48. IEA (International Energy Agency). (2013). Redrawing the energy-climate map: world energy outlook special report. OECD/IEA, Paris, France.

48a. IPCC, 2013: Summary for Policymakers. In: *Climate Change 2013: The Physical Science Basis Contribution of Working Group I to the Fifth Assessment Report of the Intergovernmental Panel on Climate Change* [Stocker, TF., D. Qin, G.-K. Plattner, M. Tignor, S.K. Allen, J. Boschung, A. Nauels, Y. Xia, V. Bex and P.M. Midgley (eds.)]. Cambridge University Press, Cambridge, UK and New York, NY, USA.

49. Jaramillo, P., Griffin, W. M. & Matthews, H. S. (2007). Comparative life-cycle air emissions of coal, domestic natural gas, LNG, and SNG for electricity generation. *Environmental Science & Technology, 41,* 6290–6296.

50. Kalliala, E. M. & Nousiainen, P. (1999). Environmental profile of cotton and polyester fabrics. *Autex Research Journal, 1,* 8–20.

51. Kalnes, T. N., Koers, K. P., Marker, T. & Shonnard, D. R. (2009). A technoeconomic and environmental life cycle comparison of green diesel to biodiesel and syndiesel. *Environmental Progress & Sustainable Energy, 28,* 111–120.

52. Keating, B. A., Carberry, P. S., Bindraban, P. S., Asseng, S., Meinke, H. & Dixon, J. (2010). Ecoefficient Agriculture: Concepts, Challenges, and Opportunities. *Crop Science, 50,* S-109-S-119.

53. Khabbaz, B. G., & Chen, G. (2010). Energy and greenhouse gas emissions of Australian Cotton: From field to fabric. *XVII World Congress of the International Commission of Agricultural and Biosystems Engineering (CIGR).* Québec City, Canada.

54. Kim, S., & Dale, B. E. (2005). Life cycle assessment of various cropping systems used for producing biofuels: Bioethanol and biodiesel. *Biomass and Bioenergy, 29,* 426–439.

55. Koknaroglu, H., Ekinci, K. & Hoffman, M. P. (2007). Cultural Energy Analysis of Pasturing Systems for Cattle Finishing Programs. *Journal of Sustainable Agriculture, 30,* 5–20.

56. Lal, R. (2004). Carbon emission from farm operations. *Environ. Int., 30,* 981–990.

57. Lansing, S., Martin, J. F., Botero, R. B., Nogueira, D.A., Silva, T., & Dias DA Silva, E. (2010). Wastewater transformations and fertilizer value when codigesting differing ratios of swine manure and used cooking grease in low-cost digesters. *Biomass and Bioenergy, 34,* 1711–1720.

58. Lijo, L., Gonzalez-Garcia, S., Bacenetti, J., Negri, M., Fiala, M., Feijoo, G., & Moreira, M. T. (2015). Environmental assessment of farm-scaled anaerobic codigestion for bioenergy production. *Waste Management, 41,* 50–59.

59. Liska, A. J., Yang, H. S., Bremer, V. R., Klopfenstein, T. J., Walters, D. T., Erickson, G. E. & Cassman, K. G. (2009). Improvements in Life Cycle Energy Efficiency and Greenhouse Gas Emissions of Corn-Ethanol. *Journal of Industrial Ecology, 13,* 58–74.

60. Martí-Herrero, J. (2011). Reduced hydraulic retention times in low-cost tubular digesters: Two issues. *Biomass and Bioenergy, 35,* 4481–4484.

61. Matsakas, L., Rova, U., & Christakopoulos, P. (2014). Evaluation of dried sweet sorghum stalks as raw material for methane production. *Biomed Res Int,* http://dx.doi.org/10.1155/2014/731731.

62. Matsuda, T., Yano, J., Hirai, Y., & Sakai, S. (2012). Life-cycle greenhouse gas inventory analysis of household waste management and food waste reduction activities in Kyoto, Japan. *International Journal of Life Cycle Assessment, 17,* 743–752.

63. Meisterling, K., Samaras, C. & Schweizer, V. (2009). Decisions to reduce greenhouse gases from agriculture and product transport: LCA case study of organic and conventional wheat. *Journal of Cleaner Production, 17,* 222–230.

64. Miranda, N. D., Tuomisto, H. L., & Mcculloch, M. D. (2015). Meta-Analysis of Greenhouse Gas Emissions from Anaerobic Digestion Processes in Dairy Farms. *Environmental Science & Technology, 49,* 5211–5219. doi: 10.1021/acs.est.5b00018.

65. Mohammad Yousefi, A. M. (2011). Economical analysis and energy use efficiency in alfalfa production systems in Iran. *Scientific Research and Essays, 6,* 2332–2336.

66. Navickas K, Venslauskas K, Zuperka V, Nekrosius A, & Kulikauskas T. (2011). Energy balance of biogas production from perennial grasses. Pages 26–27. Engineering for rural development: 10th International scientific conference: Proceedings, May 2011.

67. Navickas K, Venslauskas K, Nekrošius A, Župerka V, & Kulikauskas T. (2012). Influence of different biomass treatment technologies on efficiency of biogas production. Pages 24–25. Engineering for rural development: 11th international scientific conference: Proceedings, May 2012.

68. Ou, X., Zhang, X., Chang, S., & Guo, Q. (2009). Energy consumption and GHG emissions of six biofuel pathways by LCA in (the) People's Republic of China. *Applied Energy, 86,* S197-S208.

69. Parish, E., Dale, V., English, B., Jackson, S., & Tyler, D. (2016). Assessing multimetric aspects of sustainability: Application to a bioenergy crop production system in East Tennessee. *Ecosphere, 7,* e01206.

69a Pecorini L, Bacchi D, Burberi L, Corti A, Fredducci N (2011) *BMP* analysis and decision tools for the comparison of different management and treatment scenarios of food waste from large retailers. *Environmental Engineering and Management Journal, 12,* 77-80.

70. Phillips, C. M., Beeson, W. T., Cate, J. H., & Marletta, M. A. (2011). Cellobiose dehydrogenase and a copper-dependent polysaccharide monooxygenase potentiate cellulose degradation by Neurospora crassa. *ACS chemical biology, 6,* 1399.

71. Pimentel, D. (2003). Ethanol Fuels: Energy, balance, economics and environmental impacts are negative. *Natural Resources Research, 12,* 127–132.

72. Pimentel, D., Berardi, G. & Fast, S. (1983). Energy efficiency of farming systems- organic and conventional agriculture. *Agriculture Ecosystems & Environment, 9,* 359–372.

73. Pimentel, D. & Patzek, T. W. (2005). Ethanol Production Using Corn, Switchgrass, and Wood, Biodiesel Production Using Soybean and Sunflower. *Natural Resources Research, 14,* 65–76.

74. Pimentel, D. & Terhune, E. C. (1977). Energy and food. *Annual Review of Energy, 2,* 171–195.

75. Pires, A., Chang, N. B., & Martinho, G. (2011). Reliability-based life cycle assessment for future solid waste management alternatives in Portugal. *International Journal of Life Cycle Assessment, 16,* 316–337.

76. Reed, W., Geng, S., & Hills, F. J. (1986). Energy input and output analysis of four field crops in California. *Journal of Agronomy and Crop Science-Zeitschrift Fur Acker Und Pflanzenbau, 157,* 99–104.

77. Rennuit, C., & Sommer, S. (2013). Decision Support for the Construction of Farm-Scale Biogas Digesters in Developing Countries with Cold Seasons. *Energies, 6,* 5314–5332.

78. Renouf, M. A., Wegener, M. K. & Nielsen, L. K. (2008). An environmental life cycle assessment comparing Australian sugarcane with US corn and UK sugar beet as producers of sugars for fermentation. *Biomass and Bioenergy, 32,* 1144–1155.

79. Riva, A., D'angelosante, S., & Trebeschi, C. (2006). Natural gas and the environmental results of life cycle assessment. *Energy, 31,* 138–148.

80. Riva, C., Orzi, V., Carozzi, M., Acutis, M., Boccasile, G., Lonati, S., Tambone, F., D'imporzano, G., & Adani, F. (2016). Short-term experiments in using digestate products as substitutes for mineral (N) fertilizer: Agronomic performance, odors, and ammonia emission impacts. *Science of the Total Environment, 547,* 206–214. doi: 10.1016/jscitotenv.2015.12.156.

81. Sartori, F., LAL, R., Ebinger, M. H., & Parrish, D. J. (2006). Potential soil carbon sequestration and CO_2 offset by dedicated energy crops in the USA. *Critical Reviews in Plant Sciences, 25,* 441–472.

82. Spatari, S. Y. Z., & Maclean, H. L. (2005). Life Cycle Assessment of Switchgrass- and Corn StoverDerived Ethanol-Fueled Automobiles. *Environ. Sci. Technol, 39,* 9750–9758.

83. Schmer, m. R., Vogel, K. P., Mitchell, R. B., & Perrin, R. K. (2008). Net energy of cellulosic ethanol from switchgrass. *Proc Natl Acad Sci, 105,* 464–469.

84. Scown, C. D., Nazaroff, W. W., Mishra, U., Strogen, B., Lobscheid, A. B., Masanet, E., Santero, N. J., Horvath, A., & Mckone, T. E. (2012). Lifecycle greenhouse gas implications of US national scenarios for cellulosic ethanol production. *Environmental Research Letters, 7,* 014011.

85. Searchinger, T., Heimlich, R., Houghton, R. A., Dong, F. X., Elobeid, A., Fabiosa, J., Tokgoz, S., Hayes, D., & YU, T. H. (2008). Use of US croplands for biofuels increases greenhouse gases through emissions from land-use change. *Science, 319,* 1238–1240.

86. Singh, S., Singh, S., Pannu, C. J. S. & Singh, J. (2000). Optimization of energy input for raising cotton crop in Punjab. *Energy Conversion and Management, 41,* 1851–1861.

87. Slade, R., Saunders, R., Gross, R., & Bauen, A. Energy from biomass: the size of the global resource (2011). Imperial College Centre for Energy Policy and Technology and UK Energy Research Centre, London.

88. Somerville, C., Youngs, H., Taylor, C., Davis, S. C., & Long, S. P. (2010). Feedstocks for lignocellulosic biofuels. *Science, 329,* 790–792.

89. Spath, P. L., Mann, M. K., & Kerr, D. R. (1999). Life Cycle Assessment of Coal-fired Power Production. US Department of Energy.

90. The World Bank. (2012). *Data* [Online]. Available: http://data.worldbank.org 2012.

91. Torquati, B., Venanzi, S., Ciani, A., Diotallevi, F., & Tamburi, V. (2014). Environmental Sustainability and Economic Benefits of Dairy Farm Biogas Energy Production: A Case Study in Umbria. *Sustainability, 6,* 6696–6713.

92. Tsatsarelis, C. A. (1991). Energy requirements for cotton production in central Greece. *Journal of Agricultural Engineering Research, 50,* 239–246.

93. Tumutegyereize, P., Muranga, F. I., Kawongolo, J., & Nabugoomu, F. (2011). Optimization of biogas production from banana peels: Effect of particle size on methane yield. *African Journal of Biotechnology, 10,* 18243–18251.

94. Turner, A. J., Jacob, D. J., Benmergui, J., Wofsy, S. C., Maasakkers, J. D., Butz, A., Hasekamp, O., & Biraud, S. C. (2016). A large increase in U.S. methane emissions over the past decade inferred from satellite data and surface observations, *Geophysical Research Letters,* 43, doi: 10.1002/2016GL067987.

95. EPA (U.S. Environmental Protection Agency). (2015). "Advancing Sustainable Materials Management: Facts and Figures (2013). Assessing Trends in Material Generation, Recycling and Disposal in the United States." June 2015. Available at: https://www.epa.gov/smm/advancing-sustainable-materials-management-facts-and-figures-report.

96. EPA (U.S. Environmental Protection Agency). (2014). Inventory of U.S. greenhouse gas emissions and sinks: 1990–2012, Tech. Rep., U.S. Environ. Prot. Agency, Washington, D. C.

97. Walsh, J. J., Rousk, J., Edwards-Jones, G., Jones, D. L., & Williams, A. P. (2012). Fungal and bacterial growth following the application of slurry and anaerobic digestate of livestock manure to temperate pasture soils. *Biology and Fertility of Soils, 48,* 889–897. doi 10.1007/s00374–012–0681–0686.

98. Wang, M., Han, J., Dunn, J. B., Cai, H., & Elgowainy, A. (2012). Well-to-wheels energy use and greenhouse gas emissions of ethanol from corn, sugarcane and cellulosic biomass for US use. *Environmental Research Letters, 7,* doi:10.1088/1748–9326/7/4/045905.

99. West, T. O. & Marland, G. (2002). A synthesis of carbon sequestration, carbon emissions, and net carbon flux in agriculture: comparing tillage practices in the United States. *Agriculture Ecosystems & Environment, 91,* 217–232.

100. Worley, J. W., Vaughan, D. H., & Cundiff, J. S. (1992). Energy analysis of ethanol production fromsweet sorghum. *Bioresource Technology, 40,* 263–273.

101. Wortmann, C. S., Liska, A. J., Ferguson, R. B., Lyon, D. J., Klein, R. N., & Dweikat, I. (2010). Dryland Performance of Sweet Sorghum and Grain Crops for Biofuel in Nebraska. *Agronomy Journal, 102,* 319–326.

102. Yan, X., Tan, D. K. Y., Inderwildi, O. R., Smith, J. A. C., & King, D. A. (2011). Life cycle energy and greenhouse gas analysis for agave-derived bioethanol. *Energy & Environmental Science, 4,* 3110.

103. Yilmaz, I., Akcaoz, H., & Ozkan, B. (2005). An analysis of energy use and input costs for cotton production in Turkey. *Renewable Energy, 30,* 145–155.

104. Zentner, R. P., Lafond, G. P., Derksen, D. A., Nagy, C. N., Wall, D. D., & May, W. E. (2004). Effects of tillage method and crop rotation on nonrenewable energy use efficiency for a thin Black Chernozem in the Canadian Prairies. *Soil and Tillage Research, 77,* 125–136.

105. Zhang, S. D., Bi, X. T., & Clift, R. (2015). Life cycle analysis of a biogas-centerd integrated dairy farm-greenhouse system in British Columbia. *Process Safety and Environmental Protection, 93,* 18–30.

106. Zhang, Z.-L., Zhang, L., Zhou, Y.-L., Chen, J.-C., Liang, Y.-M., & Wei, L. (2013). Pilot-scale operation of enhanced anaerobic digestion of nutrient-deficient municipal sludge by ultrasonic pretreatment and codigestion of kitchen garbage. *Journal of Environmental Chemical Engineering, 1,* 73–78.

INDEX

R

Printed and bound by CPI Group (UK) Ltd, Croydon, CR0 4YY

23/10/2024

01777705-0018